OXFORD MEDICAL PUBLICATIONS

BLADDER CANCER

Biology, Diagnosis, and Management

BLADDER CANCER
Biology, Diagnosis, and Management

Edited by

KONSTANTINOS N. SYRIGOS

Associate Professor of Medical Oncology
University of Thessalia School of Medicine
Sotiria General Hospital
Athens, Greece

and

DONALD G. SKINNER

Professor and Chairman
Department of Urology
University of Southern California School of Medicine
USC–Norris Cancer Hospital
Los Angeles, California, USA

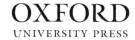

OXFORD
UNIVERSITY PRESS

OXFORD

UNIVERSITY PRESS

Great Clarendon Street, Oxford OX2 6DP

Oxford University Press is a department of the University of Oxford
and furthers the University's aim of excellence in research, scholarship,
and education by publishing worldwide in

Oxford New York

Athens Auckland Bangkok Bogotá Buenos Aires Calcutta
Cape Town Chennai Dar es Salaam Delhi Florence Hong Kong Istanbul
Karachi Kuala Lumpur Madrid Melbourne Mexico City Mumbai
Nairobi Paris São Paulo Singapore Taipei Tokyo Toronto Warsaw

and associated companies in Berlin Ibadan

Oxford is a registered trade mark of Oxford University Press

Published in the United States
by Oxford University Press, Inc., New York

British Library Cataloguing in Publication Data

Data available

Library of Congress Cataloguing in Publication Data

Bladder cancer : biology, diagnosis, and management / edited by
Konstantinos N. Syrigos and Donald G. Skinner.
(Oxford medical publications)
Includes bibliographical references and index.
1. Bladder–Cancer. I. Syrigos, Konstantinos N. II. Skinner,
Donald G. III. Series.
[DNLM: 1. Bladder Neoplasms–pathology. 2. Bladder Neoplasms–
diagnosis. 3. Bladder Neoplasms–therapy. WJ 504 B6317 1999]
RC280.B5B635 1999 616.99´462–dc21 98–50047

1 3 5 7 9 10 8 6 4 2

ISBN 0 19 263038 5

Typeset by EXPO Holdings, Malaysia

Printed in Great Britain on acid free paper by
The Bath Press, Avon

CONTENTS

CONTRIBUTORS

MURTHY ANDAVOLU, MD
Fellow in Hematology & Urology, USC-Norris Comprehensive Cancer Center Los-Angeles, CA, USA

JOHN BATTIN, MD
Department of Urology, West Virginia University School of Medicine, Morgantown, USA

MAGS M. BOWERBANK, RN BA (Hons), MMedSci
Department of Medical Oncology, St Bartholomew's Hospital, London, UK

CHARLES B. BRENDLER, MD
Professor and Chief, Department of Surgery, Section of Urology, University of Chicago, Chicago, USA

FABIO CALABRÓ, MD
Department of Medical Oncology, San Raffaele Scientific Institute, Rome, Italy

SAMUEL M. COHEN, MD, PhD
Department of Pathology & Microbiology, Eppley Institute for Research in Cancer and Allied Diseases, University of Nebraska Medical Center, 600 South 42nd Street, Box 983135, Omaha, NE 68198-3135, USA

RENZO COLOMBO, MD
Department of Urology, Scientific Institute H. San Raffaele, Milan, Italy

E. DAVID CRAWFORD, MD
Professor of Surgery, Division of Urology, University of Colorado, Denver, Colorado, USA

LUIGI FILIPPO DA POZZO, MD
Department of Urology, Scientific Institute H. San Raffaele, Milan, Italy

LOUIS J. DENIS, FACS
Chairman, Education & Training Division, EORTC, Chief, Department of Urology, Antwerp, Belgium

FRANCOIS DESGRANDCHAMPS, MD
Praticien Hospitalier, Service d'Urology, Hospital Saint-Louis, Paris, France

SUSAN S. DEVESA, ScD
National Institutes of Health, National Cancer Institute, Occupational Epidemiology Branch, Executive Plaza North, Room 418, Bethesda, USA

PAUL VAN ERPS
Education & Training Division, EORTC, Chief, Department of Urology, Antwerp, Belgium

DAVID FARRUGIA, PhD, MRCP
Department of Medical Oncology, St Bartholomew's Hospital, London, UK

CHRISTIAN T.F. FREUND, MD
Scott Department of Urology, Baylor College of Medicine, The Methodist Hospital, Houston, Texas, USA

MARTIN M. GOLDSTEIN MD
Division of Urologic Surgery, University of Rochester Medicine Center, Rochester, New York, USA

DONALD P. GRIFFITH, MD, FACS
Professor, Scott Department of Urology, Baylor College of Medicine, Houston, USA

DAVID HALL, MD
Department of Urology, West Virginia University School of Medicine, Morgantown, USA

K.J. HARRINGTON, BSc MRCP FRCR
Department of Clinical Oncology, Imperial College of Science, Technology and Medicine, Hammersmith Hospital Campus, London University, London, UK

SONNY L. JOHANSSON, MD, PhD
Department of Pathology & Microbiology, Eppley Institute for Research in Cancer and Allied Diseases, University of Nebraska Medical Center, 600 South 42nd Street, Box 983135, Omaha, NE 68198-3135, USA

GABRIEL KARATZAS, MD
Associate Professor of Surgery, Laikon General Hospital, Athens Medical School, Athens, Greece

ANASTASIOS J. KARAYIANNAKIS, MD, M.Sc.
Department of Surgery, Imperial College of Science, Technology and Medicine, Hammersmith Hospital Campus, London University, London, UK

ELIZABETH A. KINGSLEY, BSc (Hon)
Oncology Research Center, Prince of Wales Hospital, Randwick, Australia

DONALD L. LAMM, MD
Professor and Chairman, Department of Urology, West Virginia University School of Medicine, Morgantown, USA

SETH P. LERNER, MD
Assistant Professor, Scott Department of Urology, Baylor College of Medicine, The Methodist Hospital, Houston, Texas

AVIDGOR LEV, MD
Department of Urology, Scientific Institute H. San Raffaele, Milan, Italy

LUCA MARINI, MD
Department of Medical Oncology, San Raffaele Scientific Institute, Rome, Italy

EDWARD M. MESSING, MD, FACS
Division of Urologic Surgery, University of Rochester Medicine Center, Rochester, New York, USA

UNYIME O. NSEYO, MD, FACS
Professor, Department of Urology, West Virginia University School of Medicine, Morgantown, USA

R. TIMOTHY OLIVER, MD, FRCP
Professor and Chairman, Department of Medical Oncology, St Bartholomew's Hospital, London, UK

ARIA F. OLUMI, MD
Harvard Program in Urology, Brigham and Women's Hospital, Harvard Medical School, Boston, Massachusetts, USA

DIMITRIOS M. PAPAMICHAEL, MD
Department of Medical Oncology, St Bartholomew's Hospital, London, UK

MASSIMO PIGNATELLI, PhD, MRCPath
Senior Lecturer of Colorectal Pathology, Department of Histopathology, Imperial College of Science, Technology and Medicine, Hammersmith Hospital Campus, London University, London, UK

DEREK RAGHAVAN, PhD, FRACP, FACP
Professor of Medicine and Urology, Chief, Division of Medical Oncology, Associate Director for Clinical Research, USC-Norris Comprehensive Cancer Center Los-Angeles, CA, USA

JEROME P. RICHIE, MD
Professor and Chairman, Harvard Program in Urology, Brigham and Women's Hospital, Harvard Medical School, Boston, Massachusetts, USA

PATRIZIO RIGATTI, MD
Chairman, Department of Urology, Scientific Institute H. San Raffaele, Milan, Italy

JAE Y. RO, MD, PhD
Professor of Pathology, University of Texas, MD Anderson Cancer Center, Houston, Texas

NATHANIEL ROTHMAN, ScD
National Institutes of Health, National Cancer Institute, Occupational Epidemiology Branch, Executive Plaza North, Room 418, Bethesda, USA

PAMELA J. RUSSELL, MSc., PhD, Dip. Ed
Professor of Medicine, University of New South Wales, Oncology Research Center, Prince of Wales Hospital, Randwick, Australia

ANDREA SALONIA, MD
Department of Urology, Scientific Institute H. San Raffaele, Milan, Italy

PAOLA SCAVINA, MD
Department of Medical Oncology, San Raffaele Scientific Institute, Rome, Italy

KAROL SIKORA PhD, FRCP, FRCR
Professor and Chairman, Department of Clinical Oncology, Imperial College of Science, Technology and Medicine, Hammersmith Hospital Campus, London University, London, UK

DEBRA T. SILVERMAN, ScD
National Institutes of Health, National Cancer Institute, Occupational Epidemiology Branch, Executive Plaza North, Room 418, Bethesda, USA

DONALD G. SKINNER MD
Professor and Chairman, Department of Urology, University of Southern California, Norris Comprehensive Cancer Center, Los Angeles, California, USA

WALTER M. STADLER, MD
Professor, Department of Medicine, Section of Hematology/Oncology, University of Chicago, Chicago, USA

JOHN P. STEIN, MD
Assistant Professor of Urology, Department of Urology, University of Southern California, Norris Comprehensive Cancer Center, Los Angeles, California

CORA N. STERNBERG, MD, FACP
Professor and Chairman, Department of Medical Oncology, San Raffaele Scientific Institute, Rome, Italy

KONSTANTINOS N. SYRIGOS, MD, PhD
Associate Professor of Medical Oncology, and Consultant, Department of Medicine, Sotiria General
Hospital, Athens, Greece

PHEROZE TAMBOLI, MD
Fellow in Surgical Pathology, University of Texas, MD Anderson Cancer Center, Houston, Texas

ANDREW P. ZBAR, MD, FRCS, FRACS
Department of Surgery, Imperial College of Science, Technology and Medicine, Hammersmith Hospital
Campus, London University, London, UK

ALI M. ZIADA, MD
Fellow, Urologic Oncology, Division of Urology, University of Colorado, Denver, Colorado, USA

LIST OF PLATES

1. INTRODUCTION

Konstantinos N. Syrigos

In the rapidly growing field of oncology the burden of information can sometimes be overwhelming. Perhaps no disease reflects this better, than bladder cancer. Over the past decade, advances in our knowledge of the pathophysiology, diagnosis, and management of bladder cancer have been rapid. During this time the causal relationship with tobacco has been established, molecular biology has exponentially increased our knowledge, and inspired research from several centres has given us great insight into the mechanisms of bladder cancer pathogenesis, invasion, and metastasis. This has been accompanied by the development of new methods of investigation in both the experimental and clinical field. Clinical diagnostic practice has changed, while new staining techniques and interpretation have improved morphological diagnosis. Finally, novel therapeutic strategies and new approaches to palliation have been introduced.

The present volume attempts to cover extensively the area of bladder cancer based on the experience of well established scientists. The authorship is derived from an international forum and consists primarily of those who have made major contributions in the area they have been asked to discuss. As the text is particularly directed towards clinicians, efforts have been made to cover important advances in clinical and basic research with emphasis on the clinical applications. The authors have attempted to combine their clinical experience with the newest advances in the relevant sciences and to highlight the therapeutic aspects of each topic. The rationale for this policy is the perception that physicians who are acquainted with basic sciences and can use them in the evaluation and treatment of a patient are in a better position to analyse clinical problems and to help their patients.

Bladder cancer, like most oncological diseases, has increasingly become the province of many special interests, including the medical oncologist, urologist, radiotherapist, palliative care physician, and biologist. It is therefore not surprising that, in order to study the subject of bladder cancer, it is necessary to search through various sections of several oncological, urological, and surgical books, rather than turn to one work on the subject. Although we appreciate the role of books addressed to specialists, we feel strongly that there is still a major need for a comprehensive textbook on bladder cancer in this age of increasing specialization. Therefore, the purpose of this volume is to present a picture of bladder cancer in its totality and to update the subject in one volume, with emphasis on an interdisciplinary and practical approach of this disease. We have attempted to cover most aspects, giving an overview of the various specialists branches, ranging from epidemiologists and molecular biologists through oncologists and urologists to palliative care physicians and research nurses. It is our hope that physicians and researchers dealing with bladder cancer may find the presentation logical, practical, and informative. We believe that with this approach specialists associated with bladder cancer will not only get a feeling for current

practice in their own areas of interest, but will also be able to obtain sufficient information about problems presenting in their patients that involve another specialty.
Furthermore, efforts have been made to strengthen topics that are sometimes under-
appreciated and consequently underrepresented, such as the screening for bladder
cancer, the prosthetic bladder, and the role of research nurse in the management of
bladder cancer patients. Finally, management of bladder cancer is surrounded with
several controversies, regarding the role of surgery, radiotherapy, and adjuvant and
neoadjuvant chemotherapy. In this volume we attempted to present the arguments
for each approach in sequential chapters and we believe that all issues are clearly outlined and equally presented.

In conclusion, the objective of the preparation of this volume was to provide a
single, comprehensive source of information on the discipline of bladder cancer and to
furnish a platform for further investigation towards a better understanding of this
disease.

A comprehensive textbook is inevitably not fully up to date at the time of publication, and this applies particularly in these areas where advances have been more rapid.
It is therefore a tribute to our distinguished contributors and our publishers, Oxford
University Press, that this edition has appeared within 2 years of its initiation. Our
thanks are due to their staff, as well as to our contributors who have been most patient
during the gestation of the book. The editors extend their gratitude to their patients,
students, and colleagues for providing them with ongoing education, stimulus, and
purpose.

Finally, we wish to dedicate this volume to our families for their forbearance and
support throughout this project.

Athens, Greece   K. N. S.
Los Angeles, USA   D. G. S.
February 1999

2. SURGICAL ANATOMY OF THE BLADDER

Anastasios J. Karayiannakis, Andrew P. Zbar, and Gabriel Karatzas

INTRODUCTION

Surgery as the primary therapeutic modality for bladder cancer is considered in cases such as primary adenocarcinoma or squamous carcinoma, cancer consequent upon vesical schistosomiasis and bladder sarcoma, all of which have an inherent resistance to radiotherapy or chemotherapy. In transitional cell carcinoma, advanced stages (T3 and T4), as well as extensive superficial carcinoma *in situ* or multifocal recurrence following intravesical therapy are indications for surgery (1,2). The lack of durable response when radiotherapy alone is used and the failure to demonstrate improved results with preoperative radiotherapy have redefined the role of surgery as a first alternative in bladder cancer treatment (3).

Detailed knowledge of the anatomy of the bladder, pelvic lymph node drainage, seminal vesicles, prostate, uterus, and urethra is essential in order to perform radical resection, particularly in cases where normal anatomy may be obscured; most notably after prior radiation treatment, in cases of locoregional recurrence after partial cystectomy, where secondary urethrectomy is contemplated or in extended pelvic lymphadenectomy. This chapter briefly outlines the embryology and anatomy of the region as it pertains to the management of bladder cancer as well as the anatomical factors which influence surgical decision making.

EMBRYOLOGY

The urinary bladder develops early in fetal life (4). Its formation depends upon three sequential events, namely: creation of a urogenital sinus, separation of the trigone, and closure of the urachus. By the sixth week, a mesodermal septum separates the cloaca into a ventral (urogenital) sinus and the hindgut. The distal mesonephric ducts absorb into the urogenital sinus expanding and flaring open inferiorly by a process referred to as exstrophy and fuse in the mid-line as the trigone and lower ureteric orifices.

After the eighth week of development the sinus expands superiorly condensing with the pelvic mesoderm to form the dome and lateral margins of the bladder. Closure of the infra-umbilical portion of the abdominal wall and allantois is complete by the twelfth week; however, the urachus may remain patent into adult life. The trigone and posterior wall of the urethra as far as the ejaculatory ducts in the male (i.e. the most distal portion of the mesonephric ducts) are therefore mesodermal in origin whereas the remainder of the bladder is endodermal. The cranial extension of the sinus continues apically with the allantois, the intermediate portion becomes the primitive pelvic urethra and the caudal extension (the urogenital sinus proper) terminates in the urogenital membrane. In the male, the definitive urogenital sinus forms the penile urethra and in the female, the vestibule of the vagina.

Knowledge of the embryology of the bladder particularly as it applies to the terminal ureter will assist in cases where there are associated anomalies of the upper urinary tract in patients with urothelial tumours. Here, the position of the ureteric bud defines the final position of the ureteric orifice as usually in duplicated systems of the mesonephric duct the more cranial ureteric bud is carried caudally often draining the upper pole of the kidney in either an orthotopic or ectopic position. This will have implications for patients with urothelial tumours undergoing associated ureterectomy (5).

TOPOGRAPHIC ANATOMY AND MORPHOLOGY OF THE BLADDER

The bladder is largely a pelvic organ located immediately behind the pubic symphisis when empty and contracted. The full bladder rises above the symphisis and can easily be palpated or percussed suprapubically. The overdistended bladder, as in acute or chronic retention, assumes an oval outline and may bulge visibly in the lower abdomen permitting safe aspiration or suprapubic cystotomy.

The empty bladder has an apex, a superior surface, two inferolateral surfaces, a posterior or basal surface, and a neck. The apex is directed forward and ends in the fibrous cord of the urachus. The superior surface is covered by peritoneum and is in relation with loops of small bowel and the sigmoid colon in the male and with the corpus uteri and small bowel in the female. The posterior surface or basal aspect of the bladder is separated from the rectum by the seminal vesicles, the vasa deferentia, the ureters, and the rectovesical fascia in the male and by the uterine body and vaginal fornix in the female. The inferolateral surfaces relate on each side to the pubic bone and the levator ani and obturator internus muscles. The neck, which is the most inferior part of the bladder, leads to the membranous urethra (6).

An areolar connective tissue surrounds the bladder and permits distension of the bladder during filling. The prevesical space of Retzius which contains a rich venous plexus, lies between the posterior sheath of the rectus muscle, the pubic symphisis, and the bladder, and is part of the extraperitoneal space which extends from the pelvic floor to the umbilicus. The bladder lies within the visceral layers of the pelvic fascia. The condensation of this fascia forms attachments and ligaments to anchor the viscus. Anteriorly and superiorly the bladder is fixed by the median umbilical ligament which contains remnants of the urachus, attaching the dome of the bladder to the umbilicus. The lateral umbilical ligaments contain the vestiges of the fetal umbilical arteries proximal to the take off of the superior vesical artery from the main internal iliac and support the bladder against the anterior abdominal wall when it partially resides outside the pelvis. Condensations of pelvic fascia running from the levator ani muscle to the pubic bones form the puboprostatic ligament in the male and its pubovesical equivalent in the female. These ligaments effectively anchor the bladder neck. The base of the bladder is further fixed by continuity with the prostate and the urethra which are both bound in the male to the urogenital diaphragm, a musculomembranous structure attached to the ischiopubic rami and the pubic arch. When the bladder is filled the position of the neck thus remains stable.

The fascia of the bladder is either loose or dense dependent on the degree of distensibility of the region of the organ to which it is associated. It is very tenuous over the fundus of the bladder but densely adherent at the back of the trigone. Posteriorly in the female it is tough and fibrous, securing the bladder base to the cervix and the anterior vaginal fornix. In the male, at this level, it is condensed into the fascia of Denonvilliers in front of the rectal ampulla. In many cases, formed fascial bands pass laterally across the pelvic floor as the lateral ligaments of the bladder, containing the inferior vesical vascular pedicles. The urinary bladder is a hollow muscular organ which functions as a reservoir. The mucosal lining of the bladder adheres to the underlying muscular layer by a loose submucosa permitting considerable distension. When the bladder is empty, the mucosa has a wrinkled appearance but when full it is relatively smooth with few folds. In the trigone, the mucosa is firmly attached to the muscularis and therefore always appears smooth (7). The base of the trigone houses the interureteric ridge and the apex lies opposite the internal urethral orifice. The trigone is the area where the majority of bladder tumours occur.

The mucosa (urothelium) consists of several layers of relatively flat cells known as transitional cells. In normal mucosa, two distinctive types of urothelial cells are recognized: cells of the superficial layer and cells of the intermediate and basal layer. The superficial urothelial cells (umbrella cells) are terminally differentiated. These are large specialized cells with an acidophilic cytoplasm storing and secreting small amounts of neutral mucin. They have large nuclei containing condensed chromatin and inconspicuous nucleoli. These cells cover the surface and are in direct contact with urine. They are modified to preserve mucosal integrity during distension and contraction of the bladder (8). Cells comprising the intermediate and basal layers of the mucosa are small and uniform with amphophilic cytoplasm containing glycogen. They have oval nuclei which are perpendicularly oriented to the surface and which contain fine granules of evenly dispersed chromatin (9).

The basal layer of urothelium lies on a basement membrane. The estimated turnover time of normal urothelium is approximately 1 year, therefore mitotic figures are uncommon. The number of cell layers in normal urothelium varies between three and seven and although an increased number of cell layers is considered abnormal, this finding is not necessarily preneoplastic. Urothelial cell proliferation is always associated with nuclear atypia. Similarly, deeply invaginated urothelial cell nests (so-called Brunn nests) may be found. These are most commonly seen in the bladder base and are an acquired feature secondary to infection and/or chronic trauma (10). Knowledge of these cellular variants will prevent the inadvertent false cytological and histological diagnosis of malignancy.

The lamina propria of the bladder is an underlying layer of loose connective tissue containing a network of small blood vessels and a few lymphocytes. Wispy irregular muscle fibres reminiscent of a muscularis mucosae are sometimes present in this layer. Well developed muscularis mucosae analogous to that seen in the gut is found in less than 5% of bladders. Recognition of these fibres as normal and separable from the detrusor muscle is important for accurate pathological staging of invasive bladder cancer (11,12).

Beneath the lamina propria is the muscularis propria. The muscular wall of the bladder is typically described as having three layers. This is really only evident near the bladder neck. The internal longitudinal layer consists of mesh-like muscle fibres converging towards the internal urethral meatus in continuity with the urethra. The middle layer has circularly oriented fibres which are condensed anteriorly and fan out dorsolaterally. The external longitudinal layer has radially disposed muscle fibres and surrounds the bladder wall above the internal urethral meatus. The muscular structure of the rest of the bladder wall (the detrusor proper) consists of a meshwork of interconnecting muscle bundles widely separated by an interstitium containing scant collagen. The muscle bundles have no definite orientation, being longitudinal or circular and frequently altering their course in the bladder wall, weaving in and out and changing levels as well as branching and joining each other to form a well synchronized continuous muscle coat.

THE BLOOD SUPPLY OF THE BLADDER

The bladder is a highly vascular organ. The arterial supply arises from the superior, middle, and inferior vesical arteries which are branches of the hypogastric (internal iliac) artery. Small branches arise from the internal pudendal and obturator arteries also to supply the bladder. Not infrequently, there is an additional arterial supply from the pubic branch of the inferior epigastric artery which in 30% of cases represents the abnormal obturator artery. These vessels form rich anastomoses in the submucosa.

The vesical veins form a rich plexus which lies between the bladder wall proper and the adventitial layer and communicates in the male with the venous plexus of Santorini draining the penis. This joins the prostatic venous plexus and the middle rectal veins (when present) and drains into the internal iliac veins bilaterally. In the female, the vesical venous plexus communicates at the base of the bladder with a similar plexus arising at the medial end of the broad ligament, draining across the pelvic floor to the internal iliac veins.

LYMPHATIC DRAINAGE OF THE BLADDER

Knowledge of the lymphatic drainage of the bladder is vital for the proper treatment of bladder malignancy and for the conduct of pelvic lymphadenectomy. The lymphatics draining the bladder form three major bilateral collecting trunks which reach the external iliac, hypogastric, and common iliac lymph nodes.

The anterior collecting trunk drains the anterior part of the lateral bladder wall and leads to the medial group of external iliac lymph nodes. The superior collecting trunk drains the anterior part of the dome and the posterior section of the lateral bladder wall, draining into the middle group of external iliac lymph nodes. The posterior collecting trunk drains the rest of the posterosuperior bladder wall directly into the lateral group of external iliac lymph nodes by coursing along with the deferential arteries in the male and the uterine arteries in the female. These lymphatic trunks then drain into the hypogastric nodes and along the lateral sacral arteries into the lateral sacral node complex. A small group of lymphatics drain directly from this area to the common iliac lymph nodes near the sacral promontory.

NERVE SUPPLY OF THE BLADDER

The bladder receives a rich nerve supply from both divisions of the autonomic nervous system. The sympathetic nerve supply arises from the lower thoracic (T11–T12) and upper lumbar (L1–L2) segments. The sympathetic fibres descend through the lumbar splachnic nerves to join the superior hypogastric plexus, which divides into the right and left hypogastric nerves before reaching the bladder. The parasympathetic nerve supply originates from the S2 to S4 sacral segments. These fibres form the pelvic parasympathetic plexus and join the hypogastric plexus to reach the bladder as a rich vesical plexus. Branches of this vesical plexus penetrate the bladder wall and pursue a tortuous course to accommodate the stretching of the bladder during filling. The motor nerve supply to the detrusor muscle is derived mainly from the cholinergic parasympathetics, while the motor nerve supply of the trigone is derived from alpha and beta adrenergic sympathetics. Sympathetic fibres are generally detruso-inhibitory and motor to the internal urinary sphincter. The sensations of temperature, touch, and pain are transmitted in the sympathetic nerves, while those of stretch travel with the parasympathetics.

CONCLUSIONS

The technique of radical cystectomy, although standardized and associated with an acceptably low morbidity, relies on a thorough knowledge of the anatomy by the operator. This is made more difficult in patients receiving preoperative irradiation who then undergo salvage surgery. Pelvic lymphadenectomy is a frequent accompaniment of radical cystectomy, although recent reports have shown the validity of laparoscopic lymph node clearance techniques, which may be of value in the preoperative staging of patients before commencement of neo-adjuvant chemotherapy as part of bladder sparing protocols. An anatomical knowledge and intraperitoneal constraints as well as the predicted likelihood of urethral recurrence will govern the ability of the surgeon to perform orthotopic bladder substitution.

Key Points

1. Detailed knowledge of the anatomy of the bladder is essential in order to perform radical resection, particularly in cases where normal anatomy may be obscured.
2. The trigone and posterior wall of the urethra are mesodermal in origin whereas the remainder of the bladder is endodermal.
3. The arterial supply of bladder arises from the superior, middle, and inferior vesical arteries, which are branches of the hypogastric (internal iliac) artery.
4. The lymphatics draining the bladder form three major bilateral collecting trunks which reach the external iliac, hypogastric, and common iliac lymph nodes.

References

1 Skinner DG, Lieskovsky G. Management of invasive and high grade bladder cancer. In: *Diagnosis and management of genitourinary cancer* (ed. Skinner DG, Lieskovsky G).WB Saunders, Philadelphia 1988, pp. 295–312.

2 Pressler LB, Petrylak DP, Olsson CA. Invasive transitional cell carcinoma of the bladder: prognosis and management. In: *Urologic oncology* (ed. Oesterling JE, Richie JP). WB Saunders, Philadelphia 1997, pp. 275–291.

3 Gospodarowicz MK, Hawkins NV, Rawlings GA *et al.* Radical radiotherapy for muscle invasive transitional cell carcinoma of the bladder: failure analysis. *J Urol* 1989, **142**, 1448–54.

4 Kissane JM. Development and structure of the urogenital system. In: *Urological pathology* (ed. Murphy WM). WB Saunders, Philadelphia, 1989, pp. 14–16.

5 Roa-Luzuriaga JM. Renopyeloureteral duplications with extravesical dilatation of the ureters. (Bilateral case and unilateral case.) *Arch Esp Urol* 1978, **31**, 263–82.

6 Tanagho EA, Smith DR. The anatomy and function of the bladder neck. *Br J Urol* 1966, **38**, 54–61.

7 Tanagho EA, Smith DR, Meyers FH. The trigone: anatomical and physiological considerations. (1). The ureterovesical junction. *J Urol* 1968, **100**, 623–33.

8 Reuter VE. Urinary bladder and ureter. In: *Histology for pathologists* (ed. Sternberg SS). Raven Press, New York, 1992, pp. 709–19.

9 Battifora H, Eisenstein R, McDonald JH. The human urinary bladder mucosa: an electron microscopic study. *Invest Urol* 1964, **1**, 354–61.

10 Andersen JA, Hansen BF. The incidence of cell nests, cystitis cystica and cystitis glandularis in the lower urinary tract revealed by autopsies. *J Urol* 1972, **108**, 421–4.

11 Weaver MG, Abdul-Karim FW. The prevalence and character of the muscularis mucosae of the human urinary bladder. *Histopathology* 1990, **17**, 563–6.

12 Keep JC, Piehl M, MillerA, Oyasu R. Invasive carcinomas of the urinary bladder: evaluation of tunica muscularis mucosae involvement. *Am J Clin Pathol* 1989, **91**, 575–9.

3. Epidemiology of Bladder Cancer

Debra T. Silverman, Nathaniel Rothman, Susan S. Devesa

Introduction

In the United Kingdom, an estimated 12 900 cases of cancer of the urinary bladde are diagnosed and 5400 deaths from the disease occur each year (1). These account for 7.9% of all new cases of cancer among men and 3.2% of cases among women, as well as 4.4% of cancer deaths among men and 2.4% among women. In the USA, the corresponding figures are about 6.3% of all new cases among men and 2.5% among women, as well as 2.9% of cancer deaths among men and 1.5% among women (2). The lifetime risk of ever being diagnosed with bladder cancer is 3.38% among men in the USA (3). Among women, the lifetime risk is 1.18%. The lifetime risks of dying due to bladder cancer are 0.70% for men and 0.35% for women. More than 80% of bladder cancers diagnosed in the United Kingdom are histologically confirmed (4). Most of these are transitional cell carcinomas (82%); 2% are squamous cell carcinomas and 2.5% are adenocarcinomas.

Descriptive factors

International geographic variation

Internationally, incidence rates of bladder cancer among men vary more than 10-fold (4). High rates occur in western Europe and North America; relatively low rates are found in eastern Europe and several areas of Asia (Fig. 3.1). Some of the geographic variation may be the result of differing practices regarding the registration of 'benign' tumours or 'papillomas' as cancer, although rates reported by registries that include these categories are not consistently high compared with rates reported by other registries. The rankings of bladder cancer incidence rates among women are similar to those among men in North America, Oceania, and Asia, although the concordance is less in Europe.

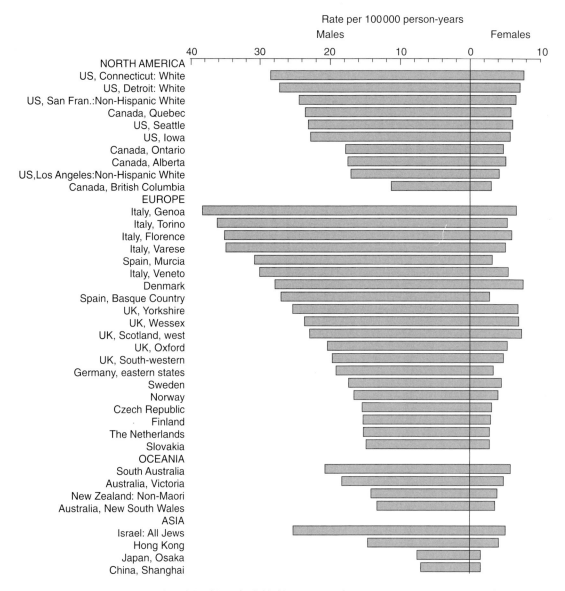

Fig. 3.1 *International variation in age-adjusted (world standard) bladder cancer incidence rates per 100 000 person-years by sex, circa 1990*

Gender and racial/ethnicity

Cancer of the bladder occurs primarily among white non-Hispanic men (Table 3.1) (5). The incidence rates among white Hispanic and black men in the US are about 50% of that among white non-Hispanics. Rates are lower yet among Asian groups, especially among Filipinos. The male/female rate ratio is 2.6 among black people, at least 3.3 among the other groups shown, and exceeds 4.0 among white non-Hispanics.

Table 3.1

BLADDER CANCER INCIDENCE BY RACIAL/ETHNIC GROUP AND SEX, US SEER PROGRAMME, 1988–92. RATES PER 100 000 PERSON-YEARS, AGE-ADJUSTED BY THE DIRECT METHOD USING THE 1970 US POPULATION STANDARD. BASED ON DATA FROM 11 SEER REGISTRIES (THE STATES OF CONNECTICUT, HAWAII, IOWA, NEW MEXICO, AND UTAH; THE METROPOLITAN AREAS OF ATLANTA, INCLUDING 10 RURAL COUNTIES, DETROIT, LOS ANGELES, SAN FRANCISCO/OAKLAND, SAN JOSE/MONTEREY, AND SEATTLE/PUGET SOUND) (74)				
Racial/ethnic group	**Males**		**Females**	
	Cases	Rate	Cases	Rate
White non-Hispanic	19 594	33.1	6694	8.1
White Hispanic	896	16.7	337	4.5
Black	877	15.2	499	5.8
Japanese	224	13.7	86	4.1
Chinese	202	13.0	69	3.7
Korean	35	10.4	16	NA
Filipino	123	8.3	33	2.1

Age-specific patterns

Incidence rates rise sharply with age, although the increases are less rapid at older ages in some populations (Fig. 3.2). About two-thirds of cases occur among persons age 65 years and older. The geographic differences apparent in the age-adjusted rates generally persist across the entire age range, with little cross-over of the age-specific rates. Excesses among males compared with females become more pronounced with increasing age.

Time trends

Incidence rates of bladder cancer among men have been rising in many areas of the world (6). From the mid-1970s to about 1990, rates increased most notably in several parts of Europe: by more than 40% in Varese, Italy; west Scotland; the eastern states of Germany; and Finland (Fig. 3.3) (4,7–9). The rates of increase in North America have not been as pronounced as in Europe. Increases in incidence rates among women have been less rapid than those among men. In parts of Oceania and Asia, rates have remained relatively low.

The observed increases in incidence may be partly explained by changes in diagnostic practice. The distinction between *in situ*

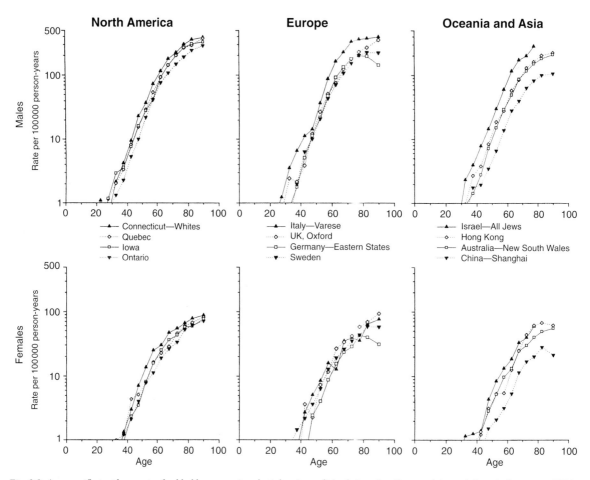

Fig. 3.2 Age-specific incidence rates for bladder cancer in selected regions of North America, Europe, Asia, and Oceania by sex, ca. 1990

and invasive disease may be difficult to make. The proportion of bladder tumours classified as 'carcinoma *in situ*' in the USA increased from less than 1% in 1969–71 to more than 7% about 1980, and considerably more in recent years (10–13). Much of the observed rise in incidence appears to be a result of an increase in the incidence of bladder cancer diagnosed at a localized stage (including *in situ*), with the rate of localized disease rising from 10.3 in 1975–78 to 11.8 in 1982–85 (11). This increase was accompanied, however, by a decrease in the incidence of unstaged bladder cancer (1.7–0.7), suggesting that some of the apparent increase in localized disease was the result of a reduction in the frequency of unstaged cases. Incidence rates of regional- and distant-stage bladder cancer remained virtually constant.

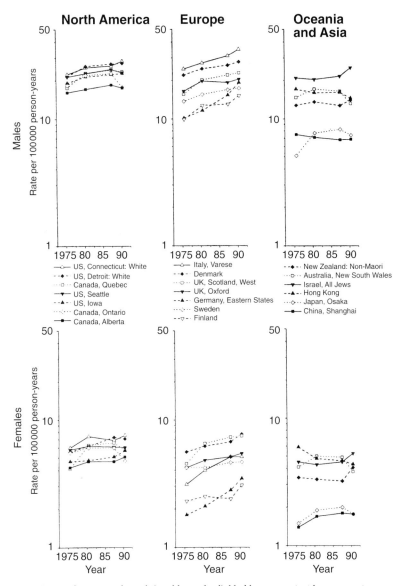

Fig. 3.3 Trends in age-adjusted (world standard) bladder cancer incidence rates in selected regions of North America, Europe, Asia, and Oceania by sex, 1973–77 to 1988–92

Stage of disease and survival

The stage of bladder cancer at diagnosis varies by age, sex, and race. The proportion localized at diagnosis in the USA declines with age from 82% among patients age 40–44 years to 70% among those 70–74 and 61% among those over 84 years (11). During 1986–93, the proportion localized at diagnosis was 76% among white men, 70% among white women, 62% among black men, and 47% among black women (Table 3.2), with the proportion distant stage ranging from 2 to 13% (3).

Five-year relative survival rates among bladder cancer patients range from 85% for white men to 54% for black women. Stage of disease at diagnosis has a substantial impact on subsequent survival. Among whites, those diagnosed with localized disease have survival rates of 90% or greater, those with regional disease have survival rates of 43–53%, in contrast to those with distant spread whose survival rates are 8% or less. Among cases diagnosed at each stage of disease, white people experience a better prognosis than black people. The relative survival rate also is higher for white men than white women for each stage of disease. Overall, black–white survival differences are only partly explained by differences in stage at diagnosis; racial disparities in survival rates persist after adjustment for stage, histological type, grade, and socio-economic status (14,15). Relative survival rates, adjusted for general population mortality, also vary by age, with higher rates at younger ages and progressively lower rates at older ages.

Table 3.2

STAGE DISTRIBUTION AND 5-YEAR RELATIVE SURVIVAL RATES (%) AMONG BLADDER CANCER PATIENTS BY RACE, SEX, AND AGE, US SEER PROGRAMME, 1986–93 (3)				
	Whites		Blacks	
	Males	Females	Males	Females
Number of cases	20 326	6714	826	441
Stage distribution (%)				
Total	100%	100%	100%	100%
Localized	76	70	62	47
Regional	17	20	24	28
Distant	2	4	6	13
Unstaged	4	6	8	13
Five-year relative survival rate (%) by stage				
Total	85.1	75.1	65.0	53.6
Localized	95.4	90.0	82.0	82.0
Regional	52.6	43.1	37.7	39.0a
Distant	7.9	4.1	5.3	0.0
Unstaged	71.0	50.6	55.2a	32.0a
Five-year relative survival rate (percent) by age at diagnosis				
<45	93.8	90.5	80.0*	NA
45–54	90.8	86.7	77.9*	49.9†
55–64	88.2	83.4	68.5	56.7*
65–74	85.4	73.7	62.8	55.9*
75+	76.6	65.6	47.5*	44.9*

* The standard error of the survival rate is between 5 and 10 percentage points. † The standard error of the survival rate is greater than 10 percentage points.

Survival among patients with bladder cancer has increased over the last several decades. During the period from 1974–76 to 1986–93, 5-year survival increased from 73.7% to 82.5% among white people and from 47.4% to 60.9% among black people (3).

RISK FACTORS

Occupation

Following a number of clinical observations and mortality surveys, the study of occupational causes of bladder cancer gained momentum in the 1950s with the identification of bladder cancer hazards in the British dyestuffs and rubber industries (16,17). During the subsequent four decades, scores of studies have suggested approximately 40 potentially high-risk occupations. Despite this effort, the relations of many of these occupations to bladder cancer risk are unclear. Observed relative risks typically have been less than two, based on a small number of exposed subjects. Further, many reported associations have not been consistently found (18). Strong evidence of increased risk is apparent for very few occupational groups.

Dyestuffs workers and dye users

In 1895, Rehn suggested that men employed in the dyestuffs industry had increased risk of bladder cancer. It was not until 1954, however, that Case showed that dyestuffs workers in England and Wales had a 10–50-fold increased risk of death from bladder cancer due to exposure to two aromatic amines, 2-naphthylamine and benzidine (16). Exposure to a third aromatic amine, l-naphthylamine, also appeared related to risk, but this elevation may have been caused by contamination with 2-naphthylamine. No excess risk was associated with exposure to aniline.

Two reports based on a cohort of dyestuffs workers in northern Italy (19,20) confirmed the increased risk from exposure to 2-naphthylamine and benzidine. A positive trend in bladder cancer mortality with increasing duration of employment was apparent; observed/expected ratios of 13, 34, and 71 were associated with employment as a dyestuffs worker for 10 years or less, 11–20 years, and more than 20 years, respectively. Dyestuffs workers involved in fuchsin and safranine T manufacturing also experienced high mortality (observed/expected = 62.5), which may have been the result of exposure to two precursors, o-toluidine and 4,4′-methylene bis(2-methylaniline). The increased risk among dyestuffs workers has also been observed in case–control studies

(21–26), with relative risks ranging from 1.7 to 8.8. Data from the United Kingdom indicate that bladder cancer risk among dyestuffs workers has been reduced since the introduction of protective measures and the subsequent banning of the industrial use of 2-naphthylamine and benzidine in 1950 and 1962, respectively (21,23).

Studies of the Italian cohort of dyestuffs workers have provided additional information on temporal patterns of risk. First, the mean time from start of exposure to death was 25 years, with a range of 12–41 years. Second, an inverse relationship between age at first exposure and risk was observed; risk was greatest for workers who started before age 25 years (observed/expected = 200.0). Third, a negative trend in relative risk with increasing time since last exposure was observed (19,20).

Users of finished dyes also may have an increased risk of bladder cancer, but the evidence is not as persuasive as that for dyestuffs manufacturing workers. Kimono painters, many of whom ingest benzidine-based dyes by licking the brush, have been found to have seven times the expected rate of bladder cancer. Coarse fishermen who use chrysoidine azo dyes to stain maggot bait have been reported to have an increased risk of bladder cancer (relative risk = 3.0 for fishermen who used bronze dyes for 5 or more years), although a more recent case–control study did not confirm this observation. Canadian dyers of cloth were reported to have a relative risk of 4.6 (26), and British textile dyers with more than 20 years employment had a relative risk of 3.4 (27). Two other studies, however, found no excess risk for dye users (18,28).

Aromatic amine manufacturing workers

Evidence that 2-naphthylamine and benzidine are human bladder carcinogens extends beyond the dyestuffs industry into the chemical industry where these aromatic amines, as well as a third bladder carcinogen, 4-aminobiphenyl, were manufactured (29). A fourfold risk was observed among 2-naphthylamine-exposed chemical workers in the USA (30). The observation of an increased risk of bladder cancer among workers involved in the commercial preparation of 4-aminobiphenyl resulted in the discontinuation of production of this aromatic amine, thus averting its widespread use (29). In a cohort of workers at a benzidine manufacturing facility, an overall excess of bladder cancer cases was apparent (SIR = 343) (31). Risk was greatest among those in the highest exposure category (SIR = 1303); little or no excess was observed for those in the low or medium exposure categories.

Corresponding to the introduction of preventive measures in the plant, a reduction in risk was observed for those first employed in 1950 or later compared with those first employed in 1945–49. In a cohort of benzidine-exposed workers in China, an overall SIR of 25 was reported, with risk ranging from 4.8 for those with low exposure to 158.4 for those with high exposure (32). Risks were elevated for both producers of benzidine (SIR = 45.7), as well as for users of benzidine-based dyes (SIR = 20.9).

Two structural analogues of benzidine, MDA (4,4′-methylene-dianiline) and MBOCA (4,4′-methylene-bis(2-chloroaniline)), are carcinogenic in animals (33), and possibly in humans, as well. MDA, a curing agent for certain resins, was associated with a threefold elevation of proportional mortality from bladder cancer (33). MBOCA, a curing agent used in the manufacture of rigid plastics, has been suggested as the exposure responsible for two non-invasive papillary tumours of the bladder in workers in a MBOCA production plant, although no invasive bladder tumours have been identified in the cohort (34). Manufacturing of another aromatic amine, 4-chloro-o-toluidine (4-C0T), has been associated with excess bladder cancer mortality in a cohort of chemical workers in Germany (relative risk = 72.7) (35). This large excess in bladder cancer mortality has been confirmed recently in another cohort of German chemical workers exposed to 4-COT (36). In New York State, a cohort of chemical workers exposed to both o-toluidine and aniline also experienced elevated risk of bladder cancer (SIR = 360), which was probably attributable to exposure to o-toluidine (37).

Rubber workers

Antioxidants containing 2-naphthylamine were used in the rubber and electric-cable manufacturing industries in Great Britain (38). Case observed that the bladder cancer mortality among British rubber workers was twice the expected level (16). This excess was observed only among rubber workers employed before 1950; 2-naphthylamine was withdrawn from use in the British rubber industry in 1949 (39).

Excess risk of bladder cancer also has been reported among rubber workers in the USA (40,41) and Italy (42), although a few studies of rubber workers found no excess (22,23,43,44). The elevation of risk reported in most American studies (45–47) is less than that reported in the British and Italian studies. There was little exposure to 2-naphthylamine in the U.S. rubber industry (45), but many workers were exposed to another antioxidant, which can be metabolized to 2-naphthylamine (29).

Leather workers

An increased risk of bladder cancer among leather workers has been observed in at least l3 studies (23,27,48–59), although no increased risk was observed in three studies of leather tanners (60–62). Most of the positive results are from case–control studies; the relative risk varied from 1.4 to 6.3. The definition of 'leather worker' was not consistent among studies. Some reported increased risks for shoe makers and shoe repairers (53,54,59), whereas others reported elevations for workers in leather products manufacturing (52) or, more broadly, for workers exposed to leather or leather products (23,51,56).

The exposure responsible for the increased risk among leather workers is not known. Cole reported that the excess was associated with jobs that involved finishing and related processes, including cutting and assembling leather pieces (51). In a large case–control study in 10 areas of the USA (56), risk was found to be slightly higher for workers with possible exposure to leather dust compared with other types of leather exposure. In addition to leather dust, leather workers also are exposed to dyes, their solvents, and unreacted intermediates (26). Bladder cancer excesses among Italian leather tannery workers have been linked to exposure to benzidine-based leather dyes. Identification of carcinogens in the leather industry may require chemical analysis of substances encountered in the industry in combination with biological monitoring of workers (56).

Painters

Bladder cancer risk has been elevated among painters in many studies (5,18,22,23,43,51,53,55,59,63–72), although a few studies have suggested no excess risk (23,73). Most of the observed relative risks have been 1.2–1.5. Jensen reported a positive trend in risk with increasing duration of employment (43); painters employed 20 years or more had a relative risk of 4.1. In a large case–control study in the USA (18), painters experienced a 50% increased risk. Among those who started working before 1930, a trend in risk with increasing duration of employment was apparent; the relative risk for such painters employed 10 years or more was 3.0. Painters may be exposed to many known or suspected carcinogens in paints (e.g. benzidine, polychlorinated biphenyls, formaldehyde, and asbestos) and solvents (e.g. benzene, dioxane, and methylene chloride) (74).

Drivers of trucks and other motor vehicles

Excess risk of bladder cancer has been observed frequently among drivers of trucks, buses, or taxi cabs (43,48,65,66,75–85), although

Table 3.3

NUMBERS OF CASES AND CONTROLS AND RELATIVE RISK ACCORDING TO DURATION OF EMPLOYMENT AS A TRUCK DRIVER OR DELIVERYMAN AMONG THOSE FIRST EMPLOYED AT LEAST 50 YEARS BEFORE OBSERVATION. DATA FROM SILVERMAN *ET AL.* (86). THE TIME OF OBSERVATION WAS THE DATE OF DIAGNOSIS FOR CASES AND THE DATE OF INTERVIEW FOR CONTROLS. MALES WITH UNKNOWN SMOKING HISTORY, DURATION OF EMPLOYMENT, OR DATE STARTED EMPLOYMENT WERE EXCLUDED

Duration of employment (years)	Cases	Controls	Relative risk*
Never any motor exhaust-related occupation	1353	2724	1.0
<5	74	129	4.2
5–9	32	45	
1.410–24	33	31	2.1
25+	22	19	2.2

(X=3.93; $P < 0.0001$)

* Relative to a risk of 1.0 for males never employed in a motor exhaust-related occupation; adjusted for age and smoking.

one Swedish study found no elevation in risk for truck drivers (68). Overall relative risks varied from 1.3 to 2.2. A positive trend in risk with increasing duration of employment was observed for drivers in most studies, with relative risks for long-term drivers ranging from 2.2 to 12.0 (43,65,76,84–86). In the largest study of bladder cancer among truck drivers, the trend in risk by duration of employment was most consistent for those first employed at least 50 years before observation (86) (Table 3.3). Although the specific exposure responsible for the elevation of risk among drivers has not been identified, one likely candidate is motor exhaust. Exhaust emissions contain polycyclic aromatic hydrocarbons (PAHs) and nitro-PAHs, which are highly mutagenic, as well as carcinogenic in laboratory animals (86).

Aluminium workers

Wigle in 1977 suggested that an elevated incidence of bladder cancer among men in the Chicoutimi census division of the Province of Quebec was the result of exposures incurred in the aluminium refining industry (87). Subsequently, increased bladder cancer mortality was observed in three cohort studies of aluminium smelter workers (88–90). The elevated risk in the aluminium industry has been associated with employment in the Soderberg potrooms (relative risk = 2.4) (91–93). Risk increased with increasing duration of employment in this department.

Table 3.4

RELATIVE RISKS PREDICTED FOLLOWING 40 YEARS OF EXPOSURE TO TAR VOLATILES. ASSUMES THAT A MINIMUM OF 10 YEARS ELAPSES BEFORE AN EFFECT OF EXPOSURE OCCURS					
BSM			**BaP**		
Concentration (mg/m^3)	Relative risk*	95% CI	Concentration (mg/m^3)	Relative risk*	95% CI
1.0	8.1	3.8–17.4	10	10.2	4.6–21.8
0.5	4.5	2.40–9.2	5	5.6	2.8–11.4
0.2	2.42	1.56–4.3	2	2.84	1.72–5.2
0.1	1.71	1.28–2.64	1	1.92	1.36–2.15
0.05	1.35	1.14–1.82	0.5	1.46	1.18–2.04
0.02	1.14	1.06–1.33	0.2	1.18	1.07–1.42
0.01	1.07	1.03–1.16	0.1	1.09	1.04–1.21

* Estimates of risk are relative to a risk of 1.0 for unexposed persons. BSM, benzene-soluble matter; BaP, benzo-[a]-pyrene.
95% CI = 95% confidence interval.

Relative risks were 1.0 for less than 1 year, 1.9 for 1–9 years, 3.0 for 10–19 years, 3.2 for 20–29 years, and 4.5 for 30 years or more (92). Armstrong used historical data on workplace exposures to better quantify exposure–response relationships (Table 3.4) (94).

Coal-tar pitch volatiles emitted from anodes in the Soderberg electrolytic reduction process may be responsible for the observed bladder cancer excess (92). The bladder carcinogens within tar volatiles are unknown, but aromatic amines (particularly 2-naphthylamine) are suspected (94).

Other occupations and exposures

Employment as a machinist has been associated with bladder cancer risk in many studies (18,95), although the increase in risk has not been consistently linked to a specific type of work. Machinists are exposed to mists from oils used as coolants and lubricants in metal machining processes (84,96). Some cutting and lubricating oils contain potentially carcinogenic PAHs (84) and nitrosamines (97).

Increased risk of bladder cancer has also been reported for many other occupational groups: metal workers, printers, chemical workers (other than those involved in manufacturing aromatic amines), hairdressers, dry cleaners, carpenters, construction workers, miners, gas workers, coke plant workers, auto mechanics, petroleum workers, railroad workers, textile workers, tailors, engineers, butchers, clerical workers, cooks and kitchen workers, food processing workers, electricians, gas station attendants, medical workers, pharmacists, glass processors, nurserymen, photographic workers, security guards and watchmen, welders, sailors, stationary firemen or furnace operators, stationary engineers, paper and pulp workers, roofers, gardeners, bootblacks, and asbestos workers (18,40,98,99). Findings for most of these occupations are not as persuasive as those discussed earlier, and require corroboration.

Strong evidence of human bladder carcinogenicity exists for occupational exposure to certain aromatic amines (29). In addition, many other occupational exposures are suspected of causing bladder cancer, including PAHs (100); diesel engine exhaust (84); leather dust (83); mineral oils (95,101); combustion and pyrolis products from natural gas and other unspecified substances (83,101); chlorinated solvents (102), particularly those used in dry cleaning (103); creosote (104); herbicides/pesticides (18,22); and asbestos (18). Further research is needed to determine the carcinogenicity of these occupational exposures.

The relation between occupation and bladder cancer risk is dynamic (18). With the elimination of bladder carcinogens from the workplace and the advent of new chemicals, changing worker exposures are generating shifts in 'high-risk occupations.' For example, risks among rubber and leather workers have diminished over time (56,39), whereas new high-risk occupations, such as truck driver and aluminium smelter worker (86,87), have emerged. Thus, occupational bladder cancer continues to be a public health problem, with risks changing over time and from population to population.

TOBACCO

Cigarettes

Cigarette smoking is well-established as a cause of bladder cancer, although the association is not as strong as that observed for smoking and several other cancers. An association between cigarette smoking and bladder cancer has been observed in more than 30 case–control studies and in more than 10 cohort studies (82,105–123). Overall, smokers appear to have two to three times the risk of non-smokers. Data from correlational studies also are consistent with a smoking-bladder cancer association. In the USA, bladder cancer mortality rates at the state level are highly correlated with per capita cigarette sales (124). Birth cohort-specific patterns of bladder cancer incidence and mortality parallel the smoking patterns of those cohorts (125,126).

Risk increases with increasing intensity of smoking (packs per day), with relative risk estimates for moderate to heavy smokers typically ranging from about 2.0 to 5.0, compared with non-smokers (82,105,107–111,113,114,117,121–123). However, the shape of the dose–response curve has varied among the studies. Some have reported a regular gradient in risk with amount smoked, whereas others have reported little change in risk from moderate to heavy smoking levels (82,105,110,113,114,117,122). Duration of smoking has been evaluated less often than intensity, but a regular duration–response relationship has been observed in most studies that investigated the issue (105,107–110,113,114,122,123).

Cessation

Cessation of cigarette smoking has been associated with a 30–60% reduction in bladder cancer risk in many studies (114). However, the pattern of change in risk in relation to time since quitting is less clear (Table 3.5). Four studies suggested that the risk of former smokers who stopped smoking for many years approximates that of non-smokers (110,122,127,128). Other studies indicate that a reduction in risk occurs within the first 2–4 years after stopping, but that risk does not continue to decline with increasing time since quitting (105,107,113,123). In most of these studies, the effect of time since quitting was not adjusted for the effects of age at starting and duration of smoking. Hartge however, estimated relative risk by length of time since quitting among intermittent former smokers (i.e. smokers who quit for at least 6 months, started again, and sub-sequently quit) with adjustment for age at starting and duration of smoking, as well as age at observation. Among all former smokers, the pattern of risk by time since quitting was weak and inconsistent (Table 3.5). When this analysis was restricted to intermittent former smokers, risk declined 50% within the first 4 years of stopping, but did not continue to decrease with increasing time since quitting. The almost immediate reduction in risk within the first few years after quitting suggests that ciga-rette smoke contains agents that act at a late stage of bladder carcinogenesis (113).

Filtration

People who smoke unfiltered cigarettes exclusively have been reported to experience about a 35–50% higher risk of bladder cancer than those who smoke filtered cigarettes exclusively (113,129). However, switching to filtered cigarettes does not

Table 3.5

RELATIVE RISKS OF BLADDER CANCER ACCORDING TO TIME SINCE QUITTING SMOKING

Ref. no.	Years since quitting	Relative risk	Comments
128	0	2.7	Risks relative to a risk of 1.0 for non-smokers, adjusted for age at observation and race
	1–3	2.9	
	4–6	1.9	
	7–10	1.4	
	11–15	1.6	
	16+	1.1	
133	0	1.0	Risks relative to a risk of l.0 for current smokers, adjusted for age at observation and lifetime cigarette consumption
	2–15	0.6	
	15+	0.5	
127	0–5	1.7	Risks relative to a risk of 1.0 for non-smokers, adjusted for age at observation
	6–15	1.0	
	16–25	1.1	
	26–35	0.9	
108	0	1.0	Risks relative to a risk of 1.0 for current smokers, adjusted for age at observation and lifetime consumption
	2–15	0.6	
	15+	0.4	

Ref. no.	Years since quitting	Relative risk		Comments
		All smokers	Intermittent smokers	
113	0	1.0	1.0	Includes women; risks relative to a risk of 1.0 for current smokers, adjusted for age at observation, sex, race, duration (all smokers); and age at observation, sex, race, duration, age started (intermittent smokers)
	1	0.9	0.7	
	2–4	0.6	0.5	
	5–9	0.8	0.4	
	10–19	0.7	0.4	
	20+	0.9	0.5	
115	0		1.0	Risks relative to a risk of 1.0 for current smokers or those who stopped less than 2 years before diagnosis/interview, adjusted for age at observation, intensity, duration
	2–4		0.6	
	5–9		0.3	
	10–19		0.2	
	20+		0.2	
137	0		1.0	Risks relative to a risk of 1.0 for current smokers, adjusted for age at observation, duration, intensity
	<3		0.4	
	3–9		0.4	
	l0+		0.6	
105	0		1.0	Risks relative to a risk of 1.0 for current smokers, adjusted for age at observation, intensity, duration, education, race, and marital status
	<6		0.7	
	7–12		0.7	
	13+		0.7	
107	0		1.6	Risks relative to a risk of 1.0 for non-smokers, adjusted for age at observation and lifetime cigarette consumption
	>1–<5		1.1	
	>5–<10		0.8	
	10+		1.4	
110	2–4		2.8	Risks relative to a risk of 1.0 for non-smokers, adjusted for age at observation and sex
	5–14		1.9	
	15+		1.0	
122	0		3.1	Risks relative to a risk of 1.0 for non-smokers, adjusted for age at observation
	1–9		1.9	
	10–19		1.5	
	20+		1.2	

Table 3.6

ESTIMATED RELATIVE RISKS OF BLADDER CANCER, ACCORDING TO USE OF FILTERED AND UNFILTERED CIGARETTES, AMONG CURRENT SMOKERS*				
	Unfiltered cigarettes/day			
Filtered cigarettes/day	None*	1–19	20–39	>40
None	2.4 (1.3–4.5)	3.13.6 (1.7–5.6)	(1.8–6.9)	
1–19	1.0 (1.4–4.1)	2.4 (1.3–5.5)	2.7 (0.8–8.5)	2.7
20–39	1.9 (1.1–3.3)	2.1 (1.2–3.7)	3.2 (1.9–5.5)	3.2 (1.5–6.7)
>40	3.0 (1.4–6.5)	2.9 (1.2–7.0)	3.6 (2.0–6.6)	3.9 (2.1–7.1)
No. of cases, controls				
None		87, 56	172, 40	61, 57
1–19	102, 29	165, 122	35, 28	8, 6
20–39	90, 48	100, 68	328, 321	26, 26
≥40	24, 21	16, 15	71, 79	73, 85

appear to reduce the excess risk (107,113,122,129) (Table 3.6). There are several possible explanations for these inconsistent findings. First, people who smoke filtered cigarettes exclusively may have different smoking histories or habits than do people who first smoked unfiltered cigarettes. For example, the latter group may start smoking earlier, or take more puffs of smoke per cigarette. Second, the effect of changing from unfiltered to filtered cigarettes may be quite small, given the small difference between the risk for smokers of only filtered cigarettes and that for smokers of only unfiltered cigarettes. Third, interview data on changing from unfiltered to filtered cigarettes may contain inaccuracies that mask a real, but small, reduction in excess risk. Fourth, smokers of only filtered cigarettes may not, in fact, have a lower risk than smokers of only unfiltered cigarettes; any observed reduction in risk may have been a chance effect.

Inhalation

Cigarette smokers who inhale deeply may have a greater risk than those who do not (107,109,130,131). Morrison observed 30–40% elevation of risk for male cigarette smokers who inhaled deeply compared with those who inhaled somewhat or not at all (132). An association between inhalation and risk has not been observed, however, in some other studies (113,133,134).

Black vs. blond tobacco

Smokers of black tobacco have a risk of bladder cancer two to three times higher than the risk in smokers of blond tobacco (109,115, 119,135–137). Three laboratory observations support this epidemiological observation. First, black tobacco has higher concentrations of aromatic amines, some of which are human bladder carcinogens, than does blond tobacco (137). Second, blood levels of 4-aminobiphenyl haemoglobin adducts, as well as adducts of several other aromatic amines, are higher for smokers of black than of blond tobacco (138). Third, the urine of smokers of black tobacco is more mutagenic than is the urine of smokers of blond tobacco (139,140).

Pipes, cigars, and smokeless tobacco

The roles of pipes, cigars, snuff, and chewing tobacco in the aetiology of bladder cancer are unclear. Evidence of increased risk is strongest for pipe smokers, particularly those who never smoked any other type of tobacco. At least 10 studies have suggested that pipe smokers experience elevated risk compared with non-smokers (relative risks typically ranged from 1.3 to 3.9) (59,108, 116,132–134,141–144), whereas five studies have suggested no association (107,111,122,145,146). A dose–response relationship has been found only rarely, although pipe smokers who inhale deeply do appear to be at greatest risk (133,141).

Weak and inconsistent relationships have been observed between bladder cancer risk and the other forms of tobacco use. For cigars, some studies have been positive (134,141–143), whereas others have shown little or no association (59,78,107,116,133,144–147). In the positive studies, relative risks for cigar smokers compared with non-smokers varied from about 1.3 to 2.5. Risks associated with the use of snuff or chewing tobacco have been assessed in a small number of studies (59,107,133,141,142,145). Of these studies, an increased risk of bladder cancer for snuff users who never smoked cigarettes has been observed in only one (143), and for users of chewing tobacco in only two (142,143).

DIETARY FACTORS

Coffee drinking

An association between coffee drinking and bladder cancer was suggested by a population-based, case–control study conducted in Massachusetts (relative risk = 1.3 for men and 2.5 for women)

(147). Since that report, many studies have evaluated this associ-ation. More than 10 studies indicated little or no overall associ-ation in either sex (112,121,143,148–155); eight studies were positive for men, but not for women (133,146,156–161); four studies were positive for women, but not for men (162–165); one study was positive for both men and women (78); and six studies suggested an overall positive association, but sex-specific risks were not examined (24,115,118,119,166,167). In most of the studies reported as positive, however, the relative risk of bladder cancer in coffee drinkers compared with non-drinkers has been less than 2. A regular dose–response relationship has been observed only infrequently (78,115,119,146,153,156,157,161), although risk was elevated among drinkers of large amounts of coffee in several studies (121,150,152,159,168,169). The weak-ness and inconsistency of the observed associations indicate that if coffee is a bladder carcinogen, it is a weak one. Alternatively, associations between coffee drinking and bladder cancer could be the result of residual confounding by smoking (152,159,170). Because cigarette smoking is both an important risk factor for bladder cancer and a strong correlate of coffee drinking, tight control for smoking is required to estimate the bladder cancer risk associated with coffee drinking alone. Although relative risk esti-mates in nearly all cited studies were adjusted for smoking, adjustment may have been inadequate if smoking categories were too broad. Confounding by smoking also could be introduced by inaccurate recall of smoking habits. In this instance, it might not be possible to control completely the effect of smoking in estimat-ing the risk of bladder cancer associated with coffee drinking.

To avoid residual confounding by smoking, the effect of coffee drinking on bladder cancer risk can be evaluated in lifelong non-smokers. Few studies, however, have had adequate numbers of non-smokers to estimate this risk with reasonable precision. Of these, some indicated no increased risk associated with coffee drinking (133,151,152,156), whereas others suggested an increased risk (118,121,143,149,154,157,159,161,165,166). Of the positive studies that distinguished between men and women in examining the coffee drinking effect, one is positive in both men and women (121), four are positive in men but not in women (149,157,159, 161), and one is positive in women but not in men (165).

ARTIFICIAL SWEETENERS

Artificial sweeteners were suggested as potential human bladder carcinogens by the results of animal experiments. The most import-ant evidence was an excess of bladder cancer in rats exposed to high doses of saccharin *in utero* and weaned to a saccharin-containing diet (171). Saccharin did not induce bladder cancer in rats or other animals fed saccharin only after birth (172).

Epidemiological studies have not substantiated a relationship between artificial sweeteners and bladder cancer. Bladder cancer mortality rates were found not to be elevated among diabetics in the USA (173) or Great Britain (174). The time trend in bladder cancer mortality in England and Wales has not appeared related to saccharin consumption (125). Bladder cancer incidence among the Danish population born during World War II, a group with higher *in utero* saccharin exposure than previous birth cohorts, was not increased in either men or women during the first 30–35 years of life (175).

Several case–control studies have provided data on the relationship between artificial sweeteners and bladder cancer. Results of most studies have been negative (24,115,119,146,148,151,153, 163–165,176–182). One study suggested a positive association in men (relative risk = 1.6) (133,183), but there was an inverse association in women (relative risk = 0.6). Moreover, a weak inverse association between use of artificially sweetened beverages and bladder cancer was apparent in both men and women. In a large US population-based, case–control study, the relative risk for subjects who had ever used artificial sweeteners was 1.0 (184). Those who reported very frequent use of artificial sweeteners appeared to have a small elevation in risk, but the dose–response pattern was irregular. A positive association was observed in two study subgroups, white male heavy smokers and non-smoking white females with no known exposure to bladder carcinogens. However, the reason for these associations is uncertain (185,186).

It is difficult to separate the effects of saccharin and cyclamates in the USA and Canada because both substances were used extensively in both countries. Studies conducted in England and Japan, however, pertain primarily to the use of saccharin (170). Results of the latter studies suggested that use of saccharin is not associated with increased bladder cancer risk.

The findings of nearly all studies indicate that the use of artificial sweeteners confers little or no excess risk of human bladder cancer. If, in fact, saccharin is a very weak carcinogen, such a low-level effect may not be detectable in epidemiological studies (185).

Alcohol drinking

Most studies that have evaluated alcohol drinking as a risk factor for bladder cancer have not supported a positive association (24, 59,118,133,146,148,151,155,186,187). Elevated risks related to the consumption of specific types of alcoholic beverages have been reported in a few studies (78,115,119,163,165,188), but these findings have not been consistent with respect to type of beverage or sex, and regular dose–response relationships have not been apparent. Thus, the positive findings are likely to be the result of chance or residual confounding by smoking.

OTHER DIETARY FACTORS

Of the dietary factors that have been evaluated in relation to bladder cancer, the most consistent evidence supports a protective effect for vegetables and fruits. Relatively high vegetable and fruit consumption has been associated with relatively low risk in most studies (108,118,119,160,167,168,179,189), but not all (190,191). Evidence of a protective effect for vegetables is stronger, however, than that for fruit (192).

The role of other dietary factors in human bladder carcinogenesis less clear. Dietary supplements of natural and synthetic retinoids inhibit bladder carcinogenesis in laboratory animals (193). However, results of epidemiological studies are inconsistent. Increasing intake of foods that contain vitamin A, particularly milk, has been associated with decreasing risk of bladder cancer in four case–control studies (143,160,167,189) and one cohort study (168), but at least two other case–control studies have not supported this relationship (165,194). The use of vitamin A supplements also has been associated with decreased risk (195). Serum levels of retinol, retinol binding protein, and carotenoids do not appear related to risk (179,194,196), although two studies reported a decreased risk associated with increased carotenoid consumption (167,181). In addition, high intake of dietary vitamin C and frequent use of vitamin C supplements were both associated with decreased risk in one study (189).

Increased bladder cancer risk also has been associated with relatively high intake of cholesterol (165), with total fat (18) and saturated fat (190), with fatty meals (108), with fried foods (168,189,195), and with relatively high pork and beef consumption (104). A nearly linear increasing trend in risk with decreasing serum levels of selenium was observed in a nested case–control study in Washington County, Maryland (196).

DRUGS

Analgesics

Heavy consumption of phenacetin-containing analgesics was first linked to cancers of the renal pelvis, ureter, and bladder by a series of case reports (197). There have been only a few case–control studies in which the relation between use of phenacetin and risk of bladder cancer has been evaluated (198–201). Fokkens reported that Dutch subjects who had a lifetime consumption of at least 2 kg had a relative risk of 4.1 compared with incidental users or non-users (198). McCredie *et al.* found a relative risk of 2.0 in Australian women age 45–85 years who had a lifetime consumption of at least 1 kg (199,200). Piper *et al.* reported a relative risk of 6.5 in US women age 20–44 years who had used phenacetin-containing compounds for at least 30 days in a year (201). Despite these fairly strong associations, a regular gradient in risk with increasing dose was demonstrated only in the Australian study (199). Further study of the relation between phenacetin and bladder cancer will be difficult because most Western countries no longer allow phenacetin-containing analgesics to be sold.

Acetaminophen was assessed as a risk factor in studies in Australia (200) and the US (201,202). Results of these studies suggest that heavy use of acetaminophen-containing analgesics does not increase risk. However, acetaminophen did not become popular until the 1970s. Thus, subjects in the two earlier studies may not have had sufficient time since initial exposure for bladder cancer to develop.

Cyclophosphamide and chlornaphazine

Cyclophosphamide, an alkylating agent that has been used to treat both malignant and non-malignant diseases since the early 1950s, has been linked to risk of bladder cancer in many case reports and case series (203,204). Cyclophosphamide has been shown to produce bladder tumours in both rats and mice (203). Patients with non-Hodgkin's lymphoma who were treated with high doses of cyclophosphamide experienced a sevenfold risk of bladder cancer in a Danish study (205). In the largest non-Hodgkin's lymphoma study to date, Travis and colleagues (206) found that cyclophosphamide-related bladder cancer is dose-dependent, with relative risks of 2.4, 6.0, and 14.5 for patients receiving cumulative doses of less than 20 g, 20–49g, and 50 g or more, respectively. Results of a study of ovarian cancer patients treated with cyclophosphamide indicated a fourfold increased risk of bladder cancer (207) . Additional groups of patients, such as long-term survivors of breast cancer who were treated with lower doses of cyclophosphamide as adjuvant chemotherapy, should be studied in order to clarify further the extent of the carcinogenic risk associated with use of this important antineoplastic drug.

In the 1960s, the antineoplastic drug chlornaphazine was linked to the development of bladder cancer (208). Chlornaphazine is related chemically to 2-naphthylamine. However, this drug was never widely used (209).

UROLOGICAL CONDITIONS

Urinary tract infection

A positive association between urinary bladder infection and risk of bladder cancer has been reported in a number of case–control studies (49,59,133,153,210–212), although two studies found no support for a causal association (213,214). In the USA, Kantor found an increased risk associated with urinary tract infections in both men and women; subjects with a history of at least three infections had a relative risk of 2, compared with those with no infections (211). In addition, bladder infection was more strongly associated with squamous cell than with transitional cell cancer, a striking parallel to the relation between schistosomiasis and squamous cell bladder cancer. The bladder infection/squamous cell carcinoma relationship also is supported by a report of increased risk of squamous cell carcinoma among young female paraplegics, a group with frequent and severe chronic urinary tract infections (53). One weakness, however, in most studies conducted to date is that information on dates of the bladder infections was not obtained. Thus, the occurrence or diagnosis of infections may have been the consequence of early bladder cancer, rather than a cause of the disease.

Urinary stasis

If carcinogens are present in urine, urinary retention or stasis might increase the risk of developing bladder cancer by increasing the duration of contact of the carcinogens with the bladder mucosa (215). Although urinary stasis has not been investigated directly as a risk factor, several findings are consistent with the hypothesis that stasis is related to risk. First, conditions that cause stasis, such as benign prostatic hypertrophy, have been associated with increased risk (210,216,217). It is uncertain, however, whether these conditions preceded the bladder cancer or were related to its diagnosis. Second, infrequent micturition and high urine concentration, both of which increase urine contact with bladder epithelium, were more prevalent in high-risk areas of Israel than in low-risk areas (218). Third, the upper hemisphere of the bladder (dome), which has less contact with urine than the rest of the bladder, is a relatively infrequent site of bladder tumours (215). Fourth, dogs exposed to 2-naphthylamine do not develop tumours in bladders that have not been in contact with urine (219). Finally, urine itself appears to be a promoter of bladder carcinogenesis in the rat (220,221).

Urine pH

In vitro and animal evidence suggests a role for urine pH in aromatic amine carcinogenesis (222–226). N-glucuronides of N-hydroxy derivatives of 2-naphthylamine, 1-naphthylamine, and 4-aminobiphenyl are hydrolysed under acidic conditions and can bind to DNA (223). Acidic urine has a similar influence on the hydrolysis of N-glucuronides of benzidine and several of its metabolites (227,228). A cross-sectional study of workers exposed to benzidine and benzidine-based dyes showed that acidic urine pH increased benzidine–DNA adduct levels in exfoliated urothelial cells (229). However, the direct influence of urine pH on bladder cancer risk in humans has not been evaluated. Diet is an important determinant of urine pH in the healthy general population (230). In particular, meat, fish, cheese, and grain products contribute to urine acidification, whereas most vegetables and fruits contribute to urine alkalinization (230). As discussed earlier, high intake of vegetables and fruits has been consistently associated with decreased bladder cancer risk in epidemiological studies (155,192). Although a role for vegetables and fruits in bladder cancer prevention has been proposed, the effect of vegetables and fruits on urine pH as a modifier of bladder cancer risk needs further evaluation.

SCHISTOSOMA HAEMATOBIUM

For nearly 90 years it has been thought that *S. haematobium* infection is related to increased risk of bladder cancer (231); results of most studies indicate that this relationship is causal (232,233). The proportional incidence of bladder cancer is high in developing countries where schistosomiasis is endemic (234). The percentage of bladder cancers that are squamous cell tumours is also much higher in endemic areas than it is in non-endemic areas. In Egypt, 70% or more of bladder cancers are squamous cell (234), compared with about 2% in the USA.

Five of six case–control studies indicated that the prevalence of schistosome infection was higher among bladder cancer patients than among controls (235–239). In series of cases from South Africa and Zambia, *S. haematobium* ova were found in higher proportions of patients with squamous cell than with transitional cell tumours (236,240). Bladder tumours have been produced in monkeys infected with *S. haematobium* (241), but these were transitional cell rather than squamous cell tumours. Squamous metaplasia has been observed in the bladders of hamsters infected experimentally with S. *haematobium* (242).

Several mechanisms by which schistosomiasis infection predisposes to bladder cancer have been suggested. First, chronic inflammation by calcific ova and urinary retention caused by infection might affect the absorption of carcinogens from the urine (243). Second, the urine of patients infected with S. *haematobium* or bacteria might have greater amounts of potentially carcinogenic nitroso compounds than that of non-infected patients (234). Third, the schistosoma antigen might depress the immunocompetence of infected patients (244).

RADIATION

Ionizing radiation causes bladder cancer, although this exposure contributes very little to bladder cancer incidence in the general population. Women who received therapeutic pelvic radiation for dysfunctional uterine bleeding appear to have a two- to fourfold risk of bladder cancer (245,246). In a large, international study of cervical cancer patients treated with radiation, high-dose radiotherapy was associated with a fourfold risk of bladder cancer (247). Higher risks were experienced by women under age 55 years when first treated, compared with those age 55 or older. Risk increased with increasing dose to the bladder. Risk also increased with time since exposure, with the relative risk reaching 8.7 for patients treated at least 20 years earlier.

Radioactive iodine (iodine-131) exposure has also been associated with elevated bladder cancer risk. A threefold risk was found among women who had a thyroid uptake procedure with iodine-131 (153). A cohort of patients treated with high dose iodine-131 for thyroid cancer also experienced excess risk (248).

Follow-up of atomic bomb survivors in Hiroshima and Nagasaki revealed a dose–response relationship between radiation exposure and bladder cancer mortality. Bladder cancer mortality also appeared to be elevated in two groups of workers at nuclear installations in the United Kingdom (249,250), but an excess was not apparent in US nuclear workers (251).

DRINKING WATER AND FLUID INTAKE

An association between by-products of chlorination in drinking water and bladder cancer risk was first suggested by ecological studies (252), and later by two case–control studies based on death certificates (253).

In seven investigations, detailed information was available on water quality and temporal aspects of exposure. These studies support the association between chlorination by-product levels in drinking water sources and bladder cancer risk. In Washington County, Maryland, residents supplied with chlorinated surface water had higher bladder cancer incidence rates than did those who consumed unchlorinated deep well water (relative risks were 1.8 and 1.6 for men and women, respectively) (254). In a subsequent nested case–control study in Washington County, bladder cancer risk was weakly associated with duration of exposure to municipal water, with a non-significant odds ratio of 1.4 for subjects with more than 40 years of exposure (255). In the NCI study conducted in 10 areas of the USA, risk increased with level of intake of beverages made with tap water (256). The gradient was restricted to subjects with at least 40 years of exposure to chlorinated surface water and was not observed among long-term consumers of non-chlorinated ground water. Among subjects whose residences were served by a chlorinated surface water source for at least 60 years, a relative risk of 2.0 was estimated for heavy consumers compared with low consumers of tap water. In a study in Massachusetts, residents of communities supplied with chlorinated drinking water experienced higher bladder cancer mortality than did those of communities exposed to water containing lower concentrations of chlorination by-products (mortality odds ratio = 1.6) (257). In a Colorado study, years of exposure to chlorinated surface water was significantly associated with increased bladder cancer risk (258). The relative risk for those exposed for more than 30 years to chlorinated surface water was 1.8 compared with subjects with no exposure. In Ontario, Canada, bladder cancer risk increased with both duration and concentration of exposure to chlorination by-products, with an odds ratio of 1.63 for subjects exposed to a trihalomethane level of at least 50 μg/l for 35 or more years (259). In an Iowa study, risk increased with duration of chlorinated-surface water use, with the odds ratio reaching 1.5 for those with at least 60 years of exposure (260). In both the Iowa and Washington County case–control studies, cigarette smoking appeared to enhance the effect of exposure to chlorination by-products. It has been suggested that the effect of chlorination by-products may, in fact, be enhanced by cigarette smoking (261).

A relation between exposure to high levels of arsenic in artesian well water and bladder cancer mortality has been suggested by surveys conducted in an endemic area of chronic arsenic toxicity, manifested by skin cancer and blackfoot disease in Taiwan (262–264). These findings have been confirmed by ecological studies in Argentina (265) and Chile and by cohort studies in Taiwan (266) and Japan (267). Ingestion of arsenic also has been associated with increased bladder cancer mortality among a cohort of patients treated with Fowler's solution (potassium arsenite) (268). In addition, biological evidence supporting the hypothesis that chronic ingestion of high levels of arsenic is carcinogenic to the bladder is provided by observations of increased micronuclei in exfoliated bladder cells of exposed individuals (269,270). In contrast, the effect of lower levels of arsenic ingestion has received little attention to date (271).

Total fluid intake may be related to bladder cancer risk, but the results have been equivocal. Increased total fluid consumption has been associated with decreased risk (210); with a positive trend in risk (108,150,161,261); and with no excess risk (59,180,260).

Hair dyes

Three lines of evidence suggest that the use of hair dyes may be associated with increased bladder cancer risk. First, hairdressers and barbers have been reported to be at elevated risk (272,273). Second, findings from mutagenicity tests and animal experiments indicate that some compounds in hair dyes are mutagens and possible bladder carcinogens (274). Third, people who dye their hair appear to excrete dye compounds in their urine (274). Results of several epidemiological studies, however, are negative (274).

Familial occurrence

Evidence for familial predisposition to bladder cancer comes mainly from clinical reports, but elevated risks among persons with bladder cancers in close relatives have been identified in a few case–control studies (78,153,275–277). In the largest case–control study to date, familial risks were especially high among those with environmental exposures, such as heavy cigarette smoking, suggesting genetic and environmental interactions. Familial occurrences provide an opportunity to identify genetic markers of susceptibility, including metabolic polymorphisms, pharmacogenetic traits, or oncogene expression.

MOLECULAR EPIDEMIOLOGY

Biological markers have become a focal point of research on bladder cancer aetiology (136,137,278). They include biomarkers of exposure, genetic susceptibility, and disease (i.e. tumour mutations).

BIOLOGICAL MARKERS OF EXPOSURE

Urinary mutagens

Investigations of urinary mutagenicity in relation to bladder cancer have focused on correlating exposure to bladder cancer risk factors with the presence of mutagens in the urine. Cigarette smoking has been found to be associated with mutagenic activity in the urine (279–280). The level of mutagenic activity has been observed to be higher for smokers of black tobacco than for smokers of blond tobacco (139). The relation of urinary mutagenic activity to the tar level of cigarettes is uncertain (140,281). Other risk factors that have been studied in relation to urinary mutagenicity include employment as a rubber worker (282), occupational exposure to benzidine (283), and cyclophosphamide exposure (284). Only one study, however, has attempted to link urinary mutagenicity directly with the risk of bladder cancer: Garner has reported an association of mutagenic urine with bladder cancer in a comparison of cases and controls, but the effect of disease status on the results is not known (285).

HAEMOGLOBIN AND DNA ADDUCTS

Haemoglobin adducts of aromatic amines have been related to cigarette smoking, but the levels of adducts have not yet been related to the occurrence of bladder cancer. Bryant found that smokers have higher levels of haemoglobin adducts of several aromatic amines, including the carcinogens 4-aminobiphenyl and 2-naphthylamine (138). The levels of adducts of 4-aminobiphenyl and 3-aminobiphenyl were correlated with the number of cigarettes smoked per day. Smokers of black tobacco had a higher mean level of haemoglobin adducts of 4-aminobiphenyl, as well as several other aromatic amines, than smokers of blond tobacco (138). Maclure has reported that the levels of the haemoglobin adduct of 4-aminobiphenyl declined after the cessation of smoking (286). Carcinogen–DNA adducts have been identified in human bladder biopsy samples (287,288) and in exfoliated urothelial cells (288,289), providing new techniques for the identification of human bladder carcinogens. Benzidine-related DNA adducts have been found in exfoliated urothelial cells of benzidine-exposed workers (290).

Biologic markers of genetic susceptibility

NAT2 phenotype/genotype

Aromatic amines must be metabolized within the host in order to exert mutagenic or carcinogenic activity (291). For many aromatic monoamines, including those found in tobacco smoke such as 4-aminobiphenyl and 2-naphthylamine, N-acetylation appears to be a detoxification pathway, with the acetylated metabolite being excreted into the urine before it can be N-oxidized to a reactive form (292). The capacity to N-acetylate is polymorphic in humans (292); slow acetylators are homozygotic for a mutated N-acetyltransferase gene (NAT2), which is responsible for decreased activity (293,294). In 1979, Lower et al. proposed that individuals with the slow acetylator phenotype might be at higher risk for aromatic amine-associated bladder cancer (295). This hypothesis was subsequently supported by results from a series of epidemiological studies that, overall, showed that individuals with the slow acetylator phenotype (296,297) or NAT2 genotype (298–300) are at greater risk of developing bladder cancer. The biological plausibility of these observations is strengthened by reports among smokers that slow acetylators have a higher mean level of the haemoglobin adduct of 4-aminobiphenyl than do rapid acetylators (301). This difference was most pronounced at low exposure levels (302).

Among persons occupationally exposed to aromatic amines, several studies have shown an excess of the slow acetylator phenotype among cases compared with controls (275,292,300,303–305), but the specific aromatic amine exposures were not well characterized. A study in Chinese workers with an increased risk of bladder cancer (32) who were exposed exclusively to benzidine did not demonstrate an excess of slow acetylators among bladder cancer cases, based on both phenotype and genotype analyses (306). In contrast, a study of bladder cancer cases who had been exposed to benzidine in Germany found a non-significant association with the slow acetylation phenotype (307). A cross-sectional study of workers in India who were currently exposed to benzidine and benzidine-based dyes showed that neither NAT2 genotype or phenotype influenced exfoliated urothelial cell benzidine–DNA adduct levels and that the predominant adduct was N-acetylated (290). These findings suggest that the association between N-acetylation and bladder cancer risk may be specific to certain aromatic amines.

Yu suggested that acetylator status may play a part in the racial/ethnic differences in bladder cancer risk (308). They found that the proportion of slow acetylators was highest among whites, intermediate among blacks, and lowest among Asians, closely paralleling the racial/ethnic variation in risk. Acetylator status also has been analysed in relation to the histological grade or the stage at diagnosis of bladder tumours (303,309,310), but the results are inconsistent.

GSTM1 null genotype

Human glutathione S-transferase M1 (GSTM1) belongs to a family of enzymes that detoxify a spectrum of reactive carcinogenic metabolites, including PAHs, by catalysing their conjugation to glutathione (311). GSTM1 is encoded by the GSTM1 gene, and is polymorphic in human populations; deficiency of this enzyme is caused by the homozygous absence of a functional GSTM1 gene (i.e. null genotype) (312). Nine studies in the general population have found that the GSTM1 null genotype is associated with elevated risk of bladder cancer (298,313–320), whereas two studies have not detected this association (299,321). Risk estimates have been modest, with most relative risks under 2.0. Two cross-sectional studies have evaluated the influence of GSTM1 genotype on urine mutagenicity (322) and haemoglobin adducts (323). Hirvonen (322) found that the GSTM1 null genotype was associated with higher urine mutagenic activity in smokers, which is thought to derive primarily from aromatic amines (323), while Yu (301) reported that the null genotype was associated with higher levels of 3- and 4-aminobiphenyl haemoglobin adducts among both smokers and non-smokers. The exact biological relationship between glutathione S-transferase M1 and aromatic amines is uncertain, however, given that glutathione conjugation is not thought to be a major detoxification pathway for these compounds.

Cytochrome P-450 enzymes

Cytochrome P-4501A2 (CYP1A2) plays an important part in the metabolic activation of several aromatic amines, including 4-aminobiphenyl and 2-naphthylamine, via N-oxidation (324).

Susceptibility to aromatic amine-induced bladder cancer may thus vary with an individual's level of CYP1A2. It is unclear, however, whether the activity of this enzyme is determined by genotype and/or by enzyme induction from environmental exposures (e.g. cigarette smoking, dietary factors, and drugs). Higher levels of 4-aminobiphenyl adducts were found in low-level smokers with rapid CYP1A2 activity, particularly among slow acetylators (325). CYP1A2 activity, as measured by 3-demethylation of theophylline, was associated with bladder cancer risk in one study (326), but uncertainty about the validity of the assay, demographic differences between cases and controls, and the potential for disease bias make interpretation of the study findings unclear. Results from case–control studies of CYP2D6 phenotype have been conflicting (327).

TUMOUR MUTATIONS

Understanding the pathogenesis of human bladder cancer at the molecular level has been evolving for a number of years. Bladder cancer appears to arise from a combination of mutations in tumour suppressor genes (e.g. *TP53*, *RB*) and oncogenes (e.g. *H-RAS*, *c-erbB*-2) (328,329). Because bladder tumours are heterogeneous with regard to their molecular characteristics, it has been hypothesized that environmental exposures may have stronger associations with subgroups of tumours defined at the cytogenetic or molecular level. A higher proportion of tumours from bladder cancer cases who smoked contained chromosome 9 alterations compared with non-smoking cases (330). An association between smoking and mutations in the TP53 gene has been suggested, but not consistently observed across studies (331,332). Occupational exposure to aromatic amines was not associated with either type or frequency of TP53 mutations in tumour samples in a study by Taylor and colleagues (333).

FUTURE RESEARCH

Bladder cancer is known to be caused by cigarette smoking, occupational exposure to certain aromatic amines, cyclophosphamide, *S. haematobium* infection, chronic ingestion of high levels of arsenic in drinking water, and ionizing radiation. It is likely that phenacetin-containing analgesics also cause the disease. The roles of a number of occupational exposures (e.g. motor exhausts), urinary tract infections, urinary stasis, urine pH, dietary factors, chlorination by-products in drinking water, chronic ingestion of low/moderate levels of arsenic in drinking water, tobacco products other than cigarettes, and genetic susceptibility deserve further study.

Cigarette smoking accounts for about 50% of bladder cancer among men and 20–30% among women (113,122,334,335). Occupational exposures have been estimated to be responsible for 10–25% of bladder cancer among men (18) and 10% among women (336), yet the exposures responsible for much of occupational bladder cancer remain unknown. Cigarette smoking and occupational exposures, however, explain only a small part of the large male excess risk of bladder cancer (335). Exploration of possible reasons for this male excess, such as gender differences in unidentified environmental risk factors, urination habits, or hormonal (337) and metabolic determinants of risk, should enhance our understanding of the aetiology of bladder cancer.

Finally, the identification of human bladder carcinogens provides an opportunity to conduct interdisciplinary studies that may help to explain the general mechanisms of carcinogenesis. Potentially useful approaches include identification of specific types of DNA adducts in human urothelial cells, evaluation of interactions between human bladder carcinogens and polymorphisms in metabolic genes, and determination of the relationship between exposure to bladder carcinogen and bladder tumour mutations.

UNRESOLVED RESEARCH ISSUES

1. Why do men have a higher risk of bladder cancer than women after all known risk factors have been taken into account?
2. What are the exposures responsible for the increased risks experienced by workers in high-risk occupations, such as painter, leather worker, and truck driver?
3. Do urinary tract infections cause bladder cancer? What role does urinary statis play in bladder carcinogenesis? Is urine pH an effect modifier of bladder cancer risk?
4. Is chronic ingestion of low/moderate levels of arsenic in drinking water a cause of bladder cancer? Are chlorination by-products in drinking water bladder carcinogens?
5. What is the role of diet in the aetiology of bladder cancer?
6. What is the influence of interindividual variation in carcinogen activation, detoxification, and DNA repair in bladder cancer aetiology?

Key Points

1. In the United Kingdom cancer of the urinary bladder accounts for 7.9% of all new cases of cancer among men and 3.2% of cases among women, as well as 4.4% of cancer deaths among men and 2.4% among women. In the USA, the corresponding figures are about 6.3% of all new cases among men and 2.5% among women, as well as 2.9% of cancer deaths among men and 1.5% among women.
2. Occupational bladder cancer continues to be a public health problem, with risks changing over time and from population to population. With the elimination of bladder carcinogens from the workplace and the advent of new chemicals, risks among rubber and leather workers have diminished over time, whereas new high-risk occupations, such as truck driver and aluminium smelter worker have emerged.
3. Cigarette smoking is well-established as a cause of bladder cancer, although the association is not as strong as that observed for smoking and several other cancers.

Acknowledgements

The authors thank Dr Kenneth Cantor for his comments on the section on drinking water and fluid intake, Ms Joan Hertel of IMS, Inc. for computer programming and figure development, and Ms Judy Lichaa and Ms Ifetayo White for clerical assistance.

References

1 Black RJ, Bray F, Ferlay J *et al.* Cancer incidence and mortality in the European Union: cancer registry data and estimates of national incidence for 1990. *Eur J Cancer* 1997, **33**, 1075–107.

2 Landis SH, Murray T, Bolden S, Wingo PA. Cancer statistics, 1998. *CA Cancer J Clin* 1998, **48**, 6–29.

3 Ries LAG, Kosary CL, Hankey BF *et al. SEER Cancer Statistics Review, 1973–94.* NIH Publ. no. 97–2789. National Cancer Institute, Bethesda, MD, 1997.

4 Parkin DM, Whelan SL, Ferlay J *et al. Cancer incidence in five continents,* Vol. VII. International Agency for Research on Cancer Scientific Publ. no. 143. International Agency for Research on Cancer, Lyon, 1997.

5 Miller BA, Kolonel LN, Bernstein L *et al. Racial/ethnic patterns of cancer in the United States 1988–92.* NIH Publ. No 96–4104. National Cancer Institute, Bethesda, MD, 1996.

6 McCredie M. Bladder and kidney carcers. In: *Trends in cancer incidence and mortality* (ed. Doll R, Fraumeni JF Jr, Muir CS). *Cancer Surveys,* 1994, 19/20, 343–68.

7 Waterhouse J, Muir C, Shanmugaratnam K *et al. Cancer incidence in five continents,* Vol. IV. International Agency for Research on Cancer Scientific Publ. no. 42. International Agency for Research on Cancer, Lyon, 1982.

8 Muir C, Waterhouse J, Mack T *et al.* (ed.) *Cancer incidence in five continents,* Vol. V. International Agency for Research on Cancer Publ. no. 88. International Agency for Research on Cancer, Lyon, 1987.

9 Parkin DM, Muir CS, Whelan SL *et al. Cancer incidence in five continents,* Vol. VI. International Agency for Research on Cancer Scientific publications. no. 120. International Agency for Research on Cancer, Lyon, 1992.

10 Cutler SJ, Young JL Jr (ed.) Third National Cancer Survey: Incidence Data. *Natl Cancer Inst Monogr* 1975, **41**, 1–454.

11 Silverman DT, Morrison AS, Devesa SS. Bladder cancer. In: *Cancer epidemiology and prevention* (ed. Schottenfeld D, Fraumeni JF Jr). Oxford University Press, New York, 1996, pp. 1156–79.

12 Lynch CF, Platz CE, Jones MP *et al.* Cancer registry problems in classifying invasive bladder cancer. *J Natl Cancer Inst* 1991, **83**, 429–33.

13 Hankey BF, Edwards BK, Ries LA *et al.* Problems in cancer surveillance: delineating in situ and invasive bladder cancer. *J Natl Cancer Inst* 1991, **83**, 384–5.

14 Hankey BF, Myers MH. Black/white differences in bladder cancer survival. *J Chronic Dis* 1987, **40**, 65–73.

15 Page WF, Kuntz AJ. Racial and socioeconomic factors in cancer survival: a comparison of Veterans Administration results with selected studies. *Cancer* 1980, **45**, 1029–40.

16 Case RAM, Hosker ME, McDonald DB *et al.* Tumours of the urinary bladder in workmen engaged in the manufacture and use of certain dyestuff intermediates in the British chemical industry. *Br J Ind Med* 1954, **11**, 75–104.

17 Case RAM, Hosker ME. Tumour of the urinary bladder as an occupational disease in the rubber industry in England and Wales. *Br J Prev Soc Med* 1954, **8**, 39–50.

18 Silverman DT, Levin LI, Hoover RN *et al.* Occupational risks of bladder cancer in the United States: I. White men. *J Natl Cancer Inst* 1989, **81**, 1472–80.

19 Decarli A, Peto J, Piolatto G *et al.* Bladder cancer mortality of workers exposed to aromatic amines: analysis of models of carcinogenesis. *Br J Cancer* 1985, **51**, 707–12.

20 Rubino GF, Scansetti G, Piolatto G *et al.* The carcinogenic effect of aromatic amines: an epidemiological study on the role of O-toluidine and 4,4'methylene bis (2-methylaniline) in inducing bladder cancer in man. *Environ Res* 1982, **27**, 241–54.

21 Boyko RW, Cartwright RA, Glashan RW. Bladder cancer in dye manufacturing workers. *J Occup Med* 1985, **27**, 799–803.

22 La Vecchia C, Tavani A. Epidemiological evidence on hair dyes and the risk of cancer in humans. *Eur J Cancer Prev* 1990, **4**, 31–43.

23 Morrison AS, Ahlbom A, Verhoek WG *et al.* Occupation and bladder cancer in Boston, USA, Manchester UK, and Nagoya. *Jpn J Epidemiol Comm Health* 1985, **39**, 294–300.

24 Najem GR, Louria DB, Seebode JJ *et al.* Life time occupation, smoking, caffeine, saccharine, hair dyes and bladder carcinogenesis. *Int J Epidemiol* 1982, **11**, 212–7.

25 Puntoni R, Bolognesi C, Bonassi S *et al.* Cancer risk evaluation in an area with a high density of chemical plants. An interdisciplinary approach. *Ann NY Acad Sci* 1988, **534**, 808–16.

26 Risch HA, Burch JD, Miller AB *et al.* Occupational factors and the incidence of cancer of the bladder in Canada. *Br J Ind Med* 1998, **45**, 361–7.

27 Antony HM. Industrial exposure in patients with carcinoma of the bladder. *J Soc Occup Med* 1974, **24**, 110,.

28 Cartwright RA, Bernard SM, Glashan RW *et al.* Bladder cancer amongst dye users. *Lancet* 1979, **2**, 1073–4.

29 International Agency for Research on Cancer. *Overall evaluations of carcinogenicity. An updating of international agency for research on cancer.* Monographs volumes. International Agency for Research on Cancer, Lyons, 1987, 1–42 (Suppl. 7).

30 Schulte PA, Ringen K, Hemstreet GP *et al.* Risk factors for bladder cancer in a cohort exposed to aromatic amines. *Cancer* 1986, **58**, 2156–62.

31 Meigs JW, Marrett LD, Ulrich FU *et al.* Bladder tumor incidence among workers exposed to benzidine: a thirty-year follow-up. *J Natl Cancer Inst* 1986, **76**, 1–8.

32 Bi W, Hayes RB, Feng P *et al.* Mortality and incidence of bladder cancer in benzidine-exposed workers in China. *Am J Ind Med* 1992, **21**, 481–9.

33 Schulte PA, Ringen K, Hemstreet GP *et al.* Occupational cancer of the urinary tract. *Occup Med: State Art Rev* 1987, **2**, 85–107.

34 Ward E, Halperin W, Thun M *et al.* Bladder tumors in two young males occupationally exposed to MBOCA. *Am J Ind Med* 1988, **14**, 267–72.

35 Stasik MJ. Carcinomas of the urinary bladder in a 4-chloro-o-toluidine cohort. *Int Arch Occup Environ Health* 1988, **60**, 21–4.

36 Popp W, Schmieding W, Speck M *et al.* Incidence of bladder cancer in a cohort of workers exposed to 4-chloro-o-toluidine while synthesizing chlordimeform. *Br J Ind Med* 1992, **49**, 529–31.

37 Ward E, Carpenter A, Markowitz S *et al.* Excess number of bladder cancers in workers exposed to ortho-toluidine and aniline. *J Natl Cancer Inst* 1991, **83**, 501–6.

38 Baus Subcommittee on Industrial Bladder Cancer: Occupational bladder cancer: a guide for clinicians. *Br J Urol* 1988, **61**, 183–91.

39 Parkes HG, Veys CA, Waterhouse JAH *et al.* Cancer mortality in the British rubber industry. *Br J Ind Med* 1982, **39**, 209–20.

40 Alderson M. *Occupational cancer.* Butterworth and Co Ltd, London, 1986.

41 International Agency for Research on Cancer. *Evaluation of the carcinogenic risk of chemicals to humans. chemicals, industrial processes and industries associated with cancer in humans*, Suppl. 4. International Agency for Research on Cancer, Lyon, 1982.

42 Negri E, Piolatto G, Pira E *et al.* Cancer mortality in a northern Italian cohort of rubber workers. *Br J Ind Med* 1989, **46**, 624–8.

43 Jensen OM, Wahrendorf J, Knudsen JB *et al.* The Copenhagen case-referent study on bladder cancer. Risks among drivers, painters and certain other occupations. *Scand J Work Environ Health* 1987, **13**, 129–34.

44 McMichael AJ, Andjelkovich DA, Tyroler HA. Cancer mortality among rubber workers. *Ann NY Acad Sci* 1976, **271**, 125–37.

45 Checkoway H, Smith AH, McMichael AJ *et al.* A case-control study of bladder cancer in the United States rubber and tire industry. *Br J Ind Med* 1981, **38**, 240–6.

46 Delzell E, Monson RR. Mortality among rubber workers III. Cause-specific mortality, 1940–78. *J Occup Med* 1981, **23**, 677–84.

47 Monson RR, Nakano KK. Mortality among rubber workers. I. White male union employees in Akron. *Ohio Am J Epidemiol* 1976, **103**, 284–96.

48 Baxter PJ, McDowall ME. Occupation and cancer in London: an investigation into nasal and bladder cancer using the Cancer Atlas. *Br J Ind Med* 1986, **43**, 44–9.

49 Brown LM, Zahm SH, Hoover RN *et al.* High bladder cancer mortality in rural New England (United States): an etiologic study. *Cancer Causes Control* 1995, **6**, 361–8.

50 Chen JG. A cohort study on the cancer experience among workers exposed to benzidine-derived dyes in Shanghai leather-tanning industry. *Chin J Prev Med* 1990, **24**, 328–31.

51 Cole P, Hoover R, Friedell G. Occupation and cancer of the lower urinary tract. *Cancer* 1972, **29**, 1250–60.

52 Decoufle P. Cancer risks associated with employment in the leather and leather products industry. *Arch Environ Health* 1979, **34**, 33–7.

53 Dolin PJ, Cook-Mozaffari P. Occupation and bladder cancer: a death-certificate study. *Br J Cancer* 1992, **66**, 568–78.

54 Garabrant DH, Wegman DH. Cancer mortality among shoe and leather workers in Massachusetts. *Am J Ind Med* 1984, **5**, 303–14.

55 Henry SA, Kennaway NM, Kennaway EL. The incidence of cancer of the bladder and prostate in certain occupations. *J Hyg* 1931, **31**, 125–37.

56 Marrett LD, Hartge P, Meigs JW. Bladder cancer and occupational exposure to leather. *Br J Ind Med* 1986, **43**, 96–100.

57 Montanaro F, Marcello C, Demers PA *et al.* Mortality in a cohort of tannery workers. *Occup Environ Med* 1997, **54**, 588–91.

58 Seniori Costantini A, Paci E, Miligi L *et al.* Cancer mortality among workers in the Tuscan tanning industry. *Br J Ind Med* 1989, **46**, 384–8.

59 Wynder EL, Onderdonk J, Mantel N. An epidemiological investigation of cancer of the bladder. *Cancer* 1963, **16**, 1388–407.

60 Edling C, Kling H, Flodin U *et al.* Cancer mortality among leather tanners. *Br J Ind Med* 1986, **43**, 494–6.

61 Mikoczy Z, Schutz A, Hagman L. Cancer incidence and mortality among Swedish leather tanners. *Occup Environ Med* 1994, **51**, 530–5.

62 Stern FB, Beaumont JJ, Halperin WE *et al.* Mortality of chrome leather tannery workers and chemical exposures in tanneries. *Scand J Work Environ Health* 1987, **13**, 108–17.

63 Barbone F, Franceschi S, Talamini R *et al.* Occupation and bladder cancer in Pordenone (north-east Italy): a case-control study. *Int J Epidemiol* 1994, **23**, 58–65.

64 Bethwaite PB, Pearce N, Fraser J. Cancer risks in painters: study based on the New Zealand Cancer Registry. *Br J Ind Med* 1990, **47**, 742–6.

65 Claude JC, Frentzel-Beyme RR, Kunze E. Occupation and risk of cancer of the lower urinary tract among men. a case-control study. *Int J Cancer* 1988, **41**, 371–9.

66 Decoufle P, Stanislawczyk K, Houten L *et al. A retrospective survey of cancer in relation to occupation.* DHEW Publ. no. (NIOSH) 77–178. US Government Printing Office, Washington, DC, 1977.

67 Guberan E, Usel M, Raymond L *et al.* Disability, mortality, and incidence of cancer among Geneva painters and electricians: a historical prospective study. *Br J Ind Med* 1989, **46**, 16–23.

68 Malker HSR, McLaughlin JK, Silverman DT *et al.* Occupational risks for bladder cancer among men in Sweden. *Cancer Res* 1987, **47**, 6763–6.

69 Matanoski GM, Stockwell HG, Diamond EL *et al.* A cohort mortality study of painters and allied tradesmen. *Scand J Work Environ Health* 1986, **12**, 16–21.

70 Myslak ZW, Bolt HM, Brockmann W. Tumors of the urinary bladder in painters: a case-control study. *Am J Ind Med* 1991, **19**, 705–13.

71 Terstegge CW, Swaen GM, Slangen JJ *et al.* Mortality patterns among commercial painters in the Netherlands. *Int J Occup Environ Health* 1995, **1**, 303–10.

72 Teschke K, Morgan MS, Checkoway H *et al.* Surveillance of nasal and bladder cancer to locate sources of exposure to occupational carcinogens. *Occup Environ Med* 1997, **54**, 443–51.

73 Englund A. Cancer incidence among painters and some allied trades. *J Toxicol Environ Health* 1980, **6**, 1267–73.

74 Miller BA, Silverman DT, Hoover RN *et al*. Cancer risk among artistic painters. *Am J Ind Med* 1986, **9**, 281–7.

75 Dubrow R, Wegman DH. Cancer and occupation in Massachusetts: a death certificate study. *Am J Ind Med* 1984, **6**, 207–30.

76 Hoar SK, Hoover R. Truck driving and bladder cancer mortality in rural New England. *J Natl Cancer Inst* 1985, **74**, 771–4.

77 Devesa SS, Silverman DT, Young JL Jr *et al*. Cancer incidence and mortality trends among whites in the United States, 1947–84. *J Natl Cancer Inst* 1987, **79**, 701–70.

78 Kunze E, Chang-Claude J, Frentzel-Beyme R. Life style and occupational risk factors for bladder cancer in Germany. A case-control study. *Cancer* 1992, **69**, 1776–90.

79 Milham S Jr Occupational mortality in Washington State, 1950–71. DHEW Publ. no. (NIOSH) 76–175-C. Washington, DC, US Government Printing Office 1976.

80 Momas I, Daures JP, Festy B *et al*. Relative importance of risk factors in bladder carcinogenesis: some new results about Mediterranean habits. *Cancer Causes Control* 1994, **5**, 326–32.

81 Porru S, Aulenti V, Donato F *et al*. Bladder cancer and occupation: a case-control study in northern Italy. *Occup Environ Med* 1996, **53**, 6–10.

82 Schifflers E, Jamart J, Renard V. Tobacco and occupation as risk factors in bladder cancer: a case-control study in southern Belgium. *Int J Cancer* 1987, **39**, 287–92.

83 Siemiatycki J, Dewar R, Nadon L *et al*. Occupational risk factors for bladder cancer: results from a case-control study in Montreal, Quebec. *Can Am J Epidemiol* 1994, **140**, 1061–80.

84 Silverman DT, Hoover RN, Albert S *et al*. Occupation and cancer of the lower urinary tract in Detroit. *J Natl Cancer Inst* 1983, **70**, 237–45.

85 Steenland K, Burnett C, Osorio AM. A case-control study of bladder cancer using city directories as a source of occupational data. *Am J Epidemiol* 1987, **126**, 2–7257.

86 Silverman DT, Hoover RN, Mason TJ *et al*. Motor exhaust-related occupations and bladder cancer. *Cancer Res* 1986, **46**, 2113–16.

87 Wigle DT. Bladder cancer: possible new high-risk occupation. *Lancet* 1977, **2**, 83–4.

88 Gibbs GW. Mortality of aluminum reduction plant workers. *1950 through 1957 J Occup Med* 1985, **27**, 761–70.

89 Rockette HE, Arena VC. Mortality studies of aluminum reduction plant workers: potroom and carbon department. *J Occup Med* 1983, **25**, 549–57.

90 Spinelli JJ, Band PR, Svirchev LM *et al*. Mortality and cancer incidence in aluminum reduction plant workers. *J Occup Med* 1991, **33**, 1150–5.

91 Theriault G, DeGuire L, Cordier S. Reducing aluminum: an occupation possibly associated with bladder cancer. *Can Med Assoc J* 1981, **124**, 419–25.

92 Theriault G, Tremblay C, Cordier S *et al*. Bladder cancer in the aluminum industry. *Lancet* 1984, **i**, 947–50.

93 Tremblay C, Armstrong B, Theriault G *et al*. Estimation of risk of developing bladder cancer among workers exposed to coal tar pitch volatiles in the primary aluminum industry. *Am J Ind Med* 1995, **27**, 335–48.

94 Armstrong BG, Tremblay CG, Cyr D *et al*. Estimating the relationship between the exposure to tar volatiles and the incidence of bladder cancer in aluminum smelter workers. *Scand J Work Environ Health* 1986, **12**, 486–93.

95 Tolbert PE. Oils and cancer. *Cancer Causes Control* 1997, **8**, 386–405.

96 Vineis P, DiPrima S. Cutting oils and bladder cancer. *Scand J Work Environ Health* 1983, **9**, 449–50.

97 Fan TY, Morrison J, Rounbehler DP *et al*. N-Nitrosodiethanolamine in synthetic cutting fluids: a part-per-hundred impurity. *Science* 1977, **196**, 70–1.

98 Matanoski GM, Elliot EA. Bladder cancer epidemiology. *Epidemiol Rev* 1981, **3**, 203–29.

99 Silverman DT, Levin LI, Hoover RN. Occupational risks of bladder cancer in the United States: II. Nonwhite men. *J Natl Cancer Inst* 1989, **81**, 1480–3.

100 Clavel J, Mandereau L, Limasset J-C *et al*. Occupational exposure to polycyclic aromatic hydrocarbons and the risk of bladder cancer: a French case-control study. *Int J Epidemiol* 1994, **23**, 1145–53.

101 Hours M, Dananche B, Fevotte J *et al*. Bladder cancer and occupational exposures. *Scand J Work Environ Health* 1994, **20**, 322–30.

102 Cordier S, Clavel J, Limasset JC *et al.* Occupational risk of bladder cancer in France: a multicentric case-control study. *Int J Epidemiol* 1997, **22**, 403–11.

103 Weiss NS. Cancer in relation to occupational exposure to perchloroethylene. *Cancer Causes Control* 1995, **6**, 257–66.

104 Steineck G, Plato N, Alfredsson L *et al.* Industry-related urothelial carcinogens: application of a job-exposure matrix to census data. *Am J Ind Med* 1989, **16**, 209–24.

105 Augustine A, Hebert JR, Kabat GC *et al.* Bladder cancer in relation to cigarette smoking. *Cancer Res* 1988, **48**, 4405–8.

106 Brownson RC, Chang JC, Davis JR. Occupation, smoking, and alcohol in the epidemiology of bladder cancer. *Am J Public Health* 1987, **77**, 1298–300.

107 Burch JD, Rohan TE, Howe GR *et al.* Risk of bladder cancer by source and type of tobacco exposure: a case-control study. *Int J Cancer* 1989, **44**, 622–8.

108 Claude J, Kunze E, Frentzel-Beyme R *et al.* Life-style and occupational risk factors in cancer of the lower urinary tract. *Am J Epidemiol* 1986, **124**, 578–86.

109 Clavel J, Cordier S, Boccon-Gibod L *et al.* Tobacco and bladder cancer in males: increased risk for inhalers and smokers of black tobacco. *Int J Cancer* 1989, **44**, 605–10.

110 D'Avanzo B, Negri E, La Vecchia C *et al.* Cigarette smoking and bladder cancer. *Eur J Cancer* 1990, **26**, 714–18.

111 Engeland A, Andersen A, Haldorsen T *et al.* Smoking habits and risk of cancers other than lung cancer: 28 years' follow-up of 26,000 Norwegian men and women. *Cancer Causes Control* 1996, **7**, 497–506.

112 Gonzalez CA, Lopez-Abente G, Errezola M *et al.* Occupation, tobacco use, coffee, and bladder cancer in the county of Mataro (Spain). *Cancer* 1985, **55**, 2031–4.

113 Hartge P, Silverman D, Hoover R *et al.* Changing cigarette habits and bladder cancer risk: A case-control study. *J Natl Cancer Inst* 1987, **78**, 1119–25.

114 International Agency for Research on Cancer. Evaluation of the Carcinogenic Risk of Chemicals to Humans. Tobacco Smoking, Vol. 38. International Agency for Research on Cancer, Lyon, 1986.

115 Iscovich J, Castelletto R, Esteve J *et al.* Tobacco smoking, occupational exposure and bladder cancer in Argentina. *Int J Cancer* 1987, **40**, 734–40.

116 Jensen OM, Wahrendorf J, Blettner M *et al.* The Copenhagen case-control study of bladder cancer: role of smoking in invasive and non-invasive bladder tumours. *J Epidemiol Community Health* 1987, **41**, 30–6.

117 McLaughlin JK, Zdenek H, Blot WJ *et al.* Smoking and cancer mortality among U.S. veterans: a 26-year follow-up. *Int J Cancer* 1995, **60**, 190–3.

118 Mills PK, Beeson L, Phillips RL *et al.* Bladder cancer in a low risk population: results from the Adventist Health Study. *Am J Epidemiol* 1991, **133**, 230–9.

119 Momas I, Daures JP, Festy B *et al.* Bladder cancer and black tobacco cigarette smoking. *Eur J Epidemiol* 1994, **10**, 599–604.

120 Nomura A, Kolonel LN, Yoshizawa CN. Smoking, alcohol, occupation and hair dye use in cancer of the lower urinary tract. *Am J Epidemiol* 1989, **130**, 1159–63.

121 Rebelakos A, Trichopoulos D, Tzonou A *et al.* Tobacco smoking, coffee drinking, and occupation as risk factors for bladder cancer in Greece. *J Natl Cancer Inst* 1985, **75**, 455–61.

122 Sorahan T, Lancashire RJ, Sole G. Urothelial cancer and cigarette smoking: findings from a regional case-controlled study. *Br J Urol* 1994, **74**, 753–6.

123 Vena JE, Freudenheim J, Graham S *et al.* Coffee, cigarette smoking, and bladder cancer in western New York. *Ann Epidemiol* 1993, **3**, 586–91.

124 Fraumeni JF Jr. Cigarette smoking and cancers of the urinary tract: geographic variation in the United States. *J Natl Cancer Inst* 1968, **41**, 1205–11.

125 Armstrong B, Doll R. Bladder cancer mortality in England and Wales in relation to cigarette smoking and saccharin consumption. *Br J Prev Soc Med* 1974, **28**, 233–40.

126 Hoover R, Cole P. Population trends in cigarette smoking and bladder cancer. *Am J Epidemiol* 1971, **94**, 409–18.

127 Cartwright RA, Adib R, Appleyard I *et al.* Cigarette smoking and bladder cancer: an epidemiological inquiry in West Yorkshire. *J Epidemiol Community Health* 1983, **37**, 256–63.

128 Wynder EL, Stellman SD. Comparative epidemiology of tobacco-related cancers. *Cancer Res* 1977, **37**, 4608–22.

129 Wynder EL, Augustine A, Kabat G et al. Effect of the type of cigarette smoked on bladder cancer risk. *Cancer* 1988, **61**, 622–7.

130 Kahn HA. The Dorn study of smoking and mortality among U.S. veterans. Report on eight and one-half years of observation. In: *Epidemiological approaches to the study of cancer and other chronic diseases* (ed. Haenszel W). NCI, US Government Printing Office, 1966, p. 1125.

131 Lopez-Abente G, Gonzalez CA, Errezola M et al. Tobacco smoking inhalation pattern, tobacco type, and bladder cancer in Spain. *Am J Epidemiol* 1991, **134**, 830–9.

132 Morrison AS. Control of cigarette smoking in evaluating the association of coffee drinking and bladder cancer. In: *Coffee and Health* (ed. MacMahon B, Sugimura T), Banbury Report 17. Cold Spring Harbor Laboratory, Cold Spring Harbor, NY, 1984, 127–36.

133 Howe GR, Burch JD, Miller AB et al. Tobacco use, occupation, coffee, various nutrients, and bladder cancer. *J Natl Cancer Inst* 1980, **64**, 701–13.

134 Lockwood K. On the etiology of bladder tumors in Kobenhavn-Frederiksberg: an inquiry of 369 patients and 369 controls. *Acta Pathol Microbiol Scand* 1961, **51** (145), 1–166.

135 De Stefani E, Correa P, Fierro L et al. Black tobacco, mate, and bladder cancer. *Cancer* 1991, **67**, 536–40.

136 Vineis P, Martone T. Molecular epidemiology of bladder cancer. *Ann 1st Super Sanita* 1996, **32**, 21–7.

137 Vineis P, Caporaso N. Tobacco and cancer: epidemiology and the laboratory. *Environ Health Perspect* 1995, **103**, 156–60.

138 Bryant MS, Vineis P, Skipper PL et al. Hemoglobin adducts of aromatic amines: associations with smoking status and type of tobacco. *Proc Natl Acad Sci USA* 1998, **85**, 9788–91.

139 Malaveille C, Vineis P, Esteve J et al. Levels of mutagens in the urine of smokers of black and blond tobacco correlate with their risk of bladder cancer. *Carcinogenesis* 1989, **10**, 577–86.

140 Mohtashamipur E, Norpoth K, Lieder F. Urinary excretion of mutagens in smokers of cigarettes with various tar and nicotine yields, black tobacco, and cigars. *Cancer Lett* 1987, **34**, 103–12.

141 Hartge P, Hoover R, Kantor A. Bladder cancer risk and pipes, cigars and smokeless tobacco. *Cancer* 1985, **55**, 901–6.

142 Mommsen S, Aagaard J. Tobacco as a risk factor in bladder cancer. *Carcinogenesis* 1983, **4**, 335–8.

143 Slattery ML, Schumacher MC, West DW et al. Smoking and bladder cancer: the modifying effect of cigarettes on other factors. *Cancer* 1988, **61**, 402–8.

144 Williams RR, Horm JW. Association of cancer sites with tobacco and alcohol consumption and socioeconomic status of patients: Interview study from the Third National Cancer Survey. *J Natl Cancer Inst* 1977, **58**, 525–47.

145 Cole P, Monson RR, Haning H et al. Smoking and cancer of the lower urinary tract. *N Engl J Med*, 1971, **284**, 129–34.

146 Wynder EL, Goldsmith R. The epidemiology of bladder cancer: a second look. *Cancer* 1977, **40**, 1246–68.

147 Cole P. Coffee drinking and cancer of the lower urinary tract. *Lancet* 1971, **i**, 1335–7.

148 Cartwright RA, Adib R, Glashan R et al. The epidemiology of bladder cancer in West Yorkshire. a preliminary report on non-occupational aetiologies. *Carcinogenesis* 1981, **2**, 343–4.

149 Ciccone G, Vineis P. Coffee drinking and bladder cancer. *Cancer Lett* 1988, **41**, 45–52.

150 Jensen OM, Wahrendorf J, Knudsen JB et al. The Copenhagen case-control study of bladder cancer. II. Effect of coffee and other beverages. *Int J Cancer* 1986, **37**, 651–7.

151 Kabat GC, Dieck GS, Wynder EL. Bladder cancer in nonsmokers. *Cancer* 1986, **57**, 362–7.

152 Morrison AS, Buring JE, Verhoek WG et al. Coffee drinking and cancer of the lower urinary tract. *J Natl Cancer Inst* 1982, **68**, 91–4.

153 Piper JM, Matanoski GM, Tonascia J. Bladder cancer in young women. *Am J Epidemiol* 1986, **123**, 1033–46.

154 Pujolar AE, Gonzalez CA, Lopez-Abente G et al. Bladder cancer and coffee consumption in smokers and nonsmokers in Spain. *Int J Epidemiol* 1993, **22**, 38–44.

155 World Cancer Research Fund in association with American Institute for Cancer Research. *Food, nutrition and the prevention of cancer: a global perspective*. Washington, DC, 1997, Chapter, 4, 338–361.

156 Bross ID, Tidings J. Another look at coffee drinking and cancer of the urinary bladder. *Prev Med* 1973, **2**, 445–51.

157 Clavel J, Cordier S. Coffee consumption and bladder cancer risk. *Int J Cancer* 1991, **47**, 207–12.

158 Fraumeni JF Jr, Scotto J, Dunham LF. Coffee drinking and bladder cancer. *Lancet* 1971, **ii**, 7735, 1204.

159 Hartge P, Hoover R, West DW, Lyon JL. Coffee drinking and risk of bladder cancer. *J Natl Cancer Inst* 1983, **70**, 1021–6.

160 Mettlin C, Graham S. Dietary risk factors in human bladder cancer. *Am J Epidemiol* 1979, **110**, 255–63.

161 Vena JE, Graham S, Freudenheim J *et al*. Drinking water, fluid intake, and bladder cancer in western New York. *Arch Environ Health* 1993, **48**, 191–8.

162 Miller CT, Neutel CI, Nair RC *et al*. Relative importance of risk factors in bladder carcinogenesis. *J Chronic Dis* 1978, **31**, 51–6.

163 Morgan RW, Jain MG. Bladder cancer: Smoking, beverages and artificial sweeteners. *Can Med Assoc J* 1974, **111**, 1067–70.

164 Simon D, Yen S, Cole P. Coffee drinking and cancer of the lower urinary tract. *J Natl Cancer Inst* 1975, **54**, 587–91.

165 Risch HA, Burch JD, Miller AB *et al*. Dietary factors and the incidence of cancer of the urinary bladder. *Am J Epidemiol* 1988, **127**, 1179–91.

166 D'Avanzo B, La Vecchia C, Franceschi S *et al*. Coffee consumption and bladder cancer risk. *Eur J Cancer* 1992, **28**, 1480–4.

167 La Vecchia C, Negri E, Decarli A *et al*. Dietary factors in the risk of bladder cancer. *Nutr Cancer* 1989, **12**, 93–101.

168 Chyou PH, Nomura AMY, Stemmermann GN. A prospective study of diet, smoking, and lower urinary tract cancer. *Ann Epidemiol*, 1993, **3**, 211–16.

169 Stensvold I, Jacobsen BK. Coffee and cancer: a prospective study of 43,000 Norwegian men and women. *Cancer Causes Control* 1994, **5**, 401–8.

170 Morrison AS, Verhoek WG, Leck I *et al*. Artificial sweeteners and bladder cancer in Manchester, UK, and Nagoya. *Jpn Br J Cancer* 1982, **45**, 332–6.

171 US Congress, Office of Technology Assessment. *Cancer testing technology and saccharin*. US Government Printing Office, Washington, DC, 1977.

172 Council on Scientific Affairs. Saccharin review on safety issues. *JAMA* 1985, **254**, 2622–4.

173 Kessler II. Cancer mortality among diabetics. *J Natl Cancer Inst* 1970, **44**, 673–86.

174 Armstrong B, Doll R. Bladder cancer mortality in diabetics in relation to saccharin consumption and smoking habits. *Br J Prev Soc Med* 1975, **29**, 73–81.

175 Jensen OM, Kamby C. Intra-uterine exposure to saccharine and risk of bladder cancer in man. *Int J Cancer* 1982, **29**, 507–9.

176 Jensen OM, Knudsen JB, Sorensen BL *et al*. Artificial sweeteners and absence of bladder cancer risk in Copenhagen. *Int J Cancer* 1983, **32**, 577–83.

177 Kessler II, Clark JP. Saccharin, cyclamate, and human bladder cancer. *JAMA* 1978, **240**, 349–55.

178 Morrison AS, Buring JE. Artificial sweeteners and cancer of the lower urinary tract. *N Engl J Med* 1980, **302**, 537–41.

179 Nomura AMY, Stemmermann GN, Heilbrun LK *et al*. Serum vitamin levels and the risk of cancer of specific sites in men of Japanese ancestry in Hawaii. *Cancer Res* 1985, **45**, 2369–72.

180 Slattery ML, West DW, Robison LM. Fluid intake and bladder cancer in Utah. *Int J Cancer* 1998, **42**, 17–22.

181 Vena JE, Graham S, Freudenheim J *et al*. Diet in the epidemiology of bladder cancer in western New York. *Nutr Cancer* 1992, **18**, 255–64.

182 Wynder EL, Stellman SD. Artificial sweetener use and bladder cancer: a case-control study. *Science* 1980, **207**, 1214–16.

183 Miller AB, Howe G. Artificial sweeteners and bladder cancer. *Lancet* 1977, **ii**, 1221–2.

184 Hoover RN, Strasser PH, Child M *et al*. Artificial sweeteners and human bladder cancer. *Lancet* 1980, **1**, 837–40.

185 Hoover R, Hartge P. Non-nutritive sweeteners and bladder cancer. *Am J Public Health* 1982, **72**, 382–3.

186 Murata M, Yakayama K, Choi BCK *et al.* A nested case-control study on alcohol, drinking, tobacco smoking, and cancer. *Cancer Detect Prev* 1996, **20**, 557–65.

187 Thomas DB, Uhl CN, Hartge P. Bladder cancer and alcoholic beverage consumption. *Am J Epidemiol* 1983, **118**, 720–7.

188 Mommsen S, Aagaard J, Sell A. An epidemiological case-control study of bladder cancer in males from a predominantly rural district. *Eur J Cancer Clin Oncol* 1982, **18**, 1205–10.

189 Bruemmer B, White E, Vaughan TL *et al.* Nutrient intake in relation to bladder cancer among middle-aged men and women. *Am J Epidemiol* 1996, **144**, 485–95.

190 Riboli E, Gonzalez CA, Lopez-Abente G *et al.* Diet and bladder cancer in Spain: a multi-centre case-control study. *Int J Cancer* 1991, **49**, 214–19.

191 Steineck G, Norell SE, Feychting M. Diet, tobacco and urothelial cancer. A 14-year follow-up of 16477 subjects. *Acta Oncol* 1988, **27**, 323–7.

192 La Vecchia C, Negri E. Nutrition and bladder cancer. *Cancer Causes Control* 1996, **7**, 95–100.

193 Hicks RM. The scientific basis for regarding vitamin A and its analogues as anti-carcinogenic agents. *Proc Nutr Soc* 1983, **42**, 83–93.

194 Tyler HA, Notley RG, Schweitzer FAW *et al.* Vitamin A status and bladder cancer. *Eur J Surg Oncol* 1986, **12**, 35–41.

195 Steineck G, Hagman V, Gerhardsson M *et al.* Vitamin A supplements, fried foods, fat and urothelial cancer. A case-referent study in Stockholm in 1985–87. *Int J Cancer* 1990, **45**, 1006–11.

196 Helzlsouer KJ, Comstock GW, Morris JS. Selenium, lycopene, tocopherol, carotene, retinol, and subsequent bladder cancer. *Cancer Res* 1989, **49**, 6144–8.

197 International Agency for Research on Cancer. *Evaluation of the carcinogenic risk of chemicals to humans. some pharmaceutical drugs*, Vol. 24. International Agency for Research on Cancer, Lyon, 1980.

198 Fokkens W. Phenacetin abuse related to bladder cancer. *Environ Res* 1979, **20**, 192–8.

199 McCredie M, Stewart JH, Ford JM *et al.* Phenacetin-containing analgesics and cancer of the bladder or renal pelvis in women. *Br J Urol* 1983, **55**, 220–4.

200 McCredie M, Stewart JH. Does paracetamol cause urothelial cancer or renal papillary necrosis? *Nephron* 1988, **49**, 296–300.

201 Piper JM, Tonascia J, Matanoski GM. Heavy phenacetin use and bladder cancer in women aged 20–49 years. *N Engl J Med* 1985, **313**, 292–5.

202 Derby LE, Jick H. Acetaminophen and renal and bladder cancer. *Epidemiology* 1996, **7**, 358–62.

203 International Agency for Research on Cancer. *Evaluation of the carcinogenic risk of chemicals to humans. some antineoplastic and immunosuppressive agents*, Vol. 26. International Agency for Research on Cancer, Lyon, 1981.

204 Levine LA, Richie JP. Urological complications of cyclophosphamide. *J Urol* 1989, **141**, 1063–9.

205 Pederson-Bjergaard J, Ersboll J, Hansen VL *et al.* Carcinoma of the urinary bladder after treatment with cyclophosphamide for non-Hodgkin's lymphoma. *N Engl J Med* 1988, **318**, 1028–32.

206 Travis LB, Curtis RE, Glimelius B *et al.* Bladder and kidney cancer following cyclophosphamide therapy for non-Hodgkinís lymphoma. *J Natl Cancer Inst* 1995, **87**, 524–30.

207 Kaldor JM, Day NE, Kittelmann B *et al.* Bladder tumours following chemotherapy and radiotherapy for ovarian cancer: a case-control study. *Int J Cancer* 1995, **63**, 1–6.

208 Thiede T, Christensen BC. Bladder tumours induced by chlornaphazine. A five year follow-up study of chlornaphazine-treated patients with polycythaemia. *Acta Med Scand* 1969, **185**, 133–7.

209 International Agency for Research on Cancer. *Evaluation of carcinogenic risk of chemicals to man. some aromatic amines, hydrazine and related substances, n-nitroso compounds and miscellaneous alkylating agents*, Vol. 4. International Agency for Research on Cancer, Lyon, 1974.

210 Dunham LJ, Rabson AS, Stewart HL *et al.* Rates, interview, and pathology study of cancer of the urinary bladder in New Orleans, Louisiana. *J Natl Cancer Inst* 1968, **41**, 683–709.

211 Kantor AF, Hartge P, Hoover RN *et al*. Urinary tract infection and risk of bladder cancer. *Am J Epidemiol* 1984, **119**, 510–5.

212 La Vecchia C, Negri E, D'Avanzo *et al*. Genital and urinary tract diseases and bladder cancer. *Cancer Res* 1991, **51**, 629–31.

213 Gonzalez CA, Errezola M, Izarzugaza I *et al*. Urinary infection, renal lithiasis and bladder cancer in Spain. *Eur J Cancer* 1991, **27**, 498–500.

214 Kjaer SK, Knudsen JB, Sorensen BL *et al*. The Copenhagen case-control study of bladder cancer. *Acta Oncol* 1989, **28**, 631–6.

215 Parkash O, Kiesswetter H. The role of urine in the etiology of cancer of the urinary bladder. *Urol Int* 1976, **31**, 343–8.

216 Fellows GJ. The association between vesical carcinoma and urinary obstruction. *Eur Urol*, Year, **4**, 187–8.

217 Mommsen S, Sell A. Prostatic hypertrophy and venereal disease as possible risk factors in the development of bladder cancer. *Urol Res* 1983, **11**, 49–52.

218 Braver DJ, Modan M, Chetrit A *et al*. Drinking, micturition habits, and urine concentration as potential risk factors in urinary bladder cancer. *J Natl Cancer Inst* 1987, **78**, 437–40.

219 McDonald DF, Lund RR. The role of the urine in vesical neoplasm. 1. Experimental confirmation of the urogenous theory of pathogenesis. *J Urol* 1954, **71**, 560–70.

220 Oyasu R, Hirao Y, Izumi K. Enhancement by urine of urinary bladder carcinogenesis. *Cancer Res* 1981, **41**, 478–81.

221 Rowland RG, Henneberry MO, Oyasu R *et al*. Effects of urine and continued exposure to carcinogen on progression of early neoplastic urinary bladder lesions. *Cancer Res* 1980, **40**, 4524–7.

222 Babu SR, Lakshmi VM, Huang GPW *et al*. Glucuronide conjugates of 4-aminobiphenyl and its N-hydroxy metabolites: pH stability and synthesis by human and dog liver. *Biochem Pharmacol* 1996, **51**, 1679–87.

223 Kadlubar FF, Miller JA, Miller EC. Hepatic microsomal N-glucuronidation and nucleic acid binding of N-hydroxy arylamines in relation to urinary bladder carcinogenesis. *Cancer Res* 1977, **37**, 805–14.

224 Kadlubar FF, Unruh LE, Flammang TJ *et al*. Alteration of urinary levels of carcinogen, N-hydroxy-2-naphthylamine, and its N-glucuronide in the rat by control of urinary pH, inhibition of metabolic sulfation, and changes in biliary excretion. *Chem Biol Interact* 1981, **33**, 129–47.

225 Kadlubar FF, Dooley KL, Teitel CH *et al*. Frequency of urination and its effects on metabolism, pharmacokinetics, blood hemoglobin adduct formation, and liver and urinary bladder DNA adduct levels in beagle dogs given the carcinogen 4-Aminobiphenyl. *Cancer Res* 1991, **51**, 4371–7.

226 Young JF, Kadlubar FF. A pharmacokinetic model to predict exposure of bladder epithelium to urinary N-hydroxyarlamine carcinogens as a function of urine pH, voiding interval and resorption. *Drug Metab Dispos* 1982, **10**, 641–4.

227 Babu SR, Lakshmi VM, Hsu FF *et al*. Role of N-glucuronidation in benzidine-induced bladder cancer in dog. *Carcinogenesis* 1992, **13**, 1235–40.

228 Babu SR, Lakshmi VM, Hsu FF *et al*. N-acetylbenzidine-N'-glucuronidation by human, dog, and rat liver. *Carcinogenesis* 1993, **14**, 2605–11.

229 Rothman N, Talaska G, Hayes RB *et al*. Acidic urine pH is associated with elevated levels of free urinary benzidine and N-acetylbenzidine and urothelial cell DNA adducts in exposed workers. *Cancer Epidemiol Biomarkers Prev* 1997, **6**, 1039–42.

230 Remer T, Manz F. Potential renal acid load of foods and its influence on urine pH. *J Am Diet Assoc* 1995, **95**, 791–7.

231 Ferguson AR. Associated bilharziosis and primary malignant disease of the urinary bladder with observations in a series of forty cases. *J Pathol Bacteriol* 1991, **16**, 76–94.

232 Badawi AF, Mostafa MH, Probert A *et al*. Role of schistosomiasis in human bladder cancer: evidence of association, aetiological factors, and basic mechanisms of carcinogenesis. *Eur J Cancer* 1995, **4**, 45–59.

233 International Agency for Research on Cancer. *Evaluation of carcinogenic risks to humans: schistosome, liver flukes and* Helicobacter pylori, Vol. 61. International Agency for Research on Cancer, Lyon, 1994.

234 Tawfik HN. Carcinoma of the urinary bladder associated with schistosomiasis in Egypt: the possible causal relationship. In: *Unusual occurrences as clues to*

cancer etiology (ed. Miller RW *et al.*). Japan Science Society Press, Tokyo, 1988, pp. 197–209.

235 Elem B, Purohit R. Carcinoma of the urinary bladder in Zambia. A quantitative estimation *Schistosoma haematobium* infection. *Br J Urol* 1974, **11**, 199–201.

236 Hinder RA, Schmaman A. Bilharziasis and squamous carcinoma of the bladder. *S Afr Med J* 1969, **43**, 617–8.

237 Gelfand M, Weinberg RW, Castle WM. Relation between carcinoma of the bladder and infestation with *Schistosoma haematobium*. *Lancet* 1967, **i**, 1249–51.

238 Mustacchi P, Shimkin MB. Cancer of the bladder and infestation with *Schistosoma hematobium*. *J Natl Cancer Inst* 1958, **20**, 825–42.

239 Vizcaino AP, Parkin DM, Boffetta P *et al.* Bladder cancer: epidemiology and risk factors in Bulawayo, Zimbabwe. *Cancer Causes Control* 1994, **5**, 517–22.

240 Bhagwandeen SB. Schistosomiasis and carcinoma of the bladder in Zambia. *S Afr Med J* 1976, **50**, 1616–20.

241 Kuntz RE, Cheever AW, Myers BJ. Proliferative epithelial lesions of the urinary bladder of nonhuman primates infected with *Schistosoma haematobium*. *J Natl Cancer Inst* 1972, **48**, 223–35.

242 El-Morsi B, Sherif M, El-Raziki ES. Experimental bilharzia squamous metaplasia of the urinary bladder in hamsters. *Eur J Cancer* 1974, **11**, 199–201.

243 Cheever AW. Schistosomiasis and neoplasia. *J Natl Cancer Inst* 1978, **61**, 13–8.

244 Mee AD. Aetiological aspects of bladder cancer in urinary bilharzia. *Saudi Med J* 1982, **3**, 123–8.

245 Inskip PD, Monson RR, Wagoner JK *et al.* Cancer mortality following radiotherapy for uterine bleeding. *Radiat Res* 1990, **123**, 331–44.

246 Wagoner JK. Leukemia and other malignancies following radiation therapy for gynecological disorders. Unpublished doctoral thesis, Harvard School of Public Health, Boston, MA, 1970.

247 Boice JD, Engholm G, Kleinerman RA *et al.* Radiation dose and second cancer risk in patients treated for cancer of the cervix. *Radiat Res* 1988, **116**, 3–55.

248 Edmonds CJ, Smith T. The long-term hazards of the treatment of thyroid cancer with radioiodine. *Br J Radiol* 1986, **59**, 45–51.

249 Inskip H, Beral V, Fraser P *et al.* Further assessment of the effects of occupational radiation exposure in the United Kingdom Atomic Energy Authority mortality study. *Br J Ind Med* 1987, **44**, 149–60.

250 Smith PG, Douglas AJ. Mortality of workers at the Sellafield plant of British Nuclear Fuels. *Br Med J* 1986, **293**, 845–54.

251 Gilbert ES, Fry SA, Wiggs LD *et al.* Analyses of combined mortality data on workers at the Hanford Site, Oak Ridge National Laboratory, and Rocky Flats Nuclear Weapons Plant. *Radiat Res* 1989, **120**, 19–35.

252 National Research Council. *Drinking Water and Health*, Vol. 3. National Academy Press, Washington DC, 1984, pp. 5–21.

253 Crump KS, Guess HA. Drinking water and cancer: Review of recent epidemiological findings and assessment of risks. *Annu Rev Public Health* 1982, **3**, 339–57.

254 Wilkins JR III, Comstock GW. Source of drinking water at home and site-specific cancer incidence in Washington County. *Maryland Am J Epidemiol* 1981, **114**, 178–90.

255 Freedman DM, Cantor KP, Lee NL *et al.* Bladder cancer and drinking water: a population-based case-control study in Washington County, Maryland (United States). *Cancer Causes Control* 1977, **8**, 738–44.

256 Cantor KP, Hoover R, Hartge P *et al.* Bladder cancer, drinking water source, and tap water consumption: a case-control study. *J Natl Cancer Inst* 1987, **79**, 1269–79.

257 Zierler S, Feingold L, Danley RA *et al.* Bladder cancer in Massachusetts related to chlorinated and chloraminated drinking water: a case-control study. *Arch Environ Health* 1988, **43**, 195–200.

258 McGeehin MA, Reif JS, Becher JC *et al.* Case-control study of bladder cancer and water disinfection methods in Colorado. *Am J Epidemiol* 1993, **138**, 492–501.

259 King WD, Marrett LD. Case-control study of bladder cancer and chlorination by-products in treated water (Ontario, Canada). *Cancer Causes Control* 1996, 7, 596–604.

260 Cantor KP, Lynch CF, Hildesheim ME *et al.* Drinking water source and chlorination byproducts. I. Risk of bladder cancer. *Epidemiology* 1998, 9, 21–8.

261 Cantor KP. Drinking water and cancer. *Cancer Causes Control* 1997, 8, 292–308.

262 Chen CJ, Chuang YC, Lin TM *et al.* Malignant neoplasms among residents of a blackfoot disease-endemic area in Taiwan: high-arsenic artesian well water and cancers. *Cancer Res* 1985, 45, 5895–9.

263 Chiang HS, Guo HR, Hong CL *et al.* The incidence of bladder cancer in the blackfoot disease endemic area in Taiwan. *Br J Urol* 1993, 71, 274–8.

264 Wu MM, Kuo TL, Hwang YH *et al.* Dose–response relation between arsenic concentration in well water and mortality from cancers and vascular diseases. *Am J Epidemiol* 1989, 130, 1123–32.

265 Hopenhayn-Rich C, Biggs ML, Fuchs A *et al.* Bladder cancer mortality associated with arsenic in drinking water in Argentina. *Epidemiology* 1996, 7, 117–24.

266 Chiou HY, Hsueh YM, Liaw KF *et al.* Incidence of internal cancers and ingested inorganic arsenic: a seven-year follow-up study in Taiwan. *Cancer Res* 1995, 55, 1296–300.

267 Tsuda T, Babazono A, Yamamoto E *et al.* Ingested arsenic and internal cancer: a historical cohort study followed for 33 years. *Am J Epidemiol* 1995, 141, 198–209.

268 Cuzick J, Sasieni P, Evans S. Ingested arsenic, keratoses, and bladder cancer. *Am J Epidemiol* 1992, 136, 417–21.

269 Moore LE, Smith AH, Hopenhayn C, *et al.* Micronuclei in exfoliated bladder cells among individuals chronically exposed to arsenic in drinking water. *Cancer Epidemiol Biomarkers Prev* 1997, 6, 31–6.

270 Warner ML, Moore LE, Smith MT *et al.* Increased micronuclei in exfoliated bladder cells of individuals who chronically ingest arsenic-contaminated water in Nevada. *Cancer Epidemiol Biomarkers Prev* 1994, 3, 583–90.

271 Bates MN, Smth AH, Cantor KP. Case-control study of bladder cancer and arsenic in drinking water. *Am J Epidemiol* 1995, 141, 523–30.

272 Clemmesen J. Epidemiological studies into the possible carcinogenicity of hair dyes. *Mutat Res* 1981, 87, 65–79.

273 Skov T, Lynge E. Cancer risk and exposures to carcinogens in hairdressers. *Skin Pharmacol* 1994, 7, 94–100.

274 Hartge P, Hoover R, Altman R *et al.* Use of hair dyes and risk of bladder cancer. *Cancer Res* 1982, 42, 4784–7.

275 Cartwright RA, Philip PA, Rogers HJ *et al.* Genetically determined debrisoquine oxidation capacity in bladder cancer. *Carcinogenesis* 1984, 5, 1191–2.

276 Kiemeney LALM, Schoenberg M. Familial transitional cell carcinoma. *J Urol* 1996, 156, 867–72.

277 Kramer AA, Graham S, Burnett WS *et al.* Familial aggregation of bladder cancer stratified by smoking status. *Epidemiology* 1991, 2, 145–8.

278 Ross RK, Jones PA, Yu MC. Bladder cancer epidemiology and pathogenesis. *Semin Oncol* 1996, 23, 536–45.

279 Menon MM, Bhide SY. Mutagenicity of urine of bidi and cigarette smokers and tobacco chewers. *Carcinogenesis* 1984, 5, 1523–4.

280 Yamasaki E, Ames BN. Concentration of mutagens from urine by absorption with the nonpolar resin XAD-2: cigarette smokers have mutagenic urine. *Proc Natl Acad Sci USA USA* 1977, 74, 3555–9.

281 Kriebel D, Henry J, Gold JC *et al.* The mutagenicity of cigarette smokers' urine. *J Environ Pathol Toxicol Oncol* 1985, 6, 157–69.

282 Falck K, Sorsa M, Vainio H. Mutagenicity in urine of workers in rubber industry. *Mutat Res* 1980, 79, 45–52.

283 DeMarini DM, Brooks LR, Bhatnagar VK *et al.* Urine mutagenicity as a biomarker in workers exposed to benzidine: correlation with urinary metabolites and urothelial DNA adducts. *Carcinogenesis* 1997, 18, 981–8.

284 Falck K, Grohn P, Sorsa M *et al.* Mutagenicity of urine of nurses handling cytostatic drugs. *Lancet* 1979, i, 1250–1.

285 Garner RC, Mould AJ, Lindsau-Smith V. Mutagenic urine from bladder cancer patients. *Lancet* 1982, ii, 389.

286 Maclure M, Bryant MS, Skipper PL *et al.* Decline of the hemoglobin adduct of 4-aminobipheryl during withdrawal from smoking. *Cancer Res* 1990, **50**, 181–4.

287 Talaska G, Schamer M, Casetta G *et al.* Carcinogen-DNA adducts in bladder biopsies and urothelial cells: a risk assessment exercise. *Cancer Lett* 1994, **84**, 93–7.

288 Talaska G, Al-Juburi AZSS, Kadlubar FF. Smoking related carcinogen-DNA adducts in biopsy samples of human urinary bladder: identification of N-(deoxyquanosin-8-yl)-4-aminobiphenyl as a major adduct. *Proc Natl Acad Sci USA USA* 1991, **88**, 5340–54.

289 Talaska G, Schamer M, Skipper P *et al.* Detection of carcinogen-DNA adducts in exfoliated urothelial cells of cigarette smokers: association with smoking, hemoglobin adducts, and urinary mutagenicity. *Cancer Epidemiol Biomarkers Prev* 1991, **1**, 61–6.

290 Rothman N, Bhatnagar VK, Hayes RB *et al.* The impact of interindividual variation in NAT2 activity on benzidine urinary metabolites and urothelial DNA adducts in exposed workers. *Proc Natl Acad Sci USA* 1996, **93**, 5084–9.

291 Morton KC, Wang CY, Garner CD *et al.* Carcinogenicity of benzine, N,N′-diacetylbenzidine, and N-hydroxy-N,N′-diacetylbenzidine for female CD rats. *Carcinogenesis* 1981, **2**, 747–52.

292 Weber WW. The acetylator gene and drug response. New York: Oxford University Press Inc 1987.

293 Blum M, Demierre A, Grant DM *et al.* Molecular mechanism of slow acetylation of drugs and carcinogens in humans. *Proc Natl Acad Sci USA* 1991, **88**, 5237–41.

294 Vastis KP, Martell KJ, Weber WW. Diverse point mutations in the human gene for polymorphic N-acetyltransferase. *Proc Natl Acad Sci USA* 1991, **88**, 6333–7.

295 Lower GM Jr, Nilsson T, Nelson CE *et al.* N-acetyltransferase phenotype and risk of urinary bladder cancer: approaches in molecular epidemiology. Preliminary results in Sweden and Denmark. *Environ Health Perspect* 1979, **29**, 71–9.

296 Dewan A, Chattopadhyay P, Kulkarni PK. N-acetyltransferase activity: a susceptibility factor in human bladder carcinogenesis. *Indian J Cancer* 1995, **32**, 15–9.

297 Hein DW. Acetylator genotype and arylamine-induced carcinogenesis. *Biochim Biophys Acta* 1988, **948**, 37–66.

298 Brockmoller J, Cascorbi C, Kerb R *et al.* Combined analysis of inherited polymorphisms in arylamine N-acetyltransferase 2, glutathione S-transferases M1 and T1, microsomal epoxide hydrolase, and cytochrome P450 enzymes as modulators of bladder cancer risk. *Cancer Res* 1996, **56**, 3915–25.

299 Okkels H, Sigsgaard T, Wolf H *et al.* Arylamine N-acetyltransferase 1 (NAT1) and 2 (NAT2) polymorphisms in susceptibility to bladder cancer: the influence of smoking. *Cancer Epidemiol Biomarkers Prev* 1997, **6**, 225–31.

300 Risch A, Wallace DMA, Bathers S *et al.* Slow N-acetylation genotype is a susceptibility factor in occupational and smoking related bladder cancer. *Hum Mol Genet* 1995, **4**, 231–6.

301 Yu MC, Ross RK, Chan KK *et al.* Glutathione S-transferase M1 genotype affects aminobiphenyl-hemoglobin adduct levels in white, black, and Asian smokers and nonsmokers. *Cancer Epidemiol Biomarkers Prev* 1995, **4**, 861–4.

302 Vineis P, Bartsch H, Caporaso N *et al.* Genetically based N-acetyltransferase metabolic polymorphism and low-level environmental exposure to carcinogens. *Nature* 1994, **369**, 154–6.

303 Cartwright RA, Glashan RW, Rogers HJ *et al.* Role of N-acetyltransferase phenotypes in bladder carcinogenesis: a pharmacogenetic epidemiological approach to bladder cancer. *Lancet* 1982, **ii**, 842–5.

304 Hanke J, Krajewska B. Acetylation phenotypes and bladder cancer. *J Occup Med* 1990, **32**, 917–18.

305 Ladero JM, Kwok CK, Jara C *et al.* Hepatic acetylator phenotype in bladder cancer patients. *Ann Clin Res* 1985, **17**, 96–9.

306 Hayes RB, Bi W, Rothman N *et al.* N-acetylation phenotype and genotype and risk of bladder cancer, in benzidine-exposed workers. *Carcinogenesis* 1993, **14**, 675–8.

307 Golka K, Prior V, Blaszkewicz M *et al.* Occupational history of genetic N-acetyltransferase polymorphism in urothelial cancer patients in Leverkusen. *Germany Scand J Work Environ Health* 1996, **22**, 332–8.

308 Yu MC, Skipper PL, Taghizadeh K *et al.* Acetylator phenotype, amino-biphenylhemoglobin adduct levels, and bladder cancer risk in white, black, and Asian men in Los Angeles, California *J Natl Cancer Inst* 1994, **86**, 712–6.

309 Hanssen HP, Agarwal DP, Goedde HW *et al.* Association of n-acetyltransferase polymorphism and environmental factors with bladder carcinogenesis. *Eur Urol* 1985, **11**, 263–6.

310 Mommsen S, Aagaard J. Susceptibility in urinary bladder cancer; acetyltransferase phenotypes and related risk factors. *Cancer Lett* 1986, **32**, 199–205.

311 Ketterer B. Protective role of glutathione and glutathione transferase in mutagenesis and carcinogenesis. *Mutat Res* 1988, **202**, 343–61.

312 Seidegard J, Vorachek WR, Pero RW *et al.* Hereditary differences in the expression of the human glutathione transferase active on trans-stilbene oxide are due to a gene deletion. *Proc Natl Acad Sci USA* 1988, **85**, 7293–7.

313 Anwar WA, Abdel-Rahman SZ, El-Zein RA *et al.* Genetic polymorphism of GSTM1, CYP2E1 and CYP2D6 in Egyptian bladder cancer patients. *Carcinogenesis* 1996, **17**, 1923–9.

314 Bell DA, Taylor JA, Paulson DF *et al.* Genetic risk and carcinogen exposure: a common inherited defect of the carcinogen-metabolism gene glutathione S-transferase M1 (GSTM1) that increases susceptibility to bladder cancer. *J Natl Cancer Inst* 1993, **85**, 1159–64.

315 Chern HD, Romkes-Sparks M, Hu JJ *et al.* Homozygous deleted genotype of glutathione S-transferase M1 increases susceptibility to aggressive bladder cancer. *Proc Am Assoc Cancer Res* 1994, **35**, 285–8.

316 Daly AK, Thomas DJ, Cooper J *et al.* Homozygous deletion of gene for glutathione S-transferase M1 in bladder cancer. *Br Med J* 1993, **307**, 481–2.

317 Katoh T, Inatomi H, Nagaoka A *et al.* Cytochrome P4501A1 gene polymorphism and homozygous deletion of the glutathione S-transferase M1 gene in urothelial cancer patients. *Carcinogenesis* 1995, **16**, 655–7.

318 Kempkes M, Golka K, Reich S *et al.* Glutathione S-transferase GSTM1 and GSTT1 null genotypes as potential risk factors for urothelial cancer of the bladder. *Arch Toxicol* 1996, **71**, 123–6.

319 Lafuente A, Pujol F, Carretero P *et al.* Human glutathione 5-transferase (GSTμ) deficiency as a marker for the susceptibility to bladder and larynx cancer among smokers. *Cancer Lett* 1993, **68**, 49–54.

320 Lin HJ, Han CY, Bernstein DA *et al.* Ethnic distribution of the glutathione transferase Mu 1–1 (GSTM1) null genotype in 1473 individuals and application to bladder cancer susceptibility. *Carcinogenesis* 1994, **15**, 1077–81.

321 Zhong S, Wyllie AH, Barnes D *et al.* Relationship between the GTSM1 genetic polymorphism and susceptibility to bladder, breast and colon cancer. *Carcinogenesis* 1993, **14**, 1821–4.

322 Hirvonen A, Nylund L, Kociba P *et al.* Modulation of urinary mutagenicity by genetically determined carcinogen metabolism in smokers. *Carcinogenesis* 1994, **15**, 813–15.

323 Bartsch H, Malaveille C, Friesen M *et al.* Black (air-cured) and blond (flue-cured) tobacco cancer risk IV. molecular dosimetry studies implicate aromatic amines as bladder carcinogens. *Eur J Cancer* 1993, **29A**, 1199–207.

324 Butler MA, Lang JF, Caporaso NE *et al.* Determination of CYP1A2 and NAT2 phenotypes in human populations by analysis of caffeine urinary metabolites. *Parmacogenetics* 1993, **2**, 116–27.

325 Landi MT, Zocchetti C, Bernucci I *et al.* Cytochrome P4501A2: enzyme induction and genetic control in determining 4-aminobiphenyl-hemoglobin adduct levels. *Cancer Epidemiol Biomarkers Prev* 1996, **5**, 693–8.

326 Lee SW, Jang IJ, Shin SG *et al.* CYP1A2 activity as a risk factor for bladder cancer. *J Korean Med Sci* 1994, **9**, 482–9.

327 Silverman DT, Morrison AS, Devesa SS. Bladder. In: *Cancer epidemiology and prevention* (ed. Schottenfeld D, Fraumeni JF Jr). Oxford University Press, New York, 1996, pp. 1142–79.

328 Cordon-Cardo C, Sheinfeld J. Molecular and immunopathology studies of oncogenes and tumor-suppressor genes in bladder cancer. *World J Urol* 1997, **15**, 113–19.

329 Reznikoff CA, Belair CD, Yeager TR *et al.* A molecular genetic model of human bladder cancer pathogenesis. *Semin Oncol* 1996, **23**, 571–84.

330 Zhang ZF, Shu XM, Cordon-Cardo C *et al.* Cigarette smoking and chromosome 9 alterations in bladder cancer. *Cancer Epidemiol Biomarkers Prev* 1997, **6**, 321–6.

331 Husgafvel-Pursiainen K, Kannio A. Cigarette smoking and p53 mutations in lung cancer and bladder cancer. *Environ Health Perspect* 1996, **104**, 553–6.

332 Spruck CH III, Rideout WM III, Olumi AF *et al.* Distinct pattern of p53 mutations in bladder cancer: relationship to tobacco usage. *Cancer Res* 1993, **53**, 1162–6.

333 Taylor JA, Li Y, He M *et al.* P53 mutations in bladder tumors from arylamine-exposed workers. *Cancer Res* 1995, **55**, 294–8.

334 D'Avanzo B, La Vecchia C, Negri E *et al.* Attributable risks for bladder cancer in northern Italy. *Ann Epidemiol* 1995, **5**, 427–31.

335 Hartge P, Harvey EB, Linehan WM *et al.* Explaining the male excess in bladder cancer risk. *J Natl Cancer Inst* 1990, **82**, 1636–40.

336 Silverman DT, Levin LI, Hoover RN. Occupational risks of bladder cancer among white women in the United States. *Am J Epidemiol* 1990, **132**, 453–61.

337 Cantor KP, Lynch CF, Johnson D. Bladder cancer, parity, and age at first birth. *Cancer Causes Control* 1992, **3**, 57–62.

4. SCREENING OF BLADDER CANCER

Martin M. Goldstein and Edward M. Messing

Bladder cancer is the fourth most common malignancy in males and eighth most common in females in the United States (1). Nearly 95% of these are transitional cell carcinomas (TCCs). Prognosis is dependent on the grade and stage at the time of presentation. Superficial tumours are relatively easily treated with local therapies and have an excellent prognosis. However, once the tumour becomes muscle invasive the prognosis is quite poor despite aggressive treatment.

Almost all bladder malignancies originate on the urothelial surface. The overwhelming majority of patients who succumb to the disease are those with metastases, and nearly all patients with metastatic disease have concomitant or prior muscle invading tumours. Nearly 90% of all patients who have TCCs that have invaded the detrusor muscle, have muscle invasion at the time of their initial diagnosis (2). If screening methods could detect bladder cancers destined to become muscle invading while they are still superficial (and therefore amenable to very successful therapy), it is likely that a significant reduction in morbidity and mortality would result.

PRINCIPLES OF SCREENING

Screening is the process by which asymptomatic people are tested to determine if they are likely to have a particular disease. Those who are deemed likely by the screening test are then evaluated further to determine if they actually have the disease. Those diagnosed are usually treated for the screened disease. The goal, of course, is to detect and treat the disease earlier than would be done if it were detected only after symptoms had occurred. The screening process is considered successful if these individuals are not only diagnosed earlier (i.e. at earlier stages), but also have decreased cause specific morbidity and/or mortality.

For a screening programme to be of value, candidate diseases must meet certain criteria (Table 4.1). The disease must be a serious health concern. It must be relatively common and occur in a population that can be defined by easily ascertainable demographics and risk factors. There must be some apparent benefit

Table 4.1

BLADDER APPROPRIATENESS OF SCREENING	
	Bladder cancer
Common problem	++
Associated morbidity and mortality from disease	++
Defined population at increased risk	++
Sensitivity of available screening test	+++
Specificity of available screening test	±
Cost of subsequent work-up	+
Do all diseases found need treatment?	+++
Effectiveness of available treatment for late-stage disease	+
Effectiveness of available treatment for early-stage disease	+++
Ability of available screening to detect the disease when still curable	+++
Relative lower morbidity and expense of treatment for early compared with advanced disease	++++
+ Represents reason to consider the disease suitable for screening: the more + the more suitable.	

(primarily for outcome, but also for disease- and treatment-related morbidity) for early treatment compared with later treatment. Additionally, the disease must have a preclinical phase of 'reasonable' duration (e.g. many months to years) during which the disease is detectable but undiagnosed because it has not yet caused symptoms, as a disease with a short preclinical course (e.g. acute infections) would necessitate unreasonably frequent screening.

How well a screening programme meets those criteria is not easy to define. Screening 'success' is based on outcome measurements. Disease specific mortality should be decreased in the screened population as compared with the unscreened population. As this is hard to prove, one would at least expect a shift towards less advanced clinical and pathological stages and a prolonged survival time after diagnosis.

The classic way to evaluate screening tests is in terms of their sensitivities, specificities, and predictive values (Table 4.2). The sensitivity of a test is its ability to designate people with the disease as positive. A test's specificity is its ability to designate people without the disease as negative. The positive predictive value (PPV) is the proportion of patients who test positively who are found to have the disease. As most patients with a negative screening test do not undergo further diagnostic examination, the true number of false-negative and true-negative results are never accurately known. PPV, however, does not rely as heavily upon these 'true' values and is therefore arguably the most valuable in comparing various screening tests.

Table 4.2

SCREENING DEFINITIONS
Sensitivity = number of people with a disease and a positive test
number of people with a disease and either a positive or negative test
or sensitivity = true positives
true positives and false negatives
Specificity = number of people without a disease and a negative test
number of people without disease and either a negative or positive test
or specificity = true negatives
true negatives and false positives
positive number of people with a positive test who have the disease
predictive = number of people with a positive test with the disease or not
value
positive true positives
or predictive = true positives and false positives
value
lead time = the interval from detection due to screening to the time at which
diagnosis would have been made without that screening (i.e. when symptoms or
signs would have provoked evaluation)
length bias sampling = the tendency of a screening test to preferentially identify
indolent disease with a long preclinical phase

A test's sensitivity can be increased at the expense of its specificity, by lowering the standards for positivity. Likewise, a test's specificity can be increased at the expense of sensitivity, by reducing the number of false-positives. This can be done by either raising the standards of positivity of the test, or by increasing the number of true-positives as compared with false-positives. The latter is accomplished by screening a population with a high prevalence of the disease, which can be achieved by selecting high risk populations for screening.

The period of time between when the disease is detected in screened individuals and when it would have been detected if the diagnosis was delayed until symptoms provoked an evaluation is the 'lead time'. Because screening detects the condition before it would normally be diagnosed, time interval survival data will favour the outcome of a screened population compared with that of an historical control unscreened population simply because of the lead time in diagnosis that screening has created, even if screened and unscreened patients eventually expire at the same age from the disease. This is called 'lead time bias'.

Length bias sampling, the tendency for screening tests to detect slower growing cancers as they are in the asymptomatic population longer than more rapidly growing ones—which quickly become symptomatic and no longer need screening to become detected—can also give an impression of increasing survival in people with screening detected cancers. These biases are important arguments against accepting the shift to earlier stages as unequivocal proof that screening improves disease outcome. (Table 4.2).

THE PROGNOSIS OF TREATED BLADDER CANCER

While TCCs exhibit a wide spectrum of biological aggressiveness ranging from low grade superficial to high grade invasive cancers, in general, they have a distinctively dichotomous behaviour. Low to moderate grade (grades I, II) superficial (stage Ta, T1) lesions frequently recur after 'complete' endoscopic resection, but rarely invade, while high grade (grade III) tumours usually are already muscle invading (stage T2+) at the time of diagnosis. It is almost exclusively the high grade TCCs that are associated with significant morbidity and mortality.

Low and moderate grade superficial TCC accounts for approximately 55% of newly diagnosed cancers. Easily treated with cystoscopic resection, they recur in approximately 50% of patients (3); however, progression to muscle invasion in subsequent recurrences is rare. High grade TCC accounts for 45% of newly diagnosed TCC. Roughly 40% of newly diagnosed high grade cancers are confined to the epithelium (Ta) or lamina propria (T1), while nearly 60% are muscle invasive (T2) or beyond when diagnosed. Moreover, the high grade superficial tumours progress to muscle invasion far more often than grade I and II TCCs do upon subsequent recurrence. Use of intravesical immunotherapy (BCG) significantly decreases the rates of recurrence and progression of superficial TCC once it is resected transurethrally, even for high grade tumours. Prior to the use of BCG, one representative study showed that stage Ta, T1 tumours progressed to muscle invasive disease 2% of the time for grade I, 11% for grade II, and 45% for grade III lesions (4). The use of intravesical BCG has reduced the subsequent progression ratios, particularly for the high grade superficial TCCs, which progress to muscle invasion roughly 25% of the time when treated with endoscopic resection and BCG.

Approximately 50% of patients with muscle invasive or more extensive disease have occult metastases at diagnosis. Nearly all patients with metastatic disease succumb from bladder cancer within 2 years despite the administration of multidrug, highly toxic, chemotherapy. Those who have muscle invasion without evidence of metastatic spread require either partial or radical cystectomy, systemic chemotherapy, and/or radiation therapy. All of these are associated with considerable morbidities and risks. Thus, screening that would permit earlier detection should not only afford patients a more favourable prognosis, it would also potentially avoid much of the morbidities associated with treating advanced disease.

RATIONALE FOR EARLY DETECTION

Excellent cure rates are achieved for stage Ta and T1 TCC, even for high grade disease. However, once the disease is muscle invasive prognosis is poor. Unfortunately, approximately 90% of patients with muscle invasive disease will be found on their initial bladder cancer presentation (2) and do not come from the pool of patients with recurrent superficial TCCs. Because all of these tumours originate in the urothelium, the opportunity exists to detect ones destined to invade muscle before they actually do so. With current detection strategies, primarily evaluating haematuria which patients note or which is discovered (and recognized) on a urinalysis done for unrelated reasons, this is not often accomplished. Because more effective therapies for metastatic TCC are not on the immediate horizon, if we are to reduce this disease's morbidity and mortality significantly, early detection strategies will need to be improved and implemented.

A common argument against screening for any chronic disease is that one may detect and treat a condition that had it not been detected, would not have led to any adverse sequelae. This has been a significant concern about screening for prostate cancer, for example. This is not the case with bladder cancer, however, which is almost never found incidentally on autopsy (5). This implies that as opposed to prostate cancer, bladder cancer's preclinical duration or potential lead time (the time interval between when it could be diagnosed if you looked for it and when it is actually diagnosed because of symptoms) is fairly brief. Put in other terms, before a patient expires, symptoms (primarily haematuria) eventually occur leading to a diagnosis. Because of TCC's rapid growth and the relatively low expense and morbidity of endoscopic resection, treatment is rarely withheld once a diagnosis is established. Therefore, patients in whom bladder cancer is detected through screening do not undergo any unnecessary tests or treatments, only earlier ones.

SCREENING FOR HAEMATURIA

Practically all bladder cancers will cause haematuria at some point (6). But, haematuria is often intermittent, even when caused by serious diseases. Thus, repeated testing for haematuria is needed—and once one specimen is positive, further evaluation should be undertaken to determine its cause. Screening for haematuria can be done by microscopic urinalysis or by using a chemical reagent strip to test for haemoglobin. 'False' positive results occur with

reagent strips in conditions such as haemoglobinuria or myo-
globinuria; in general, however, the strips are a very accurate
reflection of microscopic urinalyses in detecting haematuria (7).

The importance of complete urological examination for asymptomatic haematuria, including intravenous urography and cystoscopy,
has been known for some time. Greene in 1956 (8) and subsequently many others, have confirmed that significant lesions are
identified in 13–20% of patients who are referred for asymptomatic
microscopic haematuria, and cancer was found in 6.5–13% of
patients (9–11). Two screening studies of the general population
using haematuria home testing have been published. Messing
(12–14), Britton (15,16) and their respective colleagues solicited
from general practice patient care rosters all middle aged and elderly
men residing in geographically defined regions (South Central
Wisconsin (12–14) and Leeds, England (15) not believed to have
urological malignancies or other known causes of haematuria, and
requested them to test their urine 10–14 times at home with reagent
strips for haemoglobin. If positive even once, subjects were asked to
undergo formal urological evaluation including intravenous urography, cytology, and cystoscopy. The two studies had similar
findings. Fifteen to 20% of the screened populations had haematuria. Of those who completed the evaluation, 6–8% were found to
have urothelial cancers. Overall, 1.2–1.3% of those screened had
bladder cancer diagnosed. Noteworthy, however, is that neither
study had a prospective, randomized control population.

The Wisconsin study looked at state tumour registry data to
compare the screening participants' outcomes with those of
a contemporary, age/gender matched unscreened population.
Additionally, pathology materials from all men screened who
developed bladder cancer were compared by a referee pathologist
with materials from all men age 50 and over in Wisconsin (not
screened) who developed bladder cancer during 1 year of the
study. In both populations, roughly the same percentage had low
grade (grades I, II) superficial bladder cancers (56.8% unscreened,
52.4% screened). Approximately 45% of the cancers (43.2%
unscreened, 47.6% screened) were high grade. However, the proportion of muscle invasive tumours was significantly higher in the
unscreened population; 23.9% of all cancer registry patients
versus 4.9% of all cancers from screened patients. By 24 months
after diagnosis, 16.4% of the unscreened cases had died of bladder
cancer. In contrast none of the men participating in the screening
study in whom bladder cancer was detected has died of bladder
cancer with 4–9 years of follow up (17). It would seem, that
screening enabled the successful diagnosis of cancers destined to
become muscle invasive at preinvasive stages. Additionally, com-

pared with other diseases for which screening has been accepted as beneficial and worth the expense (e.g. mammography for breast cancer in post-menopausal women, faecal occult blood testing/or colonoscopy for colorectal cancer, and blood pressure checks for hypertension), bladder cancer screening with chemical reagent strips appears to be quite cost-effective (18).

As this was not a prospectively randomized controlled study, certain biases must be considered. Lead time bias (discussed earlier) could have contributed to the decreased mortality seen in the screened group. However, the follow up for the screened population was 4–9 years as compared with 2 years for the unscreened population. Likewise, it is unlikely that in the screened population more indolent tumours with longer preclinical durations were detected (length bias sampling), as the distribution of the grades of cancers detected in both groups were similar. The unscreened population's worse outcome could also be explained if they had received less effective therapy than the screenees. However, as the unscreened patients' outcomes paralleled those reported for contemporary optimum treatment series for similar tumour stages and grades, inferior therapy in the control population does not appear to have been involved. The control group was not randomized, however, and its subjects may have differed from the screenees in terms of their health consciousness or other risk factors. This screening method has other problems as well. While the test's sensitivity approaches 100% for cystoscopically detectable tumours (12–14,19), specificity is only 8% and the positive predictive value only 8% (although the PPV for all malignancies found is 11%, and 33% for serious diseases).

In summary, in the absence of a prospective randomized trial, the available information strongly suggests that screening with haematuria reagent strips shifts the diagnosis to an earlier non-invasive stage with a resulting decrease in mortality. However, if other screening tests could be used to reduce the number of false-positives (thereby reducing the number of negative evaluations), both cost-effectiveness and public and physician acceptance would be enhanced even further.

OTHER BLADDER CANCER SCREENING METHODS

Cytology and DNA flow cytometry

Another possible method for early detection of bladder cancer is cytological analysis of exfoliated cells found in urine. While easy to obtain, it lacks the sensitivity to be of practical use in wide-spread screening. In particular, cytology fails to pick up the well or moderately differentiated tumours. Although these low grade lesions are rarely life-threatening, if a screening modality cannot detect these cancers it would undermine the confidence of participants and physicians in the test. Flow cytometry is more sensitive than classic cytology, but likewise lacks sufficient sensitivity to detect low grade tumours.

Genetic abnormalities

Chromosomal abnormalities in bladder cancers have been identified with fluorescence *in situ* hybridization (FISH) using labelled DNA probes specific to deleted or amplified tumour marker chromosomal regions. Anomalies involving chromosomes 1, 3, 5, 7, 9, 10, 11, 13, and 17 have been reported from examining bladder cancer specimens and/or exfoliated cells (20), and identifying these anomalies by FISH is being used as an adjunct to cystoscopic examination in the follow-up of patients with histories of bladder cancer. Recently, a cosmid-directed probe for detection of small genetic anomalies in the p21 region of chromosome 9 has been used on cells collected by bladder irrigation. This has led to an important improvement in sensitivity (20), and may become a useful large-scale screening modality.

Another promising development for bladder cancer screening has been the use of microsatellite analysis of DNA in voided urine (21). Microsatellites are repeating small DNA sequences that are unique to each individual and have very low inherent mutation rates (22). With mechanisms of DNA repair disrupted in malignant cells, DNA mutations can be detected in exfoliated tumour cells found in the urine of patients with TCC. Polymerase chain reaction (PCR) is used to amplify the DNA recovered from urine on a preselected panel of microsatellite loci and chromosomal regions commonly deleted in bladder cancer. These are compared with the same loci in 'normal' DNA in peripheral white blood cells. Mao *et al.* reported that using 13 DNA markers (which included the loss of heterozygosity of chromosome 9) tumours were detected in 19 of the 20 (95%) patients with bladder cancer, where cytology was positive in only 50% (21). Equally promising results were seen using 20 microsatellite markers on patients undergoing surveillance for recurrent bladder tumours (23). Importantly, as with cytology and DNA image analyses, 'false-positive' results in patients without TCC were quite rare. This technique, however, has not been tested on populations without bladder cancer histories, in which it would be expected that only slightly over 1% would have the disease.

Marker antigens

Antibodies can be used to detect tumour-associated antigens found on exfoliated urothelial cells. When combined with cytology or image analysis, the technique of immunological staining potentially is an excellent way to detect 'pre-malignant' or malignant cells. The Lewis X blood group related antigen is normally absent from adult urothelial cells, except for occasional umbrella (superficial transitional epithelial) cells. However, bladder tumour cells have enhanced expression of the Lewis X antigen. Importantly, for screening purposes, its expression is independent of grade or tumour stage (24). Immunocytological staining for Lewis X antigen on two voided urine specimens in patients with cystoscopically evident bladder tumours (where a positive test required one of two specimens to stain positively) had a sensitivity of 95%, specificity of 85%, positive predictive value of 76%, and negative predictive value of 98% (24) in a group of patients with a high rate of bladder cancer (32%). It remains to be seen whether these excellent numbers would be obtained for a screening population with a much lower expected incidence.

The antigen M344 is expressed on approximately 70% of superficial TCCs. Staining for this antigen has been used to help increase sensitivity for the low grade superficial tumours often missed by standard cytology (25). Another antigen, DD23, is absent from normal urothelium and found on 80% of bladder tumours, regardless of grade or stage (26). A third antigen, T138, is detectable with advanced stage lesions as well as aggressive superficial cancers (27). To date, no antigen described is either extremely sensitive or tumour specific. Were these to be used for screening purposes, a combination of these antigens would likely have to be used together to increase sensitivity (28).

Growth factors, their receptors, and other biomarkers involved in urothelial carcinogenesis

Soluble factors found in urine and their receptors on urothelial cells, have been studied as possible screening tools. The expression of epidermal growth factor receptors (EGFRs) is restricted to the basal layer of transitional epithelial cells in normal and non-malignant disease state urothelium. However, in both low and high grade bladder tumours these receptors are located throughout all cell layers. Moreover, this transepithelial expression of EGFRs occurs throughout the urothelium in patients with TCC, even in regions remote from bladder tumours. The density of EGFRs in tissue also correlates with grade and aggressiveness of bladder cancer (29) and is a predictor of survival and stage progression

(30). EGF concentrations are lower in voided urine of patients with TCC (possibly due to the increased density and widespread urothelial expression of EGFRs). Measurement of EGF in voided urine and detection of EGFR on urothelial cells, already important in predicting outcome, may have additional value in screening.

Urinary autocrine motility factor (AMF) is a soluble cytokine which is present in the urine of patients with bladder cancer in higher concentrations than in healthy controls (31). It is likely to be involved with cellular motility, a property required for tumour invasion and angiogenesis. Analysis of AMF and urothelial AMF receptors may also become important future screening tools.

The Bard Bladder Tumour Antigen (BTA) test measures urinary complexes of fragmented basement membranes (presumably from enzymes originating from the tumour, which degrade the basal lamina). This commercially available test showed moderate sensitivity for grade II (71%) and exquisite sensitivity for grade III (100%) tumors as well as carcinoma *in situ* tumours. Its drawbacks are limited sensitivity for low grade tumours and a high incidence of false-positives resulting from infection or trauma (iatrogenic)(32).

The Nuclear Matrix Protein 22 test (NMP22-Matritech) is an immunoassay performed on urine collections which measures a nuclear protein that forms part of the chromatin lattices on which DNA lies. Unaffected by pyuria or trauma, this test has been shown to be effective in predicting recurrence in patients shortly after local surgical resection (TURBT) (33). It is likely to be used for surveillance primarily, and its role in screening the general population remains unclear. As with BTA, sensitivity for well and moderately differentiated TCCs is not sufficient to warrant its use as an independent screening modality.

The AuraTek FDP test, a rapid urine dipstick immunoassay test for the detection of fibrin/fibrinogen degradation products, has had similar positive results for all grades and stages of TCC. Its low cost and ease of use may make this an important instrument for bladder cancer screening; but again, its sensitivity is only 68%, low as the sole screening test. It should be noted that none of these (BTA, NMP-22, AuraTek FDP) are yet routinely used in clinical practice, let alone screening patients without bladder cancer histories. It remains to be seen how well they will perform in large populations in whom bladder cancer is present in only a small number of subjects.

SCREENING IN HIGH RISK POPULATIONS

In the general population, age and gender clearly play a part in the development of bladder cancer. Roughly 80% of newly diagnosed patients are age 60 or older, with nearly three-quarters being men. Additionally, cigarette smokers are at a far higher risk than individuals who never smoked; with former smokers also having a higher risk, intermediate between the risks of those who currently smoke and those who never have.

Many environmental and occupational exposures will also place an individual at an increased risk for the development of bladder cancer. Several studies have been undertaken to screen these high risk individuals. One study evaluated employees of the DuPont Chambers Works who produce the known carcinogens beta-naphthylamine and benzidine. Subjects used haematuria home chemical reagent strips for 14 consecutive days every 6 months (34). A high degree of protocol adherence was seen (92%) as well as a high compliance rate with repeat screening (85%) (35). Though a few new malignancies were detected, this study has not as yet been fully evaluated. These studies are limited by problems of subjects having differing degrees of exposure, changing production standards within the plant, and the possibility that the exposure itself could be affecting abnormal screening tests without leading to malignancy (false positive tests).

Another noteworthy study was conducted on subjects exposed to coal-tar-pitch using an annual voided cytology as the screening modality. Subjects screened after 1980 were compared with historical controls in the 1970s. Those subjects with cancer diagnosed after the start of screening in 1980 had a higher proportion of cancers identified at an earlier stage (77% versus 67%) and survival was improved (36). However, there are problems with this and other similar studies. There is a self-selection bias, as later individuals presented for screening earlier than their predecessors as they had heard of the possible increased risk of bladder cancer. Additionally, bladder cancer that develops after occupational exposures have an average latency period of approximately 20 years. Most workers will likely retire or move prior to completing the long-term follow up that is required.

FUTURE PERSPECTIVES FOR BLADDER CANCER SCREENING

While screening for bladder cancer seems rational and efficacious this cannot positively be proven without a randomized prospective study of screening with unscreened controls, and outcome data, with death from bladder cancer as the end-point. However, if screening is shown to save lives, then perhaps combining one or more tests with haematuria home reagent strip testing (i.e. evaluating with

Table 4.3

BLADDER CANCER DETECTION					
Test	Sensitivity	Specificity	PPV	Low-grade detection	Cost/complexity
Home haematuria	++	−	−	+	++++
Cytology	− − −	+	+	−	+++
Flow cytometry	±	+	+	−	++
Immunocytological staining with antigens	+	+	+	+	+
Growth factors and receptors?	+	−	−	+	+
Bard tumour antigen test	−	+	−	−	+
NMP-22	−	+	−	−	+
FDP test	−	+	−	−	+
Microsatellites	++	+	+	+	− −
+ favours use of this test in screening: more + the more favourable.					
− reason for not using this test in screening: more − the less favourable.					

Key Points

1. Screening is the process by which asymptomatic people are tested to determine if they are likely to have a particular disease. The screening process is considered successful if these individuals are not only diagnosed earlier (i.e. at earlier stages), but also have decreased cause-specific morbidity and/or mortality.
2. Screening that would permit earlier detection should not only afford patients a more favourable prognosis, it would also potentially avoid much of the morbidities associated with treating advanced disease.
3. Almost all bladder malignancies originate on the urothelial surface. If screening methods could detect bladder cancers destined to become muscle invading while they are still superficial (and therefore amenable to very successful and relatively innocuous therapy), it is likely that a significant reduction in morbidity and mortality would result.
4. A common argument against screening for any chronic disease is that one may detect and treat a disease that had it not been detected, would not have led to any adverse sequelae. This is not the case with bladder cancer, however, which is almost never found incidentally on autopsy.
5. In the Wisconsin home haematuria study approximately 45% of the cancers in both the screened and unscreened subjects were high grade. However, the proportion of muscle invasive tumours was significantly higher in the unscreened population; 23.9% of all unscreened cancers versus 4.9% of all screened cancers.
6. The positive predictive value is generally improved by limiting the screening program to people at high risk. Thus, it may be advantageous to restrict screening participation to people with occupational exposure to known bladder carcinogens or to men age 50 and older with smoking histories.
7. The available information strongly suggests that home haematuria screening shifts the diagnosis to an earlier non-invasive stage with a resulting decrease in mortality. However, if other screening tests could be used to reduce the number of false-positives (thereby reducing the number of negative evaluations), both cost-effectiveness and public and physician acceptance would be enhanced even further.

cystoscopy subjects who are positive on repetitive haematuria testing as their first screen who then have one or a combination of other tests also positive) may be the most cost-effective way (Table 4.3).

It should be remembered, that the efficiency of screening increases with the disease's prevalence in the screened population. For example, the positive predictive value would be improved by limiting the screening programme to people at high risk. For bladder cancer, this may mean restricting participation to people with occupational exposure to known bladder carcinogens. However, if this is done only 10–15% of people who succumb to the disease would be involved. Alternatively, limiting screening to men, age 50 and older with smoking histories, would significantly reduce the numbers to be screened and still include the considerable majority (65%) of people who eventually die from it.

CONCLUSIONS

Morbidity and mortality from bladder cancer depends directly on the stage of cancer at the time of diagnosis. For bladder cancer, survival is marginal once there is muscle invasion deep to the lamina propria; and even for the survivors, the expense, in terms of morbidity and costs, are considerable. The goal of screening is to detect the tumours in their pre-symptomatic phase and administer early treatment, presumably effecting a decrease in morbidity and mortality. While biological behaviour may make bladder cancer suitable for mass screening, it is less common than other prominent tumours for which the benefits of screening have been accepted and it is responsible for fewer deaths.

Though the debate on screening for many cancers, such as prostate cancer, is intense, screening for bladder cancer is not as intensely debated and has not been widely implemented. Although not randomized, the evidence available from the home haematuria reagent strip studies strongly suggests that screening led to an earlier stage of detection with improved survival. We await prospective randomized studies to determine further the value of mass screening for these diseases.

References

1 Parker SL, Tong T, Bolden S, Wingo PA. Cancer statistics: 1997. *CA J Clin* 1997, **47**, 5–27.
2 Kaye KW, Lange PH. Mode of presentation of invasive bladder cancer: Reassessment of the problem. *J Urol* 1992, **128**, 31–3.
3 Prout GR Jr, Barton PA, Griffin PP *et al.* Treated history of noninvasive grade I transitional cell carcinoma. *J Urol* 1992, **148**, 1413–19.
4 Heney NM, Ahmed S, Flanagan MJ *et al.* Superficial bladder cancer: Progression and recurrence. *J Urol* 1983, **130**, 1083–6.
5 Marshall VF. Current clinical problems regarding bladder tumors. *Cancer* 1956, **3**, 543–50.
6 Messing EM, Vaillancourt A. Hematuria screening for bladder cancer. *J Occup Med* 1990, **32**, 835–45.
7 Messing EM, Young TB, Hunt BB *et al.* The significance of asymptomatic microhematuria in men 50 or more years old: Findings of a home screening study using urinary dipsticks. *J Urol* 1987, **137**, 919–22.
8 Greene LF, O'Shaughnessy EJ Jr, Hendricks ED. Study of 500 patients with asymptomatic microhematuria. *JAMA* 1956, **161**, 610–13.
9 Carson CC III, Segura JW, Greene LF. Clinical importance of microhematuria. *JAMA* 1979, **241**, 149–50.
10 Golin AL, Howard RS. Asymptomatic microscopic hematuria. *J Urol* 1980, **124**, 389–91.
11 Thompson IM. The evaluation of microscopic hematuria: A population based study. *J Urol* 1987, **138**, 1189–90.
12 Messing EM, Young TB, Hunt VB *et al.* Urinary tract cancers found by home screening with hematuria dipsticks in healthy men over 50 years of age. *Cancer* 1989, **64**, 2361–7.
13 Messing EM, Young TB, Hunt VB *et al.* Home screening for hematuria: Results of a muticlinic study. *J Urol* 1992, **148**, 289–92.
14 Messing EM, Yiung TB, Hunt VB *et al.* Hematuria home screening: Repeat testing results. *J Urol* 1995, **154**, 57–61.
15 Britton JP, Dowell AC, Whelan P. Dipstick haematuria and bladder cancer in men over 60: Results of a community study. *BMJ* 1989, **299**, 1010–12.
16 Britton JP, Dowell AC, Whelan P *et al.* A community study of bladder cancer screening by the detection of occult urinary bleeding. *J Urol* 1992, **148**, 788–90.
17 Messing EM, Catalona WJ. Urethral tumors of the urinary tract. In: *Campbell's urology* (ed. Walsh PC, Retik AB, Vaughn ED, Wein AJ), 7th edn. WB Saunders, Philadelphia, in press.
18 Lawrence WF, Messing EM, Bram LL. The cost effectiveness of screening men for baldder cancer using chemical regent strips to detect microscopic hematuria. *J Urol* 1997, in press.
19 Messing EM, Vaillancourt A. Hematuria screening for bladder cancer. *J Occup Med* 1990, **32**, 838–45.
20 Wheeless LL, Reeder JE, Han R *et al.* Bladder irrigation specimens assay by fluorescence in situ hybridization to interphase nuclei. *Cytometry* 1994, **17**, 319–26.

21 Mao L, Schoenberg MP, Scicchitano M *et al*. Molecular detection of primary bladder cancer by microsatellite analysis. *Science* 1996, **271**, 659–62.

22 Brentnall TA. Microsatellite instability: Shifting concepts in tumorigenesis. *Am J Pathol* 1995, **147**, 561–3.

23 Steiner G, Scoenberg MP, Linn JF *et al*. Detection of bladder cancer recurrence by macrosatellite analysis of urine. *Nature Med* 1997, **3**, 621–4.

24 Golijanin D, Sherman Y, Shapiro A, Pode D. Detection of bladder tumors by immunostaining of the Lewis X antigen in cells from voided urine. *Urology* 1995, **46**, 173–7.

25 Bonner RB, Hemstreet GP III, Fradet Y *et al*. Bladder cancer risk assessment with quantitative fluorescence image analysis of tumor markers in exfoliated bladder cells. *Cancer* 1993, **72**, 2461–9.

26 Grossman HB, Washington RW Jr, Care TE, Liebert HB. Alterations in antigen expression in superficial bladder cancer. *J Cell Biochem* 1992, **161**, 63–8.

27 Fradet Y, Tardif M, Bourget L *et al*. Clinical cancer progression in urinary bladder tumors evaluated by multiparameter flow cytometry with monoclonal antibodies. *Cancer Res* 1990, **50**, 432–7.

28 Huland E, Huland H, Meier TH *et al*. Comparison of 15 monoclonal antibodies against tumor associated antigens of transitional cell carcinoma of the human bladder. *J Urol* 1991, **146**, 1631–6.

29 Messing EM. Clinical implications of the expression of epidermal growth factor receptors in human transitional cell carcinoma. *Cancer Res* 1990, **50**, 2530–7.

30 Mellon K, Wright C, Kelly P *et al*. Long term outcome related to epidermal growth factor receptor status in bladder cancer. *J Urol* 1995, **153**, 1919–25.

31 Guirguis R, Schiffmann E, Liu B *et al*. Detection of autocrine motility factor in urine as a marker of bladder cancer. *J Natl Cancer Inst* 1988, **80**, 1203–11.

32 D'Hallewin M, Baert L. Initial evaluation of the bladder tumor antigen test in superficial bladder cancer. *J Urol* 1996, **155**, 475–6.

33 Soloway MS, Briggman JB, Carpinigo GA *et al*. Use of the new tumor marker, urinary NMP 22, in detection of an occult or rapidly recurring transitional cell carcinoma of urinary tract following surgical treatment. *J Urol* 1996, **156**, 363–7.

34 Mason TJ, Vogler WJ. Bladder cancer screening at the Dupont Chambers Works: a new initiative. *J Occup Med* 1990, **32**, 874–7.

35 Mason TJ, Walsh WP, Lee K, Vogler WJ. New opportunities for screening and early detection of bladder cancer. *J Cell Biochem* 1992, **161**, 13–22.

36 Theriault GP, Tremblay CG, Armstrong BG. Bladder cancer screening among primary aluminum production workers in Quebec. *J Occup Med* 1990, **32**, 869–72.

5. ANIMAL MODELS FOR THE STUDY OF BLADDER CANCER

Pamela J. Russell and Elizabeth A. Kingsley

INTRODUCTION

Bladder cancer is a heterogeneous disease which occurs mostly in elderly patients. It may occur singly, but is often multifocal and presents different clinical and histopathological appearances. Over 90% of tumours are transitional cell carcinomas (TCCs), with less than 5% squamous cell carcinomas (SCCs) and 1% adenocarcinomas, but mixed tumours may also occur. Most cancers present as superficial disease (80%) and these generally respond well to treatment, while invasive disease is more difficult to treat. Currently, no markers absolutely predict the clinical outcome of individual patients, and studies of models of bladder cancer are therefore helpful for dissecting out pathways of carcinogenesis and progression as well as for treatment. Because of the paucity of well-preserved human clinical specimens for study, several such models have been developed, and these to varying extents mimic the clinical spectrum of disease in humans. Bladder tumours in animals, together with human bladder cancer cell lines, provide a basis for experimental studies of the molecular basis of processes involved in tumour formation, progression, and therapy (1–3). Available animal models include spontaneous or induced animal tumours, the growth of rodent or human bladder cancer in tissue culture, and the growth of xenografted human tumour in immunodeficient hosts. These *in vivo* systems provide the appropriate cellular milieu allowing for epithelial cell–stromal cell interactions which are crucial to the behaviour of bladder cancer cells. This chapter provides a critical appraisal of the use of the models for studies of the biological progression of bladder cancer, and highlights some recent uses of the models for testing new therapeutic strategies.

CYTOGENIC CHANGES IN BLADDER CANCER

Human ureteral cells immortalized by the expression of the SV40 virus large T antigen, or of the E6 or E7 genes of human papillomavirus (4) have provided a useful model of bladder carcinogenesis, which is tested by growing the resultant cell lines in nude mice (3,5). Studies of these lines have indicated that loss of particular chromosomes thought to harbour suppressor genes is associated with tumour formation, and this has been ratified using clinical material. Chromosomal 9 aberrations are considered to be primary events in bladder cancer (6–8), with two putative suppressor genes involved, one on 9p21 and the other on 9q34.1–2 (9,10). A prime candidate at 9p21 is the p16 gene (7) which may be inactivated through loss, mutation (11), or methylation (12), although inactivation of other chromosome 9 genes, CDKN2B and MTAP, is also common (13). One problem is that the use of cell lines has led to an over-representation of p16 changes, possibly because elevation of p16 levels occurs at senescence and cell immortalization (14). In contrast, somatic mutations of the p16 genes *in vivo* are infrequent and confined in human bladder cancer tissues to low-grade and superficial bladder cancers (15), although a higher frequency of p16 (INK4) alterations is found in bilharzia-associated bladder tumours than in other bladder tumours (16). Other major chromosome changes predicted from the model of carcinogenesis *in vitro* are loss of 3p, 18q, 13q, and 11p (4). In a different model, nine cloned sublines derived from the heterogeneous human bladder cancer cell line, UCRU-BL-17 (BL-17) (17) ranged from non-tumorigenic to invasive when grown in nude mice (18), and one of the invasive clones produced metastases in nude rats after orthotopic implantation (19). There appeared to be karyotypic evolution of the BL-17 lines with 'hotspot' changes at 1p12, 3cen–cp21 and 6cen–6q21 (20) when the cells were passaged through nude mice, and unique karyotypic features arose when two sublines showed loss of anchorage-independent growth and a change in growth *in vivo* from solid tumour to fluid-filled cyst, respectively.

BLADDER TUMOURS IN ANIMALS

Autochthonous tumours

Spontaneous

Spontaneous urothelial cancers in animals are not common, but TCCs of the bladder occur in up to 28% of male brown/Norway rats and 45% of male DA/HAN rats (21). These tumours are multifocal and papillary in type, and while invasion is sometimes seen, progression appears to occur as a continuum. These models have therefore not provided a basis for critical studies of differences between invasive and non-invasive disease which clinically, may represent two distinct entities (21,22). However, RBT tumours, which occur spontaneously in ACI rats and resemble human superficial TCC (23) have been extensively used for studies of immunotherapies, including the use of cytokines (23,24). The metastatic ability of some of these lines has allowed studies of the presence of new potential markers of progression, such as downregulation of ferritin heavy chain (ferritin H) with metastatic progression (25).

Carcinogen-induced tumours

Various environmental and industrial carcinogens have been shown to be associated with the development of bladder cancer. Estimates range from 1 to 5% of bladder cancer in the UK (26), through 11% in white American women (27) to 24% in an Italian study (28). There is a clear association between infection with *Schistosoma haematobium* (bilharzia) infection and bladder cancer, and experimental bladder cancer can be induced in schistosome-infected animals (29). This may be related to carcinogenesis associated with the infection as *S. japonicum* infection of mice causes decreased carcinogen-metabolizing hepatic activity (30). Guinea-pigs fed bracken fern develop preneoplastic lesions which after 6 months develop into papillary carcinoma, and after a year, invasive TCC and carcinoma *in situ* (CIS) with focal squamous metaplasia (31), providing a good model for studies of bladder cancer progression. Most animal models of chemical carcinogenesis have focused on rodent bladder tumours induced by arylamine chemicals (Table 5.1), which require activation to DNA-reactive metabolites, often via N-acetylation pathways (32). The ability to N-acetylate is genetically determined with an increased incidence of bladder cancer being observed in slow acetylators exposed to carcinogens (33). Insights into the importance of N-acetyltransferases to arylamine metabolism in the development of bladder cancer have been obtained by studying inbred hamsters, which are polymorphic N-acetylators (33,34) or C57BL/6 mice congenic for slow acetylation (35). Various N-nitroso compounds, such as N-butyl-N-(4-hydroxybutyl) nitrosamine (BBN) administered in the drinking water (36,37), N-[(4-(5-nitro-2-furyl)-2-thiazolyl] formamide (FANFT) (36) in the diet and N-methyl-N-nitrosourea (MNU) instilled intravesically (38), have been shown to induce bladder tumours in rodents with differences in the histopathological outcome related to dosage, lag time until tumour development, species, and strain. These formulations lead more to SCCs than TCCs of the bladder, and only rarely are metastatic deposits found. However, only TCCs, showing the full 'clinical' spectrum

Table 5.1

CHEMICALLY INDUCED BLADDER TUMOURS

Agent	Treatment	Host	Tumour type	Main uses of model
Bracken fern	Dietary	Albino rats	Epithelial hyperplasia followed by TCCs; invasion not preceded by C/S	Studies of tumour progression
	25–30% in feed for 100–150 days	Guinea-pigs	Pure TCCs; none progressed to invasion if older guinea-pigs used	Studies of tumour progression
	Dietary	Cattle	TCC as in humans and hemangiomas of bladder lining after immunosuppression	Studies of tumour progression and role of bovine papillomavirus type 2
BBN*	0.05% in water, 12 weeks	ACI rats (M**)	SCCs > TCCs	Tumour biology, keratin staining
	600 mg, 6 weeks ± retinoids	Fischer rats (F††)	Range of neoplastic changes, with TCCs and late SCCs	Tumour promotion: continuous retinoids increased tumour incidence and progression/stage
	0.05% in water, 4 weeks	Fischer rats	Preneoplastic papillary or nodular hyperplasia	Tumour promotion: uracil given mid-BBN treatment increased lesions
	0.05% in water, 9 weeks	Wistar rats (M)	TCCs	Tumour promotion: r-human growth hormone (r-HGH) potentiated tumour formation
	Dietary	Rats	Malignant TCCs	Photodynamic therapy
	0.05% in water, 4 weeks then 5% L-ascorbate in diet	Fischer 344 rats	Malignant TCCs	Cell cycle and modular biology studies
	In water	C57BL/6 mice C57B/6 × DBA/2 F_1 mice	SCCs, TCCs TCCs only	Tumour biology, chemotherapy of single or combination agents
BBN + MNU†	500 p.p.m. in water, 10 weeks, then i.p. MNU 50 mg/kg	Fischer rats (M)	TCCs	Tumour progression; MNU caused invasion; low frequency of p53 mutations, not associated with invasion
BHBN‡	0.25% in water ± disulfiram	Wistar rats (M)	TCCs	Inhibition of carcinogenesis: disulfiram inhibited tumour development
BBNOH§	28 or 44 mg/kg with or after 2-mercaptoethane (mesna)	SD rats (M)	Bladder cancer with metastases	Inhibition of carcinogenesis: mesna prolonged survival and reduced metastases
FANFT¶	Dose effects	Rats	SCCs > TCCs	Tumour biology
		Fischer rats	C/S, pleomorphic microvilli	Tumour biology
		Wistar rats	Differences in cancer development	Tumour treatment: cyclophosphamide, BCG
		Rats	NBT-II cells Cell lines: cells 'scatter' in response to growth factors	Studies of growth factor pathways, acidic and basic fibroblast growth factors, adhesion molecules
	Dietary: 0.1% *ad lib.*	C3H/He mice (F)	Range of tumours	Thio-TEPA inhibited development only, not established tumours
		C57BL/6 mice		Immunological studies

Table 5.1 continued

CHEMICALLY INDUCED BLADDER TUMOURS

Agent	Treatment	Host	Tumour type	Main uses of model
MNU	Ives[‡‡]	Wistar rats (M)	SCCs > TCCs	Tumour biology
	Ives	Wistar rats (F)	Necrosis or regression of tumours	Photodynamic therapy
	Ives	Wistar rats (F)	Methods for grading MNU tumours, SCC	T-antigen expression
	Ives	Fischer 344 rats (F)		Cytokeratin expression: CK 19 loss associated with invasion
	Ives, 1.5 mg every 2 weeks (× 4)	Fischer 344 rats	Cellular atypia, *CIS*, TCCs	Tumour biology
	Ives, 1.5 mg every 2 weeks (× 4) + oral antibiotics	Fischer rats (F)	Hyperplasia, papillary lesions, sq metaplasia	Experimental radiolabelled 5-iodo-2'deoxyuridine administration
	Ives + EGF	Fischer 344 rats (M), HBT[§§] system		Increased tumour formation
Uracil-induced urolithiasis	Given 36–103 weeks	Fischer 344 rats	More TCCs with longer treatment, high proliferating cells and invasion	Tumour progression

* N-butyl-N-(4-hydroxybutyl) nitrosamine.
† N-methyl-N-nitrosurea.
‡ N-n-butyl-N-(4-hydroxybutyl)nitrosamine
§ N-nitroso-N-butyl-N-(4-hydroxybutyl)amine
¶ N-[4-(5-nitro-2-furyl)-2-thiazolyl] formamide
** Male
†† Female
‡‡ Intravesical
§§ Heterotypically transplanted rat urinary bladder

of atypical hyperplasia, CIS, and muscle-invasive tumours are induced in Fischer, but not Copenhagen rats by a combination of intravesical MNU with oral antibiotics (39). Similarly BBN induces both SCC and TCC in C57BL/6 mice, but only TCC in C57BL/6 × DBA/2 F_1 hybrids (40). In rats, synergism occurs between low doses of several bladder carcinogens (BBN, FANFT, 2-acetylaminofluorene, and 3,3'-dichlorobenzidine) administered simultaneously or sequentially, and a multistage carcinogenesis process has been demonstrated when MNU or FANFT are used as initiators, with dietary sodium saccharin, sodium cyclamate, or tryptophan as promoters (36). These data suggest that the induction of bladder cancer is a multifactorial process.

These models have been extensively used for studying inhibition (41,42) or promotion of carcinogenic effects, for example using cyclophosphamide (43,44) or other tumorigenesis-promoting factors (45–47), possibly including the continuous presence of epidermal growth factor (EGF) in the urine (48). They have also been used for evaluating chemotherapeutic drugs and biological response modifiers (49) administered intravesically. In particular, a cell line, MBT-2, derived from a FANFT-induced tumour in C3H/HeN mice (50) has been widely used for assessment of new therapeutic strategies, such as gene therapy (see below).

Transplantable tumours

Syngeneic systems

Serial transplantation of tumours is useful experimentally but may be accompanied by a loss of heterogeneity. The characteristics and relative merits of transplantable animal tumours have been reviewed elsewhere (21,51). The FANFT-induced tumours, MBT-2 (C3H/HeN mice) and NBT-II (rats), have been used for studying biological response modifiers and new chemotherapies, as well as the role of some growth factors in bladder cancer (Table 5.1). Similarly, the mouse MD-49 tumour model has been used to study immunotherapy using KLH (52). However, there is little evidence to suggest that metastases from subcutaneous implants, the most commonly used model, arise in these systems. Metastases from NB-I rat tumours implanted under the renal capsule have been reported in 30% of animals (53), but this model does not appear to be have been widely used.

Subcutaneous xenografts

Human bladder cancer cells can be grown in immunodeficient hosts. Early work used thymectomized, irradiated, bone-marrow protected mice (54) or rats treated with anti-lymphocyte serum to

induce immunodeficiency (55). More recently, nude rodents have
been used for growing human tumours with high efficiency
(5,21,51). In particular, the use of Matrigel, a complex of extracellular matrix factors in conjunction with tumour cells, has led
to a higher tumour take rate (56). A problem with this model is
that cells do not tend to metastasize when implanted subcutaneously, a convenient site for measurement of tumour growth and
for monitoring the effects of new therapeutic agents. This is partly
overcome by the use of mice with severe combined immunodeficiency (SCIDs) (57), which has led to the development of a
subline (T24B) of the human bladder cancer cell line, T24, which
can metastasize to lungs (58).

Orthotopic models of bladder cancer

Refinement of the various methods of orthotopic implantation now
allows this system to be used routinely for a variety of applications.
Until recently, the processes of invasion and metastasis in bladder
cancer were predominantly investigated *in vitro* using reconstituted basement membranes, such as Matrigel. These studies have
highlighted the importance of adhesion molecules, proteases, and
growth factors, in particular acidic and basic fibroblast growth
factor in the invasive process (3). As with other biological aspects
of bladder cancer, it is vital that such studies be extended in an
orthotopic model. Using a syngeneic rat system, Kawamata *et al.*
(59) showed that overexpression of tissue inhibitors of matrix
metalloproteinase (TIMP1 and TIMP2) in LMC19 cells inhibited
extravasation of pulmonary metastasis but did not affect tumour
take, or local invasion. Using the same model system, it was also
demonstrated that overexpression of gelatinase A markedly accelerated the metastatic phenotype of rat MYU3L cells (60).

While induction of bladder tumours in animals by chemical
means has allowed the study of carcinogenesis and, in some cases,
chemotherapeutic agents (see above), most research leading
towards clinical applications requires models based upon human
cancer cells (19,61–63). Orthotopic models of bladder cancer
allow the study of the biology of the disease, and provide a forum
for the assessment of new methods of diagnosis and therapy, particularly intravesical approaches (3) (Table 5.2). Moreover, orthotopic implantation may be a biological necessity: over the past
decade it has become clear that malignant cells may not exhibit
their invasive and metastatic potential *in vivo* unless implanted
orthotopically (3,64–66). Many human tumour specimens and
cancer cell lines will grow only when reimplanted in their organ of
origin (67–69), while even those which grow subcutaneously in
nude mice are often encapsulated, and rarely invade or metastasize

Table 5.2

SUMMARY OF ORTHOTOPIC RODENT MODELS OF BLADDER CANCER

Model system	Type of model	Material	Method of implantation	Purpose
C$_3$Hf/HeHa mice (F*)	Syngeneic	MBT-2 cells	Intraluminal instillation following electrocautery	Nitrofurantoin inhibition of cell growth
C3H/He mice (F)	Syngeneic	MBT-2 cells	Intraluminal instillation following acid damage	Magnetic resonance imaging
C57 BL/6J mice (F)	Syngeneic	MB-49 cells	Intraluminal instillation following electrocautery	Immunotherapy with keyhole limpet haemocyanin
C3H/He mice (F)	Syngeneic	MBT-2 cells	Intraluminal instillation following acid damage	Mycobacterium cell wall treatment
BALB/c-derived Bcg inbred congenic strains, Bcgs and Bcg^r(F)	Syngeneic	MM45T cells	intraluminal instillation following acid damage	Genetic response to BCG immunotherapy
NMRI-nu/nu mice	Allogeneic	Dissociated TCC xenograft cells	Intraluminal injection following MNU‡ damage	Growth of human cancer cells
Nu/nu mice (F)	Allogeneic	RT4 cells, EJ cells	Intraluminal instillation	Development of papillary and invasive xenografts
Swiss nude mice (F)	Allogeneic	RT-10 cells	Intraluminal instillation	Transfection studies
Outbred nude mice (F)	Allogeneic	RT-10 xenograft tissue	Intact tissue transplantation	Development of metastatic model
BALB/c mice (M†)	Allogeneic	253J cells	Intramural injection	Derivation of metastatic variants
BALB/c mice (M)	Allogeneic	253J B-V cells	Intramural injection	Transfection studies
Swiss CDI mice (F)	Allogeneic	UCRU-BL-13 cells	Intramural injection	Magnetic resonance imaging
Fischer 344 rats	Syngeneic	Dissociated FANFT-induced xenografts	Intraluminal instillation following MNU damage	Development of orthotopic model
Fisher CDF rats (F)	Syngeneic	?	Intramural injection	Effects of photodynamic therapy
Fischer 344 rats (F)	Syngeneic	Ay-27 cells	Intramural injection	Positron emission tomography
Fisher CDF rats (F)	Syngeneic	Ay-27 cells	Intramural injection	Photodynamic treatment
Fisher CDF rats (F)	Syngeneic	Ay-27 cells	Intramural injection	Photodynamic treatment
Chester Beatty–Rowett × Wistar nude rats (M and F)	Allogeneic	2B8 cells	Intramural injection	Radioimmunolocalization
Chester Beatty–Rowett × Wistar nude rats (M and F)	Allogeneic	2B8 cells, BL-17/23α cells	Intramural injection	Radioimmunolocalization
Chester Beatty–Rowett × Wistar nude rats (M and F)	Allogeneic	BL-17/23α cells	Intramural injection	Radioimmunolocalization
CBH/R nu/nu hooded nude rats (F)	Allogeneic	UCRU-BL-17CL cells	Intramural injection	Radioimmunolocalization, autoradiography
Homozygous nu/nu rats (M and F)	Allogeneic	RT4 cells	Intraluminal injection with and without intramural injection	Xenograft growth with and without bladder damage

* Female.
† Male.
‡ N-methyl-N-nitrosurea.

(64,65,70). This phenomenon is not restricted to subcutaneous implantation. For instance, it has been demonstrated that while colonic carcinoma cells will invade and metastasize when injected into the gut, other malignant cells will not (70), while a variety of growth patterns was observed when renal carcinoma cells were implanted in a number of organs (71). The complex biological interactions resulting in xenograft growth, invasion, and metastasis are dramatically illustrated by a series of orthotopic experiments conducted using the human bladder cancer cell line, RT4, which was established from a low-grade non-invasive tumour (72). A suspension of RT4 cells was introduced into the bladder lumen of nude mice via a catheter (73). The take rate was approximately 50%, and the xenografts grew as superficial tumours with no evidence of invasion. When transfected with overexpressed normal or mutant HRAS gene, RT4 cells injected orthotopically produced xenografts which invaded deep into the muscularis (74) but no evidence of invasion was observed when the same cells were implanted subcutaneously. These results suggested a role for overexpressed HRAS in bladder cancer progression, and emphasized the importance of the implantation site. Another study used the 'intact tissue transplantation' orthotopic model, in which small pieces of tumour or xenograft are attached to their organ of origin, or 'onplanted', using surgical adhesive, often resulting in extensive invasion and metastasis (65). Onplanting of RT4 subcutaneous xenografts in nude mice gave rise to extensive local growth with metastasis to the lymph nodes, diaphragm, abdominal wall, omentum, pancreas, and liver (75). While the authors suggest that the contrast between their results and those achieved using a cell suspension indicates the need for cell–cell contact in the expression of the metastatic phenotype, it may also be that onplanting on the outside of the bladder allows organ colonization while circumventing the need for invasion (3).

The heterogeneous nature of bladder cancer makes necessary the development of a variety of models able to reflect the complexity of the disease (3). In particular, models involving the superficial growth of low-grade cancers exposed in the lumen of the bladder are required (21). At the present time such models are scarce, chiefly due to the lack of suitable material on which to base them. By definition, most bladder cancer cell lines are derived from high-grade, undifferentiated tumours. The RT4 line is an exception. Along with the work of Ahlering et al. (73) described above, this line forms the basis of a rat model of superficial bladder cancer developed by Oshinsky et al. (62). Because neonate rodents are less immunocompetent than adults and have less natural killer (NK) cell activity (68,76), attempts to increase the take rate of xenografts used 2–4-week-old nude rats. Injection of a cell suspension through the bladder wall into the lumen resulted in a high take rate (93%) regardless of whether the bladder was pre-damaged by electrocautery or acid-washing. A number of studies have indicated that urothelial trauma can facilitate the implantation of tumour cells (77,78). Interestingly, in contrast to the results of Ahlering et al. (73), both superficial and invasive cell growth were observed. The superficial tumours were predominantly papillary and grade I;

some were found to invade the lamina propria. Most of the muscle invasive tumours were grades II–III and undifferentiated, and contained regions of squamous dedifferentiation and necrosis. A previous study demonstrated the inability of RT4 cells to degrade basement membrane components (79). Here, invasion across the basal lamina was observed even in areas away from the site of injection, where the perforation of the lamina propria may have facilitated invasion. In the same study, RT4 cells were also injected intramurally. These xenografts also took at a rate of approximately 95%. Some remained papillary, while others became undifferentiated and invaded the muscle layers, the lymphatic system, and occasionally the surrounding viscera. No distant metastases were found. The authors suggest that the development of well-differentiated tumours within the bladder lumen and poorly differentiated tumours within the muscularis, regardless of the method of inoculation, may illustrate the role of the host tissues in cancer progression, with the urothelium retarding tumour progression and the muscularis promoting it. This study emphasizes the importance of orthotopic experimentation in the investigation of the biology of bladder cancer.

A new orthotopic model of human bladder cancer

A new model of bladder cancer has been developed by Russel and co-workers using suburothelial injection of cells in immuno-suppressed sheep. Sheep were immunosuppressed by twice daily administration of cyclosporin, and 107 cancer cells injected under the vesical mucosa during cystoscopy. Tumours were monitored by repeat cystoscopy under inhalation halothane anaesthesia, and attained a size of 1 mm^3 after approximately 3 weeks' growth. Histological examination of the xenografts demonstrated typical morphology with abundant mitoses, without necrosis, host tumour-infiltrating lymphocyte response, or fibrosis either centrally or at the submucosal interface between the ovine urothelium and the human xenograft. The development of a large animal model of human bladder cancer allows intravenous or intravesical administration of therapeutic agents under conditions closely mimicking the clinical setting, while serial biopsies can be performed cystoscopically for histological monitoring of response to therapy.

MOLECULAR BIOLOGY

As in other cancers, activation of proto-oncogenes can result in the development of bladder cancer (80,81). Somewhat paradoxically, the first account of a mutation of the HRAS gene in cancer was in the human bladder cancer cell line, T24 (82), but despite extensive searching in clinical bladder tumours, detection rates of RAS mutations at codons 12, 13, and 61, which contain more than 95% of the activating mutations seen in HRAS and KRAS, have remained relatively low [10% (83); 18% (84)]. While mutations of the *RAS* gene allow continuous signalling and hence second messenger-mediated proliferation, its transfection into RT4 human bladder cancer cells resulted in increased invasive ability when they were implanted orthotopically, as noted above (74). Wagner *et al.* (85) implanted syngeneic bladder tumours under the renal capsule of C57BL/6J mice followed by nephrectomy to allow metastases to develop. Using this model, they found a correlation between *RAS* gene activation and the ability to form tumours and metastasize. Studies in other animal models including BBN-induced F344 rat bladder tumours) (11% mutated H*RAS* at codon 61) (86), MNU-induced TCCs in rats (87), and tumours of rats induced with FANFT plus saccharin (24% mutated H*RAS*) (88) have failed to ratify any relationship between H*RAS* mutation and invasive/metastatic ability of bladder cancer cells. Despite these conflicting data, anti-RAS ribozyme expression in EJ human bladder cancer cells implanted orthotopically caused a reduced tumour take and prolonged mouse survival (89). From these data, the general consensus is that *RAS* gene activation does not play a major part in the development of bladder cancer, but may be important but not sufficient for inducing invasive/metastatic ability.

The roles of other dysregulated oncogenes in experimental models of bladder cancer, in particular, *ERBB2*, *MYC*, and *ERBB1* (which encodes the EGF receptor, EGFR), are reviewed elsewhere (3,80,90).

Many tumour suppressor genes, whose loss is associated with tumour growth, have a part in the regulation of the cell cycle. The protein (pRB) encoded by the retinoblastoma gene, *RB1*, (located on chromosome 13) controls the transition from G_1 to S phase. Cell-cycle dependent phosphorylation of pRB (91) at the end of G_1 is induced by cyclin-dependent kinases (CDKs) (92), specifically D-type cyclins in complex with CDK4 and CDK6 and cyclin E in association with CDK2 (92,93). Cyclin activity is negatively regulated by a family of proteins, p21, p16, p15, and p27. pRB phosphorylation releases the transcription factor E2F which can stimulate transcription of several cellular genes responsible for the stimulation of S phase (92,94). Mutation or loss of the RB1 gene is observed generally in high stage bladder cancers and has been associated with invasive disease, aggressiveness, and poor survival (95). Its part in animal models has not been reported.

Another tumour suppressor gene, *P53*, located on chromosome 17p, acts as 'guardian of the genome' (96) by regulating cell growth and cell death by apoptosis (97). Loss of chromosome 17p correlates well with loss of the *P53* gene in bladder cancers, and is generally seen in invasive disease (7,98), but also in a subset of *CIS* tumours (99,100) leading to the suggestion that these *CIS* tumours may progress to invasive disease via a separate pathway from those with normal *P53* (101). *P53* mutations are associated with poor prognosis, regardless of stage or therapy (102). Molecular studies of animal tumours, apart from those of human cell lines grown as xenografts in immune depressed animals, have been far more limited. *P53* mutations were not detected in bladder tumours in rats induced by BBN plus MNU (103).

P53 is effective in protecting cells against DNA damage induced by a variety of agents including ionizing radiation (104,105). Elevation of p53 protein following DNA damage allows activation of a G_1 checkpoint by induction of other genes involved with cell-cycle arrest and DNA repair including *GADD45*, *WAF1*, cyclins, and *MDM2* (106–109). In the absence of *P53*, or in cells containing *P53* mutations, the absence of cell-cycle arrest allows cells to replicate with damaged DNA, increasing the chances of accumulation of genetic defects (104,110,111). In certain tissues, p53 may induce apoptosis later after G_1 or G_2 arrest (112,113). A prediction from this model would be that in the absence of functional *P53*, cells might show increased resistance to ionizing radiation due to the loss of growth arrest and/or apoptosis. This would have implications for invasive bladder tumours which frequently carry *P53* mutations and are treated by irradiation. In cells with mutant *P53*, ionizing radiation has been shown to be associated with increased radioresistance (114–116) increased radiosensitivity, possibly due to loss of p53-dependent DNA repair (117–119) or no change in radiosensitivity (120–121). One suggestion is that any correlation between p53 function and radiosensitivity may be a tissue-specific phenomenon (121). In a recent study, we have used three human bladder cancer cell lines which differ in P53 status to dissect the molecular effects of radiation. The UCRU-BL-13 (BL-13) cell line (122) overexpresses mRNA for *MDM2*, which can bind and inactivate p53 protein (123); the BL-17 cell line (17) has a mutation in codon 280, whereas UCRU-BL-28 (124) expresses wild-type *P53* (125). Irrespective of *P53* phenotype, response to irradiation was characterized by failure to arrest in G_1 and subsequent arrest in G_2. This involved a variety of defects in p53 regulation and response, indicating that correlation of the response to irradiation and radiosensitivity with *P53* status also requires consideration of the dynamics of the response (126).

A recent study has addressed the role of cyclin D_1 overexpression in bladder carcinogenesis of rats treated with BBN and L-ascorbate (127). Despite its role in G_1 phase transition, overexpression of cyclin D_1, which was at least twofold in over 50% of tumours 18 weeks after treatment with carcinogens was found to be associated with decreased p21 expression, but p53 levels, which control cell cycling were not affected. Moreover, no *RAS* mutations were detected.

Two putative bladder cancer tumour suppressor genes have been described. We have recently shown that the *KAI1* gene (chromosome 11p11.2), which encodes a protein of the 'transmembrane 4 Superfamily' and suppresses metastasis formation by rat prostate Dunning AT6.1 cells (128) is downregulated in invasive and high-grade bladder tumours (129). Animal studies to determine the role of the KAI1 protein *in vivo* are currently being undertaken in our laboratory. The gelsolin gene, on chromosome 9, is also underexpressed in bladder cancer compared with normal bladder cells (130). Its introduction into UMUC-2 human bladder cancer cells reduced their tumorigenicity in nude mice.

GROWTH FACTORS AND RECEPTORS

In many cancers, progression is associated with a shift from paracrine growth stimulation to autocrine regulation of cellular growth. This is also the case in bladder cancer. A large number of growth factor pathways appear to be important in regulating the growth of bladder cancer cells (3,90). Of these, the two most important appear to be the EGF and the insulin-like growth factor (IGF-I) axes.

USE OF MODELS FOR THE DEVELOPMENT OF NEW BLADDER CANCER THERAPIES

Human bladder cancer cell lines have provided the most used model for evaluating new chemotherapeutic agents and for determining possible modes of resistance in bladder cancer (131–134). However, animal models and human bladder cancer cell lines grown in nude mice have also been used to trial new chemotherapeutic regimens, biological response modifiers, and photodynamic therapy (Table 5.2). A syngeneic rat orthotopic model has used to study the biodistribution and photodynamic effects of chloro-aluminium sulphonated phthalocyanine (135) and 5-aminole-vulinic acid-induced protoporphyrin IX (136), when administered both intravenously and intravesically. Studies of tumours grown orthotopically have until recently been hampered by an inability to obtain kinetic data on tumour measurements, and outcomes have had to rely on histological analysis at the end of the experiments. A recent breakthrough for this work is the ability to use magnetic resonance imaging (MRI) longitudinally to measure the kinetics of orthotopic bladder tumour growth in nude mice after systemic or intravesical treatments. A comparison was made of the efficacy of standard doxorubicin and liposome-encapsulated doxorubicin in nude mice carrying human BL-13 xenografts (63). The MRI images obtained indicated that in this model the normal clinical course of bladder cancer is followed. The xenografts responded to the chemotherapy at a rate similar to that observed clinically, a result which again illustrates the importance of orthotopic experiments, as subcutaneous BL-13 xenografts do not respond to doxorubicin (137). MRI has also been used successfully in syngeneic orthotopic models, to study the effects of immunotherapy with intravesical tumour necrosis factor alpha (TNFα) (138), mycobacterium cell wall (139), and bacille Calmette-Guérin (BCG) (140).

IMMUNOTHERAPY

The MBT-2 tumour line has been extensively used to study new immunotherapeutic approaches, including the use of cytokines (141). Intravesical therapy with BCG, an attenuated strain of *Mycobacterium bovis*, has proved to be the most effective form of immunotherapy in the clinical setting. Its effectiveness, as shown using the orthotopic bladder tumour model, depends on the uptake and processing of the BCG antigens by bladder tumour cells, as well as on the immune response induced in the host, and in particular, the development of delayed-type hypersensitivity (DTH) which is associated with CD4+ T-helper (Th) cells, but requires co-operation with CD8+ cytolytic cells (CTLs) (141). This DTH response results in cytokine production and macrophage invasion, and the antitumour activity requires both activated T cells and macrophages (141). Studies using BALB/c.CD2 (CD2) mice have indicated that MM45T bladder tumours respond to intravesical BCG in BALB/c but not CD2 mice, which differ in their expression of the Bcg gene. These studies indicate that genetic regulation of macrophages may also play a part in BCG response (140). This has implications for patient selection for BCG therapy. Studies *in vitro* indicated that BCG plus interferon-alpha (IFNα2b) were more effective than either alone in killing a variety of human bladder cancer cell lines, although the sensitivity of the lines varied greatly (142), leading to a phase I clinical trial. The MBT-2 line has also been used to determine the possible role of different immune cell populations in the killing of bladder tumours. Complete remission of MBT-2 tumours grown in C3H/He mice following treatment with a combination of inter-leukin-2 (IL-2) and cyclophosphamide was associated with high levels of natural killer (NK) cells (143), and bropirimine, which activates NK cells has been shown to be effective against trans-planted MBT-2 and human KoTCC-1 cells *in vivo* (144). On the other hand, lymphokine activated killer (LAK) cells appear to mediate cytolysis of bladder cancer cells through a process which involves binding of LAK cells to the adhesion molecule, ICAM-1, expressed on bladder cancer cells (145). The expression of ICAM-1 can be upregulated by treatment with either interferon-gamma (IFNγ) or TNFα (145).

The size and capacity of the rat bladder, as compared with the mouse, makes a rat-based model desirable for the study of new methods of diagnosis and therapy of bladder cancer (19,62). One such method is the intravesical administration of monoclonal antibodies (MAbs), which have been labelled with radioisotopes, drugs, or toxins. Superficial bladder cancer represents an excellent target for MAb-based therapies, as intravesical administration via a catheter can circumvent most of the problems associated with systemic delivery, such as exposure of normal tissues, catabolism of the MAb by the mononuclear phagocyte system, and the pro-duction of a human antimouse antibody response, which in com-bination can reduce the amount of antibody reaching the target tissue to as little as 0.0007% injected dose per gram (146). An orthotopic nude rat model of superficial bladder cancer has been developed by Russell and co-workers, specifically for the study of the localization of radiolabelled MAbs. CBH/R *nu/nu* hooded nude rats are pre-irradiated with 700 rads from a cobalt source, and human bladder cancer cells injected intramurally. Although some xenografts remain confined to the muscularis, a significant pro-portion grow through the rat urothelium and are exposed within the lumen. After palpable tumours develop, the rats are injected intraluminally with radiolabelled MAb. The animals are killed 24 h later. Biodistribution studies indicate that specific localiza-tion of MAbs can occur following intravesical administration. Using the human bladder cancer cell line, BL-17/5 (formally known as BL-17/23α) as a target, a maximum uptake of 3.3% injected dose per gram was achieved, and a maximum xenograft/normal bladder ratio of 40 : 1 (147,148). These figures are well in excess of any reported from the clinical trials conducted using intravesical MAb administration. Many factors may contribute to this difference. BL-17/5 is a subline of BL-17, a cell line derived from a high-grade metastatic cancer (17). As such, it may not be sufficiently representative of the superficial cancers being targeted in the clinical trials. The choice of MAb is of course critical, but a number of biological considerations also require investigation, including the distribution of the target antigen (superficial expression versus even distribution) and the ultrastructure of the tumour, both of which could play vital roles in the uptake of the MAb. Some of these issues have been investigated by concurrent autoradiography and histology of BL-17 xenografts after injection of ^{125}I-labelled MAb into the bladder (149). Erratic antibody uptake, with a maximum of 0.47% injected dose per gram and an 11.3 : 1 xenograft/normal bladder ratio, was related to the site of xenograft growth. Where the target xenografts were exposed in the lumen of the bladder, the antibody had penetrated the tissue to approximately 12 cell layers. In contrast, where the rat urothelium overlay the human cells, minimal antibody deposition was observed. These results again emphasize the need for orthotopic models with superficial xenograft growth. The model of Russell and co-workers is currently being developed further in order to compare the binding and penetration of antibody fragments and single chains against that of intact MAb.

Gene therapy for bladder cancer

Various strategies have been devised to kill tumour cells using gene therapy approaches. Orthotopic growth of tumours in animals offers an excellent model system in which to test these approaches, especially given the ability to measure tumour volume by MRI (63). Genes can be delivered directly *in vivo* using either physical methods or viral vectors. Alternative programmes which require *in vitro* manipulation of either resected tumour cells, tumour infiltrating lymphocytes, or fibroblasts, which are engineered to express cytokines, have been widely used, but may be more difficult to apply in the clinic (141). Physical methods of transfection (e.g. the use of cationic lipids) are suitable for local gene delivery such as might be required in immune enhancement strategies. Viral vector systems can potentially provide both local and systemic gene delivery and the different properties of individual vectors suggests their suitability for particular purposes. Adenovirus (Ad) vectors can infect both dividing and non-dividing cells (whereas retroviruses do not) to achieve efficient transient expression of genes. For cancer therapy involving cell killing and immune approaches, stable integration and long-term expression of therapeutic genes may not be necessary. However, to achieve specificity after systemic delivery, adenovirus particle infectivity should be restricted to target cells, either by altering viral tropism or by introducing specificity at the level of therapeutic gene expression following viral entry into the cell by the use of specific promoters. Both recombinant *Vaccinia* virus and adenovirus vectors have been successfully used to transfer encoded genes into orthotopically implanted MBT-2 and MB-49 bladder tumours after intravesical installation (150,151). In bladder cancer, an additional delivery system is also available. Recombinant BCG organisms have been developed that actively secrete cytokine products or serve as depots for biologically relevant antigens (152). The phagocytosis of BCG by bladder cancer cells would ensure that the genes of interest are delivered to the tumour cells.

One gene therapy strategy is repair of a genetic lesion, such as mutation or deletion of a tumour suppressor gene or overexpression of an oncogene by introduction of a wild-type gene or an inhibitory anti-sense RNA, respectively. Such an approach has been shown to be far more efficient than expected because it causes apoptotic cell death, resulting in substantial tumour regression or tumour growth delay (153). Retrovirally introduced wild-type *P53* in human bladder cancer cell lines, BIU-87 and EJ, *in vitro* prevented their ability to grow in nude mice (154). While *P53* can be efficiently delivered via adenovirus vectors administered intravesically (151), its effects on tumours growing in the bladder have not been reported. Two other relevant gene therapy approaches for bladder cancer are those which enhance anti-tumour immunity and those which effect cell killing via enzyme-directed prodrug therapy (EPT). Combinations of both approaches may be even more effective (155) given that the immune response is stimulated at the site of cell killing, seeding immune cells which can migrate to metastatic sites. The combination of EPT with immune-enhancing strategies should theoretically control both local and metastatic disease. Enhanced anti-tumour immunity is based in part on the production of CTLs. Th cells secrete chemical messages or cytokines, such as IL-2, which can activate CTLs to kill tumour cells directly, but this requires two signals. T cells given the first signal, but not the second become anergic. Many tumour cells express tumour-associated antigens (TAA), which interact with the Th-cell receptor complex in association with major histocompatibility complex (MHC) class 2 molecules which are present on antigen-presenting cells (APC), such as macrophages or dendritic cells, to provide the first signal. However, tumour cells may fail to elicit Th cells because they do not express costimulatory molecules which are required to interact with the APC molecular complex to provide the second signal. Hence, novel anticancer vaccines can theoretically be prepared by engineering the tumour cells to express such molecules. In the mouse, costimulators include B7–1, B7–2 or integrin/adhesion molecules; human equivalents are currently being cloned. Attempts to stimulate the immune system optimally to reject established tumours and metastatic foci have involved injection of autologous APC treated *ex vivo* with peptides derived from tumour antigens. Alternatively, the expression of cytokine genes such as IL-2, TNF, and IFN in tumour cells which are engineered *ex vivo* and reinjected has been shown to bypass the need for Th cells in mice. Introduced cytokine genes have been used in several formats to stimulate immune responses in tumour systems (156). MBT-2 mouse bladder tumours transfected with and producing IL-2 or GM-CSF failed to grow, and inoculation of mice with the transfectant resulted in the induction of immunity in the recipients capable of protecting the mice from further tumour challenge (157). Moreover, treatment of mice with established intravesical MBT-2 tumours was effective in curing some animals.

The EPT approach relies on expressing a gene encoding an enzyme which can activate a prodrug to a toxic metabolite. This approach was initially applied successfully to the treatment of brain tumours in rodents; retrovirus-producing cells expressing a toxin gene under the long terminal repeat promoter were injected into the brain, allowing transduction of glioma cells. The perceived advantage of EPT systems is derived from a so-called 'bystander' effect. Comprehensive cell killing is achieved without the need to express the enzyme in all cells. As normal neural cells of the brain are non-dividing and resistant to retrovirus infection, subsequent injection of prodrug resulted in almost complete tumour regression without effects on normal brain (158). This approach is now in clinical trials (159). To date, the most widely used toxin gene has been the herpesvirus thymidine kinase gene (HSVtk) but a wide variety of enzymes currently used in antibody-mediated systems for prodrug activation may also be adapted for gene therapy (160). HSVtk phosphorylates ganciclovir (GCV) which can then disrupt DNA synthesis, thereby destroying proliferating cells. However, other mechanisms may also operate. Using adenoviruses, the HSVtk gene, expressed under the control of a non-specific Rous sarcoma virus (RSV) promoter, has been shown with GCV treatment to suppress growth of MBT-2 bladder cells implanted subcutaneously in syngeneic mice *in vivo*. Toxic effects included hepatitis.

Concluding remarks

The above review indicates the importance of using orthotopic implantation for studies of bladder cancer. Not only does this enable the use of intravesical therapies, but the biology of the disease is much more reflective of that which occurs in the clinic. New models that provide a spectrum of disease, and present superficial and invasive diseases as distinct entities are needed in order to provide information about the molecular changes which allow the development of invasive disease. Such knowledge could provide new treatment regimens, based on inhibiting the particular changes which occur. The future will allow the testing of new strategies based on treatments such as the use of MAbs, used in conjunction with other treatments which reduce tumour bulk or gene therapy, including local delivery of corrective or suicidal genes together with upregulation of the immune response. Such treatments may inhibit local recurrence and more distant disease. Models which allow intravesical delivery are essential if they are to provide accurate predictive information for patients with bladder cancer.

Points of controversy

1. Pathways to invasion: Do tumours with chromosome 9 deletions have a separate molecular pathway from those with P53 mutations/loss?
2. Orthotopic implantation: the biology of bladder cancers grown subcutaneously and orthotopically is very different. Future studies should use orthotopic implantation if they are to impact on clinical disease.
3. Do changes in cell cycling (e.g. loss of *RB1* or *P53* or increased cyclin D function) alter the response of bladder cancer cells to radiation? Can these changes be used to select patients for radiation therapy?
4. How critical is the role of genetic inheritance of macrophage genotype in the response to BCG therapy? Should patients be screened?
5. Can new therapies, such as radioimmunotherapy using MAbs or gene therapy prevent tumour recurrence?
6. Should such therapies be given concomitantly with standard treatments or at a different time?

References

1 Raghavan D, Shipley WU, Garnick MB *et al.* Biology and management of bladder cancer. *N Engl J Med* 1990, **322**, 1129–38.
2 Raghavan D, Huben R. Management of bladder cancer. *Curr Probl Cancer* 1995, **19**, 5–63.
3 Russell PJ, Glaves D. Experimental models of bladder cancer. In: *Principles and practice of genitourinary oncology* (ed. Raghavan D, Scher HI, Liebel SA, Lange PH). Lippincott-Raven Publishers, Philadelphia, 1997, pp. 195–206.
4 Reznikoff CA, Kao C, Messing EM *et al.* A molecular genetic model of human bladder carcinogenesis. *Semin Cancer Biol* 1993, **4**, 143–52.
5 Russell PJ, Raghavan D, Philips J, Wills EJ. The biology of urothelial cancer. In: *The management of bladder cancer* (ed. Raghavan D). Edward Arnold Publishers, London, 1988, pp. 1–41.
6 Miyao N, Tsai YL, Lerner SP *et al.* Role of chromosome 9 in human bladder cancer. *Cancer Res* 1993, **53**, 4066–70.
7 Cairns P, Mao L, Merlo A *et al.* Rates of p16 (MTS1) mutations in primary tumors with 9p loss. *Science* 1994, **265**, 415–17.
8 Stadler WM, Sherman J, Bohlander SK *et al.* Homozygous deletions within chromosomal bands 9p21–22 in bladder cancer. *Cancer Res* 1994, **54**, 2060–3.
9 Orlow I, Lianes P, Lacombe L *et al.* Chromosome 9 allelic losses and microsatellite alterations in human bladder tumors. *Cancer Res* 1994, **54**, 2848–51.
10 Simoneau AR, Spruck CH III, Gonzales-Zulueta M *et al.* Evidence for two tumor suppressor loci associated with proximal chromosome 9p to q and distal chromosome 9q in bladder cancer and the initial screening for GAS1 and PTC mutations. *Cancer Res* 1994, **56**, 5039–43.
11 Williamson MP, Elder PA, Shaw ME *et al.* P16 (CDKN2) is a major deletion target at 9;21 in bladder cancer. *Hum Mol Genet* 1995, **4**, 1569–77.
12 Gonzalez-Zulueta M, Bender CM, Yang AS *et al.* Methylation of the 5′ CpG island of the p16/CDKN2 tumor suppressor gene in normal and transformed human tissues correlates with gene silencing. *Cancer Res* 1995, **55**, 4531–5.
13 Stadler WM, Olopade OI. The 9p21 region in bladder cancer cell lines: large homozygous deletion inactivate the CDKN2, CDKN2B and MTAP genes. *Urol Res* 1996, **24**, 239–44.

14 Reznikoff CA, Yeager TR, Belair CD *et al*. Elevated p16 at senescence and loss of p16 at immortalization in human papillomavirus 16, E6, but not E7, transformed human uroepithelial cells. *Cancer Res* 1996, **56**, 2886–90.

15 Miyamoto H, Kubota Y, Fujinami K *et al*. Infrequent somatic mutations of the p16 and p15 genes in human bladder cancer: p16 mutations occur only in low-grade and superficial bladder cancers. *Oncol Res* 1995, **7**, 327–30.

16 Tamimi Y, Bringuier PP, Smit F *et al*. Homozygous deletions of p16 (INK4) occur frequently in bilharziasis-associated bladder cancer. *Int J Cancer* 1996, **68**, 183–7.

17 Russell PJ, Jelbart ME, Wills E *et al*. Establishment and characterization of a new human bladder cancer cell line showing features of squamous and glandular differentiation. *Int J Cancer* 1988, **41**, 74–82.

18 Brown JL, Russell PJ, Philips J *et al*. Clonal analysis of a bladder cancer cell line: an experimental model of tumour heterogeneity. *Br J Cancer* 1990, **61**, 369–76.

19 Russell PJ, Ho Shon I, Boniface GR *et al*. Growth and metastasis of human bladder cancer xenografts in the bladder of nude rats: a model for intravesical radioimmunotherapy. *Urol Res* 1991, **19**, 207–13.

20 Brown JL, Lukeis R, Palavidis Z *et al*. Karyotypic analysis of a heterogeneous human transitional cell carcinoma of the bladder. *Cancer Genet Cytogenet* 1994, **72**, 116–25.

21 Schalken JA, Van Moorselaar RJA, Bringuer PP, DeBruyne FMJ. Critical review of the models to study the biologic progression of bladder cancer. *Semin Surg Oncol* 1992, **8**, 274–8.

22 Jones PA, Droller MJ. Pathways of development and progression in bladder cancer: new correlations between clinical observations and molecular mechanisms. *Semin Urol* 1993, **11**, 177–92.

23 Van Moorselaar RJ, Hendriks BT, Borm G *et al*. Inhibition of rat bladder tumor (RBT323) growth by tumor necrosis factor alpha and interferon-gamma in vivo. *J Urol* 1992, **148**, 458–62.

24 Cornel EB, Van Oosterwijk E, de Streek JD *et al*. High energy shock waves induced increase in the local concentration of systemically given TNF-alpha. *J Urol* 1994, **152**, 2164–6.

25 Vet JA, Van Moorselaar RJ, Debruyne FM, Schalken JA. Differential expression of ferritin heavy chain in a rat transitional cell carcinoma progression model. *Biochim Biophys Acta* 1997, **1360**, 39–44.

26 Wallace DMA. Review: Occupational urothelial cancer. *Br J Urol* 1988, **61**, 75–182.

27 Silverman DT, Hoover RN, Albert S, Graff KM. Occupation and cancer of the lower urinary tract in Detroit. *J Natl Cancer Inst* 1983, **70**, 237–45.

28 Vineis P. Black (air-cured) and blond (flue-cured) tobacco and cancer risk. I. Bladder cancer (Review). *Eur J Cancer* 1991, **27**, 1491–3.

29 Badawi AF, Mostafa MH, O'Connor PJ. Involvement of alkylating agents in schistosome-associated bladder cancer: the possible basic mechanisms of induction. *Cancer Lett* 1992, **63**, 171–88.

30 Ishii A, Matsuoka H, Aji T *et al*. Parasite infection and cancer: with special emphasis on *Schistosoma japonicum* infections (Trematoda). *Mutat Res* 1994, **305**, 273–81.

31 Bringuier PP, Piaton E, Berger N *et al*. Bracken-fern-induced bladder tumors in guinea pigs, a model for human neoplasia. *Am J Pathol* 1995, **147**, 858–68.

32 Lower GM Jr. Concepts in causality: chemically induced human urinary bladder cancer. *Cancer* 1982, **49**, 1056–66.

33 Hein DW, Trinidad A, Yerokun T *et al*. Genetic regulation of acetyltransferases in the Syrian inbred hamster: a model for man. *Progr Clin Biol Res* 1990, **340B**, 115–24.

34 Yerokun T, Kirlin WG, Trinidad A *et al*. Identification and kinetic characterization of acetylator genotype dependent and independent arylamine carcinogen N-acetyltransferases in hamster bladder cytosol. *Drug Metab Disposition* 1989, **17**, 231–7.

35 Nerurkar PV, Schut HA, Anderson LM *et al*. DNA adducts of 2-amino-3-methylimidazo [4,5-f] quinoline (IQ) in colon, bladder, and kidney of congenic mice differing in Ah responsiveness and N-acetyltransferase genotype. *Cancer Res* 1995, **55**, 3043–9.

36 Cohen SM. Multi-stage carcinogenesis in the urinary bladder. *Food Chem Toxicol* 1985, **23**, 21–8.

37 Herman CJ, Vegt PDJ, Debruyne FMJ *et al.* Squamous and transitional elements in rat bladder carcinomas induced by N-butyl-N-4-hydroxybutyl-nitrosamine (BBN). A study of cytokeratin expression. *Am J Pathol* 1985, **120**, 419–26.

38 Hicks RM, Wakefield J. Rapid induction of bladder cancer in rats with N-methyl-N-nitrosourea. *J Histol Chem Biol Int* 1972, **5**, 139–52.

39 Steinberg GD, Brendler CB, Ichikawa T *et al.* Characterization of an N-methyl-N-nitrosourea-induced autochthonous rat bladder cancer model. *Cancer Res* 1990, **50**, 6668–74.

40 Moon RC, Detrisac CJ, Thomas CF, Kelloff GJ. Chemopreventiation of experimental bladder cancer. *J Cell Biochem* 1992, **161**, 134–8.

41 Berger MR, Schmahl D. Delayed development of bladder cancer in male SD rats induced with N-nitroso-N-(4-hydroxybutyl) amine following concomitant administration of sodium 2-mercaptoethane sulfonate. *Cancer Lett* 1986, **32**, 313–21.

42 Samma S, Uchida K, Seidenfeld J, Oyasu R. Effects of alpha-difluromethylornithine on the development of deeply invasive urinary bladder carcinomas in mice. *Urol Res* 1990, **18**, 277–80.

43 Adolphs HD, Thiele J, Kiel H. Effect of intralesional and systemic BCG-application or a combined cyclophosphamide BCG treatment on experimental bladder cancer. *Urol Res* 1979, **7**, 71–8.

44 Hicks RM. Effect of promoters on incidence of bladder cancer in experimental animal models. *Environ Health Perspectives* 1983, **50**, 37–49.

45 Uchida K, Samma S, Momose H *et al.* Stimulation of urinary bladder tumorigenesis by carcinogen-exposed stroma. *J Urol* 1990, **143**, 618–21.

46 Kawai K, Yamamoto M, Kameyama H, Rademaker A, Oyasu R. Enhancement of rat urinary bladder tumorigenesis by lipopolysaccharide-induced inflammation. *Cancer Res* 1993, **53**, 5172–5.

47 Lina BAR, Hollanders VMH, Kuijpers MHM. The role of alkylizing and neutral potassium salts in urinary bladder carcinogenesis in rats. *Carcinogenesis* 1994, **15**, 523–7.

48 Fujimoto K, Tannaka Y, Rademaker A, Oyasu R. Epidermal growth factor-responsive and -refractory carcinomas initiated with N-methyl-N-nitrosurea in rat urinary bladder. *Cancer Res* 1996, **56**, 2666–70.

49 Morales A, Pang AS. Prophylaxis and therapy of an experimental bladder cancer with biological response modifiers. *J Urol* 1986, **135**, 191–3.

50 Murphy WM, Soloway MS. The effect of thio-TEPA on developing and established mammalian bladder tumors. *Cancer* 1980, **45**, 870–5.

51 Raghavan D, Debruyne F, Herr H *et al.* Experimental models of bladder cancer: a critical review. *Prog Clin Biol Res* 1986, **221**, 171–208.

52 Swerdlow RD, Ratliff TL, La Regina M *et al.* Immunotherapy with keyhole limpet hemocyanin: efficacy and safety in the MB-49 intravesical murine bladder tumor model. *J Urol* 1994, **151**, 1718–22.

53 Drago JR, Nesbitt JA. NB rat bladder cancer model: evaluation of the subrenal capsular assay system. *J Surg Oncol* 1987, **36**, 5–7.

54 Kovnat A, Armitage M, Tannock I. Xenografts of human bladder cancer in immune-deprived mice. *Cancer Res* 1982, **42**, 3696–703.

55 Lacy PE, Davie JM, Finke EH. Transplantation of insulin-producing tissue. *Am J Med* 1981, **70**, 589–94.

56 Kerbel RS, Cornil I, Theodorescu D. Importance of orthotopic transplantation procedures in assessing the effects of transfected genes on human tumor growth and metastasis. *Cancer Metastasis Rev* 1991, **10**, 201–15.

57 Williams SS, Alosco TR, Croy BA, Bankert RB. The study of human neoplastic disease in severe combined immunodeficient mice. *Lab Anim Sci* 1993, **43**, 139–46.

58 Xie X, Brunner N, Jensen G *et al.* Comparative studies between nude and scid mice on the growth and metastatic behaviour of xenografted human tumors. *Clin Exp Metastasis* 1992, **10**, 201–10.

59 Kawamata H, Kawai K, Kameyama S *et al.* Over-expression of tissue inhibitor of matrix metalloproteinases (TIMP1 and TIMP2) suppresses extravasation of pulmonary metastasis of a rat bladder carcinoma. *Int J Cancer* 1995, **63**, 680–7.

60 Kawamata H, Kameyama S, Kawai K *et al.* Marked acceleration of the metastatic phenotype of a rat bladder carcinoma cell line by the expression of human gelatinase A. *Int J Cancer* 1995, **65**, 568–75.

61 Huland E, Arndt R, Huland H. Human transitional cell carcinoma in the NMRI-nu/nu mouse bladder: a new animal model for the in vivo use of monoclonal antibodies and cytotoxic agents. *Cancer Res* 1986, **46**, 2488–9.

62 Oshinsky GS, Chen Y, Jarrett T *et al.* A model of bladder tumor xenografts in the nude rat. *J Urol* 1995, **154**, 1925–9.

63 Mazurchuk R, Glaves D, Raghavan D. Magnetic resonance imaging of response to chemotherapy in orthotopic xenografts of human bladder cancer. *Clin Cancer Res* 1997, **3**, 1635–41.

64 Fidler IJ. Critical factors in the biology of human cancer metastasis: Twenty-eighth G.H.A. Clowes Memorial Award lecture. *Cancer Res* 1990, **50**, 6130–8.

65 Kubota T. Metastatic models of human cancer xenografted in the nude mouse: the importance of orthotopic transplantation. *J Cell Biochem* 1994, **56**, 4–8.

66 Togo S, Shimada H, Kubota T *et al.* Host organ specifically determines cancer progression. *Cancer Res* 1995, **55**, 681–4.

67 Sharkey FE, Fogh J. Considerations in the use of nude mice for cancer research. *Cancer Metastasis Rev* 1984, **3**, 341–60.

68 Fidler IJ. Rationale and methods for the use of nude mice to study the biology and therapy of human cancer metastasis. *Cancer Metastasis Rev* 1986, **5**, 29–49.

69 DeVore DP, Houches DP, Overjera AA *et al.* Collagenase inhibitors retarding invasion of a human tumor in nude mice. *Exp Cell Biol* 1980, **48**, 367–73.

70 Wang WR, Sordat B, Piguet D, Sordat M. Implantation site and expression of the invasive phenotype. In: *Immune-deficient animals* (ed. Sordat B). Karger, Basel, 1984, pp. 239–45.

71 Naito S, Von Eschensach AC, Giavazzi R, Fidler IJ. Growth and metastasis of tumor cells isolated from a human renal cell carcinoma implanted into different organs of nude mice. *Cancer Res* 1986, **46**, 4109–15.

72 Rigby CC, Franks LM. A human tissue culture cell line from a transitional cell tumor of the urinary bladder: growth, chromosome pattern, and ultrastructure. *Br J Cancer* 1970, **24**, 746–54.

73 Ahlering TE, Dubeau L, Jones PA. A new in vivo model to study invasion and metastasis of human bladder carcinoma. *Cancer Res* 1987, **47**, 6660–5.

74 Theodorescu D, Cornil I, Fernandez BJ, Kerbel RS. Overexpression of normal and mutated forms of HRAS induces orthotopic bladder invasion in a human transitional cell carcinoma. *Proc Natl Acad Sci USA* 1990, **87**, 9047–51.

75 Fu X, Hoffman RM. Human RT-4 bladder carcinoma is highly metastatic in nude mice and comparable to ras-H-transformed RT-4 when orthotopically onplanted as histologically intact tissue. *Int J Cancer* 1992, **51**, 989–91.

76 Hanna N. Expression of metastatic potential of tumor cells in young nude mice is correlated with low levels of natural killer cell-mediated cytotoxicity. *Int J Cancer* 1980, **26**, 675–80.

77 Soloway MS, Masters S. Urothelial susceptibility to tumor cell implantation: influence of cauterization. *Cancer* 1980, **46**, 115–63.

78 See WA, Chapman PH. Heparin prevention of tumor cell adherence and implantation on injured urothelial surfaces. *J Urol* 1987, **138**, 182–6.

79 Weiss RE, Liu BCS, Ahlering T *et al.* Mechanisms of human bladder tumor invasion: role of protease cathepsin. *Br J Urol* 1990, **144**, 798–804.

80 Russell PJ, Brown J, Grimmond SM, Raghavan D. Molecular biology of bladder cancer. *Br J Urol* 1990, **65**, 121–30.

81 Sidransky D, Messing E. Molecular genetics and biochemical mechanisms in bladder cancer. *Urol Clin North Am* 1992, **4**, 629–39.

82 Reddy EP, Reynolds RK, Santos E, Barbacid M. A point mutation is responsible for the acquisition of transforming properties by the T24 human bladder carcinoma oncogene. *Nature* 1982, **300**, 149–52.

83 Knowles MA, Williamson M. Mutation of H-ras is infrequent in bladder cancer: confirmation by single-strand conformation polymorphism analysis designed restriction fragment length polymorphisms, and direct sequencing. *Cancer Res* 1993, **53**, 133–9.

84 Burchill SA, Neal DE, Lunec J. Frequency of H-ras mutations in human bladder cancer detected by direct sequencing. *Br J Urol* 1994, **73**, 516–21.

85 Wagner HE, Joyce AD, Summerhayes IC. Urothelial cancer metastases after implantation of tumor cells under the kidney capsule. *Helv Chir Acta* 1993, **59**, 803–7.

86 Fujita J, Ohuchi H, Ito N *et al.* Activation of H-ras oncogene in rat bladder tumors induced by N-butyl-N-(4-hydroxybutyl) nitrosamine. *J Natl Cancer Inst* 1988, **80**, 37–43.

87 Yura Y, Azuma M, Uchida K *et al.* Ras gene alterations in invasive and non-invasive rat bladder cancer induced by N-methyl-N-nitrosurea. *Br J Cancer* 1991, **64**, 10–14.

88 Mann AM, Asamoto M, Chlapowski FJ *et al.* Ras involvement in cells transformed with 2-amino-4-(5-nitro-2-furyl) thiazole (ANFT) in vitro and with N-[4-(5-nitro-2-furyl)-s-thiazoyl] formamide in vivo. *Carcinogenesis*, 1992, **13**, 1651–5.

89 Eastham JA, Ahlering TE. Use of an anti-ras ribozyme to alter the malignant phenotype of a human bladder cancer cell line. *J Urol* 1996, **156**, 1186–8.

90 Cairns P, Liu BCS, Sidransky D. Molecular biology of bladder cancer. In: *Principles and practice of genitourinary oncology* (ed. Raghavan D, Scher HI, Leibel SA, Lange PH). Lippincott-Raven Publishers, Philadelphia, 1997, pp. 223–30.

91 Cordon-Cardo C. Mutation of cell cycle regulators—biological and clinical implications for human neoplasia. *Am J Pathol* 1995, **147**, 545–60.

92 Weinberg RA. Retinoblastoma protein and cell cycle control. *Cell* 1995, **81**, 323–30.

93 Hunter T, Pines J, Cyclin and cancer II. Cyclin D and CDK inhibitors come to age. *Cell* 1994, **79**, 573–82.

94 Huber HE, Goodhart PJ, Huang PS. Retinoblastoma protein reverses DNA binding by transcription factor E2F. *J Biol Chem* 1994, **269**, 6999–7005.

95 Cordon-Cardo C, Wartinger D, Petrylak D *et al.* Altered expression of the retinoblastoma gene product: prognosis indicator in bladder cancer. *J Natl Cancer Inst* 1992, **84**, 1251–6.

96 Lane DP. Cancer. p53, guardian genome. *Nature* 1992, **358**, 15–16.

97 Shaw P, Bovey R, Tardy S *et al.* Induction of apoptosis by wild-type p53 in a human colon tumor derived cell line. *Proc Natl Acad Sci USA* 1992, **89**, 4495–9.

98 Sidransky D, Von Eschenbach A, Tsai YC *et al.* Identification of p53 gene mutations in bladder cancers and urine samples. *Science* 1991, **252**, 706–9.

99 Fujimoto K, Yamada Y, Okajima E *et al.* Frequent association of p53 mutation in invasive bladder cancer. *Cancer Res* 1992, **52**, 1393–8.

100 Dalbagni G, Presti JC, Reuter VE *et al.* Genetic alterations in bladder cancer. *Lancet*, 1993, **342**, 469–71.

101 Spruck CH III, Ohneseit PF, Gonzalez-Zulueta M *et al.* Two molecular pathways to transition cell carcinoma of the bladder. *Cancer Res* 1994, **54**, 784–8.

102 Esrig D, Elmajian D, Groshen S *et al.* Accumulation of nuclear p53 and tumor progression in bladder cancer. *N Engl J Med* 1994, **331**, 1259–64.

103 Ozaki M, Shibata MA, Takahashi S *et al.* Lack of involvement of p53 gene mutations in N-methyl-N-nitrosourea-induced bladder tumor progression in N-butyl-N-(4-hydroxybutyl) nitrosamine-treated rats and no suppression by indomethacin. *Cancer Lett* 1997, **115**, 249–55.

104 Kastan MB, Onyekwere O, Sidransky D *et al.* Participation of p53 protein in the cellular response to DNA damage. *Cancer Res* 1991, **51**, 6304–11.

105 Hall PA, McKee PH, Menage HD *et al.* High levels of p53 protein in UV-irradiated normal human skin. *Oncogene* 1993, **8**, 203–7.

106 El-Deiry WS, Tokino T, Velculescu VE *et al.* WAF1, a potential mediator of p53 tumor suppression. *Cell* 1993, **75**, 817–25.

107 El-Deiry WS, Harper JW, O'Connor PM *et al.* WAF1/CIP1 is induced in p53-mediated G1 arrest and apoptosis. *Cancer Res* 1994, **54**, 1169–74.

108 Price BD, Park SJ. DNA damage increases the levels of MDM2 messenger RNA in wtp53 human cells. *Cancer Res* 1994, **54**, 896–9.

109 Waga S, Hannon GJ, Beach D, Stillman B. The p21 inhibitor of cyclin-dependent kinases controls DNA replication by interaction with PCNA. *Nature* 1994, **369**, 574–8.

110 Lowe SW, Schmitt EM, Smith SW *et al.* P53 is required for radiation induced apoptosis in mouse thymocytes. *Nature* 1993, **362**, 847–9.

111 Nelson WG, Kastan MB. DNA strand breaks: the DNA template alterations that trigger p53-dependent DNA damage response pathways. *Mol Cell Biol* 1994, **14**, 1815–23.

112 Clarke AR, Gledhill S, Hooper ML *et al.* P53 dependence of early apoptotic and proliferative responses within the mouse intestinal epithelium following gamma-irradiation. *Oncogene*, 1994, **9**, 1767–73.

113 Symonds H, Krall L, Remington L *et al.* P53-dependent apoptosis suppresses tumor growth and progression in vivo. *Cell* 1994, **78**, 703–11.

114 Lee JM, Bernstein A. P53 mutations increase resistance to ionizing radiation. *Proc Natl Acad Sci USA* 1993, **90**, 5742–6.

115 McIlwrath AJ, Vasey PA, Ross GM, Brown R. Cell cycle arrests and radiosensitivity of human tumor cell lines: dependence on wild-type p53 for radiosensitivity. *Cancer Res* 1994, **54**, 3718–22.

116 Xia F, Wang X, Wang YH *et al.* Altered p53 status correlates with differences in sensitivity to radiation-induced mutation and apoptosis in two closely related human lymphoblast lines. *Cancer Res* 1995, **55**, 12–15.

117 Biard DS, Martin M, Rhun YL *et al.* Concomitant p53 gene mutation and increased radiosensitivity in rat lung embryo epithelial cells during neoplastic development. *Cancer Res* 1994, **54**, 3361–4.

118 Kawashima K, Mihara K, Usuki H *et al.* Transfected mutant p53 gene increases X-ray-induced cell killing and mutation in human fibroblasts immortalized with 4-nitroquinole 1-oxide but does not induce neoplastic transformation of the cells. *Int J Cancer* 1995, **61**, 76–9.

119 Smith ML, Chen IT, Zhan Q *et al.* Involvement of the p53 tumor suppressor in repair of uv-type DNA damage. *Oncogene* 1995, **10**, 1053–9.

120 Brachman DG, Beckett M, Graves D *et al.* P53 mutations does not correlate with radiosensitivity in 24 head and neck cancer cell lines. *Cancer Res* 1993, **53**, 3667–9.

121 Slichenmyer WJ, Nelson WG, Slebos RJ, Kastan MB. Loss of a p53-associated G1 checkpoint does not decrease cell survival following DNA damage. *Cancer Res* 1993, **53**, 4164–8.

122 Russell PJ, Wass J, Lukeis R *et al.* Characterization of cell lines derived from a multiply aneuploid human bladder transitional-cell carcinoma, UCRU-BL-13. *Int J Cancer* 1989, **44**, 276–85.

123 Momand J, Zambetti GP, Olson DC *et al.* The mdm-2 oncogene forms a complex with the p53 protein and inhibits p53-mediated transactivation. *Cell* 1992, **69**, 1237–45.

124 Russell PJ, Palavidis Z, Philips J *et al.* Establishment and characterization of a new human bladder cancer cell line, UCRU-BL-28. *J Urol* 1993, **150**, 1038–44.

125 Ribeiro JCC, Barnetson AR, Fisher R *et al.* Radiosensitivity is independent of p53 status in three human bladder cancer cell lines. *Int J Rad Biol* 1997, **72**, 11–20.

126 Ribeiro JCC, Hanley J, Russell PJ. Studies of X-irradiated bladder cancer cell lines showing differences in p53 status: absence of a p53-dependent cell cycle checkpoint pathway. *Oncogene*, 1996, **13**, 1269–78.

127 Lee CCR, Yamomoto S, Wanibuchi H *et al.* Cyclin D1 overexpression in rat two-stage bladder carcinogenesis and its relationship with oncogenes, tumor suppressor genes and cell proliferation. *Cancer Res* 1997, **57**, 4765–76.

128 Dong JT, Lamb WP, Rinker-Schaeffer CW *et al.* Kai 1, a metastasis suppressor gene for prostate cancer on chromosome 11p11.2. *Science* 1995, **268**, 884–6.

129 Yu Y, Yang JL, Markovic B *et al.* Loss of Kai1 mRNA expression in both high grade and invasive human bladder cancers. *Clin Cancer Res* 1997, **3**, 1045–9.

130 Tanaka M, Mullauer L, Ogiso Y *et al.* Gelsolin: a candidate for suppressor of human bladder cancer. *Cancer Res* 1995, **55**, 3228–32.

131 Saika T, Tsushima T, Nasu Y *et al.* Histopathological study of metallothionein in bladder cancer and renal cell carcinoma. *Jpn J Urol* 1992, **83**, 636–42.

132 Xu BH, Gupta V, Singh SV. Mitomycin C sensitivity in human bladder cancer cells: possible role of glutathione and glutathione transferase in resistance. *Arch Biochem Biophys* 1994, **308**, 164–70.

133 Kotoh S, Naito S, Yokomizo A *et al.* Increased expression of DNA topoisomerase I gene and collateral sensitivity to camptothecin in human cisplatin-resistant bladder cancer cells. *Cancer Res* 1994, **54**, 3248–52.

134 Hasegawa S, Abe T, Naito S *et al.* Expression of mutidrug resistance-associated protein (MRP), MDR1 and DNA topoisomerase II in human multidrug-resistant bladder cancer cell lines. *Br J Cancer* 1995, **71**, 907–13.

135 Bachor R, Flotte T, Scholtz M *et al.* Comparison of intravenous and intravesical administration of chloro-aluminium sulfonated phthalocyanine for photodynamic treatment in a rat bladder cance model. *J Urol* 1992, **147**, 1404–10.

136 Iinuma S, Bachor R, Flotte T, Hasan T. Biodistribution and phototoxicity of 5-aminolevulinic acid-induced PpIX in an orthotopic rat bladder tumor model. *J Urol* 1995, **153**, 802–6.

137 Glaves D, Murray MK, Raghavan D. Novel bi-functional anthracycline/nitrosurea chemotherapy: analysis in a pre-clinical model of anthracycline-resistant disease. *Clin Cancer Res* 1996, **2**, 1315–19.

138 Chin J, Kadhim S, Garcia B *et al.* Magnetic resonance imaging for detecting and treatment monitoring of orthotopic murine bladder tumor implants. *J Urol* 1991, **145**, 1297–301.

139 Chin J, Kadhim SA, Batislam E *et al.* Mycobacterium cell wall: an alternative to intravesical bacillus Calmette Guérin (BCG) therapy in orthotopic murine bladder cancer. *J Urol* 1996, **156**, 1189–93.

140 Kadhim SA, Chin JL, Batislam E *et al.* Genetically regulated response to intravesical Bacillus Calmette Guerin immunotherapy of orthotopic murine bladder tumor. *J Urol* 1997, **158**, 646–52.

141 Ratliff T, Lattime EC, Williams RD. Immunology of bladder cancer. In: *Principles and practice of genitourinary oncology* (ed. Raghavan D, Scher HI, Leibel SA, Lange PH). Lippincott-Raven Publishers, Philadelphia, 1997, pp. 239–48.

142 Pryor K, Stricker P, Russell P *et al.* Antiproliferative effects of bacillus Calmette-Guérin (BCG) and Interferon alpha 2b on human bladder cancer cell lines in vitro. *Cancer Immunol Immunother* 1995, **41**, 309–16.

143 Wada S, Ikemoto S, Terade T *et al.* Combined therapy of interleukin 2 with cyclophosphamide or bacillus Calmette-Guerin against implanted bladder cancer cells in mice. *Urologia Intis* 1991, **47**, 104–7.

144 Tahara M, Nomura S, Takahashi M *et al.* In vitro direct antiproliferative activity and in vivo antitumor activity of bropirimine against bladder cancer. *Jpn J Cancer Chemother* 1996, **23**, 1039–44.

145 Campbell SC, Tanabe K, Alexander JP *et al.* Intercellular adhesion molecule-1expression by bladder cancer cells: functional effects. *J Urol* 1994, **151**, 1385–90.

146 Kunkler RB, Kockelbergh RC. The therapeutic potential of monoclonal antibodies for bladder cancer. *Br J Urol* 1995, **75**, 9–17.

147 Russell PJ, Plomley J, Ho Shon I *et al.* Monoclonal antibodies for intravesical radioimmunotherapy of human bladder cancer. *Cell Biophys* 1993, **22**, 27–47.

148 Russell PJ, Davis K, Kingsley E *et al.* Preclinical studies of monoclonal antibodies for intravesical radioimmunotherapy of human bladder cancer. *Cell Biophys* 1994, **24/25**, 155–61.

149 Kingsley EA, Yu Y, Hanley JR *et al.* Monoclonal antibody binding to, and penetration of, human bladder cancer xenografts grown orthotopically in a nude rat model. *Antibody Immunoconj Radiopharm* 1995, **8**, 32–5.

150 Lee SS, Eisennlohr LC, McCue PA *et al.* Intravesical gene therapy: in vivo gene transfer using recombinant Vaccinia virus vectors. *Cancer Res* 1994, **54**, 3325–8.

151 Werthman PE, Drazan KE, Rosenthal JT *et al.* Adenoviral p53 gene transfer to orthotopic and peritoneal murine bladder cancer. *J Urol* 1996, **155**, 753–6.

152 Jacobs WR Jr, Snapper SB, Lugosi L, Bloom BR. Development of BCG as a recombinant vaccine vehicle. *Curr Top Microbiol Immunol* 1990, **155**, 153–60.

153 Eastham JA, Hall SJ, Sehgal I *et al.* In vivo gene therapy with p53 or p21 adenovirus for prostate cancer. *Cancer Res* 1995, **55**, 5151–5.

154 Li M, Gu FL, Li WB *et al.* Introduction of wild-type p53 gene downregulates the expression of H-ras gene and suppresses the growth of bladder cancer cells. *Urol Res* 1995, **23**, 311–14.

155 Chen SHC, Chen XHL, Wang Y *et al.* Combination gene therapy for liver metastasis of colon carcinoma in vivo. *Proc Natl Acad Sci USA* 1995, **92**, 2577–81.

156 Golumbek P, Lazenby A, Levitsky H *et al.* Treatment of established renal cancer by tumor cells engineered to secrete interleukin-4. *Science* 1991, **254**, 713–16.

157 Connor J, Bannerji R, Saito S *et al.* Regression of bladder tumors in mice treated with IL-2 gene-modified tumor cells. *J Exp Med* 1993, **147**, 545–60.

158 Culver KW, Ram Z, Wallbridge S *et al.* In vivo gene transfer with retroviral vector-producer cells for treatment of experimental brain tumors. *Science* 1992, **256**, 1550–2.

159 Culver K, Van Gilder J, Link C *et al.* Gene therapy for the treatment of malignant brain tumors with in vivo tumor transductionwith the herpes simplex thymidine kinase gene/ganciclovir system. *Hum Gene Ther* 1994, **5**, 343–79.

160 Deonarain MP, Spooner RA, Epenetos AA. Genetic delivery of enzymes for cancer therapy. *Gene Ther* 1995, **2**, 235–44.

6. The pathology of bladder cancer

Sonny L. Johansson and Samuel M. Cohen

Introduction

Tumours of the lower urinary tract comprise approximately 10% of all male cancers and less than half of that figure in females. The incidence has been rising and over 50 000 new cases are diagnosed annually in the United States. In Sweden, 23% more cases were diagnosed in 1994 compared with 1983 (1). In Europe and the United States more than 90% of the tumours are of urothelial (transitional cell) origin. Transitional cell is a misnomer, but because it is so widely used in the literature and in clinical practice it can be used synonymously with urothelial, a term which we prefer. Approximately 5% of bladder tumours are squamous cell carcinomas (SCCs) and 1% adenocarcinomas, the remainder comprising uncommon variants of bladder carcinoma and various sarcomas such as rhabdomyosarcoma and leiomyosarcoma (2) (Table 6.1).

Papilloma

Inverted papilloma is a distinct, uncommon benign bladder tumour. In a prospective study of all bladder tumours diagnosed in a region of western Sweden with a population of 1.6 million individuals during 1987–1988, 12 of 713 bladder tumours were inverted papillomas (1.7%) (3). There is a male to female ratio of 5 to 1 and the peak incidence is in the sixth decade (4). The tumour, originally described by Paschkis in 1927 (5) and labelled inverted papilloma by Potts and Hirst 1963 (6), is usually 1–2 cm in diameter with a polypoid or nodular appearance and a smooth surface. Histologically, the tumour is composed of anastomosing cords of bland urothelial cells appearing to involve the lamina propria. These tumours usually show no anaplasia. Typically, the cords display a palisading pattern of cells and cystic spaces are common (Figs 6.1 and 6.2). The urothelial lining is usually preserved and can be thinner than normal, normal, or slightly hyperplastic. Kunze *et al.* described what they considered a variant of inverted papilloma with features of hypertrophic cystitis glandularis containing mucin-producing, tall columnar cells (4).

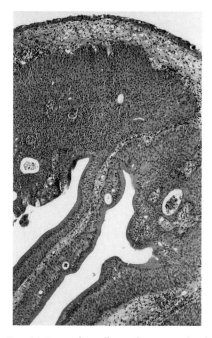

Fig. 6.1 *Inverted papilloma showing cords of blend urothelial cells with peripheral palisading and small cystic spaces (H&E, × 105)*

Table 6.1

CLASSIFICATION OF URINARY BLADDER TUMOURS AND TUMOUR-LIKE LESIONS

I. Epithelial neoplasms
Urothelial (transitional cell) neoplasms
    Papilloma
        Inverted
        Everted
    Urothelial carcinoma
        Papillary
        Non-papillary (solid)
    Carcinoma *in situ* and possible precursor lesions
    Variants of transitional cell carcinoma
        Transitional cell carcinoma, nested type
        Lymphoepithelioma-like carcinoma
    Micropapillary carcinoma
    Sarcomatoid carcinoma
Squamous cell carcinoma
    Conventional type
    Verrucous type
Villous adenoma
Adenocarcinoma
    Papillary, glandular, mucinous, signet ring cell and clear cell carcinoma types (and mixtures)
Small cell carcinoma (neuroendocrine carcinoma)
Mixed carcinoma

II. Carcinosarcoma

III. Sarcomas
Rhabdomyosarcoma
Leiomyosarcoma

IV. Lymphoma

V. Paraganglioma

VI. Tumour-like lesions
    Pseudosarcoma
    Polypoid cystitis
    Amyloid

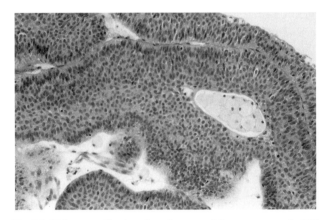

Fig. 6.2 Higher magnification of another area of the same tumour (× 210)

Mitoses are usually absent and if present the tumour is likely to represent a urothelial carcinoma with an inverted pattern. The behaviour of inverted papilloma is benign, and transurethral resection of the bladder (TURB) tumour is usually curative. In some cases the patients develop urothelial cancer elsewhere in the bladder or in the urinary tract, and it is possible that similar aetiological factors which induce bladder cancer may also produce inverted papilloma (7). An increasing number of cases of inverted papilloma with recurrence have been reported. Some of these cases may recur because of incomplete resection, but in most cases the tumour is probably an urothelial carcinoma with an inverted pattern (2).

The strict definition of everted papilloma is that of a papillary tumour lined by no more than seven layers of urothelial cells, which do not display any appreciable anaplasia and have umbrella cells on the surface (8) (Figs 6.3 and 6.4). In our experience this tumour is solitary, benign and very rare, comprising less than 1% of all bladder tumours. One of the authors (S.L.J.) has seen only five cases in over 20 years of a busy uropathological practice. The lesion is often (but not always) seen in younger individuals and does not seem to be associated with recurrence or increased risk for subsequent bladder cancer. However, some experienced urological pathologists have advocated the extension of the diagnosis of papilloma to include all WHO grade I tumours (9–11) (see discussion below).

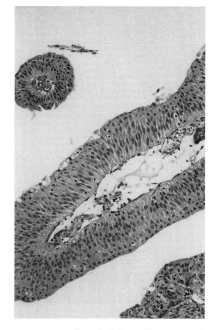

Fig. 6.3 Everted urothelial papilloma. Note the fibrovascular core and the normal appearing urothelial cells. (H&E, ×210)

UROTHELIAL CARCINOMA

Urothelial carcinoma may appear as papillary or non-papillary tumours, and more than one lesion is present in approximately 25% of the patients, predominantly in individuals with papillary tumours. The majority of bladder tumours, 70–80%, show a papillary configuration reminiscent of seaweed by cystoscopic examination (Fig. 6.5 and Plate 1). The non-papillary tumours are sessile, nodular, or ulcerated masses. Approximately 60% of the tumours are located in the lateral or posterior walls while 20% appear in the trigone.

Papillary tumours are often associated with recurrence (57–85%), but seldom invade or metastasize. Patients with low-grade papillary tumours most often undergo transurethral resection of the tumour with a curative aim.

The role of the pathologist is to transmit the following diagnostic and prognostic information to the urologist:

(1) classification of the tumour (histological type) (Table 6.1);

(2) growth pattern (papillary, non-papillary, or both);

(3) tumour grade;

(4) tumour stage; and

(5) angiolymphatic invasion.

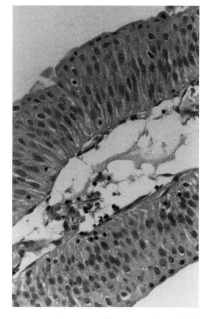

Fig. 6.4 Higher power of Fig. 6.3. The urothelial cells lack appreciable atypia. (H&E, ×400)

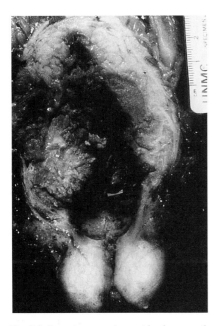

Fig. 6.5 Cystectomy specimen with a large papillary urothelial carcinoma

Other important prognostic factors include tumour size and multiplicity, mitosis density, tentacular invasion, and associated carcinoma *in situ*.

GRADING

The first system for grading bladder tumours was described by Broders in 1922 and was based on the percentage of tumour cells that looked like normal urothelial cells and thus were differentiated. The system included four grades (12). Several grading systems have subsequently been proposed, all of which include four or five grades (Table 6.2). The most widely used is the one adopted by WHO in 1973 (13). Other grading systems include the original and modified Bergkvist system (14,15) and the one proposed by Murphy *et al.* in the third series of Armed Forces Institute of Pathology fascicles (10).

The WHO grading system from 1973 includes three grades of urothelial carcinoma plus undifferentiated carcinoma. The system is simple but lacks well defined histological or cytological criteria. Grade 1 represents the most well differentiated tumour displaying the least degree of cellular anaplasia. Grade 3 tumours show the worst cellular anaplasia that still can be recognized as urothelial in origin. The original Bergkvist system gives more detailed criteria for malignancy grading based on the degree of deviation from the normal cellular pattern (14). The modified Bergkvist system, proposed by Dr C. Busch and co-workers, divides the large and heterogeneous grade 2 group into grades 2A and 2B. Grade 1 represents a pattern with predominant order and almost no variation and slight nuclear atypia and enlargement. In grade 2A the impression of order is predominant but variation has occurred, such as nuclear enlargement and variation in nuclear hyperchromasia. In grade 2B the impression of disorder predominates (Figs 6.6–6.10) (15,16).

Table 6.2

HISTOLOGICAL GRADING SYSTEMS FOR UROTHELIAL TUMOURS		
WHO (13)	**Malmström *et al.* (15)**	**Murphy *et al.* (10)**
Papilloma	Papilloma	Papilloma
Grade 1	Grade 1	Papilloma
	Grade 2A	
Grade 2	Grade 2B	Low grade
Grade 3	Grades 3–4	High grade

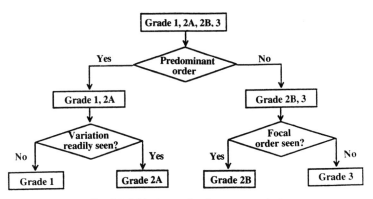

Fig. 6.6 Subjective grading by pattern analysis

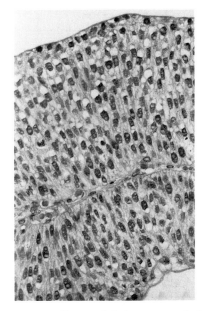

Fig. 6.7 Papillary urothelial tumour, grade 1. (H&E, ×400)

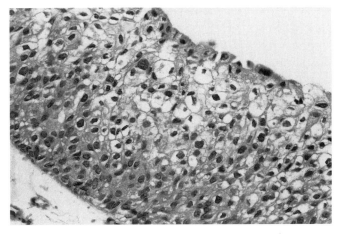

Fig. 6.9 Papillary urothelial carcinoma, grade 2B. (H&E, ×450)

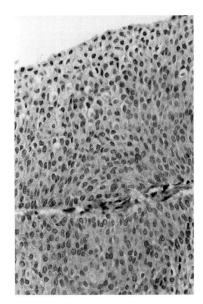

Fig. 6.8 Papillary urothelial tumour, grade 2A. (H&E, ×400)

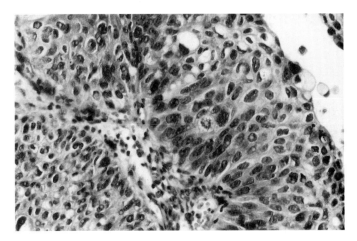

Fig. 6.10 Papillary urothelial carcinoma, grade 3. (H&E, ×450)

The WHO system can be easily translated into the modified Bergkvist system. Thus, WHO grade 1 corresponds to Bergkvist grades 1 and 2A. WHO grade 2 corresponds to Bergkvist grade 2B and WHO grade 3 to Bergkvist grade 3. Although grading is a powerful predictor of prognosis in most studies, it is subjective, and reproducibility may be lower than 50% when different pathologists review the sections (17,18). Oms reported a study involving six pathologists grading 57 cases of urothelial carcinoma. The percentage of cases diagnosed as grade 3 varied between 19 and 44%, which is disturbing in view of the prognostic importance of histological grade and its influence on treatment (19). More promising objective computer-based grading methods using object based and textural analysis are being developed (16,20).

Because of the fact that at least 20% of bladder tumours are grade 1 and that these tumours do not invade or metastasize, it seems inappropriate to classify these tumours as carcinoma. Recognizing this fact, Dr. F.K. Mostofi arranged for a meeting of a WHO panel in Washington, DC, in October 1997. The meeting was preceded by a workshop organized by Dr Mostofi and attended by urological pathologists with a special interest in bladder cancer as well as some urologists. The meeting was followed by another meeting in March 1998, in Boston with 40 urological pathologists from around the world with special interest and knowledge of bladder tumours. On both occasions there was consensus (>80%) that the present WHO system needs to be revised and that the WHO grade 1 tumour should not be called carcinoma. The replacement term proposed was papillary neoplasm of low malignant potential. In a prospective study of all cases of bladder tumours in a Swedish area of 1.6 million individuals, 255 of 680 patients had lesions that were WHO grade 1, stage Ta (37.5%). Ninety-five cases were modified Bergkvist grade 1 and 160 grade 2A. The recurrence rate was 35% in grade 1 and 71% in grade 2A ($P < 0.001$). No patient with grade 1 tumour progressed to an invasive lesion and only six with a grade 2A tumour progressed (3.8%) (unpublished data). When the WHO classification was used, the progression rate was 2.4% (six of 255) further supporting the need for new terminology for grade 1 urothelial carcinoma.

BLADDER CANCER STAGING

To stratify adequately patients for treatment, clinical and pathological staging is critical. The principal international staging system used is that of the AJCC/UICC, which we strongly recommend for use by all (21) (Table 6.3). The presence of carcinoma

Table 6.3

PATHOLOGICAL STAGING OF CARCINOMA OF THE URINARY BLADDER	
AJCC stage	**Level of invasion**
Ta	Non-invasive papillary carcinoma
Tis	Carcinoma *in situ*
T1	Tumour invades the lamina propria
T2	Tumour invades the muscularis propria (detrusor muscle)
T2a	Superficial muscularis propria
T2b	Deep muscularis propria
T3	Tumour invades perivesical tissue
T3a	Microscopically
T3b	Macroscopically (extravesical mass)
T4	Invasion of adjacent structures
T4a	Prostate, uterus, vagina
T4b	Pelvic wall, abdominal wall
N1–N3	Lymph node metastasis
N1	Regional node <2 cm
N2	Regional node 2–5 cm
N3	Regional node >5 cm
M	Distant metastasis

in situ (CIS) should be stated in the report as well as the presence or absence of muscularis propria in the biopsy specimen. By tradition, clinicians have long been using the term superficial cancer for Ta and T1 papillary urothelial carcinoma. This is a bad term as the behaviour and survival is different for Ta and T1 tumours (22). The 5-year survival is over 90% for patients with Ta tumours and 75% for T1 tumours.

One of the recent controversies in bladder cancer is whether T1 tumours should be substaged in relation to the level of the muscularis mucosa. The existence of a muscularis mucosa (MM) was described by Dixon and Gosling in 1983 (23). This tunica muscularis mucosa varies in its development within a given bladder and may be formed as a continuous (rarely) or interrupted layer (24). The latter is generally the rule; it consists of thin wisps of smooth muscle fibres. It is present approximately one-third to one-half way between the urothelium and the muscularis propria. (Fig. 6.11) This level is also populated with arteries of relatively large calibre, which are oriented parallel to the mucosal surface and are closely associated with the fibres of the muscularis mucosa. They can be used as a landmark if the fibres are absent. Younes *et al*. subclassified T1 tumours into T1a (above), T1b (at the level of), and T1c (beyond the MM). T1a and T1b had a 5-year survival rate of 75% as compared with 11% for T1c (25). Hasui *et al*. found that T1 tumours infiltrating to the level or below the

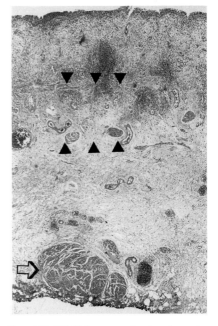

Fig. 6.11 TURB fragment showing the region of the muscularis mucosa with larger vessels (Gehveen arrowheads) and muscularis (open arrow) propria. (H&E, ×21)

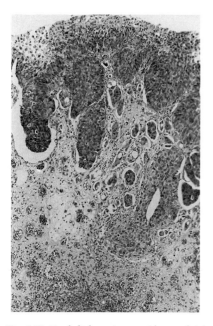

Fig. 6.12 Urothelial carcinoma with superficial invasion into the lamina propria and retraction artefact. (H&E, × 100)

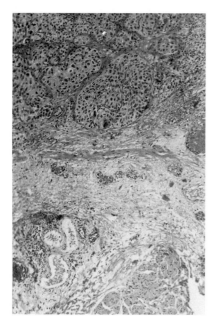

Fig. 6.13 Urothelial carcinoma infiltrating to the level of muscularis mucosa. (H&E, ×100)

MM (classified as T1b) had a progression rate of 53.5% (15 of 28) compared with 6.7% in the more superficial (T1a) tumours (four of 60) ($P < 0.01$) (26). Angulo *et al.* found similar results in a larger series of patients (27). They reported that subdividing T1 tumours was prognostically important and should be done whenever possible, but they were able to do so in only 58% of the cases. In contrast, Platz *et al.*, reviewing slides from 77 T1 patients, found that microstaging of bladder cancer was technically difficult in cases derived from different urologists and laboratories and did not yield prognostically significant separation (28). We performed a prospective study of 701 bladder tumours of which we found 121 to be stage T1. We were able to subdivide 90% of the cases into T1a and T1b (above the level of MM or below the MM) (Figs 6.12 and 6.13). The high success rate is probably related to the fact that all patients were treated by TURB by a limited number of experienced urologists who used a minimum of cautery effect. Further, all tumours were primary tumours and had not been biopsied before. Patients with stage T1b, grade 3 tumours had a significantly higher progression rate and an almost double risk of dying from bladder cancer compared with patients with stage T1a, grade 3 tumours (3). We also found that T1b patients treated only with TURB had a poor prognosis while T1b patients treated with cystectomy had an excellent prognosis (3). Although we recognize that subclassification of T1 tumours may be difficult because of problems of specimen orientation, tangential cutting and crush and cautery artefacts, we agree with Younes *et al.*, Hasui *et al.*, and Angulo *et al.* that it should be done whenever possible (25–27).

Non-papillary tumours comprise 20–30% of all bladder tumours, with muscle invasion present in 90% of these patients. Associated (secondary) CIS is common, and 20% of the patients have a history of papillary carcinoma. The 5-year survival rate has been reported to vary between 20 and 50%. The treatment of patients with muscle invasive disease is influenced by the extent of carcinoma. Perivesical extension may result in unresectability. Of particular importance is the involvement of the prostate by tumour. The incidence of prostatic involvement is approximately 50% in patients with muscularis propria invasion (29,30) and especially high if the patients have multifocal CIS. Prostatic involvement represents stage 4 disease irrespective of degree of involvement. It has been suggested that prostatic involvement by urothelial carcinoma should be subclassified as follows (31):

(1) confined to the prostatic urethral mucosa;

(2) prostatic ducts and acini (non-invasive); and

(3) with invasion of prostatic stroma.

Clearly, radical therapy is indicated in patients with invasion of prostatic stroma (32–34).

UROTHELIAL DYSPLASIA AND CARCINOMA IN SITU

The most severe degree of dysplasia of the urothelium, CIS, was first reported by Melicow in 1952 who described markedly atypical cells in the bladder mucosa adjacent to bladder cancer (35). It can occur without associated bladder tumours (so-called primary CIS), but this is very uncommon and usually is seen in men over 50 (2). Usually, it is associated with synchronous or metachronous bladder tumours. The frequency is highest in patients with high-grade tumours (35,36). The mucosa appears red and velvety by cystoscopy (Fig. 6.14 and Plate 2). Urothelial dysplasia is usually associated with nuclear abnormalities; the epithelium may be of normal thickness or hyperplastic. Morphologic criteria (up to 10) have been used, such as changes in the number of urothelial cell layers, disturbance in polarity, mitosis, nuclear crowding, nuclear clearing, increased nuclear size, changes in chromatin pattern, nuclear irregularity, prominent nucleoli, and mucosal denudation (37,38). The terms mild, moderate and severe dysplasia have been used (37), and Mostofi and Sesterhenn proposed CIS grades 1, 2, and 3 for mild, moderate, and severe dysplasia/CIS (39). Owing to poor reproducibility, it has not been possible to gain national or international acceptance for either of these classifications. Furthermore, a panel of urologists expressed deep concern that use of the terms CIS grades 1 and 2 may result in unwarranted aggressive treatment (40). We feel that it is possible to identify where the entire urothelium or part of it is replaced by malignant cells and label such lesions CIS (Fig. 6.15). The abnormal urothelium shows marked lack of cellular cohesion often resulting in very few or no malignant cells or only denuded mucosa (41). The tumour cells may be large or may have scanty or relatively abundant cytoplasm. In the pagetoid type, neoplastic cells are present among benign cells (42) (Fig. 6.16). Epithelial abnormalities with features less than severe dysplasia/CIS can appropriately be labelled dysplasia or atypia of unknown significance (Fig. 6.17). The term dysplasia is used differently in Europe, where atypia is synonymous with the term dysplasia used in the United States. Patients with bladder tumours, especially high grade, should undergo random (selected site) biopsies (mapping). Careful examination of cystectomy specimens have revealed that CIS may often be extensive, with involvement of prostatic urethra, prostate, and ureters (35,41).

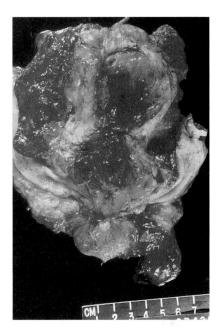

Fig. 6.14 Cystectomy specimen with carcinoma in situ. Note the reddish velvety mucosal surface

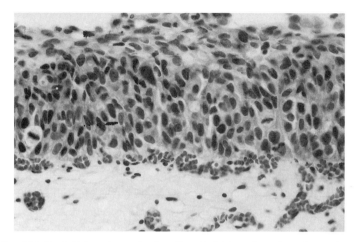

Fig. 6.15 *Urothelial carcinoma* in situ. *Note the high-grade nuclear abnormalities.* (*H&E, ×450*)

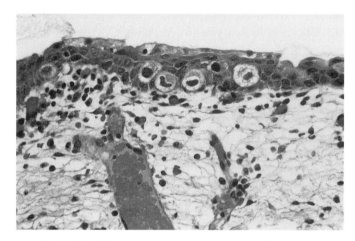

Fig. 6.16 *Urothelial carcinoma* in situ, *pagetoid type. (H&E, ×450)*

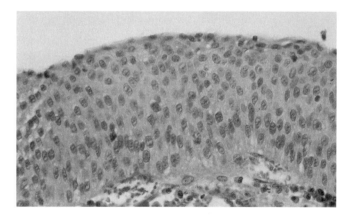

Fig. 6.17 *Hyperplastic urothelium showing dysplasia of unknown significance. (H&E, ×450)*

Additional prognostic factors

Although grade and stage have been shown to be the major prognostic factors in bladder cancer, a number of other factors have shown an influence on prognosis in various studies. One of the earliest markers discovered was vascular invasion. In a study of patients with Ta and T1 tumours, we found that patients with T1 tumours who had lymphatic invasion had a poor prognosis. Thus, of 10 such patients, seven died within 6 years from widespread metastases (22). Bell *et al.* reported that the 5-year survival of patients with or without vascular invasion was 29 and 57%, respectively. However, their study was not limited to T1 tumours (43). Two recent studies using immunohistochemical methods to visualize vascular endothelium did not show vascular invasion to be of prognostic value (44,45). These methods also revealed that it is difficult to determine the presence or absence of vascular invasion on haematoxylin and eosin stained (H&E) sections, and what was called vascular invasion in the past often was retraction artefact.

The presence of blood group antigens (A, B, H, and the Lewis antigen) on the surface of epithelial cells depends on the individual's secretor status. Some 85% of the population are secretors and express A, B, or H in their normal urothelium. The loss of these antigens and the Lewis antigen in bladder cancer patients has been reported to correlate with progression and poorer prognosis, but such markers have not proven superior to grade and stage and are not used in the routine evaluation of bladder cancer (46–49). Human chorionic gonadotrophin (HCG) is demonstrated in bladder cancer cells and in serum of some patients with bladder cancer. Increased serum levels have been found to predict metastatic disease (50,51). Expression is mainly seen in high-grade tumours and has been found to correlate with prognosis in one study while another study showed no correlation (52,53).

Cellular proliferation can be determined by several different methods, such as measurement of S-phase fraction by flow cytometry, mitosis count, and immunohistochemistry for Ki-67 or proliferating cell nuclear antigen (PCNA). All of these methods have, in various studies, shown a correlation with grade and stage and often with prognosis (54–60). Lipponen *et al.* (1993) and Vasko *et al.* (1995) reported that mitosis count is a significant prognostic factor independent of stage and grade (61,62).

Epidermal growth factor (EGF) is normally present in the urine. Expression of the EGF receptor (EGFR) has been found to correlate with grade and stage and outcome. In low-stage disease it correlates with recurrence and progression, and in higher stage it correlates with outcome (63–65). However, in a multivariate analysis it was not independent of stage (66).

The HER-2 (c-erbB-2) oncogene is expressed in many cancers including bladder cancer, and some studies show a positive correlation with grade and stage and outcome while others do not (67–72). The overall impression is that c-erbB-2 expression is of questionable clinical value in managing patients with bladder cancer.

The role of p53 protein is to stop cell proliferation and to allow for repair of damaged DNA. Inactivation of the p53 suppressor gene, located on chromosome 17, results in cell proliferation. Mutation of p53 is seen to a variable degree in many different cancers including bladder cancer. The mutated p53 has a prolonged half life and the protein can be demonstrated by immunohistochemistry. Lipponen (73) reported on the prognostic significance of p53 expression except in superficial bladder cancer, but found that it was not a predictor of survival independent of grade and stage. In contrast, Sarkis *et al.* and Serth *et al.* in multivariate analyses found that expression of p53 was a significant predictor for progression and relapse in stages Ta and T1 bladder cancer (74,75). Fossa and associates (53) failed to demonstrate any significant difference in the prognosis of p53-negative and p53-positive muscle invasive bladder cancer. In contrast, Esrig *et al.* (76), in a study of 243 patients with bladder cancer treated by radical cystectomy, found that the overexpression of p53 significantly correlated with recurrence and crude survival and was independent of grade and pathological stage.

Defects in the short or long arms of chromosome 9 or both are frequently low-grade, non-invasive papillary tumours (77). High-grade invasive tumours in contrast have a defect in chromosome 17, representing an abnormality in the p53 gene (78). Abnormalities on chromosome 9 are uncommon in high-grade, stage Ta and T1 tumours or CIS. A few patients with concomitant low-grade papillary carcinoma and CIS have been studied, and chromosome 9 abnormalities were identified in the former and p53 abnormalities in the latter (79). Based on these differences, these authors suggested the possibility of two different pathways in the development of non-invasive bladder cancer. P53 mutations seem to be an early event in CIS as they were found in CIS patients without a previous history of bladder cancer. Furthermore the patients did not have any loss of material on either chromosome 9 or 17. In patients with superficial bladder cancer, chromosome 9 alterations are sufficient for tumours to develop, but progression of these tumours are likely to require additional changes on chromosome 9, 17, or others (79). Chromosomal alterations involving chromosomes 3, 5, 7, 8, 10, 11, and 13 have also been identified, especially in high-grade invasive bladder cancer, probably representing progression of malignancy associated with genetic instability of DNA (77,80).

VARIANTS OF BLADDER CANCER

In 1994, Amin *et al.* reported 18 patients with micropapillary carcinoma of the bladder (81). The surface of the tumour often had a micropapillary pattern, and the invasive component showed a micropapillary pattern strongly resembling papillary serous carcinoma of the ovary (Fig. 6.18). All patients in their series had vascular invasion and 10 of 18 had CIS. The prognosis was poor with only seven patients alive without disease after a mean follow-up of 44.8 months (range 6–96 months). In the other 11 patients, follow-up was a mean of 47 months (6–96 months). In a prospective study, we found the incidence of micropapillary carcinoma to be 0.7% of all bladder cancer. We studied 20 patients with a mean age of 69 years and a sex ratio (male/female) of 2.3 : 1. Lymphatic invasion was present in 15 (identified by immunoperoxidase staining with antibodies against factor VIII) and CIS was present in 13. Virtually all tumours stained with antibodies against CK 7, CK 20 and CD 15 (LeuM l). Thirty-five per cent were positive for CA 125 (in males and females). Coexistent conventional urothelial carcinoma was seen in 18 of 20 cases. All but five patients presented with stage T3a or higher. Only five patients survived 5 years, one of whom succumbed to the disease after 7 years. Thus, it is important to recognize this micropapillary pattern as aggressive therapy is needed to improve prognosis (82).

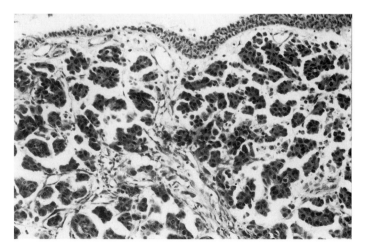

Fig. 6.18 Micropapillary carcinoma showing features reminiscent of papillary serous carcinoma of the ovary. Prominent retraction artefact is present. (H&E, ×225)

Bladder carcinoma resembling lymphoepithelioma of the nasopharynx is rare. We found an incidence of 0.4% of bladder cancers in a prospective study (83). Of the 23 cases so far published in the literature, 15 were males and nine females. The tumours are composed of sheets of nests with large pale cells. The tumour cells are organized in a syncytial pattern and have conspicuous nucleoli. The background has an abundant lymphoid stroma (Fig. 6.19). Owing to the presence of prominent lymphoid cells the tumour may be misdiagnosed as lymphoma or severe cystitis. The tumours are classified as having focal lymphoepithelioma like pattern (<50%), predominant (>50%) or pure (84). Of the 23 published cases, nine were pure, eight predominant, and six focal lymphoepithelial pattern. The other elements usually comprised high-grade urothelial carcinoma. The tumour cells marked with pankeratin (Mak-6) and CK7, while only one of nine tumours studied was positive for CK 20. The majority of the lymphocytes intermixed between the tumour cells mark as T lymphocytes; B cells were mainly present at the periphery of the tumour cells, often as B-cell nodules (83). Hybridization to Epstein–Barr virus-coded ribonucleic acid was negative in 20 cases reported. The tumour is usually high stage; all but four of the 23 reported cases were muscle invasive. The prognosis is good except in patients classified as focal lymphoepithelial carcinoma, which has a prognosis similar to urothelial carcinoma of similar stage.

The nested variant of urothelial carcinoma, a term coined by Murphy and Deana, (85) was first described by Stern in 1979 (86) and later by Talbert and Young (1989) who referred to this entity as carcinoma with deceptively bland features (87). This invasive

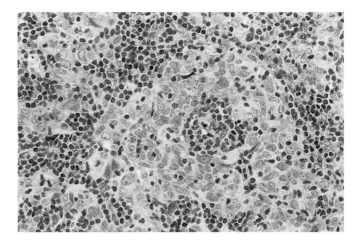

Fig. 6.19 Lymphoepithelial-like carcinoma showing pale tumour cells in a syncytial pattern mixed with lymphocytes. (H&E, ×450)

carcinoma is characterized by a distinctive growth pattern with small nests of bland, benign-appearing urothelial cells resembling von Brunn nests or cystitis cystica (Fig. 6.20). Rare tumour cells may show more dysplastic features. Some tumours may have a tubular or microcystic pattern (87) (Fig. 6.21). The differential diagnosis includes nephrogenic metaplasia, paraganglioma, and exuberant von Brunn nests or cystitis cystica. In the 23 cases hitherto reported, only one patient was a female. The mean age was 68 years, identical to conventional urothelial carcinoma. Drew *et al.* reported an aggressive behaviour in 60% of the patients, similar to high-grade conventional urothelial carcinoma (88).

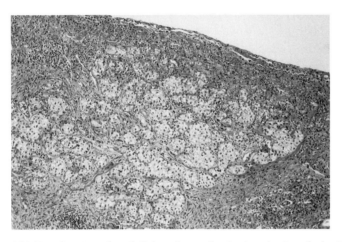

Fig. 6.20 *Nested variant of urothelial carcinoma showing invasion into the lamina propria. Note the bland appearance of the tumour. (H&E, × 112)*

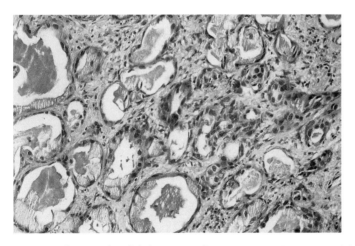

Fig. 6.21 *Nested variant of urothelial carcinoma showing a microcystic pattern reminiscent of nephrogenic metaplasia. Note the presence of more atypical cells. (H&E, × 225)*

Sarcomatoid carcinoma is a rare bladder tumour composed of malignant spindle cells surrounding islands of carcinoma, usually urothelial or SCC (Fig. 6.22). Sarcomatoid areas, which may totally dominate, may resemble malignant fibrous histiocytoma or leiomyosarcoma, and epithelial differentiation may be lacking in limited biopsy material. However, some of the spindle cells usually stain positive with keratin antibodies, which is confirmatory. Ultrastructural examination will also show epithelial differentiation. We reserve the term carcinosarcoma for tumours showing both carcinomatous and sarcomatous differentiation (by electron microscopy or immunohistochemistry), especially when heterologous elements are present (chondro-, osteo-, rhabdomyo- or liposarcoma). Sarcomatoid sarcomas most often present as a bulky polypoid mass in older men. The tumour is usually high stage and the 5-year survival is less than 30% (10).

Carcinosarcomas are most often seen in males (sex ratio 3 : 1) and present as large polypoid masses. The mean age at presentation is 62 years. The tumours contain a mixture of malignant epithelial elements, most often urothelial, but SCC, adenocarcinoma, small cell carcinoma, and undifferentiated carcinoma may also be seen. These elements are mixed with sarcomatous elements, usually heterologous (chondro-, osteo-, lipo-, or rhabdomyosarcomatous). The prognosis is poor; most deaths have been a result of local growth rather than metastasis. Metastasis may display both epithelial and mesenchymal elements (10).

SCC must be sufficiently differentiated to have some combination of intercellular bridges, individual cell keratinization, and keratin pearls. Non-keratinizing areas are often impossible to

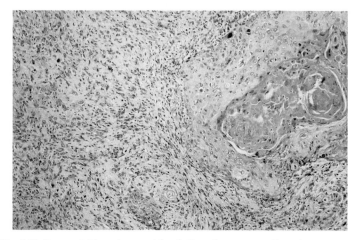

Fig. 6.22 Sarcomatoid carcinoma with spindle and squamous cell carcinoma components. (H&E, ×112)

differentiate from high-grade urothelial carcinoma, and Murphy *et al.* stated that the distinction between mixed urothelial and SCC in any particular case may be arbitrary (10). Other individuals are more dogmatic, stating that the diagnosis of SCC should be restricted to pure tumours without identifiable urothelial carcinoma (2). We disagree with such a strict definition, and feel that if the main part of the tumour shows malignant squamous elements it should be called SCC. These different definitions may explain why the incidence of SCC has varied in different series between 3 and 8%, or even higher, in the Western world (2,10). The male to female ratio is 1.7 : 1 and most cases are diagnosed in the sixth decade or later. In areas of endemic schistosomiasis, SCC comprises two-thirds of all bladder cancer. Additional risk factors include chronic bladder infection, in dwelling catheters, bladder calculi, infected diverticuli, and keratinizing squamous metaplasia (89) (Fig. 6.23 and Plate 3). The conventional type of SCC is a nodular or plaque-like, often ulcerated lesion. The histological features are identical to SCC elsewhere in the body and most tumours are of grades 2 or 3. The majority of patients present with high-stage disease and the 5-year survival is 25% or less.

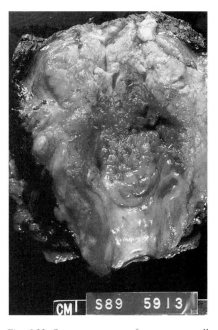

Fig. 6.23 *Gross appearance of a squamous cell carcinoma which developed in a quadriplegic woman with an indwelling catheter for 24 years*

The verrucous variant of SCC was originally described in the oral cavity and is rarely found in the bladder except in patients with schistosomiasis, where approximately 3% of the bladder tumours are of the verrucous type (10). The tumour is cauliflower-like. The histological features include well differentiated squamous epithelium without significant dysplasia lining church spire-like fibrovascular cores. The tumour is well circumscribed with pushing borders. If the biopsies are superficial it is virtually impossible to diagnosis this tumour. Verrucous carcinoma is locally aggressive but does not metastasize.

Bladder tumours with a histological appearance of villous or tubulovillous adenoma of the colon have been described, with four cases reported (2). We recently encountered a case occurring in a 47-year-old man with a non-functioning bladder. He developed mucosuria and a large polypoid mass was seen on cystoscopy. The biopsy was suggestive of villous adenoma. A cystectomy was performed and a 7 cm villous adenoma was found involving the intramural part of the ureter with associated intestinal metaplasia in the bladder mucosa (Fig. 6.24). Three of the four reported cases have been in males. Three of the patients were treated with TURB and one with cystectomy. No recurrence occurred during a follow-up period of 14–16 months. Murphy *et al.* consider villous tumours as a glandular neoplasm, histologically and indistinguishable from villous and tubulovillous adenomas and carcinomas of the colon. They recognize that these neoplasms are difficult to classify but

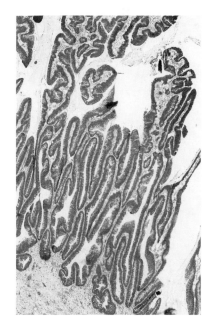

Fig. 6.24. *Villous adenoma indistinguishable from its colonic counterpart. (H&E, ×40)*

consider them particularly well differentiated forms of adeno-carcinoma (10).

Adenocarcinoma comprises approximately 1% of bladder tumours, and like other types of bladder cancer has a male pre-dominance. There is a close embryological relationship between the cloaca and the bladder but the normal urothelium is devoid of intestinal metaplasia. These changes are considered by many to be a precursor lesion developing in a setting of chronic inflamma-tion and infection such as schistosomiasis. Other predisposing factors include non-functioning bladder and extrophy of the bladder. Approximately one-third of adenocarcinomas occur in the urachus and are characterized by location in the dome, epi-centre in the wall of the bladder, and lack of intestinal metaplasia. Furthermore, a primary tumour elsewhere must be excluded. Primary adenocarcinoma is usually solitary. The majority of the lesions are glandular, some of which are indistinguishable from colon cancer; other patterns include papillary, mucinous, signet ring cell type, and clear cell adenocarcinoma (Fig. 6.25). More than one pattern is often seen (90). The differential diagnosis includes bladder involvement by colonic, gynaecological or pro-static carcinoma, and metastatic carcinoma. Prostatic carcinoma is almost invariably positive for prostatic acid phosphatase and prostate-specific antigen (PSA), whereas adenocarcinomas of the bladder are almost uniformly negative for these markers (2). The prognosis is dependent on tumour size, stage and tumour type. The 5-year survival varies between 6% and 61% in different studies. Grignon reported better survival in non-urachal com-pared with urachal carcinoma while we did not find any signi-ficant difference in our study (91).

Primary small cell carcinoma of the urinary bladder with histo-logical features indistinguishable from its pulmonary counterpart was first reported in 1981 (92), and has since been reported with increasing frequency (2). In a prospective study of bladder tumours we found the incidence of small cell carcinoma to be 0.7% (93). So far more than 130 cases have been reported. We found a male to female sex ratio of 2.7 : 1 with a mean age of 71 years. The tumour lacks specific gross pathological features and can occur anywhere in the bladder. The tumour can have an oat cell pattern with a relatively uniform cell population, scant cytoplasm, and hyperchromatic nuclei with dispersed chromatin usually lacking or having inconspicuous nucleoli. The tumour cells of the intermediate type have more cytoplasm, and it is not unusual to see cells that are more spindly (Fig. 6.26). Nuclear moulding is prominent in both types, mitosis is frequent, and necrosis often extensive. Dense core granules have been found in

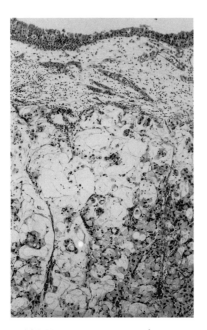

Fig. 6.25 Mucinous carcinoma with signet ring cell differentiation arising in the dome of the bladder. Note the normal appearing urothelium. (H&E, ×100)

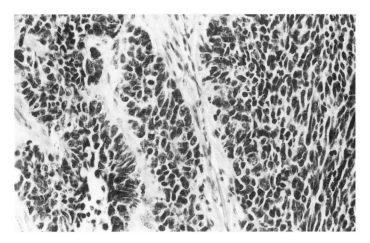

Fig. 6.26 Small cell carcinoma showing focal spindle cells. (H&E, × 450)

most cases examined by electron microscopy, and immunohisto-chemistry also displays evidence of neuroendocrine different-iation. Thus, staining with antibodies against neuron-specific enolase is usually positive. Some cases express synaptophysin and chromogranin. Staining for cytokeratin is positive in most cases. The differential diagnosis includes lymphoma, which usually can be determined on routine histological examination, but some-times cytokeratin and lymphoid immunohistochemical markers are needed. In our series (93), 10 of 25 cases were pure oat cell type, four pure intermediate cell type and 11 mixed with either urothelial carcinoma, SCC or adenocarcinoma, or more than one of these components (Fig. 6.27). Five of 18 patients with localized

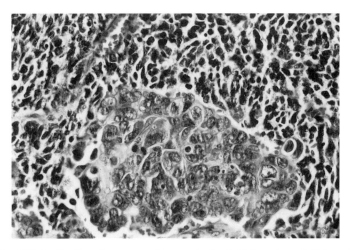

Fig. 6.27 Small cell carcinoma, oat cell type, mixed with high-grade urothelial carci-noma. (H&E, × 450)

disease (stages T2–T4) survived 5 years (28%). All received radiation treatment with various surgical procedures: transurethral resection in three cases, partial bladder resection in one, and cystectomy in one. Similar survival results (29%) were reported in a literature review by Angulo *et al.* in 1996 (94). Thus, patients with small cell carcinoma of the bladder fare better than patients with small cell carcinoma of the lung. Angulo *et al.* reported one patient with metastatic disease who was treated with systemic chemotherapy. The patient died after 5 months because of myocardial infarction, but an autopsy revealed no residual tumour in the bladder or in the lymph node metastasis (94).

Tumours comprised of two or more histologically distinctive epithelial components are referred to as mixed carcinomas and comprise approximately 4–6% of urothelial carcinomas. The most common appearance is that of high-grade urothelial carcinoma mixed with squamous carcinoma or adenocarcinoma. The criteria for distinguishing mixed carcinomas from urothelial carcinomas with small foci of squamous or glandular differentiation are not well defined. The tumours are generally high-stage lesions and the behaviour is related to the fact that these are high-stage and high-grade tumours (10).

Leiomyosarcoma is a rare tumour, although it is the most common mesenchymal malignancy of the bladder in adults. The morphological criteria separating leiomyoma from leiomyosarcoma in the urinary bladder has not been well established. Walker *et al.* stated that 'it seems prudent to label leiomyosarcoma a smooth muscle neoplasm demonstrating infiltrative, destructive invasion of the vesical musculature' (95). In contrast, the designation of leiomyoma should be reserved for circumscribed smooth muscle tumours with minimal cytological atypia and virtually no mitotic activity. Leiomyosarcomas are usually large tumours with a polypoid appearance. The cut surface is either that of a myxoid tumour or shows a 'fish flesh' appearance. The tumours are composed of fascicles of spindle cells with cigar-shaped nuclei crossing each other at 90° angles. The frequency of mitosis is variable as is the degree of nuclear pleomorphism. Some neoplasms are markedly myxoid. The tumours generally express vimentin and muscle specific actin while desmin reactivity is variable. The differential diagnosis includes sarcomatoid carcinoma and carcinosarcoma as well as pseudosarcoma. The individual cells of pseudosarcoma are more spindle-shaped with little pleomorphism, and mitotic figures are rare. Leiomyosarcoma is treated by partial cystectomy or radical cystectomy depending upon the size and location of the tumour. The 5-year survival has been reported to be 67% (2).

Rhabdomyosarcoma of the urinary bladder is a tumour predominantly of childhood, with most cases diagnosed before the age of 5. Tumours often appear as polypoid, multiple grape-like masses or as a large solitary mass. The trigone is the most common location. Histologically, the tumours most often show features of embryonal rhabdomyosarcoma with a cambium layer composed of rhabdomyoblasts located below the urothelium. Below this more condensed cambium layer is a more dispersed cell population scattered in a loose myxoid stroma. Many of these cells are rhabdomyoblasts. Institution of combination therapy (surgery, radiation, and chemotherapy) through the Intergroup Rhabdomyosarcoma Study has resulted in marked improvement in the prognosis, with relatively few children dying from their disease (96).

Paraganglioma comprises 0.1% of all bladder neoplasms; some 200 cases have been described (2,10). It has been reported to occur from childhood to old age. The most characteristic symptoms include bursting headache and anxiety, a pounding sensation, blurred vision, sweating, and even syncope, usually associated with urination. Hypertension is present in most individuals. Elevated catecholamines or their metabolites are increased in the urine. Typically, the tumours are composed of nests of cells (zellballen) separated by a prominent sinusoidal vascular network. The individual tumour cells are uniform and polygonal, showing amphophilic pale cytoplasm (Fig. 6.28). Focally nuclear pleomorphism with bizarre cells may be identified but malignant behaviour is seen in less than 20% of the tumours. The tumours lack immune reactivity for cytokeratin and epithelial membrane antigen while they stain positive with antibodies to neuroendocrine markers such as neuron-specific enolase and chromogranin.

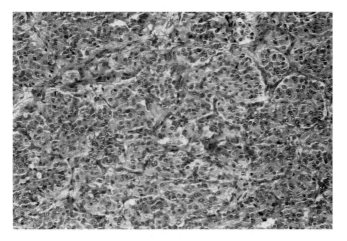

Fig. 6.28 Paraganglioma showing characteristic cell balls. (H&E, ×225)

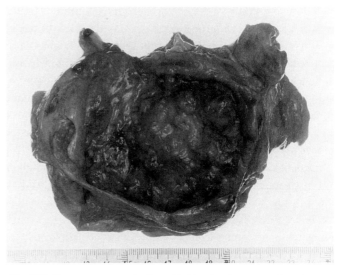

Fig. 6.29 Gross appearance of urinary bladder showing metastatic melanoma

Malignant lymphoma of the bladder is rare as a primary tumour, with only some 30 cases described in the literature. There is a marked female preponderance (male to female ratio 1 : 6.5). The vast majority of bladder lymphomas were non-Hodgkin lymphomas, B-cell type (97).

Extravesical tumours usually involve the urinary bladder by direct extension from adjacent organs, including the prostate, uterus, and rectum. Distant mestatases only comprise 2.3% of the cases (98). In a comprehensive review by Goldstein (99), melanoma (Fig. 6.29 and Plate 4) was the most common tumour metastatic to the bladder, followed by gastric carcinoma, breast, kidney, and lung cancer. The majority of metastases to the bladder are incidental findings at autopsy. Most cases with secondary involvement of the bladder are adenocarcinoma of the prostate, which generally has characteristic histology. In difficult cases immunohistochemical examination with antibodies against prostatic specific antigen and prostatic acid phosphatase may be needed.

TUMOUR-LIKE LESIONS

Polypoid (or papillary) cystitis is a reactive mucosal lesion, which in the overwhelming majority of cases is associated with the use of an indwelling catheter (100). Typically, the lesions are located in the posterior wall or dome of the bladder, areas predominantly irritated by the tip of the catheter. By cystoscopy the lesions are either bullous, polypoid, or papillary, and often haemorrhagic. Papillary lesions by cystoscopy may be indistinguishable from low-grade papillary tumour. By light microscopy a true fibrovascular core is lacking in polypoid cystitis, the umbrella cells are preserved, and there is no dysplasia of the urothelium. Microabscesses are often present in the urothelium (100). Furthermore polypoid cystitis is reversible. It will regress and disappear when the catheter is removed (101).

Pseudosarcoma is a lesion with many names including inflammatory pseudotumour, pseudomalignant spindle cell proliferation, pseudosarcomatous fibromyxoid tumour, and postoperative spindle cell nodule. We prefer the name pseudosarcoma as the lesion mimics a sarcoma and may occur spontaneously, or it may develop subsequent to or concomitant with mucosal damage caused by instrumentation to the bladder (biopsies, TURB), chronic inflammation, or other bladder tumours (102). The lesions are generally poorly circumscribed and composed of spindle cells or strap cells in a myxoid or oedematous background with thin walled blood vessels and scattered inflammatory cells. Some lesions are virtually identical to nodular fasciitis while in others there are more cellular, tight fascicles present. Nuclear enlargement and eosinophilic nucleoli are characteristic of reactive atypia. The reactive nature of the lesion is further emphasized by the presence of inflammatory cells, such as eosinophils and lymphocytes, which are present in a vascular myxoid matrix reminiscent of granulation tissue. Mitoses are rare and abnormal mitoses are not present. The spindle cells express vimentin, often express smooth muscle actin and muscle-specific actin, and sometimes express cytokeratin; staining for epithelial membrane antigen is negative. Thus, immunohistochemistry is not helpful in differentiating pseudosarcoma from the main differential diagnosis, namely leiomyosarcoma (102).

Amyloidosis is most often of primary type and associated with gross, painless haematuria in 85% of the patients. The lesion will often appear as nodular and therefore frequently is mistaken for bladder tumour by the cystoscopist. Histological deposits of amyloid can be seen in the lamina propria in association with veins and arteries and sometimes in the muscularis propria. The amyloid is best visualized by Congo red stain and examination in birefringent light (10).

Points of controversy

1. Everted urothelial papilloma, does it exist? Yes, but it is extremely rare.
2. Introducing new terminology for WHO grade 1 bladder carcinoma is crucial as the overwhelming majority of tumours behave in a benign fashion. The suggested term is papillary urothelial tumour of low malignant potential.
3. Subclassification of T1 tumours into T1a and T1b, is it worth doing? Yes, it should be done whenever possible.

References

1 Cancer Incidence in Sweden, The National Board of Health and Welfare, Centre for Epidemiology, Stockholm 1993–94.
2 Grignon D. Neoplasms of the urinary bladder. In: *Urologic surgical pathology* (ed. Bostwick DC, Eble JN). Mosby, New York, 1997, pp. 184–302.

3 Holmang S, Hedelin H, Anderstrom C *et al.* The importance of the depth of invasion in stage T1 bladder carcinoma: a prospective cohort study. *J Urol* 1997, **157**, 800–3.

4 Kunze E, Schauer A, Schmitt M. Histology and histogenesis of two different types of inverted papillomas. *Cancer* 1983, **51**, 348–58.

5 Paschkis R. Uber Adenoma der Harnblase. *Z Urol Nephrol*, 1927, **21**, 313–15.

6 Potts IF, Hirst E. Inverted papilloma of the bladder. *J Urol* 1963, **90**, 175–81.

7 Anderstram C, Johansson S, Pettersson S. Inverted papilloma of the urinary tract. *J Urol* 1982, **127**, 1132–4.

8 Koss LG. Tumors of the Urinary Bladder, Second Series Fascicle, Washington, DC, 1974, Armed Forces Institute of Pathology.

9 Jordan AM, Weingarten J, Murphy WM. Transitional cell neoplasms of the urinary bladder: can biologic potential be predicted from histologic grading? *Cancer* 1987, **60**, 2766–74.

10 Murphy WM, Beckwith JB, Farrow GM. *Tumors of the kidney, bladder, and related structures*, Third Series, Fascicle. Armed Forces Institute of Pathology, Washington, DC, 1994.

11 Reuter VE, Melamed MR. The lower urinary tract. In: *Diagnostic surgical pathology* (ed. Sternberg SS). Raven Press, New York, 1994.

12 Broders ACI. Epithelioma of the genitourinary organs. *Ann Surg*, 1922, **75**, 574.

13 Mostofi FK, Sobin HL, Torloni H. *Histologic typing of urinary bladder tumors*. World Health Organization, Geneva, 1973.

14 Bergkvist A, Ljungqvist A, Moberger D. Classification of bladder tumors based on the cellular pattern. *Acta Chir Scand*, 1965, **130**, 378–84.

15 Malmstram PU, Busch C, Norlen BJ. Recurrence, progression and survival in bladder cancer. *Scand J Urol Nephrol*, 1987, **21**, 185–95.

16 Choi HK, Vaski J, Bengtsson E *et al.* Grading of transitional cell bladder carcinoma by texture analysis of histological sections. *Anal Cell Pathol* 1994, **6**, 327–43.

17 Abel PD, Henderson D, Bennett MK *et al.* Differing interpretations by pathologists of the pT category and grade of transitional cell cancer of the bladder. *Br J Urol* 1988, **62**, 339–42.

18 Robertson AJ, Swanson Beck J, Burnett RA *et al.* Observer variability in histopathological reporting of transitional cell carcinoma and epithelial dysplasia in bladders. *J Clin Pathol* 1990, **43**, 17–21.

19 Ooms ECM, Anderson WAD, Alons CL *et al.* Analysis of the performance of pathologists in the grading of bladder tumors. *Hum Pathol* 1983, **14**, 140–3.

20 Jarkrans T, Vask J, Bengtsson E *et al.* Grading of transitional cell bladder carcinoma by object based image analysis of histological sections. *Anal Cell Pathol* 1995, **8**, 135–58.

21 AJCC. *Cancer Staging Manual*, 5th edn. Lippincott–Raven Publisher, Philadelphia, 1997.

22 Anderstrom C, Johansson S, Nilsson S. The influence of lamina propria invasion on the prognosis of patients with bladder tumors. *J Urol* 1980, **124**, 23–6.

23 Dixon JS, Gosling JA. Histology and fine structure of the muscularis mucosae of the human urinary bladder. *J Anat*, 1983, **136**, 265–71.

24 Ro JY, Ayala AG, El-Naggar A. Muscularis mucosa of urinary bladder. Importance for staging and treatment. *Am J Surg Pathol*, 1987, **11**, 668–72.

25 Younes M, Sussman J, True LD. The usefulness of the level of the muscularis mucosae in the staging of invasive transitional cell carcinoma of the urinary bladder. *Cancer* 1990, **66**, 543–8.

26 Hasui Y, Osada Y, Kitada S, Nishi S. Significance of invasion to the muscularis mucosae on the progression of superficial bladder cancer. *Urology*, 1994, **43**, 782–6.

27 Angulo JD, Lopez JI, Grignon DJ, Sanchez-Chapado M. Muscularis mucosa differentiates two populations with different prognosis in stage T1 bladder cancer. *Urology*, 1995, **45**, 47–53.

28 Platz CE, Cohen MB, Jones MP *et al.* Is microstaging of early invasive cancer of the urinary tract possible or useful? *Mod Pathol* 1996, **9**, 1035–9.

29 Mahadevia PS, Koss LG, Tar IJ. Prostatic involvement in bladder cancer: prostate mapping in 20 cystoprostatectomy specimens. *Cancer* 1986, **58**, 2096–102.

30 Wood DP Jr, Montie JE, Pontes JE *et al.* Transitional cell carcinoma of the prostate in cystoprostatectomy specimens removed for bladder cancer. *J Urol* 1989, **141**, 346–51.

31 Hardeman SW, Soloway MS. Transitional cell carcinoma of the prostate: diagnosis, staging and management. *World J Urol* 1988, **6**, 170–3.

32 Matzkin H, Soloway MS, Hardeman S. Transitional cell carcinoma of the prostate. *J Urol* 1991, **146**, 1207–12.

33 Hardeman SW, Perry A, Soloway MS. Transitional cell carcinoma of the prostate following intravesical therapy for transitional cell carcinoma of the bladder. *J Urol* 1988, **140**, 289–92.

34 Wishnow KI, Ro JY. Importance of early treatment of transitional cell carcinoma of prostatic ducts. *Urology*, 1988, **32**, 11–15.

35 Melicow MM. Histological study of vesical urothelium intervening between gross neoplasms in total cystectomy. *J Urol* 1952, **68**, 261.

36 Wolf H, Rosenkilde-Olsen P, Fischer A *et al*. Urothelial atypia concomitant with primary bladder tumour. *Scand J Urol Nephrol*, 1987, **21**, 33–6.

37 Nagy GK, Frable WJ, Murphy WM. Classification of premalignant urothelial abnormalities: a Delphi study of the National Bladder Cancer Collaborative Group A. *Pathol Ann*, 1982, **17**, 219–33.

38 Murphy WM, Soloway MS. Developing carcinoma (dysplasia of the urinary bladder). *Pathol Ann*, 1982, **17**, 197–217.

39 Mostofi FK, Sesterhenn IA. Pathology of epithelial tumors and carcinoma in situ of bladder. *Prog Clin Biol Res* 1984, **162A**, 55–74.

40 Friedell GH, Soloway MS, Hilgar AG. Summary of workshop on carcinoma in situ of the bladder. *J Urol* 1986, **136**, 1047–8.

41 Farrow GM, Utz DC, Rife CC. Morphological and clinical observations of patients with early bladder cancer treated with total cystectomy. *Cancer Res* 1976, **36**, 2495–501.

42 Orozco RE, Vander Zwaag R, Murphy WM. The pagetoid variant of urothelial carcinoma in situ. *Hum Pathol* 1993, **24**, 1199–202.

43 Bell JT, Burney SW, Friedell GH. Blood vessel invasion in human bladder cancer. *J Urol* 1971, **105**, 675–8.

44 Larsen MP, Steinberg GD, Brendler CB *et al*. Use of *Ulex europaeus* agglutinin I (UEAI) to distinguish vascular and pseudovascular invasion in transitional cell carcinoma of bladder with lamina propria invasion. *Mod Pathol* 1990, **3**, 83–8.

45 Ramani P, Birch BRP, Harland SJ *et al*. Evaluation of endothelial markers in detecting blood and lymphatic channel invasion in pT1 transitional carcinoma of bladder. *Histopathology*, 1991, **19**, 551–4.

46 Cordon-Cardo C, Reuter VE, Lloyd KO *et al*. Blood group-related antigens in human urothelium: enhanced expression of precursor Le^X and Le^Y determinants in urothelial carcinoma. *Cancer Res* 1988, **48**, 4113–20.

47 Malmstrom PU, Busch C, Norlhn BJ, Andersson B. Expression of ABH blood group isoantigen as a prognostic factor in transitional cell bladder carcinoma. *Scand J Urol Nephrol*, 1988, **22**, 265–70.

48 Malmstrom PU, Norlhn BJ, Andersson B, Busch C. Combination of blood group ABH antigen status and DNA-ploidy as an independent prognostic factor in transitional cell carcinoma of the urinary bladder. *Br J Urol* 1989, **64**, 49–55.

49 Pauwels RPE, Schapers RFM, Smeets AWGB *et al*. Blood group isoantigen deletion and chromosomal abnormalities in bladder cancer. *J Urol* 1988, **40**, 959–63.

50 Iles RK, Jenkins BJ, Oliver RTD *et al*. Beta human chorionic gonadotrophin in serum and urine: a marker for metastatic urothelial cancer. *Br J Urol* 1989, **64**, 241–4.

51 Iles RK, Chard T. Human chorionic gonadotropin expression by bladder cancers; biology and clinical potential. *J Urol* 1991, **145**, 453–8.

52 Seidal T, Breborowicz J, Malmstrom PU, Busch C. Immunoreactivity to human chorionic gonadotropin in urothelial carcinoma: correlation with tumor grade stage and prognosis. *J Urol Pathol* 1993, **1**, 397–9.

53 Fossa SD, Berner AA, Jacobsen AB *et al*. Clinical significance of DNA-ploidy and S-phase fraction and their relation to p53 protein, c-erbB-2 protein and HCG in operable muscle invasive bladder cancer. *Br J Cancer* 1993, **68**, 572–8.

54 Farsund T, Hoestmark JG, Laerum OD. Relation between flow cytometric DNA distribution and pathology in human bladder cancer. *Cancer* 1984, **54**, 1771–7.

55 Lipponen PK, Collan Y, Eskelinen MJ *et al*. Comparison or morphometry and DNA flow cytometry with standard prognostic factors in bladder cancer. *Br J Urol* 1990, **65**, 589–97.

56 Bush C, Price P, Norton J *et al.* Proliferation in human bladder carcinoma measured by Ki-67 antibody labelling: its potential clinical importance. *Br J Cancer* 1991, **64**, 357–60.

57 Melamed MR. Flow cytometry for detection and evaluation of urinary bladder carcinoma. *Semin Surg Oncol*, 1992, **8**, 300–9.

58 Jacobsen A, Pettersen EO, Amellem N *et al.* The prognostic significance of deoxyribonucleic acid flow cytometry in muscle invasive bladder carcinoma treated with preoperative irradiation and cystectomy. *J Urol* 1992, **147**, 34–7.

59 Mulder AH, Van Hootegem JCSP, Sylvester R *et al.* Prognostic factors in bladder carcinoma: histologic parameters and expression of a cell cycle-related nuclear antigen Ki-67. *J Pathol* 1992, **166**, 37–43.

60 Al-Abadi H, Nagel R. Deoxyribonucleic acid content and survival rates of patients with transitional cell carcinoma of the bladder. *J Urol* 1994, **15**, 37–42.

61 Lipponen PK, Nordling S, Eskelinen MJ *et al.* Flow cytometry in comparison with mitotic index in predicting disease outcome in transitional cell bladder cancer. *Int J Cancer* 1993, **53**, 42–7.

62 Vaskò J, Malmstram PU, Taube A *et al.* Towards an objective method of mitosis counting and its prognostic significance in bladder cancer. *J Urol Pathol* 1995, **3**, 315–8.

63 Neal DE, Sharples L, Smith K *et al.* The epidermal growth factor receptor and the prognosis of bladder cancer. *Cancer* 1990, **65**, 1619–25.

64 Messing EM. Clinical implications of the expression of epidermal growth factor receptors in human transitional cell carcinoma. *Cancer Res* 1990, **50**, 2530–4.

65 Wood DP Jr, Fair WR, Chaganti RSK. Evaluation of epidermal growth factor receptor DNA amplification and mRNA expression in bladder cancer. *J Urol* 1992, **147**, 274–7.

66 Nguyen PL, Swanson PE, Jaszcz W *et al.* Expression of epidermal growth factor receptor in invasive transitional cell carcinoma of the urinary bladder. *Am J Clin Pathol* 1994, **101**, 166–76.

67 Asamoto M, Hasegawa R, Masuko T *et al.* Immunohistochemical analysis of c-erbB-2 oncogene product and epidermal growth factor receptor expression in human urinary bladder carcinomas. *Acta Pathol Jpn*, 1990, **40**, 322–6.

68 Swanson PE, Frierson HF Jr, Wick MR. c-erbB-2 (HER-2/neu) oncopeptide immunoreactivity in localized, high grade transitional cell carcinoma of the bladder. *Mod Pathol* 1992, **5**, 531–3.

69 Ye DW, Zheng JF, Qian SX *et al.* Correlation between the expression of onco-genes *ras* and C-erbB-2 and the biological behavior of bladder tumors. *Urol Res* 1993, **21**, 39–43.

70 Lipponen P. Expression of c-erbB-2 oncoprotein in transitional cell bladder cancer. *Eur J Cancer* 1993, **29**, 749–52.

71 Lee SE, Chow NH, Chi YC *et al.* Expression of c-erbB-2 protein in normal and neoplastic urothelium: Lack of adverse prognostic effect in human urinary bladder cancer. *Anticancer Res* 1994, **14**, 317–24.

72 Mellon JK, Lunec J, Wright C *et al.* C-erbB-2 in bladder cancer: Molecular biology, correlation with epidermal growth factor receptors and prognostic value. *J Urol* 1996, **155**, 321–4.

73 Lipponen PK. Over-expression of p53 nuclear oncoprotein in transitional-cell bladder cancer and its prognostic value. *Int J Cancer* 1993, **53**, 365–8.

74 Sarkis AS, Dalbagni G, Cordon-Cardo C *et al.* Nuclear over-expression of p53 protein in transitional cell bladder carcinoma: a marker for disease progression. *J Natl Cancer Inst* 1993, **85**, 53–9.

75 Serth J, Kuczyk MA, Bokemeyer C *et al.* p53 Immunohistochemistry as an independent prognostic factor for superficial transitional cell carcinoma of the bladder. *Br J Cancer* 1995, **71**, 201–5.

76 Esrig D, Elmajian D, Groshen S *et al.* Accumulation of nuclear p53 and tumor progression in bladder cancer. *N Engl J Med* 1994, **331**, 1259–64.

77 Miyao N, Tsai YC, Lerner SP *et al.* Role of chromosome 9 in human bladder cancer. *Cancer Res* 1993, **53**, 4066–70.

78 Olumi AF, Tsai YC, Nicholas PW *et al.* Allelic loss of chromosome 17p distin-guishes high grade from low grade transitional cell carcinomas of the bladder. *Cancer Res* 1990, **50**, 7081–3.

79 Spruck CH, Ohneseit F, Gonzalez-Zuleta M *et al.* Two molecular pathways to transitional cell carcinoma of the bladder. *Cancer Res* 1994, **54**, 784–91.

80 Knowles MA, Elder PA, Williamson M *et al.* Allelotype of human bladder cancer. *Cancer Res* 1994, **54**, 531–8.

81 Amin MB, Ro JY, El-Sharkawy T *et al.* Micropapillary variant of transitional cell carcinoma of the urinary bladder. Histologic pattern resembling ovarian papillary serous carcinoma. *Am J Surg Pathol* 1994, **18**, 1224–32.

82 Johansson SL, Borghede G, Holmang S. Micropapillary carcinoma of bladder. *Mod Pathol* 1997, **10**, 794–9.

83 Holmang S, Borghede G, Johansson SL. Bladder carcinoma with lympho-epithelioma-like differentiation: a report of 9 cases. *J Urol* 1998, **159**, 779–82.

84 Amin BM, Ro JY, Lee KM *et al.* Lymphoepithelioma-like carcinoma of the urinary bladder. *Am J Surg Pathol*, 1994, **18**, 466–73.

85 Murphy WM, Deana DG. The nested variant of transitional cell carcinoma: A neoplasm resembling proliferation of Brunn's nests. *Mod Pathol* 1992, **5**, 240–3.

86 Stern JB. Unusual benign bladder tumor of Brunn nest origin. *Urology*, 1979, **14**, 288–9.

87 Talbert ML, Young RH. Carcinomas of the urinary bladder with deceptively benign-appearing foci. *Am J Surg Pathol* 1989, **13**, 374–81.

88 Drew PA, Furman J, Civantos F, Murphy WM. The nested variant of transitional cell carcinoma: An aggressive neoplasm with innocuous histology. *Mod Pathol* 1996, **9**, 989–94.

89 Johansson SL, Cohen SM. The etiology of bladder cancer. *Semin Surg Oncol*, 1997, **13**, 291–8.

90 Johansson SL, Anderstrom CRK. Primary adenocarcinoma of the urinary bladder and urachus. In: *Textbook of uncommon cancers* (ed. Williams CJ, Krikorian JG, Green MR, Raghavan D). John Wiley, Chichester, 1988.

91 Anderstrom C, Johansson SL, Von Schultz L. Primary adenocarcinoma of the urinary bladder, a clinicopathologic and prognostic study. *Cancer* 1983, **52**, 1273–9.

92 Cramer SF, Aikawa M, Cebelin M. Neurosecretory granules in small cell carcinoma of the urinary bladder. *Cancer* 1981, **47**, 724–30.

93 Holmang S, Borghede G, Johansson SL. Primary small cell carcinoma of the bladder: a report of 25 cases. *J Urol* 1995, **153**, 1820–4.

94 Angulo JC, Lopez JI, Sanchez-Chapado M *et al.* Small cell carcinoma of the urinary bladder. *J Urol Pathol*, 1996, **5**, 1–4.

95 Walker AN, Mills SE, Young RH. Mesenchymal and miscellaneous other primary tumors of the urinary bladder. In: *Pathology of the urinary bladder* (ed. Young RH). Churchill Livingstone, New York, 1989.

96 Hays DM, Raney RB Jr, Lawrence W Jr *et al.* Bladder and prostatic tumors in the Intergroup Rhabdomyosarcoma Study (IRS-1): results of therapy. *Cancer* 1982, **50**, 1472–82.

97 Ohsawa M, Aozasa K, Horiuchi K, Kanamaru A. Malignant lymphoma of bladder. *Cancer* 1993, **72**, 1969–74.

98 Melicow MM. Tumors of the urinary bladder: a clinicopathological analysis of over 2500 specimens and biopsies. *J Urol* 1955, **74**, 498–511.

99 Goldstein AG. Metastatic carcinoma to the bladder. *J Urol* 1967, **98**, 209–11.

100 Ekelund P, Johansson SL. Polypoid cystitis: a catheter associated lesion of the human bladder. *Acta Pathol Microbiol Scand*, 1979, **87A**, 179–82.

101 Ekelund P, Anderstrom C, Johansson SL, Larsson P. The reversibility of catheter associated polypoid cystitis. *J Urol* 1983, **13**, 456–9.

102 Lundgren L, Aldenborg F, Angervall L, Kindblom LG *et al.* Pseudosarcomatous spindle cell proliferation in the urinary bladder of adults. *Hum Pathol* 1994, **25**, 181–4.

7. NON-TRANSITIONAL CELL CARCINOMA OF THE BLADDER

Mahul B. Amin, Pheroze Tamboli, and Jae Y. Ro

The most common carcinomas of the urinary bladder, up to 90%, arise from the urothelium and are referred to as urothelial or transitional cell carcinomas (TCC). While transitional cell carcinomas predominantly occur in organs lined by urothelium, the other carcinomas of the urinary bladder are also seen at diverse sites in the body. The other carcinomas include squamous cell carcinoma and its variants, adenocarcinoma and its variants, and undifferentiated carcinomas such as small cell carcinoma, lymphoepithelioma-like carcinoma, and giant cell carcinoma (Table 7.1). In this chapter

Table 7.1

HISTOLOGICAL VARIANTS OF TRANSITIONAL CELL CARCINOMA (TCC) AND OTHER CARCINOMAS OF THE URINARY BLADDER

I. Histological variants of transitional cell carcinoma
A. Histological variants containing or exhibiting
  1. Squamous differentiation
  2. Glandular differentiation
  3. Deceptively benign features
    a. Nested pattern (resembling von Brunn's nests)
    b. Small tubular pattern
    c. Microcysts
    d. Endophytic growth pattern
B. Distinctive histological variants
  1. Micropapillary variant of TCC
  2. Sarcomatoid carcinoma
C. Undifferentiated carcinoma*
  1. Small cell carcinoma
  2. Lymphoepithelioma-like carcinoma
  3. Giant cell carcinoma
  4. Undifferentiated carcinoma, not otherwise specified (NOS)

II Squamous cell carcinoma
A. Variant
  1. Verrucous carcinoma
  2. Sarcomatoid carcinoma

III Adenocarcinoma
A. Anatomical variants
  1. Bladder mucosa
  2. Urachal
B. Histological variants
  1. Typical intestinal type (enteric)
  2. Mucinous (including colloid)
  3. Signet ring cell
  4. Clear cell
  5. Sarcomatoid carcinoma

* Refers to tumours that are undifferentiated by light microscopy.

we discuss the pathology of non-transitional cell carcinomas of the urinary bladder and the histological variants of transitional cell carcinoma.

HISTOLOGICAL VARIANTS OF TRANSITIONAL CELL CARCINOMA

The term 'histological variant' is used here to describe a distinctively different morphological pattern that is seen in both papillary and non-papillary TCC. Recognition of these histological variants is important because some are associated with a clinical outcome different from that of conventional TCC and may require a different therapeutic approach; awareness of some of the unusual patterns may be critical in avoiding diagnostic misinterpretations. Two general rules need to be followed when dealing with histological variants: First, the 'histological variant' should be documented in the pathology report because metastatic tumours usually exhibit the same distinctive histological pattern, knowledge of which facilitates making the association between the metastasis and the primary tumour. Second, the possibility that the 'histological variant' morphology represents a metastasis should always be considered and ruled out, as the pattern of the variant tumours is different from that of conventional TCC.

Squamous and glandular differentiation

Squamous differentiation, seen in both papillary and non-papillary tumours, is found in up to 20% of TCC and is more commonly seen with invasive tumours. The clinical significance of squamous differentiation in transitional cell tumours is uncertain. Squamous differentiation has been associated with poor response to radiation therapy and to systemic chemotherapy [1,2]. Frazier *et al.* reported an unfavourable prognosis in patients with squamous differentiation, who had undergone radical cystectomy [3].

Glandular differentiation is also seen in both papillary and non-papillary TCC but less commonly so than squamous differentiation [4]. In addition, mucin-positive cells have been reported in 14%, 49%, and 63% of grades I, II, and III tumours, respectively [5]. The clinical significance of glandular differentiation and mucin positivity remains uncertain, but one study has shown it to be associated with a poor response to chemotherapy [6]. Recognizing these two patterns is important in order not to confuse TCC with squamous cell carcinoma or adenocarcinoma when these metaplastic changes are extensive.

'Deceptively bland' patterns of non-papillary transitional cell carcinoma

The 'deceptively bland' patterns of TCC are the variants that mimic non-neoplastic conditions such as cystitis cystica, von Brunn's nests, nephrogenic adenoma, and/or benign neoplasms, such as inverted papilloma. The deceptively bland variants of TCC include TCC with tubules, microcystic TCC, nested TCC, and TCC with an endophytic growth pattern. The main reason for awareness of these variants is to avoid under-diagnosis and to prescribe appropriate therapy, as these variants of TCC may be diagnostically confused with the aforementioned lesions. It is difficult to draw meaningful conclusions about the biological potential of these tumours because the number of cases that could possibly be included in this category is limited, and the clinical information on these variants is sparse. The nested variant of TCC, however, is known to pursue an aggressive course, with proclivity for metastatic disease (7,8).

Transitional cell carcinoma with tubules

This consists of small nests of cells and bland-appearing tubules, some of which may be dilated, a pattern that tends to mimic nephrogenic adenoma (8). Some tubules may be lined by urothelium, a feature which helps distinguish these tumours from nephrogenic adenoma, in which the tubules are lined by flattened, cuboidal, or columnar cells.

Microcystic transitional cell carcinoma

Variably sized cysts within nests of invasive TCC may be confused with cystitis cystica, especially in superficial biopsies where its invasive character may not be apparent (9,10). Variation in shape and size of the cysts, nuclear atypia, and presence of muscularis propria invasion help identify this variant.

Nested transitional cell carcinoma

A packed arrangement of small nests of tumour cells, which may mimic von Brunn's nests, with bland cytological features characterizes this histological variant (8,11). The presence of larger sized nests, irregularly shaped, closely packed, or irregularly distributed nests, focal nuclear atypia, stromal reaction, and muscularis propria invasion help to distinguish nested TCC from von Brunn's nests. All reported cases have behaved in a persistent and aggressive fashion (8,11).

Transitional cell carcinoma with an endophytic growth pattern

A broad-front pattern, i.e. broad, pushing tongues of neoplastic urothelium extending into the lamina propria, may be seen as the exclusive endophytic growth pattern. This pattern of lamina propria invasion may be observed in some large papillary TCC that possess not only a prominent exophytic component, but also 'invade' the lamina propria in a pushing fashion much like that of cutaneous and mucosal verrucous carcinoma. The downward projections are usually bulbous with regular contours, but in some cases narrow tentacular extensions may be seen. These bulbous projections may appear as rounded nests when cut tangentially.

The endophytic pattern may exhibit another morphological variation of cords and nests of neoplastic cells extensively involving the lamina propria; this is referred to as the inverted papilloma-like pattern (12,13). Often the cords are elongated and regular, forming slender trabeculae, that occasionally interanastomose. Helpful features to recognize carcinoma include: the often variable thickness of the cords and trabeculae, with transition into nests and solid areas, and cytological atypia which varies from that of WHO grade I to WHO grade III TCC. The nests generally have smooth contours and also vary in size and shape, occasionally with microcystic and rarely with macrocystic areas (14).

In some cases, the inverted papilloma-like and broad-front patterns may coexist. Tumours with an exophytic papillary component usually show continuity with the endophytic portion, and transition from the exophytic to the endophytic component may be seen in some cases as undulating gyriform cords of cells that subsequently dip into the lamina propria. The downward projection is so pronounced in some examples that the base of the tumour lies on the muscularis propria. The mere depth of this extension into the bladder wall may be enough to merit a diagnosis of invasion in a strict sense. We believe, however, that these tumours should be considered non-invasive if the basement membrane is intact at the light-microscopic level. The likelihood of metastasis of tumours with these histological characteristics is infinitesimally small because the basement membrane is not breached, except if the pattern is accompanied by true stromal invasion (14–16). In about 50% of tumours with broad-front growth, there is focal, unequivocally destructive invasion into the lamina propria or muscularis propria. It is important to distinguish the innocuous broad-front, pushing incursion into the lamina propria from destructive stromal invasion because the latter bestows on the neoplasm the ability to metastasize (14). Distinction between broad-front incursion into the lamina propria and true invasion in transurethral resection of bladder tumour (TURBT) specimens is further complicated by tangential sectioning, crush artefact, and thermal injury.

Micropapillary transitional cell carcinoma

This relatively rare histological variant comprises 0.6–1% of all TCC. It is predominantly seen in men, with a male-to-female ratio of 5 : 1, significantly higher than the 3 : 1 ratio seen with conventional TCC. This tumour tends to be aggressive: more than 95% of patients present with muscularis propria invasive disease, 44% have metastatic disease, and 17% have local extension (17).

Histologically, micropapillary TCC has a characteristic architecture superficially resembling papillary serous carcinoma of the ovary (17). The micropapillary pattern may be focal, extensive (>90%), or be the exclusive pattern, and it may be seen as the non-invasive or invasive component. The surface component is composed of thin, delicate filiform papillae, which in cross-section appear as glomeruloid bodies. The invasive component shows tight papillary clusters, which may be present in clear spaces created by retraction artefact, mimicking vascular invasion. This feature is quite characteristic of the invasive component and is also retained in the histological appearance of the metastases. Awareness of these retraction spaces or lacunae is important so as not to over-diagnose the presence of vascular invasion, an ominous sign in invasive TCC regardless of stage. Focal vascular invasion is very common. Psammoma bodies are exquisitely rare, in contrast to ovarian papillary serous carcinoma.

In the series by Amin *et al.* (18), cases were high-grade, high-stage, and had recognizable conventional TCC; more than 50% of patients had TCC *in situ*, and glandular differentiation was also seen in some (17). Stage at presentation and the proportion of the micropapillary component seemed to be important in determining prognosis. The presence of micropapillary TCC in a superficial biopsy lacking muscularis propria should prompt another biopsy, so as not to miss muscularis propria invasion. A metastatic tumour of the peritoneum, mesentery, or abdominal lymph nodes with a micropapillary architecture should alert one to the possibility of the primary tumour's origin in the urinary bladder, especially in the absence of an ovarian tumour.

Sarcomatoid carcinoma

Sarcomatoid carcinoma is a rare variant, which usually represents dedifferentiation of a conventional TCC, and is more common than primary sarcomas of the urinary bladder. The key to this diagnosis is the presence of both carcinomatous and sarcomatous components (18–21). The sarcomatous element exhibits a prominent spindle cell component that may resemble leiomyosarcoma,

fibrosarcoma, or malignant fibrous histiocytoma (18–21). Heterologous differentiation in the form of rhabdomyosarcoma, chondro-
sarcoma, and osteosarcoma may be evident, but it does not have
any prognostic significance. A storiform pattern, areas of myxoid
degeneration, and tumour giant cells may also be present. The
sarcomatoid areas tend to merge with foci of carcinoma that
may include TCC, squamous cell carcinoma, adenocarcinoma, and
small cell carcinoma (20). If no recognizable carcinomatous component is found, a cytokeratin immunohistochemical stain or
ultrastructural studies may be required to confirm the epithelial
nature of the tumour. Differential diagnosis includes sarcoma,
pseudosarcomatous fibromyxoid tumour, postoperative spindle
cell nodule, and malignant melanoma.

Sarcomatoid carcinomas usually present at an advanced stage
and consequently have a poor prognosis (18–20,22,23). Compared
stage for stage with conventional TCC, however, there is no difference in the rate of survival.

UNDIFFERENTIATED CARCINOMAS OF THE URINARY BLADDER

Small cell carcinoma

Small cell carcinoma is an undifferentiated carcinoma which is
usually seen in the lungs, but can rarely occur in the urinary
bladder, accounting for approximately 0.5% of bladder carcinoma
(24–30). The histogenesis of small cell carcinoma remains uncertain, but it is postulated to originate from multipotential stem
cells like the neuroendocrine cells found in normal urothelium.

Histologically, it is composed of small uniform cells with
scant cytoplasm and round to spindled hyperchromatic nuclei
(Fig. 7.1). The nuclear chromatin is finely dispersed, nucleoli are
absent or inconspicuous, and usually there is brisk mitotic activity
(31). The Azzopardi phenomenon, i.e. encrustation of the elastica
of blood vessels with DNA debris, has been identified in some
cases, and necrosis is a common feature (26). Angiolymphatic
invasion is commonly present. The tumour cells variably stain
with neuron-specific enolase, chromogranin, and synaptophysin
immunohistochemical stains, confirming their neuroendocrine
differentiation. Some tumours demonstrate a typical dot-like
pattern of pan-cytokeratin staining, which is also characteristic
of neuroendocrine carcinoma. Ultrastructural studies have shown
the presence in some tumours of neurosecretory dense core
granules (26).

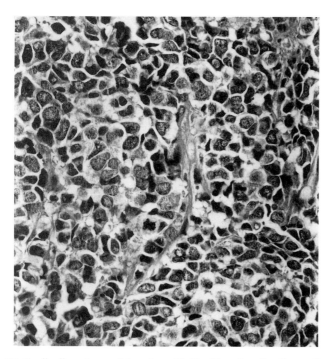

Fig. 7.1 Small cell carcinoma of the urinary bladder. Nest of small uniform cells with scant cytoplasm and round hyperchromatic nuclei

The tumours may be present in a pure form or combined with TCC, adenocarcinoma, or squamous cell carcinoma. Metastases from another site, such as small cell carcinoma of the lung, must be ruled out before primary small cell carcinoma of the urinary bladder is diagnosed. The presence of a conventional TCC component, including Transitional Carcinoma *in situ* (TCIS), supports a primary origin in the bladder. The differential diagnosis includes direct extension into the bladder by a small cell carcinoma of the prostate, metastatic small cell carcinoma from other sites, and lymphoma.

Small cell carcinoma of the bladder is an aggressive tumour and usually presents with high-stage disease. More than 50% of patients succumb to the disease, with a mean survival time of 7 months (25–30). Patients receiving systemic chemotherapy, similar to that used for such tumours of the lung, survive longer, with up to 46% 5-year survival as opposed to 20% without chemotherapy (29,32–34). This fact is one of the most important reasons for recognizing this distinct tumour.

Lymphoepithelioma-like carcinoma

Lymphoepithelioma-like carcinoma of the bladder has a morphological appearance similar to the nasopharyngeal neoplasm of the

same name. It is a rare neoplasm, with only 23 cases reported
to date, belonging to the undifferentiated spectrum of urinary
bladder epithelial neoplasia (35–38). Lymphoepithelioma-like
carcinoma of the bladder is not associated with the Epstein–Barr
virus, unlike its nasopharyngeal counterpart (39). It is seen as
diffuse sheets of malignant cells having indistinct cytoplasmic
borders and large vesicular nuclei with prominent nucleoli, and
a pathognomonic extensive lymphocytic infiltrate (Fig. 7.2).
Finding a dense lymphoid infiltrate in a bladder biopsy or transurethral resection (TUR) specimen should provoke a search for
neoplastic cells, because this tumour may be misinterpreted as
chronic cystitis or malignant lymphoma. Also included in the differential diagnosis is small cell carcinoma of the urinary bladder
or prostate and poorly differentiated TCC with a lymphoid
stroma. Accurate distinction between these differential diagnostic
considerations is essential as therapy and outcome may differ.
Tumours presenting in a pure form or with a predominant
lymphoepithelioma-like pattern have responded well to chemotherapy and are associated with more favourable outcome than
conventional TCC (35–38). The three cases reported by Dinney
et al. were treated with methotrexate, vinblastine, doxorubicin,
and cisplatin chemotherapy alone, and showed a favourable
response (36).

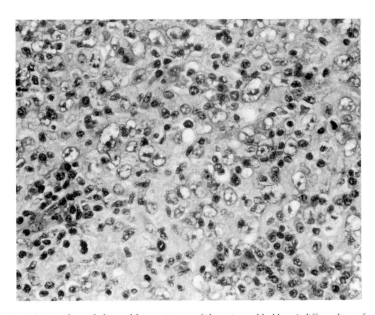

*Fig. 7.2 Lymphoepithelioma-like carcinoma of the urinary bladder. A diffuse sheet of
malignant cells, having indistinct cytoplasmic borders, large vesicular nuclei, and
prominent nucleoli, with a lymphocytic infiltrate*

Giant cell carcinoma

This is another undifferentiated carcinoma which resembles its namesakes found at other sites. It is composed of a prominent giant cell component, i.e. poorly cohesive cells with abundant cytoplasm and multiple nucleoli, and a population of smaller mononuclear cells (13). Their epithelial origin can be confirmed by the use of a cytokeratin immunohistochemical stain. Other poorly differentiated elements such as spindle cells are almost always present in addition to the giant cells. It is important to distinguish these tumours from TCC with osteoclast-like giant cells and TCC with syncytiotrophoblasts, as giant cell carcinoma is an anaplastic carcinoma with uniformly poor prognosis.

SQUAMOUS CELL CARCINOMA OF THE URINARY BLADDER

Squamous cell carcinoma of the bladder is uncommon except that, in geographic locations where schistosomiasis is endemic it accounts for 73% of all bladder cancers (40); whereas in regions without schistosomiasis, it accounts for only about 5% of all urinary bladder tumours (41–45). Significant predisposing factors for developing squamous cell carcinoma include chronic infection and inflammation, keratinizing squamous metaplasia; hypercalcaemia (46) and inappropriate secretion of antidiuretic hormone (47) have rarely been associated with it.

Keratinizing squamous metaplasia, the most likely precursor to squamous cell carcinoma, occurs in response to chronic irritation and inflammation. It frequently precedes squamous cell carcinoma, especially in areas of endemic schistosomiasis (40,48). The metaplastic epithelium tends to persist, and over time it may show dysplastic changes that culminate in squamous cell carcinoma. As this form of metaplasia is a marker for squamous cell carcinoma, patients with the condition need to be followed closely in the event they develop squamous cell carcinoma. In a study of 78 patients with squamous metaplasia, Benson *et al.* reported synchronous squamous cell carcinoma in 22%; more importantly, an additional 20% of patients developed squamous cell carcinoma at a later date, with a mean of 11 years and a maximum of 30 years (49).

Squamous cell carcinoma is more common in women than TCC, with a male-to-female ratio of about 1.2–2 : 1 (43,44,50,51). The age distribution is similar to that seen for conventional TCC.

The gross appearance of squamous cell carcinoma is variable; tumours tend to be large and may be sessile, papillary, polypoid, or nodular. Foci of necrosis and grey-white keratin debris are common. Ulceration and haemorrhage may be present. The microscopic features are similar to those of squamous cell carcinoma at other sites (Fig. 7.3), the majority of tumours being well or moderately differentiated, often with abundant keratin production. These tumours usually invade the muscularis propria (52,53). Some cases have been associated with condyloma acuminatum (54,55). Rare cases of verrucous carcinoma have also been reported, more commonly in patients with schistosomiasis (40,55–58).

The main differential diagnostic consideration is TCC with squamous differentiation. The presence of any neoplastic transitional cell component, including carcinoma *in situ*, should be ruled out before a diagnosis of pure squamous cell carcinoma is made. Other considerations are keratinizing squamous dysplasia, which lacks the full thickness nuclear atypia and invasive features of squamous cell carcinoma, and a squamous cell carcinoma extending from the cervix or vagina. Verrucous carcinoma may be confused with condyloma acuminatum, especially if the entire lesion is not biopsied.

The prognosis of squamous cell carcinoma is poor, with 5-year survival ranging from 7.4% to 50% (50,59–61) and 10-year survival approaching 5% (59). Patients are more apt to die of local recurrence than metastases, in contradistinction to TCC (50,60,62).

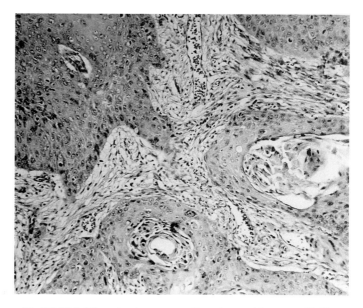

Fig. 7.3 Well differentiated squamous cell carcinoma of the urinary bladder

Adenocarcinoma of the urinary bladder

Adenocarcinoma of the urinary bladder varies in frequency from 0.5% to 2% of all bladder cancers (45,63,64). These tumours may be categorized as those arising from the urinary bladder proper and those arising form the urachus. We will first briefly discuss the putative precursor lesions of adenocarcinoma and then discuss the bladder and urachal varieties.

Precursor lesions

The putative precursor lesions include cystitis glandularis (intestinal type) and nephrogenic adenoma.

Cystitis glandularis with intestinal metaplasia

Intestinal metaplasia is manifest as goblet cells or colonic-type glands. This lesion may be focal or diffuse; the latter usually occurs in patients with chronic irritative bladder problems like stones or long-term catheterization. The diffuse form, especially if it is persistent or extensive, is associated with adenocarcinoma and is considered to be a precursor lesion (65–70). Cystitis glandularis of the typical type, i.e. without intestinal-type epithelium, is not associated with an increased risk of adenocarcinoma.

Nephrogenic adenoma (or nephrogenic metaplasia)

This has been considered by some to be a precursor lesion because of its propensity for recurrence and its morphological similarities to clear cell adenocarcinoma of the urethra and urinary bladder (71). Its association with adenocarcinoma is weak at best, and we seriously doubt its neoplastic potential.

Adenocarcinoma of the urinary bladder proper

This tumour accounts for about 60–80% of all urinary bladder adenocarcinomas, the rest being of urachal origin (72).

In gross appearance, the tumour varies from papillary to exophytic to sessile, and may have a mucoid or gelatinous appearance/consistency. It is usually infiltrative, with areas of ulceration and haemorrhage. Uncommonly, with signet ring cell carcinomas, there may be diffuse thickening of the bladder wall resembling linitis plastica of the stomach.

Adenocarcinoma forms a variety of histological patterns, including enteric (resembling colonic adenocarcinoma) (Fig. 7.4), mucinous or colloid (with abundant extracellular mucin), signet

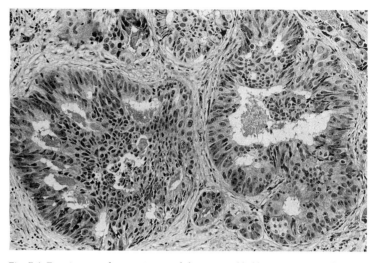

Fig. 7.4 *Enteric-type adenocarcinoma of the urinary bladder, reminiscent of colonic adenocarcinomas*

ring cell, clear cell (73), mixed (two or more patterns), and not otherwise specified (NOS) (74). NOS and enteric are the commonest subtypes seen. That diffuse signet ring cell carcinoma may not show any surface change cystoscopically or pathologically, is an important fact to remember when examining superficial biopsy samples (75,76). Intestinal metaplasia of the adjoining urothelium is commonly present.

The differential diagnosis includes TCC with glandular differentiation, metastatic adenocarcinoma, nephrogenic adenoma, villous adenoma, and florid cystitis glandularis. Ruling out a metastasis or direct local extension of a colonic adenocarcinoma is imperative before a diagnosis of primary enteric-type adenocarcinoma of the urinary bladder is made, because of the nearly identical histology of the two tumours. Likewise, with signet ring cell carcinoma, metastases from the gastrointestinal tract, and metastatic lobular carcinoma of the breast need to ruled out.

Adenocarcinomas generally have a poor prognosis, with crude survival rates of 17% at 5 years and 11% at 10 years (77).

Adenocarcinoma of the urachus

Adenocarcinomas arising from the urachus need to be distinguished from those of the urinary bladder proper, based on a number of clinical and pathological features. The most important criteria for establishing the urachus as the site of origin are: location of the tumour in the dome of the bladder with the epicentre in the muscular wall of the bladder rather than the mucosa;

absence of intestinal metaplasia of the uninvolved urothelium; the presence of urachal remnants; sharp demarcation between tumour and normal urothelium; and exclusion of metastases from another site (72,78,79).

The clinical, gross, histological, and immunohistochemical features of urachal adenocarcinomas do not differ significantly from those of non-urachal ones. Mucinous adenocarcinomas are the most common subtype seen, with the enteric type next, and those with signet ring cell pattern being the least common (75,77,80). Some tumours exhibit mixed differentiation with squamous and glandular components. Urachal tumours have a different pattern of local spread in that they sometimes extend along the urachal tract and may even involve the abdominal wall.

The main reason for identifying urachal adenocarcinoma is because of surgical considerations—partial cystectomy or *en bloc* resection with umbilectomy being important options. Urachal adenocarcinomas are also resistant to radiation therapy (81). The staging system of these adenocarcinomas is the same as for all other urinary bladder cancers (77,82). As all these cancers arise in the muscular wall and are staged as muscularis propria invasive tumours, Sheldon *et al.* proposed a separate staging system, whose clinical utility has not yet been established (81). The prognosis of these tumours, compared with that of non-urachal ones, is still controversial; some studies have reported better prognosis (64,77,83), some worse (72,84,85) and some have shown no difference (86,87).

References

1 Martin JE, Jenkins BJ, Zuk RJ, Blandy JP, Baithun SI. Clinical importance of squamous metaplasia in invasive transitional cell carcinoma of the bladder. *J Clin Pathol* 1989, **42**, 250–3.

2 Akdas A, Turkeri L. The impact of squamous metaplasia in transitional cell carcinoma of the bladder. *Int J Urol Nephrol* 1990, **23**, 333–6.

3 Frazier HA, Robertson JE, Dodge RK, Paulson DF. The value of pathologic factors in predicting cancer-specific survival among patients treated with radical cystectomy for transitional cell carcinoma of the bladder and prostate. *Cancer* 1993, **71**, 3993–4001.

4 Grace DA, Winter CD. Mixed differentiation of primary carcinoma of the urinary bladder. *Cancer* 1968, **21**, 1239–43.

5 Donhuijsen K, Schmidt U, Richter HJ, Leder LD. Mucoid cytoplasmic inclusions in urothelial carcinomas. *Hum Pathol* 1992, **23**, 860–4.

6 Logothetis CJ, Dexeus FH, Chong C, Sella A, Ayala AG, Ro JY, Pilat S. Cisplatin, cyclophosphamide and doxorubicin chemotherapy for unresectable urothelial tumors: The MD Anderson experience. *Urology* 1989, **141**, 33–7.

7 Amin MB, Murphy WM, Reuter VE, Weiss MA, Ro JY, Ayala AG, Eble JN, Young RH. Controversies in the pathology of transitional cell carcinoma of the urinary bladder. Part I. In: *ASCP reviews in pathology* (ed. Rosen PP, Fechner RE). ASCP Press, Chicago, 1996, pp. 1–39.

8 Talbert WM, Young RH. Carcinoma of the urinary bladder with deceptively benign appearing foci: A report of three cases. *Am J Surg Pathol* 1989, **13**, 374–81.

9 Young RH, Zuckerberg LR. Microcystic transitional cell carcinomas of the urinary bladder: report of 4 cases. *Am J Clin Pathol* 1991, **96**, 635–9.

10 Paz A, Rath-Wolfson L, Lask D, Koren R, Manes A, Mukamel E, Gal R. The clinical and histological features of transitional cell carcinoma of the bladder with microcysts: analysis of 12 cases. *Br J Urol* 1997, **79**, 722–5.

11 Murphy WM, Deana DG. The nested variant of transitional cell carcinoma: A neoplasm resembling proliferation of Brunn's nests. *Mod Pathol* 1992, **5**, 240–3.

12 Paulsen JC, Metawalli N, Wu B, Nochomovitz L. Transitional cell carcinoma of urinary bladder with features of inverted papilloma. *Modern Pathol* 1988, **11**, 710–8.

13 Young RH, Eble JN. Unusual forms of carcinoma of the urinary bladder. *Hum Pathol* 1991, **22**, 948–65.

14 Amin MB, Gomez JA, Young RH. Urothelial transitional cell carcinoma with endophytic growth patterns: A discussion of patterns of invasion and problems associated with assessment of invasion in 18 cases. *Am J Surg Pathol* 1997, **21**, 1057–68.

15 Koss LG. Mapping of the urinary bladder: Its impact on the concepts of bladder cancer. *Hum Pathol* 1979, **10**, 533–48.

16 Brawn PN. The origin of invasive carcinoma of the bladder. *Cancer* 1982, **50**, 515–19.

17 Amin MB, Ro JY, El-Sharkawy T, Lee KW, Troncoso P, Silva EG, Ordonez NG, Ayala AG. Micropapillary variant of transitional cell carcinoma of the urinary bladder. Histologic pattern resembling ovarian papillary serous carcinoma. *Am J Surg Pathol* 1994, **18**, 1224–32.

18 Young RH, Wick MR, Mill SE. Sarcomatoid carcinoma of the urinary bladder: A clinicopathological analysis of 12 cases and review of literature. *Am J Clin Pathol* 1988, **90**, 653–61.

19 Young RH. Carcinosarcoma of urinary bladder. *Cancer* 1987, **59**, 1333–9.

20 Ro JY, Ayala AG, Wishnow K, Ordonez NG. Sarcomatoid bladder carcinoma: clinicopathological and immunohistochemical study of 44 cases. *Surg Pathol* 1988, **1**, 359–74.

21 Lopez-Beltran A, Pacelli A, Rothenberg HJ, Wollan PC, Zincke H, Blute ML, Bostwick DG. Carcinosarcoma and sarcomatoid carcinoma of the bladder: clinicopathological study of 41 cases. *J Urol* 1998, **159**, 1497–503.

22 Torenbeek R, Blomjous CEM, de Bruin PC, Newling DW, Meijer CJ. Sarcomatoid carcinoma of the urinary bladder: clinicopathologic analysis of 18 cases with immunohistochemical and electron microscopic findings. *Am J Surg Pathol* 1994, **18**, 241–9.

23 Lahoti C, Schinellar R, Rangwala AF, Lee M, Mizrachi H. Carcinosarcoma of urinary bladder: report of five cases with immunohistologic study. *Urology* 1994, **43**, 389–93.

24 Podesta AH, True LD. Small cell carcinoma of the urinary bladder: Report of 5 cases with immunohistochemistry and review of the literature with evolution of prognosis according to stage. *Cancer* 1989, **64**, 710–804.

25 Blomjous CER, Vos W, De Voogt H, Van der Valk P, Meijer CJ. Small cell carcinoma of the urinary bladder: A clinicopathologic, morphometric, immunohistochemical and ultrastructural study of 18 cases. *Cancer* 1989, **64**, 1347–57.

26 Grignon DJ, Ro JY, Ayala AG, Shum DT, Ordonez NG, Logothetis CJ, Johnson DE, Mackay B. Small cell carcinoma of the urinary bladder. A clinicopathologic analysis of 22 cases. *Cancer* 1992, **69**, 527–36.

27 Lopez JI, Angulo JC, Toledo JD. Small cell carcinoma of the urinary bladder: a clinicopathological study of six cases. *Br J Urol* 1994, **73**, 43–9.

28 Yu DS, Chang SY, Wang J, Yang TH, Cheng CL, Lee SS, Ma CM. Small cell carcinoma of the urinary tract. *Br J Urol* 1990, **66**, 590–5.

29 Angulo JC, Lopez JI, Sanchez-Chapado M. Small cell carcinoma of the urinary bladder: a report of two cases with complete remission and a comprehensive literature review with emphasis on therapeutic decision. *J Urol Pathol* 1996, **5**, 9–28.

30 Abbas F, Civantos F, Benedetto P, Soloway MS. Small cell carcinoma of the bladder and prostate. *Urology* 1995, **46**, 617–30.

31 Ali SZ, Reuter VE, Zakowski MF. Small cell neuroendocrine carcinoma of the urinary bladder. A clinicopathologic study with emphasis on cytologic features. *Cancer* 1997, **79**, 356–61.

32 Oesterling JE, Brendler CB, Burgers JK, Marshall FF, Epstein JI. Advanced small cell carcinoma of the bladder: Successful treatment with combined

radical cystoprostatectomy and adjuvant methotrexate, vinblastine, doxorubicin and cisplatin chemotherapy. *Cancer* 1990, **65**, 1928–36.

33 Mackey JR, Au HJ, Hugh J, Venner P. Genitourinary small cell carcinoma: determination of clinical and therapeutic factors associated with survival. *J Urol* 1998, **159**, 1624–9.

34 Cheng DL, Unger P, Forscher CA, Fine EM. Successful treatment of metastatic small cell carcinoma of the bladder with methotrexate, vinblastine, doxorubicin and cisplatin therapy. *J Urol* 1995, **153**, 417–19.

35 Amin MB, Ro JY, Lee KM, Ordonez NG, Ayala AG. Lymphoepithelioma-like carcinoma of the urinary bladder. *Am J Surg Pathol* 1994, **18**, 466–73.

36 Dinney CPN, Ro JY, Babaian RJ, Johnson DE. Lymphoepithelioma of the bladder: a clinicopathological study of 3 cases. *J Urol* 1993, **149**, 840–1.

37 Jones EC. Lymphoepithelioma-like carcinoma of the urinary bladder: A diagnostic challenge with biological and therapeutic implications. *Adv Anat Pathol* 1995, **2**, 159–64.

38 Holmang S, Borghede G, Johansson SL. Bladder carcinoma with lymphoepithelioma-like differentiation: a report of 9 cases. *J Urol* 1998, **159**, 779–82.

39 Gulley ML, Amin MB, Nicholls JM, Banks PM, Ayala AG, Srigley JR, Eagan PA, Ro JY. Epstein-Barr virus is detected in undifferentiated nasopharyngeal carcinoma but not in lymphepithelioma-like carcinoma of the urinary bladder. *Hum Pathol* 1995, **26**, 1207–14.

40 El-Bolkainy MN, Mokhtar NM, Ghoneim MA, Hussein MH. The impact of schistosomiasis on the pathology of bladder carcinoma. *Cancer* 1981, **48**, 2643–8.

41 Wolf H, Olsen PR, Fischer A, Hojgaard K. Urothelial atypia concomitant with primary bladder tumour. Incidence in a consecutive series of 500 unselected patients. *Scand J Urol Nephrol* 1987, **21**, 33–8.

42 Sarma KP. Squamous cell carcinoma of the bladder. *Int Surg* 1970, **53**, 313–19.

43 Rous SN. Squamous cell carcinoma of the bladder. *J Urol* 1978, **120**, 561–2.

44 Faysal MH. Squamous cell carcinoma of the bladder. *J Urol* 1981, **126**, 598–9.

45 Groeneveld AE, Marszalek WW, Heyns CF. Bladder cancer in various population groups in the greater Durban area of KwaZulu-Natal, South Africa. *Br J Urol* 1996, **78**, 205–8.

46 Eddeland A, Hedelin H. Bladder cancer associated with hypercalcaemia. A case report. *Scand J Urol Nephrol* 1980, **14**, 211–13.

47 Kaye SB, Ross EJ. Inappropriate anti-diuretic hormone (ADH) secretion in association with carcinoma of the bladder. *Postgrad Med J* 1977, **53**, 274–6.

48 Khafagy MM, El-Bolkainy MN, Mansour MA. Carcinoma of the bilharzial urinary bladder, a study of the associated mucosal lesions in 86 cases. *Cancer* 1972, **30**, 150–9.

49 Benson RCJ, Swanson SK, Farrow GM. Relationship of leukoplakia to urothelial malignancy. *J Urol* 1984, **131**, 507–11.

50 Bessette PL, Abell MR, Herwig KR. A clinicopathologic study of squamous cell carcinoma of the bladder. *J Urol* 1974, **112**, 66–7.

51 Costello AJ, Tiptaft RC, England HR, Blandy JP. Squamous cell carcinoma of bladder. *Urology* 1984, **23**, 234–6.

52 Newman DM, Brown JR, Jay AC, Pontius EE. Squamous cell carcinoma of the bladder. *J Urol* 1968, **100**, 470–3.

53 Rundle JSH, Hart AJL, McGeorge A, Smith JS, Malcolm AJ, Smith PM. Squamous cell carcinoma of the bladder. A review 114 patients. *Br J Urol* 1982, **54**, 522–6.

54 Bruske T, Loch T, Thiemann O, Wirth B, Janig U. Panurothelial condyloma acuminatum with development of squamous cell carcinoma of the bladder and renal pelvis. *J Urol* 1997, **157**, 620–1.

55 Walther M, O'Brien DP III, Birch HW. Condylomata acuminata and verrucous carcinoma of the bladder: case report and literature review. *J Urol* 1986, **135**, 362–5.

56 Holck S, Jorgensen L. Verrucous carcinoma of urinary bladder. *Urology* 1983, **22**, 435–7.

57 Wyatt JK, Craig I. Verrucous carcinoma of urinary bladder. *Urology* 1980, **16**, 97–9.

58 Oida Y, Yasuda M, Kajiwara H, Onda H, Kawamura N, Osamura RY. Double squamous cell carcinomas, verrucous type and poorly differentiated type, of the urinary bladder unassociated with bilharzial infection. *Pathol Int* 1997, **47**, 651–4.

59 Johnson DE, Schoenwald MB, Ayala AG, Miller LS. Squamous cell carcinoma of the bladder. *J Urol* 1976, **115**, 542–4.

60 Swanson DA, Liles A, Zagars GK. Preoperative irradiation and radical cystectomy for stages T2 and T3 squamous cell carcinoma of the bladder. *J Urol* 1990, **143**, 37–40.

61 Ghoneim MA, el-Mekresh MM, el-Baz MA, el-Attar IA, Ashamallah A. Radical cystectomy for carcinoma of the bladder: critical evaluation of the results in 1,026 cases. *J Urol* 1997; **158**, 393–9.

62 Sakkas JL. Clinical pattern and treatment of squamous cell carcinoma of the bladder. *Int Surg* 1966, **45**, 71–6.

63 Jacobo E, Loening S, Schmidt JD, Culp DA. Primary adenocarcinoma of the bladder: a retrospective study of 20 patients. *J Urol* 1977, **117**, 54–6.

64 Thomas DG, Ward AM, Williams JL. A study of 52 cases of adenocarcinoma of the bladder. *Br J Urol* 1971, **43**, 4–15.

65 Young RH, Parkhurst EC. Mucinous adenocarcinoma of bladder. Case associated with extensive intestinal metaplasia of urothelium in patient with nonfunctioning bladder for twelve years. *Urology* 1984, **24**, 192–5.

66 Elem B, Alam SZ. Total intestinal metaplasia with focal adenocarcinoma in a schistosoma-infested defunctioned urinary bladder. *Br J Urol* 1984, **56**, 331–43.

67 Shaw JLG, Imbriglia JE. Transition of cystitis glandularis to primary adenocarcinoma of the bladder. *J Urol* 1958, **79**, 815.

68 Lin JI, Yong HS, Tseng CH, Marsidi PS, Choy C, Pilloff B. Diffuse cystsitis glandularis associated with adenocarcinomatous change. *Urology* 1980, **15**, 411–15.

69 Kittredge WE, Collett AJ, Morgan C. Adenocarcinoma of the bladder associated with cystitis glandularis: A case report. *J Urol* 1964, **91**, 145.

70 Edwards PD, Hurm RA, Jaeschke WH. Conversion of cystitis glandularis to adenocarcinoma. *J Urol* 1972, **108**, 568–70.

71 Molland EA, Trott PA, Paris AM, Blandy JP. Nephrogenic adenoma: a form of adenomatous metaplasia of the bladder. A clinical and electron microscopical study. *Br J Urol* 1976, **48**, 453–62.

72 Mostofi FK, Thomas RV, Dean AL. Mucous adenocarcinoma of the urinary bladder. *Cancer* 1955, **8**, 741–58.

73 Humphrey PA. Clear cell neoplasms of the urinary tract and male reproductive system. *Semin Diagn Pathol* 1997, **14**, 240–52.

74 Loening SA, Jacobo E, Hawtrey CE, Culp DA. Adenocarcinoma of the urachus. *J Urol* 1978, **119**, 68–71.

75 Grignon DJ, Ro JY, Ayala AG, Johnson DE. Primary signet ring cell carcinoma of the urinary bladder. *Am J Clin Pathol* 1991, **95**, 13–20.

76 Saphir O. Signet-ring cell carcinoma of the urinary bladder. *Am J Pathol* 1955, **31**, 223–31.

77 Grignon DJ, Ro JY, Johnson DE, Ordonez NG. Primary adenocarcinoma of the urinary bladder: A clinicopathologic analysis of 72 cases. *Cancer* 1991, **67**, 2165–72.

78 Jones WA, Gibbons RP, Correa RJ Jr, Cummings KB, Mason JT. Primary adenocarcinoma of bladder. *Urology* 1980, **15**, 119–22.

79 Abenoza P, Manivel C, Fraley EE. Primary adenocarcinoma of urinary bladder. Clinicopathologic study of 16 cases. *Urology* 1987, **29**, 9–14.

80 Pallesen G. Neoplastic Paneth cells in adenocarcinoma of the urinary bladder: A first case report. *Cancer* 1981, **47**, 1834–7.

81 Sheldon CA, Clayman RV, Gonzalez R, Williams D, Fraley EE. Malignant urachal lesions. *J Urol* 1984, **131**, 1–8.

82 Wilson TG, Pritchett TR, Lieskovsky G, Warner NE, Skinner DG. Primary adenocarcinoma of bladder. *Urology* 1991, **38**, 223–6.

83 Anderstrom C, Johansson SL, von Schultz L. Primary adenocarcinoma of the urinary bladder: A clinicopathologic and prognostic study. *Cancer* 1983, **52**, 1273–80.

84 Kakizoe T, Matsumoto K, Andoh M, Nishio Y, Kishi K. Adenocarcinoma of urachus: Report of 7 cases and review of the literature. *Urology* 1983, **21**, 360–6.

85 Dandekar NP, Dalal AV, Tongaonkar HB, Kamat MR. Adenocarcinoma of bladder. *Eur J Surg Oncol* 1997, **23**, 157–60.

86 Nocks BN, Heney NM, Daly JJ. Primary adenocarcinoma of the urinary bladder. *Urology* 1983, **21**, 26–9.

87 Fuselier HA Jr, Brannan W, Ochsner MG, Matos LH. Adenocarcinoma of the bladder seen at Ochsner Medical Institutions. *South Med J* 1978, **71**, 804–6.

8. THE BIOLOGY OF BLADDER CANCER

Walter M. Stadler and Charles B. Brendler

INTRODUCTION

Bladder cancer is predicted to develop in 54 500 Americans in 1997 and lead to 11 700 deaths in the same year (1). The death rate from this disease has slowly been declining over the last 2 decades, probably due to improvements in the diagnosis and therapy of localized disease (2). None the less, for certain sub-groups the risk of developing progressive muscle invasive disease is significant and approximately one-half of these patients will go on to develop metastatic disease (3). Furthermore, the treatment options available for metastatic bladder cancer are woefully limited, and less than 5% of patients with metastatic disease who are treated with the standard methotrexate, vinblastine, adria-mycin, and cisplatin (MVAC) chemotherapy regimen are long-term survivors (4,5). There thus continues to be a need for better diagnosis of localized disease, better prognostic and predictive markers of future disease activity, and better treatment options for those who develop metastatic disease. These improvements will likely arise directly from some of the new knowledge regard-ing the biology of bladder oncogenesis that has been elucidated over the last several years.

In this sense, investigators interested in studying bladder cancer have been direct beneficiaries of the revolution in modern biologi-cal and molecular biological technique, which allow the detailed analysis of small clinical samples. Because all stages of bladder cancer are easily accessible for biopsy and because urothelial cells are continually shed in the urine, unique opportunities for analysing molecular alterations in this disease exist. Furthermore, several investigators have described *in vitro* and animal model systems in which therapeutic and diagnostic strategies for bladder cancer can be tested. Bladder cancer has thus been and will likely continue to be one of the first human tumours in which 'transla-tional research' from laboratory to patient care and vice versa is realized.

In this chapter we describe some of the molecular events, espe-cially the early events, in urothelial oncogenesis and their poten-tial clinical applications. Specifically, we focus on the possible uses of these molecular alterations as predictive markers and therapeutic targets. These descriptions are not meant to be an exhaustive review of the literature, but rather an attempt to synthesize some of the current data in a context that will stimulate further clinical and basic science research.

PATHWAYS FOR BLADDER ONCOGENESIS

Any description of the molecular pathways in bladder oncogenesis must be firmly grounded in clinical and pathological data. Typical descriptions of tumour development rely on a linear series of events, perhaps best elucidated by Vogelstein and colleagues in their description of colon cancer development (6). These descriptions were a major intellectual achievement because they described clearly the multiple events that were required for development of the full malignant phenotype and helped categorize the various genetic events involved such as inactivation of tumour suppressor genes, activation of oncogenes, and the involvement of a 'molecular gatekeeper'. Clinical experience, however, suggests that this linear pathway is an oversimplification. In bladder cancer, carcinoma *in situ* (CIS) and Ta lesions are both confined to the epithelial surface, but have vastly different natural histories. In addition, squamous cell carcinoma has a different set of epidemiological risk factors than the more common transitional cell histology. These differences almost certainly reflect differences in the underlying molecular pathology as well.

Figure 8.1 is a model of urothelial oncogenesis that reflects some of these complexities. This is likely to still be a simplification, but it gives us a context in which to examine the described molecular alterations. This model allows us to generate hypotheses, testable in clinical trials, regarding the potential clinical utility of certain alterations. Although the model depicts development of adenocarcinomas and squamous carcinomas, most research has concentrated on the more common transitional cell carcinoma. The remainder of the discussion, unless otherwise noted, will thus focus on transitional cell carcinoma as well.

This model also helps describe the critical difference between a prognostic and a predictive molecular marker. A prognostic marker is one that is associated with a particular clinical state, for example nodal metastasis (a 'box' in Fig. 8.1). A predictive marker, on the other hand, is a molecular alteration that leads to or produces a particular clinical state (an 'arrow' in Fig. 8.1). By necessity, predictive markers will also be correlated with a clinical

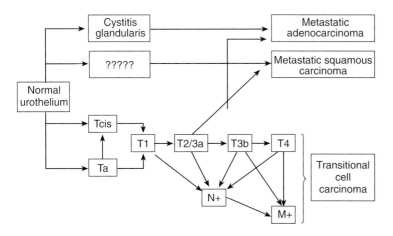

Fig. 8.1 Clinical progression in bladder cancer. Normal urothelium can become malignant along several pathways. Subsequent progression leads to several well recognized clinical states (represented by boxes). The arrow's width is an indication of the probability that one clinical state will lead to another. For example the risk of developing T1 disease is much higher in patients with Tcis than in patients with Ta disease. Abbreviations: Ta: papillary tumour, Tcis: carcinoma in situ, T1: carcinoma invasive into lamina propria, T2/3a: carcinoma invasive into muscle, T3b: carcinoma invasive into perivesicle fat, T4: carcinoma invasive into surrounding tissue, N+: carcinoma in lymph nodes, M+: carcinoma in distant sites. See Chapter 11 for definition of T stages

state, but paradoxically the correlation may be weaker than that for a prognostic marker. Retrospective studies are adequate for exploring various alterations as potential prognostic markers, but only prospective clinical studies can determine whether an alteration is in fact a predictive marker. In our example of nodal metastasis, a predictive marker is an alteration that if present in a truly localized tumour leads to a high probability of subsequent nodal metastasis. If such a marker proves to be an independent risk factor in a multivariant analysis, it becomes clinically even more useful. Only a few molecular alterations in bladder cancer have shown clinical utility in such an analysis. Even more difficult to demonstrate and the true test of a predictive marker's utility would be a differential change in the tumour's natural history following a clinical intervention that is dependent on the marker's alteration. Thus, in the nodal metastasis example, resection of a localized tumour with an alteration in the predictive marker would decrease the risk of subsequent nodal disease, whereas resection of a localized tumour without an alteration in the predictive marker would not improve the risk of subsequent nodal disease. In the subsequent sections of this chapter we shall emphasize the demonstrated and potential prognostic and predictive utility of the molecular alterations in bladder cancer.

CHROMOSOME 9 DELETIONS AND p16 INACTIVATION—THE INITIATING EVENT(S)?

The most common genetic lesion in bladder cancer is hemizygous deletion of chromosome 9. This was first described in cytogenetic studies and subsequently confirmed in DNA studies using Southern blotting techniques and markers recognizing restriction length polymorphisms (RFLP) (7–10). These early studies were limited by the lack of sufficient markers covering the entire chromosome and the requirement for large amounts of DNA making analysis of small localized tumours difficult or impossible. More detailed analysis using polymerase chain reaction (PCR) technology and microsatellite repeats suggested that an entire chromosome 9 allele was most commonly deleted and that this occurred in 30–75% of clinical tumours, including small localized papillary cancers (11,12). The exact frequency of deletions was not clear because minimal amounts of contaminating normal tissue in the PCR reaction can obscure a deletion in the tumour material. These observations, however, suggested that inactivation of one or more tumour suppressor genes on chromosome 9 was critical to bladder oncogenesis.

Subsequent studies showed that some tumours have losses only on the short arm and some only on the long arm of chromosome 9 (12). It was thus suggested that at least two chromosome 9 tumour suppressor genes are inactivated in bladder cancer. The candidate gene(s) on the long arm remain to be identified, but the CDKN2AA (p16INK4A) gene was rapidly identified as the 9p tumour suppressor candidate.

The first clue which led to this discovery was that the short arm hemizygous deletions centred on band 9p21. At the same time, mapping studies in bladder and other cell lines revealed a series of homozygous deletions in this region (13,14). These latter observations were initially considered by some investigators to be artefacts of cell culture because they had difficulty confirming homozygous deletions in primary tumours. In retrospect, this initial difficulty was probably due to PCR amplification of chromosome 9 material from surrounding normal tissue, because with technical improvements homozygous chromosome 9 deletions were detected in primary bladder cancer specimens (15–18).

Using cell lines from a variety of malignancies, two research groups showed that the minimal common region of 9p21 homozygous deletions centred on the previously described CDKN2AA gene (19,20). The additional discovery of inactivating point mutations in this gene in primary tumours and tumour cell lines led these groups to propose that CDKN2A was the 9p21 tumour suppressor gene. Further studies revealed that some tumours had altered methylation patterns in upstream regulatory regions of this gene and that this led to loss of CDKN2A expression (21). Finally, germline deletion of CDKN2A in mice predisposes them to tumour formation (22). As a result of these studies, most investigators now believe that CDKN2A is an important tumour suppressor gene, and its inactivation is important in the malignant transformation of several normal tissues including normal urothelium.

CDKN2A encodes the p16 cell cycle inhibitory protein which inhibits the cdk4 and cdk6 cyclin dependent kinases (23). As a result, p16 overexpression leads to G_1 cell cycle arrest (Fig. 8.2).

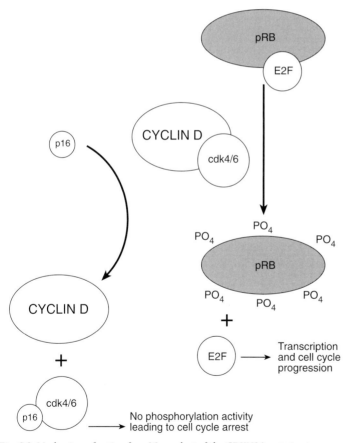

Fig. 8.2 *Mechanism of action for p16, product of the CDKN2A putative tumour sup-pressor gene. p16 binds to and inhibits the function of cdk4 and cdk6. In the absence of p16, these two kinases bind to cyclin D and are activated to phosphorylate a number of key regulatory proteins, including pRb. In its phosphorylated form, pRb no longer binds E2F, and as a result this transcription factor can then stimulate expression of genes critical for cell cycle progression*

In the simplest view, inactivation of p16 would allow a cell to continue cycling, thus producing a tumour. However, an alternatively spliced CDKN2A variant and the closely related p15, p18, and p19 proteins also inhibit the cell cycle in a similar manner, but do not appear to be tumour suppressor genes (24). The p16 protein must thus have some unique biological properties. More recently, we and others have suggested that p16 is important in cellular senescence (22,25–27). Senescence is an irreversible growth arrest that occurs in all cultured normal cells thus preventing the generation of immortal cell lines (28). It has generally been considered to be the cellular homologue of ageing. It has also been argued that senescence is a defence against the accumulation and propagation of carcinogenic mutations, and that escape from senescence and resultant immortalization is a critical step in oncogenesis. Loss of p16 expression may thus contribute to the ability of a urothelial cell to proliferate indefinitely. While this property may not lead to the full malignant phenotype, the analogy to continuously growing, recurrent Ta tumours is intriguing and further detailed studies on p16 expression in normal, hyperplastic, and low-grade Ta urothelium are eagerly awaited.

While some of the studies on the biological implications of p16 expression are ongoing, the observed 9p21 chromosomal deletions can be considered a marker for bladder cancer diagnosis. Fluorescent in situ hybridization (FISH) provides a unique tool for detecting these deletions. In this method a DNA probe is fluorescently labelled and can then be hybridized to intact cells. Using a bank of bladder wash specimens, Reeder et al. recently showed that FISH detected chromosome 9 deletions have a greater than 90% sensitivity for diagnosing bladder cancer (29). This is more sensitive than a battery of PCR assays (which included assays for 9p21 losses) in bladder wash specimens that were also reported to have a high sensitivity for detecting cancer (30). Interestingly, the study on FISH detected losses revealed that some patients with a history of bladder cancer, but no clinically detectable disease, still had 9p21 chromosomal deletions in their exfoliated urothelial cells. This suggests that 9p21 deletions, and perhaps p16 inactivation, may be a pre-malignant event and may be a clinically useful marker for detecting patients at risk for developing bladder cancer. In addition, these studies raise the issue of whether chromosome 9 deletions could be used as an intermediate marker for chemoprevention studies. Further prospective clinical trials are clearly needed.

One other important implication of the 9p deletions is that they often encompass a gene encoding an enzyme in the purine nucleotide salvage pathway, methylthioadenosine phosphorylase (31). Although this gene is not vital to cell survival, its deletion may make cells more sensitive to certain anti-metabolites and suggests therapeutic options that may be more toxic to bladder cancer than normal cells (32,33).

pRB INACTIVATION—AN ALTERNATIVE TO p16 INACTIVATION?

RB1 was first hypothesized to be a tumour suppresser gene by genetic analysis of familial retinoblastoma (34). Subsequent cloning of the gene confirmed Knudson's 'two-hit' hypothesis and was instrumental in stimulating the current explosion of research in cancer genetics (35). Additional studies revealed that point mutations of RB1 occurred in a wide variety of spontaneous malignancies, including bladder cancer (36,37). Another important advance occurred when it was recognized that a number of gene products from tumour viruses, including E7 from human papilloma virus and large T from the SV40 virus, bound and inactivated the RB1 gene product pRB (38). Inactivation of RB1 by point mutations or tumour viruses leads to release of E2F, an important DNA transcription factor critical for cell cycle progression. As depicted in Fig. 8.2, normal pRB phosphorylation, which is inhibited by p16, also results in E2F release. Thus, loss of p16 would lead to the accumulation of phosphorylated pRB and a resultant increase in free E2F levels. Functionally, this is equivalent to inactivation of pRB by point mutations or tumour viruses, and one would predict that p16 and pRb inactivation would be complementary. In support of this hypothesis, p16 alterations are rarely observed in tumours or tumour cell lines in which pRb is inactivated, and pRb alterations are rarely observed in tumours or tumour cell lines in which p16 is inactivated (39–41).

In fact, in most tumour systems, including bladder cancer, p16 is markedly upregulated when pRb is inactivated (39). This has been hypothesized to be a manifestation of a physiological feedback loop in a normal cell in which phosphorylated pRB induces p16 in order to prevent uncontrolled and continuous cell cycle progression. Although there is some experimental support for this hypothesis, we have challenged this view using an *in vitro* model system of bladder cancer development (Fig. 8.3). In this model, normal human urothelial cells (HUC) are immortalized with either the E7 or the E6 oncoprotein from an oncogenic human papilloma virus (42). E7 inactivates pRb and E6 inactivates p53 (see below).

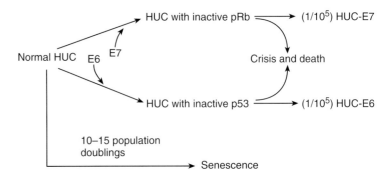

Fig. 8.3 An in vitro model system for bladder cancer (42). Normal human urothelial cells (HUC) can be cultured for approximately 10–15 doublings prior to senescence. Transformation with the E6 or E7 oncoproteins of human papilloma virus (HPV) 16 (which bind and inactivate p53 and pRb respectively) leads to escape from senescence and generation of an immortal cell line at a rate of 1/105 cells. Karyotypic and genetic analysis of the immortalized cells reveals alterations reminiscent of those found in primary bladder cancers suggesting that in vitro immortalization and in vivo oncogenesis are analogous

We showed that E7 transformation of normal HUC does not lead to elevated p16, but, as in the case of untransformed normal urothelial cells, p16 becomes elevated when these cells approach senescence ('crisis') (25). Unlike normal cells, a minority of E7 transformed cells escape senescence and form an immortal cell line in which high levels of p16 expression are maintained. As *in vitro* immortalization may mimic *in vivo* oncogenesis, these data suggest that inactivation of the p16/pRB pathway is critical in oncogenesis, and that at least one component of the pathway must be inactivated for successful tumour formation. Further support for this hypothesis comes from N-butyl-N-(4-hydroxybutyl)nitrosamine (BBN) induced rat bladder tumours (43). This animal model closely recapitulates the pathological development of human bladder tumours. Recently, it was reported that cyclin D_1 is over-expressed in a majority of the induced papillomas which appear to be a relevant precursor lesion (44). The net biological effect of such an alteration is predicted to be activation of cdk4 and/or cdk6, hyperphosphorylation of pRB, and subsequent release of E2F. This alteration is thus functionally equivalent to p16 inactivation in human tumours.

If pRB alterations can substitute for p16 alterations in primary bladder cancer, then they should also be observed in early stage cancers. Although this has been reported in a number of studies, it has also been observed that pRB loss is correlated with stage, grade, and an increased risk of recurrence, progression, and death (36,37). Similar correlations have not been made for tumours with p16 inactivation. Whether the apparent more aggressive nature of tumours with pRb as opposed to p16 inactivation is due to the direct biological effects of pRB or due to associated genetic alterations remains to be determined. It is notable that the E7 immortalized urothelial cells invariably also harbour 20q chromosomal amplifications (45). Although similar 20q amplifications have been observed in primary bladder cancers, the relationship to pRB alterations and prognosis has not been determined (46). These observations suggest that pRB alterations in superficial tumours may be a predictive marker for subsequent progression, but there have been no adequate clinical trials to address this issue.

p53 INACTIVATION-GENOMIC INSTABILITY AND CLINICAL AGGRESSIVENESS

The P53 tumour suppressor gene is the most commonly inactivated gene in human malignancy. Alterations are found in 20–60% of bladder cancers and are correlated with stage, grade, recurrence, progression, and survival (47–49). P53 inactivation may also be the first true predictive marker in bladder cancer, because its inactivation in CIS, which is presumably confined to the epithelial layer, is correlated with subsequent progression and death (49,50). If this is confirmed in prospective studies, we may be able to identify a group of patients with CIS who could be treated conservatively (i.e. those who do not have p53 alterations).

Before further discussing the biological and clinical implications of p53 inactivation in bladder cancer, a number of important technical comments regarding detection of these alterations must be made. The vast majority of P53 mutations in human tumours are point mutations that lead to an increased protein half-life. Thus, under certain conditions, mutant but not normal p53 products can be detected in primary tumours by immunohistochemistry. Using the 1801 antibody, studies have shown that immunohistochemical detection of p53 in greater than 10–20% of tumour cells is highly correlated with mutations as detected by sequencing (51,52). It needs to be stated, however, that some tumours inactivate p53 by mechanisms that would lead to absent or decreased protein levels. These include gene deletion, point mutations that lead to frame shifts and markedly shortened protein products that may not carry the immunogenic epitopes, and inactivation by tumour virus oncoproteins such as E6, which leads to increased destruction and thus lower protein levels. Also, normal p53 is upregulated by a number of relevant cellular insults including radiation therapy and some chemotherapeutic agents

(53,54). Thus, the significance of detectable p53 in tumours following such manipulation remains unclear. Finally, different techniques for antigen retrieval or different antibodies may make the immunohistochemistry sensitive enough to detect even normal p53. Therefore, sequencing remains the gold standard for detection of p53 abnormalities in primary bladder tumours.

Despite these caveats, it is clear that alteration of p53 is a prognostic indicator in bladder cancer. Recent developments in understanding the biology of p53 help explain this observation. As stated, a number of DNA damaging agents, most notably radiation, induce p53. In some cells, such as cultured normal human urothelial cells, the radiation induced p53 leads only to cell cycle arrest (through induction of p21) and presumably repair of the DNA damage (through induction of GADD45 and other DNA repair enzymes) (53,54). In other cells, induction of p53 leads to programmed cell death (apoptosis), likely by activation of pro-apoptotic proteins such as bax and downregulation of anti-apoptotic proteins such as bcl-xL and bcl-2. Whether a cell proceeds down the apoptotic pathway depends on cell type, degree of DNA damage, and alterations in any of the regulating proteins. p53 is thus felt to be the most critical protein in regulating the G_1 checkpoint or restriction point in cycling cells. This restriction point, first hypothesized by Pardee, is the point in the G_1 phase of the cell cycle in which a cell must decide whether to proceed to S phase and DNA synthesis (55). A similar checkpoint has been hypothesized to be present in late G_2 in which a cell must decide whether to proceed to M phase and mitosis. Some preliminary evidence suggests that p53 may be important in the regulation of this G_2 checkpoint as well. As a result, cells in which p53 has been inactivated are unable to respond appropriately to DNA damage and continue to replicate mutated and altered DNA.

It has thus been hypothesized that the highly aneuploid nature of many aggressive bladder cancers is the result of p53 inactivation. In support of this concept, it has been shown that E6 immortalized normal human urothelial cells have a very aneuploid and unstable karyotype whereas E7 immortalized normal human urothelial cells have a near diploid and stable karyotype (42). Presumably, the genomic instability leads to an increased gene mutation rate, some of which will lead to a cellular growth advantage and thus be selected for further tumour development.

Although p53 mutations may lead to biologically aggressive tumour behaviour, the lack of appropriate checkpoint regulation may also cause these tumours to be more susceptible to certain therapeutic approaches (56,57). Space considerations prevent a full discussion of this phenomenon, but *in vitro* investigations have shown that such an approach may be valid, and further clinical studies are awaited.

ACTIVATION OF THE EPIDERMAL GROWTH FACTOR PATHWAY—ESCAPE FROM GROWTH CONTROL

The recognition that the tumorigenic properties of some retroviruses are due to transduction and activation of normal cellular genes was a major step in understanding the genetic basis of malignancy (58). Subsequent research revealed that many of these oncogenes are important constituents of the growth factor signalling pathway. One such gene, v-erb-B, was first identified in the avian erythroblastosis virus, but was soon recognized to be a homologue of the epidermal growth factor receptor (EGFR) (59). Epidermal growth factor (EGF) is a amino acid peptide growth factor found in high concentrations in the urine (60). When bound to EGFR, the intrinsic tyrosine kinase activity of the receptor is activated; then, through a kinase cascade whose details are still being elucidated, cell division and growth are stimulated (61).

The concentration of EGF in the urine of patients with bladder cancer is well within the range required for stimulating the growth of tumour cell lines, including bladder cancer cell lines, although the concentration is actually lower than that in the urine of normal individuals (62). *In vitro* experiments, however, reveal that malignant urothelial but not normal urothelial cells respond to exogenous EGF, despite the fact that both express the EGF receptor (63). Potential differences in the signalling cascade between normal and malignant urothelium have not yet been explored, but immunohistochemical studies reveal that the degree of EGFR expression correlates with bladder cancer stage and prognosis (64). More detailed immunohistochemical studies have also shown that in normal individuals only the basal layer of urothelium expresses EGFR, whereas in malignant urothelium and histologically normal urothelium in individuals with bladder tumours EGFR is expressed diffusely throughout all urothelial layers (65–68). These observations suggest that EGFR expression may be a premalignant change in the oncogenic pathway and perhaps may even be an intermediate marker for chemopreventive studies. These studies also suggest that EGFR overexpression may be a predictive marker for subsequent invasive disease. Neither of these possibilities has been adequately addressed in prospective clinical trials.

EGFR may not only be a useful biological marker, but also a reasonable therapeutic target. Recently, a number of compounds that inhibit the receptor kinase activity of EGFR have been described (69). Growth inhibition of orthotopic human bladder cancer in nude mice treated with one of these inhibitors has also been reported (70). As such, further clinical development of these compounds to determine their effectiveness in human superficial and advanced bladder cancer is underway.

It should be noted that activation of the EGFR signalling pathway can occur through other ligands such as transforming growth factor (TGF)-alpha, which is also detectable in the urine (71). In addition, other membrane tyrosine kinases that presumably activate the growth factor signalling cascade are overexpressed or activated in bladder carcinomas. The most well studied is probably ERB-B2 (also known as HER2-neu). This protein is overexpressed in 20–30% of bladder tumours and has been correlated with stage, grade, and outcome (72). Activation, or inadequate control, of growth factor signalling pathways is thus a common theme in bladder cancer and is probably a major cause of proliferative activity in bladder cancer. As in the case of EGFR signalling these other signalling pathways may also be attractive therapeutic targets.

SUMMARY AND CONCLUSIONS

It has been argued that more than 25 years of intensive laboratory research has not led to significant impacts on cancer mortality, especially for the common adult tumours (73). There is, however, little dispute that there have been major advances in understanding the biology of carcinogenesis and in understanding the fundamental alterations in cancer cells that lead to the malignant phenotype. Although further advances in this basic understanding are no doubt forthcoming, one of the major challenges for the new millennium is to translate these findings into practical clinical applications that will benefit patients and lead to lower mortality rates. It is our contention that bladder cancer is a disease in which these goals can be met in the near future.

We have discussed some of the molecular events leading to bladder cancer including chromosome 9 and CDKN2A deletions, TP53 and RB1 inactivations, and EGFR overexpression. This is far from an exhaustive list and ignores important additional genetic alterations including 3p chromosomal deletions, 20q chromosomal amplifications, and inactivation of a number of genes and proteins thought to be important in the development of metastatic disease. We have chosen to discuss this limited set of alterations because of the extensive experimental and clinical data available for each one. We have attempted to demonstrate potential clinical applications and have pointed out clinical trials in progress or suggested clinical trials which could alter our approach to patients with this disease. We hope that this summary will stimulate further research that will allow the tremendous advances in understanding basic urothelial oncogenesis to lead to equally dramatic advances in patient care.

Key Points

1. The most common genetic lesion in bladder cancer is hemizygous deletion of chromosome 9 (30–75%). CDKN2A, the 9p21 tumour suppressor gene, encodes the p16 cell cycle inhibitory protein which inhibits the cdk4 and cdk6 cyclin-dependent kinases. As a result, p16 overexpression leads to G_1 cell cycle arrest Inactivation of p16 would allow a cell to continue cycling, thus producing a tumour.
2. p53 mutation may lead to biologically aggressive tumour behaviour and is a prognostic indicator in bladder cancer
3. ERB-B2 (also known as HER2-neu), is overexpressed in 20–30% of bladder tumours.

References

1 Parker SL, Tong TBS, Wingo PA. Cancer statistics. *CA* 1997, **47**, 5–27.
2 Hankey BF, Silverman DT. *SEER cancer statistics review.* NIH Publ. no. 93–2789. National Cancer Institute, Bethesda, 1993.
3 Koch MO, Smith JA. Natural history and surgical management of superficial bladder cancer (stages Ta/T1/CIS). In: *Comprehensive textbook of genitourinary oncology* (ed. Vogelzang NJ, Scardino PT, Shipley WU, Coffey DS). Williams & Wilkins 1996, pp. 405–15.
4 Loehrer PJ, Einhorn LH, Elson PJ *et al.* A randomized comparison of cisplatin alone or in combination with methotrexate, vinblastine, and doxorubicin in patients with metastatic urothelial carcinoma: a cooperative group study. *J Clin Oncol* 1992, **10**, 1066–73.
5 Saxman SB, Propert KJ, Einhorn E *et al.* Long term follow up of phase III intergroup study of cisplatin alone or in combination with methotrexate, vinblastine, and doxorubicin in patients with metastatic urothelial carcinoma: A cooperative group study. *J Clin Oncol* 1997, **15**, 2564–9.
6 Fearon ER, Vogelstein B. A genetic model for colorectal tumorigenesis. *Cell* 1990, **61**, 759–67.
7 Knowles MA, Elder PA, Williamson M *et al.* Allelotype of human bladder cancer. *Cancer Res* 1994, **53**, 1230–2.
8 Habuchi T, Ogawa O, Kakehi Y *et al.* Accumulated allelic losses in the development of invasive urothelial cancer. *Int J Cancer* 1993, **53**, 579–84.
9 Smeets W, Pauwels R, Laarakkers L *et al.* Chromosomal analysis of bladder cancer III. Nonrandom alterations. *Cancer Genet Cytogenet* 1987, **29**, 29–41.
10 Tsai YC, Nichols PW, Hiti AL *et al.* Allelic losses of chromosomes 9, 11, and 17 in human bladder cancer. *Cancer Res* 1990, **50**, 44–7.
11 Cairns P, Shaw ME, Knowles MA. Initiation of bladder cancer may involve deletion of a tumour suppressor gene on chromosome 9. *Oncogene* 1994, **8**, 1083–5.
12 Ruppert JM, Tokino K, Sidransky D. Evidence for two bladder cancer suppressor loci on human chromosome 9. *Cancer Res* 1993, **53**, 5093–5.
13 Stadler WM, Sherman J, Bohlander SK *et al.* Homozygous deletions within chromosomal bands 9p21–22 in bladder cancer. *Cancer Res* 1994, **54**, 2060–3.
14 Olopade OI, Bohlander SK, Pomykala H *et al.* Mapping of the shortest region of overlap of deletions of the short arm of chromosome 9 associated with human neoplasia. *Genomics* 1992, **14**, 437–43.
15 Williamson MP, Elder PA, Shaw ME *et al.* P16 (CDKN2) is a major deletion target at 9p21 in bladder cancer. *Hum Mol Genet* 1995, **4**, 1569–77.
16 Cairns P, Polascik TJ, Eby Y *et al.* Frequency of homozygous deletions at p16/CDKN2 in primary human tumors. *Nature Genet* 1995, **11**, 210–12.
17 Orlow I, Lacombe L, Hannon GJ *et al.* Deletion of the p16 and p15 genes in human bladder tumors. *J Natl Cancer Inst* 1995, **87**, 1524–9.
18 Gonzalez-Zulueta M, Shibata A, Ohneseit PF *et al.* High frequency of chromosome 9p allelic loss and CDKN2 tumor suppressor gene alterations in squamous cell carcinoma of the bladder. *J Natl Cancer Inst* 1995, **87**, 1383–93.
19 Kamb A, Gruis NA, Weaver-Feldhaus J *et al.* A cell cycle regulator potentially involved in genesis of many tumor types. *Science* 1994, **264**, 436–40.
20 Nobori T, Miura K, Wu DJ *et al.* Deletions of the cyclin-dependent kinase-4 inhibitor gene in multiple human cancers. *Nature* 1994, **368**, 753–6.

21 Herman JG, Merlo A, Mao L *et al.* Inactivation of the CDKN2/p16/MTS1 gene is frequently associated with aberrant DNA methylation in all common human cancers. *Cancer Res* 1995, **55**, 4525–30.

22 Serrano M, Lee HW, Chin L *et al.* Role of the INK4A locus in tumor suppression and cell mortality. *Cell* 1996, **85**, 27–37.

23 Serrano M, Hannon GJ, Beach D. A new regulatory motif in cell-cycle control causing specific inhibition of cyclin D/CDK4. *Nature* 1993, **366**, 704–7.

24 Sherr CJ. Cancer cell cycles. *Science* 1996, **274**, 1672–7.

25 Reznikoff CA, Yeager T, Belair CD *et al.* Elevated p16 in senescent human uroepithelial cells is retained upon E7 but not E6 induced immortalization. *Cancer Res* 1996, **56**, 2886–90.

26 Hara E, Smith R, Parry D *et al.* Regulation of p16CDKN2 expression and its implications for cell immortalization and senescence. *Mol Cell Biol* 1996, **16**, 859–67.

27 Rogan EM, Bryan TM, Hukku B *et al.* Alterations in p53 and p16ink4 expression and telomere length during spontaneous immortalization of Li–Fraumeni syndrome fibroblasts. *Mol Cell Biol* 1995, **15**, 4745–53.

28 Campisi J. Replicative senescence: An old lives tale? *Cell* 1996, **84**, 497–500.

29 Reeder JE, Morreale JF, O'Connell MJ *et al.* Loss of the CDKN2/p16 locus detected in bladder irrigation specimens by fluorescence in situ hybridization. *J Urol* 1997, **158**, 1717–21.

30 Mao L, Schoenberg MP, Scicchitano M *et al.* Molecular detection of primary bladder cancer by microsatellite analysis. *Science,*Year, **271**, 659–62.

31 Stadler WM, Olopade OI. The 9p21 chromosomal region in bladder cancer. Large homozygous deletions inactivate the CDKN2, CDKN2B, and MTAP genes. *Urol Res* 1996, **24**, 239–44.

32 Chen ZH, Olopade OI, Savarese TM. Expression of methylthioadenosine phosphorylase cDNA in p16-, MTAP- malignant cells: restoration of methylthioadenosine phosphorylase-dependent salvage pathways and alterations of sensitivity to inhibitors of purine de novo synthesis. *Mol Pharmacol* 1997, **52**, 903–11.

33 Hori H, Tran P, Carrera CJ *et al.* Methylthioadenosine phosphorylase cDNA transfection alters sensitivity to depletion of purine and methionine in A549 lung cancer cells. *Cancer Res* 1996, **56**, 5653–8.

34 Francke U. Retinoblastoma and chromosome 13. *Cytogenet Cell Genet* 1976, **16**, 131–4.

35 Knudson AG. Mutation and cancer: statistical study of retinoblastoma. *Proc Natl Acad Sci USA* 1971, **68**, 820–3.

36 Cordon-Cardo C, Wartinger D, Petrylak D *et al.* Altered expression of the retinoblastoma gene product: Prognostic indicator in bladder cancer. *J Natl Cancer Inst* 1992, **84**, 1251–6.

37 Logothetis DJ, Xu HJ, Ro JY *et al.* Altered expression of retinoblastoma protein and known prognostic variables in locally advanced bladder cancer. *J Natl Cancer Inst* 1992, **84**, 1256–61.

38 DeCaprio JA, Ludlow JW, Figge J *et al.* SV40 large tumor antigen forms a specific complex with the product of the retinoblastoma susceptibility gene. *Cell* 1988, **54**, 275–83.

39 Yeager T, Stadler WM, Belair C *et al.* Increased p16 levels correlate with pRb alterations in human urothelial cells. *Cancer Res* 1995, **55**, 493–7.

40 Otterson GA, Kratzke RA, Coxon A *et al.* Absence of p16INK4 protein is restricted to the subset of lung cancer lines that retains wildtype RB. *Mol Cell Biol* 1994, **14**, 7256–64.

41 Aagaard L, Lukas J, Bartkova J *et al.* Aberrations of p16Ink4 and retinoblastoma tumour-suppressor genes occur in distinct sub-sets of human cancer cell lines. *Int J Cancer* 1995, **61**, 115–20.

42 Reznikoff CA, Belair C, Savelieva E *et al.* Long-term genome stability and minimal genotypic and phenotypic alterations in HPV16, E7-, but not E6-, immortalized human uroepithelial cells. *Genes Dev* 1994, **8**, 2227–40.

43 Fukushima S, Imaida K, Sakata T *et al.* Promoting effects of sodium l-ascorbate on two-stage urinary bladder carcinogenesis in rats. *Cancer Res* 1983, **43**, 4454–7.

44 Lee CCR, Yamamoto S, Wanibuchi H *et al.* Cyclin D1 overexpression in rat two-stage bladder carcinogenesis and its relationship with oncogenes, tumor suppressor genes and cell proliferation. *Cancer Res* 1997, **57**, 4765–76.

45 Savelieva E, Belair CD, Newton MA *et al*. 20q gain associates with immortalization: 20q13.2 amplification correlates with genome instability in human papillomavirus 16, E7 transformed human uroepithelial cells. *Oncogene* 1997, **14**, 551–60.

46 Kallioniemi A, Kallioniemi OP, Citro G *et al*. Identification of gains and losses of DNA sequences in primary bladder cancer by comparative genomic hybridization. *Genes Chromosomes Cancer* 1995, **12**, 213–9.

47 Esrig D, Elmajian D, Groshen S *et al*. Accumulation of nuclear p53 and tumor progression in bladder cancer. *N Engl J Med*, 1994, **331**, 1259–64.

48 Sarkis AS, Bajorin DF, Reuter VE *et al*. Prognostic value of p53 nuclear overexpression in patients with invasive bladder cancer treated with neoadjuvant MVAC. *J Clin Oncol* 1995, **13**, 1384–90.

49 Sarkis AS, Dalbagni G, Cordon-Cardo C *et al*. Association of p53 nuclear overexpression and tumor progression in carcinoma in situ of the bladder. *J Urol* 1994, **152**, 388–92.

50 Vet JAM, Witjes JA, Marras SAE *et al*. Predictive value of p53 mutations analyzed in bladder washings for progression of high-risk superficial bladder cancer. *Clin Cancer Res* 1996, **2**, 1055–61.

51 Esrig D, Spruck CH III, Nichols PW *et al*. P53 nuclear protein accumulation correlates with mutations in the p53 gene, tumor grade, and stage in bladder cancer. *Am J Pathol* 1993, **143**, 1389–97.

52 Cordon-Cardo C, Dalbagni G, Saez GT *et al*. P53 mutations in human bladder cancer: genotypic versus phenotypic patterns. *Int J Cancer* 1994, **5**, 347–53.

53 Levine AJ. P53, the cellular gatekeeper for growth and division. *Cell* 1997, **88**, 323–31.

54 Harris CC. Structure and function of the p53 tumor suppressor gene: Clues for rational cancer therapeutic strategies. *J Natl Cancer Inst* 1996, **88**, 1442–55.

55 Pardee AB. A restriction point for control of normal animal cell proliferation. *Proc Natl Acad Sci USA* 1974, **71**, 1286–90.

56 Powell SN, DeFrank JS, Connell P *et al*. Differential sensitivity of p53 (–) and p53 (+) cells to caffeine-induced radiosensitization and override of G2 delay. *Cancer Res* 1995, **55**, 1643–8.

57 Fan S, Smith ML, Rivet DJ *et al*. Disruption of p53 function sensitizes breast cancer MCF-7 cells to cisplatin and pentoxifylline. *Cancer Res* 1995, **55**, 1649–54.

58 Cooper GM. In: *Oncogenes* (ed.), Jones and Bartlett Boston 1995.

59 Downdard J, Yarden Y, Mayes E *et al*. Close similarity of epidermal growth factor receptor and v-erb-B oncogene protein sequences. *Nature* 1984, **307**, 521–4.

60 Messing EM. Growth factors and bladder cancer: clinical implications of the interactions between growth factors and their urothelial receptors. *Semin Surg Oncol* 1992, **8**, 285–92.

61 Khazaie K, Shirrmacher V, Lechtner RB. EGF receptor in neoplasia and metastasis. *Cancer Metastasis Rev* 1993, **12**, 255–74.

62 Messing EM, Murphy-Brooks N. Recovery of epidermal growth factor in voided urine of patients with bladder cancer. *Urology* 1994, **44**, 502–6.

63 Messing EM, Reznikoff CA. Normal and malignant human urothelium: in vitro effects of epidermal growth factor. *Cancer Res* 1987, **47**, 2230–5.

64 Mellon K, Wright C, Kelly P *et al*. Long term outcome related to epidermal growth factor receptor status in bladder cancer. *J Urol* 1995, **153**, 919–25.

65 Witjes JA, Umbas R, Debruyne FM, Schalken JA. Expression of markers for transitional cell carcinoma in normal bladder mucosa of patients with bladder cancer. *J Urol* 1995, **154**, 2185–9.

66 Wagner U, Sauter G, Moch H *et al*. Patterns of p53, erbB2 and EGFR expression in premalignant lesions of the urinary bladder. *Hum Pathol* 1995, **26**, 970–8.

67 Limas C, Bair R, Bernhart P, Reddy P. Proliferative activity of normal and neoplastic urothelium and its relation to epidermal growth factor and transferrin receptors. *J Clin Pathol* 1993, **46**, 810–6.

68 Messing EM. Clinical implications of the expression of epidermal growth factor receptors in human transitional cell carcinoma. *Cancer Res* 1990, **50**, 2530–7.

69 Fry DW, Nelson JM, Slintak V *et al*. Biochemical and antiproliferative properties of 4-[ar (alk)ylamino]-pyridopyrimidines, a new chemical class of potent and specific epidermal growth factor receptor tyrosine kinase inhibitor. *Biochem Pharmacol* 1997, **54**(8), 877–87.

70 Dinney CPN, Parker C, Dong Z *et al*. Therapy of human transitional cell carcinoma of the bladder by oral administration of the epidermal growth factor
receptor protein tyrosine kinase inhibitor 4,5-dianilophthalimide. *Clin Cancer
Res* 1997, **3**, 161–8.

71 Katoh M, Inagaki H, Kurosawa-Ohsawa K *et al*. Detection of transforming
growth factor alpha in human urine and plasma. *Biochem Biophys Res Commun*
1990, **167**, 1065–72.

72 Sato K, Moriyama M, Mori S *et al*. An immunohistologic evaluation of c-erbB-2
gene product in patients with urinary bladder carcinoma. *Cancer* 1992, **70**,
2493–8.

73 Bailar JC, 3rd Gornik HL. Cancer undefeated. *N Engl J Med* 1997, **336**, 1569–74.

9. THE ROLE OF ADHESION MOLECULES IN THE BIOLOGY OF BLADDER CANCER

K.N. Syrigos, K.J. Harrington, and M. Pignatelli

INTRODUCTION

It is now widely recognized that shedding and subsequent reimplantation of neoplastic cells within the bladder may, at least in part, be responsible for the high recurrence rates of bladder cancer. There is a growing body of evidence suggesting that alterations in the adhesion properties of neoplastic cells may play a pivotal role in the development and progression of the malignant phenotype in a range of tumour types including bladder cancer. Adhesion molecules are intimately involved in the control of such processes as morphological differentiation, cellular proliferation, and invasion and colonization of distant organs (1). Reduced cell-matrix adhesion allows neoplastic cells to circumvent the control of differentiation induced by the normal extracellular environment, while loss of the intercellular adhesion allows malignant cells to escape from their site of origin, degrade the extracellular matrix, acquire a more motile and invasive phenotype, and finally invade and metastasize (2). In bladder cancer in particular desquamation of single cells or whole sheets from the underlying lamina propria requires interruption of tight junctions between neighbouring cells and reorganization of intermediate filaments (3).

In addition to participate in tumour invasiveness and metastasis, cell adhesion is fundamental for the establishment and maintenance of multicellular organisms: the normal development and function of tissues is governed by the interactions of cells with each other and with their acellular environment, as they are mediated by adhesion. Furthermore, interactions between the cytoskeleton and the adhesion molecules regulate or significantly contribute to a variety of functions, including signal transduction, cell growth, differentiation, site-specific gene expression, morphogenesis, immunological function, cell motility, wound healing, and inflammation (4). It is thus hardly surprising that the molecular mechanisms of cell adhesion consists a field of intensive study over the last decade. To date, a diverse system of transmembrane glycoproteins have been identified to make the cell extracellular matrix adhesion (substrate adhesion molecules, SAMs) and the intercell adhesion (cell–cell adhesion molecules, CAMs) (5). Most of these receptors have been characterized and at present, the main families of adhesive molecules are: the cadherins, the integrins, the members of the immunoglobulin superfamily, and the selectins. These adhesion molecules are genetically and biochemically distinct, although in some instances, they are functionally related (6). This chapter presents recent data regarding the role of selected CAMs and SAMs in the pathogenesis of bladder cancer and their clinical exploitation as biomarkers of this malignant disease.

CADHERINS

The cadherins are the prime mediators of cell–cell adhesion, achieved via homotypic interactions: a cadherin molecule on one cell binds to a cadherin molecule of the same type on another cell to form a homodimer (7). Functionally, the cadherins appear to be the most important adhesion molecules as, when they are normally expressed, the inactivation of other CAMs seems to have little effect on cell biology (8).

The cadherin family consists of more than 16 molecules that although they are encoded by different genes, they comprise a distinct group of phylogenetically and structurally related molecules. They require the presence of calcium in order to function normally, being rapidly degraded by protease action in the absence of this ion. Alterations in the expression of the cadherins are a necessary step for the progression of a malignant tumour, as loss (transient or permanent) of a functional intercellular adhesion junction is a requirement for tumour cells to invade locally, to escape from the primary site, and to metastasize to distant organs (2,9).

E-cadherin is a transmembrane protein with an extracellular amino terminal end that binds a single calcium ion and a carboxy terminal cytoplasmic tail which interacts with cytoskeletal proteins through the catenin complex (10). The catenin complex consists of α-catenin, β-catenin, γ-catenin, and p120. The E-cadherin–catenin complex is found at sites of cell–cell contact known as the adherens junction or zonula adherens and their formation is a prerequisite for normal functioning of E-cadherin, as dysfunctional catenin complex leads to defective E-cadherin activity: reversible downregulation of E-cadherin function through phosphorylation of catenins has been shown to cause adherens junction destabilization (11). Finally, it seems that E-cadherin functions as a tumour-suppressor gene, as loss of expression, and/or abnormal function of E-cadherin leads to loss of cell polarity and derangement of normal tissue architecture.

The role of catenins is currently under investigation and it seems that, in addition to adhesion, they are involved in several cell functions. α-catenin plays an important part in linking the E-cadherin–catenin complex to the actin cytoskeleton (12). β-catenin is involved in organogenesis and tissue morphogenesis playing an important part in normal development and tissue function, as it is demonstrated by the *in utero* death of β-catenin gene knockout mice. It also plays a critical part in regulating cadherin-mediated cell recognition and adhesion (13). γ-catenin, which shares very high sequence homology with β-catenin, is present in the zonula adherens junction and may function within the desmosomal plaque (14). The p120 protein, which was originally identified as a substrate of *src* and several other receptor tyrosine kinases, binds directly to the cytoplasmic domain of E-cadherin and participates in the modulation of E-cadherin-mediated cell adhesion.

Both β- and γ-catenins have been shown to interact with the adenomatous polyposis coli (APC) tumour suppressor gene product (15,16). *In vitro* studies have demonstrated that wild-type APC downregulates β-catenin levels, thus interfering with cadherin-mediated adhesion (17). APC mutations occur in the early stages of development of adenomatous polyps both in the stomach and the colon, while the wild-type APC gene is also expressed in normal bladder (18). As a dynamic equilibrium exists between E-cadherin–catenin complexes, APC–catenin complexes and free pools of catenins, factors influencing these interactions may alter the stoichiometry in favour of the motility (APC–catenin) rather than the adhesive (E-cadherin–catenin) complex (19,20), permitting some cells to escape from the primary site and invade locally or metastasize.

Several *in vitro* studies of human bladder cancer cell lines have demonstrated a correlation between abnormal E-cadherin expression and an aggressive phenotype. Loss of E-cadherin expression is associated with loss of cellular differentiation and increased cellular invasiveness and infiltration in collagen gel assays (21,22), while transfection of these cell lines with E-cadherin cDNA is able to suppress this invasiveness (22).

Investigation of the expression of E-cadherin in histopathological material from human bladder cancers, has demonstrated that aberrant E-cadherin expression correlates with lack of differentiation, muscle invasion and distant metastasis (23,24). Loss of normal E-cadherin expression has also been shown to correlate with decreased recurrence-free and overall survival, although multivariate analysis suggests that it has no independent prognostic value over the grade and stage of the tumour (25–27). Increased levels of soluble E-cadherin can be detected in the serum of patients with bladder cancer and their role in the follow-up of these patients is currently under investigation, with very promising preliminary results: they correlate with advanced grade and with the number of superficial lesions, while patients with elevated serum E-cadherin levels have an increased risk of having recurrent disease at the follow-up cystoscopy (28). Soluble forms of E-cadherin have also been detected in the urine of patients with bladder cancer and they may reflect shedding from the urinary epithelium, as part of the normal turnover of this molecule (29).

With regard to the catenins, loss of membranous α-, β-, and γ-catenin immunoreactivity has been associated with advanced tumour grade and stage, whereas loss of normal membranous γ-catenin has also been associated with a worse prognosis of bladder cancer patients. In addition, the presence of multiple abnormalities in the E-cadherin–catenin complex was correlated with advanced grade and stage as well as with poor survival of bladder cancer patients (27,30,31).

A number of possible mechanisms have been proposed to account for the documented reduction in E-cadherin function in bladder cells undergoing malignant transformation. These include suppression or mutation of the E-cadherin gene (9), translation disorder (22), allelic loss of 16q (32), or finally increased protease-mediated degradation (33). Nevertheless, one should bear in mind that the commonly observed heterogeneous pattern of E-cadherin expression might be caused either by tumour heterogeneity or by unstable expression of E-cadherin *in vivo* (34).

In conclusion, loss of the normal, membranous E-cadherin–catenin complex immunoreactivity occurs frequently in transitional bladder carcinomas and correlates with high grade, advanced stage, and poor prognosis. As the catenins function as a whole in the establishment of close cellular contacts, bladder tumours with abnormal expression of all four components are endowed with an invasive and metastatic phenotype, suggesting a multistep progress of the malignant transformation. The involvement of APC with the catenins, together with the tumour suppressor function of E-cadherin suggest a role for these proteins in bladder tumorigenesis. Study of the interactions of these proteins with the adhesion and signalling pathways will contribute to our better understanding of this fundamental area of bladder cancer biology.

INTEGRINS

The integrins are transmembrane glycoproteins with a molecular weight of 100–140 kDa. They are composed of non-covalently associated $\alpha\beta$ heterodimers, made up of different combinations of

15 α and nine β chains. This allows for the formation of a vast array of different integrin molecules which, by virtue of the fact that the ligand binding site contains regions derived from both α and β chains, can interact with a wide variety of different molecules. Integrins are expressed by every cell type derived from the three primary germ layers and their presence is required for the maintenance of normal tissue architecture (5,35). The majority of known integrins are SAMs, functioning as receptors for extracellular matrix proteins including collagens, laminin, vitronectin, thrombospondin, von Willebrand factor, and fibronectin (5). Some integrins bind to a single, specific ligand [e.g. $\alpha_6\beta_1$ to laminin (36) and $\alpha_5\beta_1$ to fibronectin (37)], while others have overlapping ligand specificities (e.g. $\alpha_1\beta_1$ binds laminin and collagen, $\alpha_3\beta_1$ binds laminin, collagen, and fibronectin) (38). In some cases a particular integrin may exhibit different specificities when expressed on different cell types, while certain integrins (e.g. $\alpha_4\beta_1$ and $\alpha_v\beta_2$) can function both as a SAM and a CAM (6,37). It is obvious, therefore, that the range of integrin–ligand interactions is very complex, even in the normal state.

With regard to the bladder, immunohistochemical studies have shown that normal human urothelium expresses integrins $\alpha3$, αV, β_1, and β_4. Their presence in the urothelial basement membrane provides the molecular basis for the impermeability of the bladder wall (38). The most commonly expressed integrin in the normal human bladder, $\alpha_6\beta_4$, is found in the basolateral surface of the basal layer and in the lamina propria. It is also coexpressed with collagen VII within the desmosomal anchoring complex. Altered expression of $\alpha_6\beta_4$ has been reported as an early event in the development of bladder cancer (39–41), with cells showing loss of normal polarization of expression in addition to expression on suprabasal cells. This loss of normal localization of $\alpha_6\beta_4$ expression may predispose bladder cancer cells to invade locally and to metastasize. This hypothesis is supported by the observation that the degree of derangement of expression is positively correlated with poorly differentiated and advanced tumours (41).

In conclusion, expression of integrins in bladder cancer is aberrant, downregulated and with a progressive loss of its expression from the normal urothelium to invasive bladder cancer. This abnormal expression is correlated with a more aggressive phenotype, local invasion, and metastasis.

IMMUNOGLOBULIN SUPERFAMILY (IgSF)

These molecules share the immunoglobulin structural homology unit which consists of a length of 70 to 110 amino acids forming β-pleated sheets. Each unit is stabilized by a disulphide cross-link between the β-strands (42). The members of this family include the intercellular cell adhesion molecules (ICAMs), the major histocompatibility molecules, the T-cell receptor, the platelet-derived growth factor receptor, the colony-stimulating factor-1 receptor, as well as the deleted in colon cancer (DCC) gene product. They mediate either homotypic or heterotypic adhesion and can function either as CAMs or SAMs. With regard to bladder cancer, the expression of some of the members of this family has been investigated and has been shown to be deranged.

Intercellular cell adhesion molecules

While untreated superficial bladder carcinoma cells do not express ICAM-1, this adhesion molecule is re-expressed after immunotherapy with bacille Calmette-Guérin (BCG), or interferon gamma (IFN-γ) (43,44).The ICAM-1 that is produced can be detected in urine of these patients and has been correlated with the response of the tumour to immunotherapy (43). It seems that this molecule can render bladder tumour cells vulnerable to non-antigen specific cytotoxicity mediated by activated lymphocytes (43). ICAM-1 is also involved in cell-mediated lysis of bladder cancer cells by promoting binding of lymphokine-activated killer (LAK) cells (44). Finally, *in vitro* experiments have shown that cells in which abnormal ICAM-1 expression was not corrected by IFN-γ treatment had a more aggressive phenotype. Therefore, it seems that abnormal ICAM-1 expression facilitates avoidance of immunological surveillance (44).

C-CAM-1, another member of this family, acts as a tumour suppressor in human bladder tissue and its expression is downregulated in bladder cancer cells (45).

Allelic loss at the DCC gene (five chromosome 18q loci) has been confirmed in 36% of bladder cancers. This loss has been associated with muscle invasive disease and increased recurrence rate (46,47). Further studies are needed to estimate accurately whether or not DCC loss is causal of disease progression in bladder cancer.

The oncofetal protein carcinoembryonic antigen (CEA), a 180 kDa transmembrane glycoprotein, is also a member of the IgSF, which has been shown to act as an accessory adhesion molecule mediating Ca^{2+}-independent homotypic aggregation. CEA is a normal cell product that is overexpressed by adenocarcinomas, primarily of the colon, breast, and lung. Where it functions as a CAM, CEA has also a role as an accessory SAM.

There have been several studies detailing the expression of CEA by transitional carcinoma cells, both *in vivo* and *in vitro*. These studies have yielded conflicting results. Positive staining for CEA has been demonstrated in 10–80% of cases, by various researchers (48). CEA expression was not correlated with grade or stage, although this finding is not universally accepted (49,50). A shift to cytoplasmic rather than membranous staining is found progressively more frequent in advanced grade and stage of the disease (48,51). Soluble serum or urine elevations of CEA are less frequent (52), while no correlation has been established between urine or serum CEA levels and CEA tissue expression (51).

In conclusion, it seems that CEA expression by bladder cancer cells is sporadic, with questionable clinical significance.

SELECTINS

Selectins are transmembrane glycoproteins which mediate heterotypic interactions between blood cells and endothelial cells (6,52). As these molecules are primarily expressed by endothelial cells and mainly involved in inflammatory processes, it is not surprising that no reports are available of the expression of selectins in bladder cancer.

CONCLUSIONS

From the above presentation it is obvious that multiple and diverse cell adhesion molecules take part in intercellular and cell–matrix interactions of bladder cancer. The progression of bladder cancer is a multistep process where some adhesive molecules play a pivotal role in the development of recurrences, invasion, and distant metastasis. In addition, recent data implicate some of these molecules in cell signalling and tumour suppression, with important consequences in the tumour growth.

Large studies are now in progress to validate the use of selected adhesion molecules as molecular tools for the diagnosis and assessment of bladder cancer. Furthermore, knowledge of the expression of some of them may provide us with crucial information regarding the response to treatment, the disease-free and overall survival of the bladder cancer patients. With regard to treatment in particular, some adhesive molecules have been considered as potential targets for immunotherapy, while studies are in progress to establish whether normal expression of the adhesive molecules restored by gene transfer or biological therapy can induce a less invasive and metastatic phenotype of bladder cancer.

It is therefore obvious that this field consists a challenging area of research and further knowledge will contribute to a more dynamic approach of diagnosis, prognosis, and treatment of bladder cancer.

Key Points

1. Aberrant expression of the E-cadherin–catenin complex in bladder cancer correlates with lack of differentiation, muscle invasion, and distant metastasis. Loss of normal complex expression has been shown to correlate with decreased recurrence-free and overall survival, although multivariate analysis suggests that it has no independent prognostic value over the grade and stage of the tumour.
2. Expression of integrins in bladder cancer is aberrant, downregulated and with a progressive loss of its expression from the normal urothelium to invasive bladder cancer. This abnormal expression is correlated with a more aggressive phenotype, local invasion, and metastasis.
3. Abnormal ICAM-1 expression facilitates avoidance of immunological surveillance, while C-CAM-1 acts as a tumour suppressor in human bladder tissue and its expression is downregulated in bladder cancer cells.

References

1 Albelda SM. Role of integrins and other cell adhesion molecules in tumor progression and metastasis. *Lab Invest* 1993, **68**, 4–17.

2 Takeichi M. Cadherins in cancer: implications for invasion and metastasis. *Curr Opin Cell Biol* 1993, **5**, 806–11.

3 Jezernik K. Desquamation of urinary bladder epithelial cells. *Pflugers Arch* 1996, **431**, 249–50.

4 Tuckwell DS, Weston SA, Humphries MJ. Integrins: a review of their structure and mechanisms of ligand binding. *Symp Soc Exp Biol* 1993, **47**, 107–36.

5 Edelman GM, Crossin KL. Cell adhesion molecules: implications for a molecular histology. *Annu Rev Biochem* 1991, **60**, 155–90.

6 Hynes RO, Lander AD. Contact and adhesive specificities in the associations, migrations, and targeting of cells and axons. *Cell* 1992, **68**, 303–22.

7 Takeichi M. Cadherin cell adhesion receptors as a morphogenetic regulator. *Science* 1991, **251**, 1451–5.

8 Duband JL, Dufour S, Hatta K *et al.* Adhesion molecules during somitogenesis in the avian embryo. *J Cell Biol* 1987, **104**, 1361–74.

9 Behrens J, Frixen U, Schipper J *et al.* Cell adhesion in invasion and metastasis. *Semin Cell Biol* 1992, **3**, 169–78.

10 Ozawa M, Kemler R. Molecular organization of the uvomorulin-catenin complex. *J Cell Biol* 1992, **116**, 989–96.

11 Shibamoto S, Hayakawa M, Takeuchi K *et al.* Tyrosine phosphorylation of beta-catenin and plakoglobin enhanced by hepatocyte growth factor and epidermal growth factor in human carcinoma cells. *Cell Adhes Commun* 1994, **1**, 295–305.

12 Hirano S, Kimoto N, Shimoyama Y *et al.* Identification of a neural alpha-catenin as a key regulator of cadherin function and multicellular organization. *Cell* 1992, **70**, 293–301.

13 Knudsen KA, Wheelock MJ. Plakoglobin, or an 83-kD homologue distinct from beta-catenin, interacts with E-cadherin and N-cadherin. *J Cell Biol* 1992, **118**, 671–9.

14 Ozawa M, Nuruki K, Toyoyama H, Ohi Y. Cloning of an alternative form of plakoglobin (gamma-catenin) lacking the fourth armadillo repeat. *J Biochem Tokyo* 1995, **118**, 836–40.

15 Su LK, Vogelstein B, Kinzler KW. Association of the APC tumor suppressor protein with catenins. *Science* 1993, **262**, 1734–7.

16 Tsao J, Shibata D. Further evidence that one of the earliest alterations in colorectal carcinogenesis involves APC. *Am J Pathol* 1994, **145**, 531–4.

17 Munemitsu S, Albert I, Rubinfeld B, Polakis P. Deletion of an amino-terminal sequence beta-catenin in vivo and promotes hyperphosporylation of the adenomatous polyposis coli tumor suppressor protein. *Mol Cell Biol* 1996, **16**, 4088–94.

18 Midgley CA, White S, Howitt R *et al.* APC expression in normal human tissues. *J Pathol* 1997, **181**, 426–33.

19 Hulsken J, Birchmeier W, Behrens J. E-cadherin and APC compete for the interaction with beta-catenin and the cytoskeleton. *J Cell Biol* 1994, **127**, 2061–9.

20 Rubinfeld B, Souza B, Albert I *et al.* The APC protein and E-cadherin form similar but independent complexes with alpha-catenin, beta-catenin, and plakoglobin. *J Biol Chem* 1995, **270**, 5549–55.

21 Behrens J, Mareel MM, Van-Roy FM, Birchmeier W. Dissecting tumor cell invasion: epithelial cells acquire invasive properties after the loss of uvomorulin-mediated cell-cell adhesion. *J Cell Biol* 1989, **108**, 2435–47.

22 Frixen UH, Behrens J, Sachs M *et al.* E-cadherin-mediated cell-cell adhesion prevents invasiveness of human carcinoma cells. *J Cell Biol* 1991, **113**, 173–85.

23 Fujisawa M, Miyazaki J, Takechi Y *et al.* The significance of E-cadherin in transitional-cell carcinoma of the human urinary bladder. *World J Urol* 1996, **14**, S12–5.

24 Del Ross JS, -Rosario AD, Bui HX *et al.* Expression of the CD44 cell adhesion molecule in urinary bladder transitional cell carcinoma. *Mod Pathol* 1996, **9**, 854–60.

25 Syrigos KN, Krausz T, Waxman J *et al.* E-cadherin expression in bladder cancer using formalin-fixed, paraffin-embedded tissues: correlation with histopathological grade, tumour stage and survival. *Int J Cancer* 1995, **64**, 367–70.

26 Lipponen PK, Eskelinen MJ. Reduced expression of E-cadherin is related to invasive disease and frequent recurrence in bladder cancer. *J Cancer Res Clin Oncol* 1995, **121**, 303–8.

27 Shimazui T, Schalken JA, Giroldi LA *et al*. Prognostic value of cadherin-associated molecules (alpha-, beta-, and gamma-catenins and p120cas) in bladder tumors. *Cancer Res* 1996, **56**, 4154–8.

28 Griffiths TR, Brotherick I, Bishop RI *et al*. Cell adhesion molecules in bladder cancer: soluble serum E-cadherin correlates with predictors of recurrence. *Br J Cancer* 1996, **74**, 579–84.

29 Banks RE, Porter WH, Whelan P *et al*. Soluble forms of the adhesion molecule E-cadherin in urine. *J Clin Pathol* 1995, **48**, 179–80.

30 Syrigos KN, Harrington K, Waxman J, Krausz T, Pignatelli M. Altered γ-catenin expression correlates with poor survival in patients with bladder cancer. *J Urol*, 1998, **160**, 1889–93.

31 Syrigos KN, Karayiannakis A, Syrigou EI, Harrington K, Pignatelli M Abnormal expression of p120 correlates with poor survival in patients with bladder cancer. *Eur J Cancer*, 1998, **34**, 2037–40.

32 Tsuda H, Zhang WD, Shimosato Y *et al*. Allele loss on chromosome 16 associated with progression of human hepatocellular carcinoma. *Proc Natl Acad Sci USA* 1990, **87**, 6791–4.

33 Katayama M, Hirai S, Kamihagi K *et al*. Soluble E-cadherin fragments increased in circulation of cancer patients. *Br J Cancer* 1994, **69**, 580–5.

34 Shiozaki H, Oka H, Inoue M *et al*. E-cadherin mediated adhesion system in cancer cells. *Cancer* 1996, **77**, 1605–13.

35 Hynes RO. The impact of molecular biology on models for cell adhesion. *Bioessays* 1994, **16**, 663–9.

36 Sonnenberg A, Linders CJ, Modderman PW *et al*. Integrin recognition of different cell-binding fragments of laminin (P1, E3, E8) and evidence that alpha 6 beta 1 but not alpha 6 beta 4 functions as a major receptor for fragment E8. *J Cell Biol* 1990, **110**, 2145–55.

37 Elices MJ, Osborn L, Takada Y *et al*. VCAM-1 on activated endothelium interacts with the leukocyte integrin VLA-4 at a site distinct from the VLA-4/fibronectin binding site. *Cell* 1990, **60**, 577–84.

38 Wilson CB, Leopard J, Cheresh DA, Nakamura RM. Extracellular matrix and integrin composition of the normal bladder wall. *World J Urol* 1996, **14**, S30–7.

39 Grossman HB, Washington RW Jr, Carey TE, Liebert M. Alterations in antigen expression in superficial bladder cancer. *J Cell Biochem* 1992, **161** (Suppl.), 63–8.

40 Liebert M, Washington R, Wedemeyer G *et al*. Loss of co-localization of alpha 6 beta 4 integrin and collagen VII in bladder cancer. *Am J Pathol* 1994, **144**, 787–95.

41 Liebert M, Washington R, Stein J *et al*. Expression of the VLA beta 1 integrin family in bladder cancer. *Am J Pathol* 1994, **144**, 1016–22.

42 Hunkapiller T, Hood L. Diversity of the immunoglobulin gene superfamily. *Adv Immunol* 1989, **44**, 1–63.

43 Jackson AM, Alexandroff AB, McIntyre M *et al*. Induction of ICAM 1 expression on bladder tumours by BCG immunotherapy. *J Clin Pathol* 1994, **47**, 309–12.

44 Nouri AM, Hussain RF, Dos-Santos AV, Oliver RT. Defective expression of adhesion molecules on human bladder tumour and human tumour cell lines. *Urol Int* 1996, **56**, 6–12.

45 Campbell SC, Tanabe K, Alexander JP *et al*. Intercellular adhesion molecule-1 expression by bladder cancer cells: functional effects. *J Urol* 1994, **151**, 1385–90.

46 Brewster SF, Gingell JC, Browne S, Brown KW. Loss of heterozygosity on chromosome 18q is associated with muscle-invasive transitional cell carcinoma of the bladder. *Br J Cancer* 1994, **70**, 697–700.

47 Miyamoto H, Shuin T, Ikeda I *et al*. Loss of heterozygosity at the p53, RB, DCC and APC tumour suppressor gene loci in human bladder cancer. *J Urol* 1996, **155**, 1444–7.

48 Takashi M, Murase T, Mitsuya H *et al*. Immunohistochemical localization of epithelial membrane antigen, carcinoembryonic antigen and secretory component in urinary bladder cancer *Hinyokika Kiyo* 1986, **32**, 541–52.

49 Casetta G, Cavallini A, Piana P *et al*. Immunohistochemical determination of antigen 19–9 (CA 19–9) in transitional carcinoma of the bladder. *Minerva Urol Nefrol* 1992, **44**, 169–72.

50 Wolf H. Prognostic factors in bladder carcinoma. *Scand J Urol Nephrol* 1991, **138**, 153–60.
51 Jakse G, Rauschmeier H, Rosmanith P, Hofstadter F. Determination of carci-noembryonic antigen in tissue, serum and urine in patients with transitional cell carcinoma of the urinary bladder. *Urol Int* 1983, **38**, 121–5.
52 Bevilacqua M, Butcher E, Furie B *et al.* Selectins: a family of adhesion recep-tors. *Cell* 1991, **67**, 233–7.

10. CLINICAL PRESENTATION AND INVESTIGATION OF BLADDER CANCER

John P. Stein and Donald G. Skinner

INTRODUCTION

Approximately 75–85% of patients with primary transitional cell carcinoma of the bladder present with low-grade tumours confined to the superficial mucosa. The risk of superficial recurrence in those patients with bladder tumours confined to the mucosa is 75%, with the majority of these cancers amenable to initial transurethral resection and selected administration of intravesical immuno- or chemotherapy (1–4). However, 20–40% of all patients with transitional cell carcinoma of the bladder will either initially present with, or develop an invasive carcinoma of the bladder. Furthermore, it has been reported that nearly 50% of these patients treated locally for invasive bladder cancer die of metastatic disease within 2 years of therapy (3). This obviously underscores the need to have a clear understanding of the clinical presentation of patients with bladder cancer, as well as the appropriate investigation (radiographic and cystoscopic evaluation) of this disease. Only with a better understanding of the clinical presentation and appropriate staging of this disease will the urologist be able to diagnose and effectively treat bladder cancer at an early curable stage in the hope of providing patients the best possible survival.

This chapter will review the clinical presentation of patients with bladder cancer. In addition, as treatment schemes and prognosis of patients with bladder cancer are based on the accurate clinical staging of the disease, the appropriate laboratory, radiographic, and cystoscopic evaluation of patients with bladder cancer will be discussed.

CLINICAL PRESENTATION

The average age of diagnosis for transitional cell carcinoma of the bladder is 69 years for males and 71 years for women (6). Interestingly, in contrast to almost all other urological malignancies, bladder cancer has rarely been reported as an incidental finding at autopsy (5,6). This is in direct contrast to prostate cancer and even renal cell carcinoma, in which autopsy discovered tumours are more common than the clinical diagnosis of the tumour. This observation suggests that prior to death, most patients with bladder cancer are diagnosed with the disease. This may also imply that the preclinical latency period (time prior to diagnosis) is relatively short, suggesting that this tumour progresses quickly enough to cause signs or symptoms which lead to the diagnosis of the disease. Furthermore, this supports the notion that all patients with bladder cancer should be treated appropriately for the disease based on their physiology age and not chronological age. We have recently evaluated our extensive experience with invasive bladder cancer in the elderly population (greater than 80 years) and emphasize that elderly patients can, and should be treated with excellent outcomes based on their overall medical condition and not necessarily their strict chronological age (7).

The most common finding in patients with bladder cancer is haematuria. Nearly 80% of patients present with some form of haematuria, which may be visible (gross) or discovered on routine urinalysis (microscopic) (8,9). The haematuria seen in patients with bladder cancer is classically painless and may be intermittent. Furthermore, while the degree of haematuria does not correlate with the extent of the disease, simply the presence of haematuria requires urological evaluation. This may be particularly important in patients over 50 years of age or with a known predisposing factor for bladder cancer. Known predisposing risk factors for bladder cancer include: those with a smoking history, those with a known exposure to industrial carcinogens, or those who have had indwelling catheters in their bladder for an extended period of time.

Irritative bladder or voiding symptoms are the second most common form of presentation seen in about 25% of patients with bladder cancer. Irritative voiding symptoms may include urinary urgency, frequency, and dysuria and are usually seen in patients with carcinoma *in situ* (CIS) or with an invasive bladder tumour (10,11). Furthermore, patients with irritative voiding symptoms and bladder cancer generally have associated haematuria. Although irritative voiding symptoms are more commonly suggestive of bacterial or interstitial cystitis, the physician must always consider a bladder tumour in any patient with irritative voiding symptoms without an obvious bladder infection.

Although uncommon, patients with bladder cancer may also present with symptoms of bladder outlet obstruction including: urinary retention, pelvic fullness, suprapubic pain or discomfort, with a suprapubic or pelvic mass. Ipsilateral flank pain may occur secondary to ureteral obstruction. Less commonly, when bilateral ureteral obstruction is present the patient may present with flank pain or renal insufficiency. Evidence of advanced or metastatic disease may present with constitutional symptoms including anorexia, weight loss, and generalized weakness. Patients with bone metastases may present with bone pain or even anaemia if there is extensive bone involvement.

The physical examination is usually unremarkable in most patients with bladder cancer. Patients with superficial bladder cancer confined to the mucosa or the submucosa generally have a normal physical examination. A careful physical examination is always necessary to exclude coexistent pathology. All patients should undergo a careful bimanual pelvic examination to determine the presence of a palpable mass, as well as any induration or fixation of contiguous organs or the pelvic side wall. In the female patient, the vaginal examination allows evaluation of the entire urethra and vagina. Patients with large or advanced bladder tumours may have abdominal tenderness, a bladder mass, or induration on physical examination.

RADIOGRAPHIC EVALUATION

An excretory urogram (intravenous pyelogram, IVP) is usually performed first to evaluate the upper urinary tract radiographically. This test should be performed prior to cystoscopy. Radiographic abnormalities of the upper urinary tract may include a cortical defect, hydronephrosis, a poorly or non-functional kidney, and a filling defect identified anywhere along the collecting system (calyces, renal pelvis, or ureter). Any filling defect or abnormality identified on the IVP, or if the entire upper urinary tract is not well visualized, can then be further assessed at the time of cystoscopy with retrograde ureteropyelography. Patients allergic to intravenous contrast material, or with a history of renal insufficiency may alternatively undergo an ultrasonography of the kidneys followed by bilateral retrograde ureteropyelography at cystoscopy. This ensures complete radiographic evaluation of the upper urinary tract and will identify any synchronous upper urinary tract urothelial tumours, which occur in about 5% of patients with bladder cancer (12).

Bladder filling defects are identified in only 50% of patients with bladder tumours on IVP (13). Large tumours are more easily identified and are characterized by non-specific filling defects of the bladder wall. In addition, non-symmetrical bladder wall expansion during the filling phase of the IVP may also suggest a bladder wall tumour (14). Other causes for a bladder filling defect include a blood clot, a bladder fold in a non-distended bladder, or the result of extrinsic compression from an adjacent organ. To improve the diagnostic evaluation of the bladder, IVP images should be obtained during early bladder filling, along with a distended bladder film, and a postevacuation film.

Bladder tumours associated with ipsilateral hydronephrosis, generally suggest an invasive lesion of the bladder (15,16). In fact, Hatch and Barry found ureteral obstruction to be associated with muscle invasion in over 90% of patients with transitional cell carcinoma and hydronephrosis (15).

We recently performed a retrospective analysis of 415 consecutive patients who underwent radical cystectomy for invasive bladder cancer at out institution from 1983 through 1993 (16). We evaluated the specific variable of hydronephrosis (unilateral and bilateral) as determined by preoperative radiographic imaging studies with regard to pathological stage and clinical outcome. Of these patients, 299 patients (72%) demonstrated no preoperative evidence of hydronephrosis, 94 patients (23%) had unilateral hydronephrosis, and 22 patients (5%) had bilateral hydronephrosis. All patients were uniformly treated and pathologically staged. A significant correlation between hydronephrosis and advanced cancer stage ($P < 0.0001$), and decreased patient survival ($P < 0.0001$) was identified. Of the 116 patients with either unilateral or bilateral hydronephrosis, 86% had muscle invasive tumours or greater (pathological stage >P2). Of the 94 patients with unilateral hydronephrosis, 83% demonstrated bladder tumours with pathological evidence of muscle invasion of the bladder (>P2). This confirms previous reports that patients presenting with unilateral hydronephrosis and bladder cancer generally have muscle invasive tumours. Furthermore, when evaluating patients with bladder cancer who present with bilateral hydronephrosis, over 90% of patients demonstrated advanced disease pathologically, with extension outside the bladder (>P3b, or lymph node positive disease). Moreover, the 5-year survival for patients with no hydronephrosis was 62%, compared with 45% and 30% for those with unilateral and bilateral hydronephrosis, respectively.

These data obviously suggest that patients with unilateral hydronephrosis have muscle invasive tumours, while those patients presenting with bilateral hydronephrosis have a more ominous prognosis. Obviously, the presence of hydronephrosis (unilateral or bilateral) as determined by preoperative radiographic imaging is an important piece of clinical information, which may help dictate therapy and provide prognostic information.

URINARY CYTOLOGY

Urinary cytology should be performed in all patients diagnosed or suspected to have bladder cancer. The evaluation of a voided urine specimen for exfoliated cancer cells may be particularly useful in patients with high-grade bladder tumours, or when CIS is present (16). The limitations of urinary cytology are due to the normal cytological appearance of well-differentiated tumours cells, and the fact that well-differentiated tumours cells are more cohesive and less commonly shed into the urine. Cytological results have been disappointing in patients with low-grade bladder tumours with an overall sensitivity of about 30% (17). In addition, about 20% of high-grade tumours or CIS will have a false negative urinary cytology. Moreover, a negative voided urinary cytology does not exclude the presence of a bladder tumour. In fact, because most low-grade bladder tumours have a normal urinary cytology, a positive urinary cytology in the context of a low-grade bladder tumour should raise the suspicion of a concomitant high-grade tumour. Even in the face of a normal radiographic evaluation, a positive urinary cytology should alert the physician to a bladder tumour somewhere along the urinary tract.

Ideally, urinary cytology should not be obtained from a first-voided morning specimen; rather from a well hydrated patient to optimize the appearance of the cancer cell. Cellular degeneration occurs in urine that has remained in the bladder for an extended period of time and should be avoided (18). Other factors that may artefactually alter the urinary cytology result include: urinary tract infection, indwelling catheters, bladder instrumentation, radiation therapy, and intravesical immuno- or chemotherapy. To improve the accuracy and sensitivity of urinary cytology, saline bladder washings may be employed (19). This mechanical action (barbotage) enhances tumour cell shedding and provides better cytological evaluation. A cytology specimen obtained by barbotage has been reported to be positive in 10% of patients with grade I bladder tumours, 50% of those with grade II tumours, and 90% of those with grade III tumours (20).

Recently, a urine antibody test for bladder tumour antigen (BTA, Bard Diagnostic Sciences, Redmond, WA, USA) has been developed to improve and add to the diagnostic capabilities of routine urinary cytology. The BTA test is an assay for the qualitative detection of bladder tumour antigen in the urine (21). The antigen is composed of basement membrane complexes that have been isolated and characterized from the urine of patients with bladder cancer. In a large, well designed, prospective, multicentre trial involving 499 patients, the BTA test was found to be more sensitive than urine cytology; the BTA was found to have an overall sensitivity of 40% compared with only 16% for urine cytology in detecting recurrent bladder cancer in patients with low-grade and low-stage tumours(21). Its sensitivity for low-grade tumours is approximately 30%. When stratified by stage, the BTA assay was more sensitive for Ta tumours than urinary cytology (31% versus 4%) and T1 tumours (48% versus 22%). Furthermore, for grade 2 tumours, the BTA assay was also more sensitive. Clearly, further evaluation of this assay is needed to define its true role in the initial evaluation of patients with bladder cancer. However, because the BTA test is a simple, rapid and an inexpensive adjunct to cystoscopy, and the fact that it is more sensitive than routine urinary cytology for low-grade and low-staged tumours, it may be an attractive method along with urinary cytology for the initial evaluation and surveillance of patients with bladder cancer.

CYSTOSCOPY

The diagnosis of bladder cancer is ultimately made on cystoscopic examination of the bladder, and pathological evaluation of the resected tumour specimen. When a bladder tumour is suspected from previous radiographic imaging studies, or identified cysto-scopically, or abnormal cells reported on urinary cytology, a careful bimanual examination is first performed. This should be performed in the lithotomy with good pelvic relaxation under general anaesthesia. This helps to determine the presence, extent, and fixation of a palpable bladder mass. If a bladder tumour is palpable prior to resection, then bimanual examination should also be performed following resection of the bladder tumour. The presence of a palpable bladder mass after transurethral resection implies extravesical tumour extension. Conversely, resolution of any induration or a palpable mass following complete trans-urethral resection suggests a more superficial tumour confined to the bladder.

Cystoscopic evaluation begins with careful inspection of the entire urethra, prostate, and bladder neck. Examination of the bladder should be comprehensive and methodical. Mapping of the entire bladder should be performed prior to resection or biopsy of any bladder tumours. The number, location, size, and configuration (papillary, flat, sessile, or nodular) of all tumours, and any associated mucosal abnormalities should be accurately recorded. Furthermore, retrograde pyelography should be first performed when the upper urinary tract has not been adequately evaluated, or is suspicious for a concomitant lesion seen on previous radiographic imaging studies. If an upper urinary tract lesion is identified, ipsilateral ureteral cytology, saline lavage, brushing biopsy, or even ureteroscopy may be performed for complete evaluation.

Only once the entire urinary tract has been completely evaluated (either radiographically or endoscopically) should transurethral resection or deep biopsy of the tumour be performed. This is important to establish a pathological diagnosis with determination of tumour grade and depth of tumour invasion. The accurate pathological determinants of the resected bladder tumour are critical in the clinical staging and treatment decision process of the patient with bladder cancer. Care must be taken during resection or biopsy to ensure an accurate histological evaluation. The use of excess cautery should be minimized to preserve the architectural structure of the tissue and avoid cautery artefact.

Directed bladder biopsies of adjacent and normal appearing bladder mucosa remote from the primary tumour should also be performed in conjunction with transurethral resection. Mucosal biopsies are best performed with the use of cold cup biopsy forceps. Mucosal biopsies should include (in addition to suspicious lesions) four uniform sites: lateral to both ureteral orifices, the trigone, and the dome of the bladder (Fig. 10.1). Biopsies need not be deep as only the mucosa requires histological examination. The results of these biopsies are an important adjunct that may influence treatment decisions particularly in the presence of low-grade superficial tumours. The presence of CIS associated with a low-grade tumour is known to increase the recurrence rate and may warrant early institution of intravesical immuno- or chemotherapy (22). In addition, transurethral biopsy of the prostatic urethra and stroma should be performed for complete staging purposes in men; nearly 30% of men with CIS will have prostatic involvement with tumour, which may also alter treatment recommendations (23).

The ideal method to resect a bladder tumour is, first, to resect the superficial portion followed by resection of the deeper portion along with a portion of the muscularis propria. These specimens should be submitted separately to the pathologist. Care must be taken during the resection of any tumour to prevent a bladder perforation and potential tumour spill. To minimize bladder perforations, resection of the tumour is best performed with the continuous-flow resectoscope while the bladder is only partially distended or filled. In addition, resection must be performed with the patient completely paralysed under general anaesthesia. It

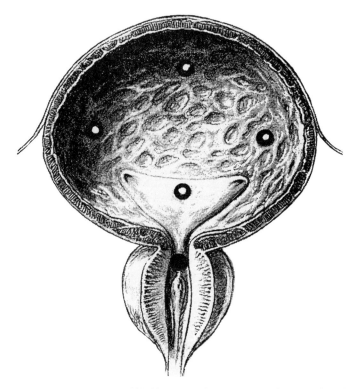

Fig. 10.1 *Suggested location of bladder mucosa biopsy: trigone, dome, and lateral to both ureteral orifices*

should be kept in mind that resecting bladder tumours on the lateral bladder wall may stimulate a obturator nerve reflex with violent contraction of the adductor muscles of the thigh and possible bladder perforation. Once the tumour is completely resected the site should be fulgurated.

Complete resection of an obvious invasive bladder tumour (broad-based, sessile), particularly when radical cystectomy is anticipated, should be avoided. Bladder tumours that encroach or involve a ureteral orifice can be completely resected. However, fulgeration of the ureteral orifice following resection should be avoided. If resection of a ureteral orifice is necessary, placement of a stent may be prudent to prevent acute ureteral obstruction secondary to oedema. Care must also be taken when a bladder tumour is identified in a bladder diverticulum. These tumours should be biopsied rather than resected. This reduces the risk of perforation of the thinned wall diverticuli which by definition lack any muscularis propria. Furthermore, patients with bladder tumours located in a bladder diverticulum are probably best treated with radical cystectomy and therefore an extensive resection is unnecessary; only a tissue diagnosis is required.

STAGING

The need for and the development of a staging system for bladder cancer was based on the observation that the extent of bladder wall invasion and tumour grade were important in determining the prognostic differences between various tumours. The American Joint Committee on Cancer (AJCC) is currently the most commonly used clinical and pathological staging system for bladder cancer (24). This staging system takes into account bladder tumours (T), includes the status and extent of the lymph node involvement (N), and the presence of metastases (M) and is described in detail elsewhere (Chapter 12). Prognostic differences exist between each of these clinical stages and currently determine appropriate treatment schemes. However, despite our best efforts there is still considerable clinical staging errors in patients with bladder cancer; nearly 30–40% of patients being understaged and 10–20% of patients being overstaged (25,26).

The clinical staging of a bladder tumour may also help dictate the extent of imaging techniques performed. Patients with superficial tumours treated conservatively (observation or intravesical therapy) rarely require elaborate staging studies such as computed tomography (CT) or bone scan imaging. However, patients with invasive tumours, or those undergoing more aggressive forms of therapy (cystectomy) may warrant these additional imaging studies when indicated.

Complete clinical staging should evaluate the most common metastatic sites for bladder cancer including the lungs, liver, and bone. A chest X-ray should be performed on all patients. A CT scan of the chest is only obtained when pulmonary metastases are suspected either by history, or because of an abnormal chest X-ray. In addition, liver function tests, and serum alkaline phosphatase should be obtained routinely on all patients with bladder cancer. All patients with an elevated serum alkaline phosphatase or with complaints of bone pain should undergo a bone scan. A CT scan of the abdomen/pelvis should be performed in patients with suspected metastases, elevated liver functions tests, a bladder tumour associated with ipsilateral or bilateral hydronephrosis, or in patients with a T4 primary bladder tumour; the results of which may impact upon the decision for neoadjuvant therapy. A CT scan of the abdomen and pelvis may also provide some clinical information regarding the pelvic and retroperitoneal lymph nodes as well as the presence of any liver lesions. However, a CT scan of the pelvis strictly for staging of the primary bladder tumour should not routinely be performed as it is neither sensitive nor specific enough to evaluate the degree of primary bladder wall tumour invasion (27). There is general agreement that CT scanning cannot differentiate between superficial and invasive bladder tumours owing to the similar density values of tumour and normal bladder wall. Furthermore, the evaluation of a bladder tumour extravesical extension with CT scanning is also poor. CT scanning cannot detect microscopic infiltration of the tumour beyond the bladder wall. It should be understood that benign perivesical changes (scar formation following previous operation or transurethral resection) cannot be differentiated from tumour growth on the imaging study (28). This is particularly true following a transurethral resections of a bladder tumour, or following irradiation therapy where oedema and artefactual changes in the bladder wall make interpretation difficult. One must keep in mind the limitations of CT scanning in the clinical staging of patients of the primary bladder tumour (29).

Commonly, CT scanning is performed to evaluate the regional (pelvic) and the retroperitoneal lymph nodes as well. However, CT scanning of the abdomen and pelvis may be limited in accuracy because it can detect only obvious gross extravesical tumour extension, and large (>2 cm) pelvic or retroperitoneal lymph nodes (30,31). Furthermore, a reactive or an enlarged pelvic or retroperitoneal lymph node (particularly following resection of a bladder tumour) is not diagnostic of tumour involvement. CT scanning can simply detect only the presence of enlarged lymph nodes; neither the internal architecture nor the pathological contents are revealed.

We believe the diagnostic value of CT scanning staging in patients with bladder cancer must be carefully considered. If the clinical investigation suggests an operable bladder tumour, it is not unreasonable to proceed and pathologically stage the patient with a pelvic lymphadenectomy and radical cystectomy. However, despite the limitations of CT scanning, some will argue that it is not unreasonable to perform an abdominal and pelvic CT scan; which is more sensitive than physical examination in grossly evaluating the regional and metastatic extent of the disease. Furthermore, proponents for neoadjuvant chemotherapy in the treatment of invasive bladder cancer may also argue there is a role for CT scanning of the abdomen and pelvis for staging purposes (32).

Magnetic resonance imaging (MRI) studies currently plays a small part in the evaluation of patients with bladder cancer. The resolution of the pelvic and retroperitoneal lymph nodes and anatomy is not as good as CT scanning. However, MRI may have a part in the evaluation of suspected bone metastases as it appears to be more sensitive than both CT and bone scans for this purpose.

MOLECULAR MARKERS

The optimal management of bladder cancer requires the detection, precise clinical staging, as well as the true assessment of the tumour's biological potential. Currently, histological evaluation (including determination of tumour grade and stage) are the primary prognostic variables which dictate treatment strategies for patients with bladder cancer. Although these two conventional histopathological variables provide a certain degree of stratification of a tumour's biological potential, there remains a significant degree of tumour heterogeneity even within various prognostic subgroups of bladder cancer. This makes the accurate and reliable prediction of the tumour's aggressiveness difficult. The future of clinical staging, with a more accurate determination of the aggressiveness of a specific bladder tumour may ultimately involve the application of various molecular or prognostic tumour markers. The ability to predict better an individual tumour's true biological potential would in turn facilitate treatment selection decisions and identify those patients who may benefit from adjuvant therapy or more aggressive therapy, and also identify these patients who may require less aggressive treatment strategies.

Advances in molecular biology have led to the discovery of certain suspected tumour markers which may influence cancer development and progression. Currently, the molecular marker best understood, and most well studied is the p53 tumour suppressor gene.

The p53 gene is located on chromosome 17p13 and encodes for a 53-kDa protein. The p53 gene functions as a tumour suppressor gene. Specifically, the p53 protein plays a vital part in the regulation of the cell cycle (34). When DNA damage occurs, the level of p53 protein increases causing cell cycle arrest. This allows for the repair of DNA and prevents propagation of the DNA defect. Mutations in the p53 gene result in the production of an abnormal and usually dysfunctional protein product with a prolonged half-life compared with the wild-type protein. Consequently, this abnormal protein accumulates in the cell nucleus and can be detected by immunohistochemical staining. Several studies have demonstrated that nuclear accumulation of p53 protein as determined by immunohistochemical staining correlates with gene mutations as detected by DNA sequence analysis (35,36).

Mutations in the p53 gene are the most common genetic defect in human tumours (33). Approximately 50–60% of invasive bladder tumours demonstrate p53 gene abnormalities. Furthermore, it has been shown that p53 alteration, as determined by immunohistochemical techniques, is an important prognostic indicator for bladder cancer progression (37–40). Increased p53 immunoreactivity has been found in higher grade and stage bladder cancers and is associated with increased disease progression and decreased disease-specific survival (37).

Our group evaluated p53 nuclear reactivity in 243 patients with invasive bladder cancer who were uniformly treated by radical cystectomy (37). We found that immunohistochemical detection of the p53 protein in tumour nuclei provided important prognostic information in this group of patients with bladder cancer. Patients with an increased p53 expression (altered p53) were found to have a significantly increased risk of disease recurrence and a significantly decreased overall survival when compared with those patients with a wild-type p53 (unaltered p53). This association was independent of tumour grade, pathological stage, and lymph node status and was strongest in patients with organ confined tumours (P1, P2, P3a). Furthermore, nuclear accumulation of p53 was found to be the only independent predictor of disease progression in a multivariable analysis of p53 status, histological grade and pathological stage in the overall group of patients.

Similar results were found by Lipponen and associates in 212 patients with primary bladder cancer who were evaluated for p53 immunoreactivity (39). Increased p53 nuclear reactivity was found to be a significant adverse prognostic factor in patients with muscle invasive bladder cancers. Increased tumour grade, as well as tumour progression were associated with increased p53 expression. In another study, Sarkis and associates evaluated p53 expression in 11 patients with muscle invasive bladder tumours treated with neoadjuvant chemotherapy (40). They found that increased p53 nuclear reactivity was significantly associated with disease progression and cancer specific death when compared with those patients without increased p53 nuclear reactivity.

Based on an accumulating amount of evidence supported by a number of independent studies, p53 determination appears to be an important prognostic tumour marker for bladder cancer progression. In general, increased expression of p53 as determined by immunohistochemical methods is more commonly seen in higher grade and invasive bladder tumours. Furthermore, increased p53 immunoreactivity is associated with a higher likelihood of disease progression and cancer-specific death. Patients diagnosed with bladder tumours with p53 alterations may have a higher incidence of tumour recurrence and disease progression which may therefore warrant an early and aggressive form of therapy. On the contrary, patients with bladder tumours demonstrating no evidence of p53 alterations may be treated in a more conservative fashion.

Key Points

1. Elderly patients can, and should be treated with excellent outcomes based on their overall medical condition and not necessarily their strict chronological age.
2. The most common findings in patients with bladder cancer is haematuria (80%) and irritative bladder or voiding symptoms (25%). Although uncommon, patients with bladder cancer may also present with urinary retention, pelvic fullness, suprapubic pain or discomfort, and with a suprapubic or pelvic mass.
3. Bladder tumours associated with ipsilateral hydronephrosis, generally suggest an invasive lesion of the bladder, while those patients presenting with bilateral hydronephrosis have a more ominous prognosis.
4. Urinary cytology should be performed in all patients diagnosed or suspected to have bladder cancer and it may be particularly useful in patients with high-grade bladder tumours, or when CIS is present.
5. The diagnosis of bladder cancer is ultimately made on cystoscopic examination of the bladder, and pathological evaluation of the resected tumour specimen.

Incorporating molecular markers in the clinical evaluation and staging of bladder cancer is currently in its infancy. However, the application of various molecular markers (p53), in addition to clinical staging in patients with bladder cancer, may provide valuable additional prognostic information with therapeutic implications. It is very possible that this form of research may one day become an integral component of clinical staging and dictate therapeutic management schemes.

References

1　Parker SL, Tong T, Bolden S, Wing PA. *Cancer statistics 1996. CA* 1996, **46**, 8–11.
2　Crawford ED, Davis MA. Nontransitional cell carcinomas of the bladder. In: *Genitourinary cancer management* (ed. De Kernian JB, Paulson DF). Lea & Febiger, Philadelphia, 1987, 95–105.
3　Skinner DG, Lieskovsky G. Management of invasive and high-grade bladder cancer. In: *Diagnoses and management of genitorurinary cancer* (ed. Skinner DG, Lieskovsky G), Vol. 1. WB Saunders, Philadelphia, 1988, 295–312.
4　Droller MJ. Individualizing the approach to invasive bladder cancer. *Contemp Urol* 1990, **July/August**, 54–61.
5　Resseguie LT, Nobrega FT, Farrow GM *et al.* Epidemiology of renal and ureteral cancer in Rochester, Minnesota, 1950–74, with special reference to clinical and pathologic features. *Mayo Clin Proc* 1978, **53**, 503–10.
6　Kishi K, Hirota T, Matsumoto K *et al.* Carcinoma of the bladder: A clinical and pathological analysis of 87 autopsy cases. *J Urol* 1981, **125**, 36–9.
7　Figueroa AF, Stein JP, Dickinson M *et al.* Radical cystectomy in the elderly patient: an updated experience with 404 patients. *Cancer* 1998, **83**, 141–7.
8　Fitzpatrick JM. Superficial bladder cancer: natural history, evaluation and manggement. *AUA Update Ser* 1989, **8**, 82–7.
9　Wallace DM, Harris DL. Delay in treating bladder tumors. *Lancet* 1965, **i**, 332.
10　Utz DC, Hanash KA, Farrow GM *et al.* The plight of the patient with carcinoma in situ of the bladder. *J Urol* 1970, **103**, 160–4.
11　Farrow GM. Clinical observations in 69 cases of an in situ carcinoma of the bladder. *Cancer Res* 1977, **37**, 2794–8.
12　Oldbring J, Glifberg I, Mikulowski P *et al.* Carcinoma of the renal pelvis and ureter following bladder carcinoma. Frequency, risk factors and clinicopathological findings. *J Urol* 1989, **141**, 1311–3.
13　Hillman BJ, Silvert M, Cook G *et al.* Recognition of bladder tumors by excretory urography. *Radiology* 1981, **138**, 319–23.
14　Dershaw DD, Panicek DM. Imaging of invasive bladder cancer. *Semin Oncol* 1990, **17**, 544–50.
15　Hatch TR, Barry JM. The value of excretory radiography in staging bladder cancer. *J Urol* 1986, **135**, 49.
16　Badalament RA, Fair WR, Whitmore WF *et al.* The relative value of cytometry and cytology in the management of bladder cancer. *Semin Urol* 1988, **6**, 22–30.
17　Zein T, Wajsman Z. Evaluation of bladder washings and urine cytology in the diagnosis of bladder cancer and its correlation with selected biopsies of the bladder mucosa. *J Urol* 1984, **132**, 670–5.
18　Koshikawa T, Leyh H, Schenck U. Difficulties in evaluating urinary specimens after local mitomycin therapy of bladder cancer. *Diagn Cytopathol* 1989, **5**, 117–21.
19　Matzkin H, Moinuddin S *et al.* Value of urine cytology versus bladder washing in bladder cancer. *Urology* 1992, **39**, 201.
20　Soloway MS, Morrison DA. Modalities used in the diagnosis, staging and evaluation of bladder cancer. *AUA Update Ser* 1985, **4**, 1–7.
21　Sarosdy MF, De Vere White RW. Results of a multicenter trial using the BTA test to monitor for and diagnose recurrent bladder cancer. *J Urol* 1995, **154**, 379–83.
22　Smith G, Elton RA, Beynon LL *et al.* Prognostic significance of biopsy result of normal-looking mucosa in cases of superficial bladder cancer. *Br J Urol* 1983, **55**, 665–9.

23 Grabstalt H. Prostatic biopsy in selected patients with carcinoma in situ of the bladder: Preliminary report. *J Urol* 1984, **132**, 1117–9.

24 American Joint Committee on Cancer (AJCC). *Cancer staging manual*, 5th edn. J.B. Lippincott-Raven, Philadelphia, 1997.

25 Skinner DG. Current state of classification and staging of bladder cancer. *Cancer Res* 1977, **37**, 2838–41.

26 Skinner DG, Tift JP, Kaufman JJ. High dose, short course preoperative radiation therapy and immediate single stage radical cystectomy with pelvic node dissection in the management of bladder cancer. *J Urol* 1982, **127**, 671–4.

27 Nishimura K, Hida S. The validity of magnetic resonance imaging (MRI) in the staging of bladder cancer: Comparison with computed tomography (CT) and transurethra ultrasonography (US). *Jpn J Clin Oncol* 1988, **18**, 217–21.

28 Sager EM, Talle K, Fossa S *et al.* The role of CT in demonstrating perivesical tumor growth in the preoperative staging of carcinoma of the urinary bladder. *Radiology* 1983, **146**, 443–6.

29 Lantz EJ, Hattery RR. Diagnostic imaging of urothelial cancer. *Urol Clin North Am* 1984, **11**, 567–83.

30 Nurmi M, Kateyuo K, Puntala P. Reliability of CT in preoperative evaluation of bladder carcinoma. *Scand J Urol Nephrol* 1988, **22**, 125–8.

31 Voges GE, Tauschke E, Stockle M *et al.* Computerized tomography: An unreliable method for accurate staging fo bladder tumors in patients who are candidates for radical cystectomy. *J Urol* 1989, **142**, 972–4.

32 Scher HI, Yagoda A, Herr HW *et al.* Neoadjuvant M-VAC (methotrexate, vinblastine, doxorubicin and cisplatin) effect on the primary bladder lesion. *J Urol* 1988, **139**, 470–4.

33 Hollstein M, Sidransky D, Vogelstein B *et al.* P53 mutations in human cancers. *Science* 1991, **253**, 49–53.

34 Lane DP. Cancer: p53, guardian of the genome. *Nature* 1992, **358**, 15–17.

35 Esrig D, Spruck CH III, Nichols PW *et al.* P53 nuclear protein accumulation correlates with mutations in the p53 gene, tumor grade, and stage in bladder cancer. *Am J Pathol* 1993, **143**, 1389–97.

36 Dalbagni G, Cordon-Cardo C *et al.* Tumor suppressor alterations in bladder cancer. *Surg Oncol Clin North Am* 1995, **4**, 231.

37 Esrig D, Elmajian D *et al.* Accumulation of nuclear p53 and tumor progression in bladder cancer. *N Engl J Med* 1994, **331**, 1259.

38 Cordon-Cardo C, Dalbagni G, Saez GT *et al.* P53 mutations in human bladder cancer: genotypic versus phenotypic patterns. *Int J Cancer* 1994, **56**, 347–53.

39 Lipponen PK. Over-expression of the p53 nuclear onocprotein in transitional cell carcinoma of the bladder and its prognostic value. *Int J Cancer* 1993, **53**, 365–9.

40 Sarkis AS, Dalbagni G, Cordon-Cardo C *et al.* Nuclear over-expression of p53 protein in transitional cell bladder carcinoma: a marker for disease progression. *J Natl Cancer Inst* 1993, **85**, 53–9.

11. Prognostic factors in the management of invasive bladder cancer

John P. Stein and Donald G. Skinner

Introduction

The optimal management of invasive bladder cancer requires the early detection and accurate assessment of the tumour's true biological potential. Histological evaluation, including determination of tumour grade and stage, have been and continue to be the primary variables which provide prognostic information and help dictate treatment strategies for patients with bladder cancer. Although these two conventional histopathological variables (grade, stage) provide a certain degree of stratification of a tumour's biological potential, there remains a significant degree of tumour heterogeneity even within various subgroups. This makes the accurate and reliable prediction of the tumour's aggressiveness difficult. Furthermore, the ability to predict precisely an individual tumour's true biological potential would in turn facilitate better treatment selection decisions for patients who may benefit from adjuvant therapy, and also identify patients who may require less aggressive treatment strategies.

Conventional tumour grade and stage remain the primary prognostic determinants in patients with invasive bladder cancer; however, intense research efforts are being made to identify and characterize better the different types of bladder cancer and their varying biological potential. Our understanding of tumour biology has evolved rapidly over the past decade which has been prompted by advances in molecular biology, immunology, and cytogenetics. This increase in knowledge has provided an opportunity to identify and evaluate novel tumour markers which may provide some additional prognostic information beyond general histology and gross DNA content, in order to distinguish better the potential behaviour of an individual tumour. This has led to the discovery of various molecular prognostic markers which are only now beginning to be applied in a clinical manner (translational research).

Transitional cell carcinoma of the bladder has generally been viewed as two different disease processes; superficial (non-invasive) and invasive bladder cancers. The desire to predict which superficial tumours will recur or progress, and which invasive tumours will metastasize has led to the development of a variety of bladder cancer prognostic markers. Superficial bladder tumours are generally thought to be more of a locally proliferative, recurrent process, but can maintain the potential to become invasive and even metastatic. The use of molecular markers may help guide decision making processed in the treatment of superficial bladder cancer (1). The ability to stratify superficial tumours with invasive or metastatic capabilities, to those superficial tumours unlikely to become invasive or clinically threatening would obviously be of great clinical benefit. Superficial bladder tumours that maintain a more malignant phenotype may be better treated with early aggressive intravesical therapy, or even cystectomy. On the other hand, muscle invasive bladder cancer is notorious for its potential clinical virulence, and is ideally treated with surgical extirpation (2). Despite this aggressive form of therapy, there remains a significant incidence of recurrence and disease progression in some patients, who may ultimately benefit from some adjuvant form of chemotherapy. In this chapter we will discuss routine conventional prognostic indices (tumour grade and stage), as well as more novel prognostic markers (molecular) and comment on their potential clinical application in bladder cancer today.

PATHOLOGICAL STAGE

Currently, radical cystectomy provides the optimal result with regards to accurate pathological staging, prevention of local recurrence, and overall survival in patients with bladder cancer. In contemporary series, the best long-term survival rates for invasive bladder cancer have been achieved with radical cystectomy (3,4–6). In the male, radical cystectomy includes removal of the prostate and seminal vesicles and regional lymph nodes; in the female, it includes removal of the cervix, uterus, ovaries, and if necessary the anterior vaginal wall, as well as the regional lymph nodes. Complete histological evaluation of the radical cystectomy specimen along with the regional lymph nodes provides accurate evaluation of the extent of the primary bladder tumour (p-stage), the degree of tumour differentiation (grade), and the status of the regional lymph nodes; all important factors which may influence the decision for adjuvant therapy based upon pathological criteria.

The natural history of high-grade invasive bladder tumours suggests that invasive bladder tumours tend to invade progressively from their superficial origin in the mucosa, to the lamina propria, and sequentially into the muscularis propria, perivesical fat, and contiguous pelvic organs; with an increasing incidence of lymph node involvement at each site (6–8). Despite recent advances in radiographic imaging techniques, error in clinical staging of the primary bladder tumour is common (9,10). Radical cystectomy, however, provides accurate pathological staging of the primary bladder tumour and regional lymph nodes.

Pathological staging of the primary bladder tumour has been, and remains today the most clinically important and useful prognostic variable regarding clinical outcomes (recurrence and survival) in patients treated for bladder cancer (8,11–15) The most commonly employed pathological staging system for bladder cancer is the TNM system proposed by the American Joint Committee on Cancer (15).

We have recently evaluated our extensive long-term experience with radical cystectomy in the treatment and management of invasive transitional cell carcinoma of the bladder (16). A comprehensive computerized bladder cancer database has been developed and maintained to provide clinical and demographic information on these patients, pathological characteristics of the radical cystectomy specimen, and clinical outcome (recurrence and survival) results in these patients.

Between July 1971 and June 1997, a total of 994 patients undergoing radical cystectomy with bilateral pelvic lymphadenectomy with the intent to cure for bladder cancer were evaluated. The pathological characteristics of the cystectomy specimens and long-term follow-up were analysed. Of these 994 patients; 802 (80%) were men, and 182 (20%) were women. The median age at cystectomy was 64 years with a range of 22–93 years. All patients were treated uniformly with *en bloc* radical cystectomy and pelvic lymphadenectomy with a median follow-up of 8.19 years. The two treatment variables in this group of patients were the use of a high-dose, short course of preoperative radiation therapy to 86 patients between 1971 and 1978 (4) and adjuvant chemotherapy in selected patients from 1978 to the present (17). The most significant prognostic variable in this group of patients was the primary pathological stage of their bladder tumour, and the status of the regional lymph nodes.

The pathological stage of the 994 patients include:

- 58 patients with P0 (6%)—no evidence of tumour
- 97 patients with Pis disease only (10%)—carcinoma *in situ*
- 38 patients with Pa disease (4%)—non-invasive papillary carcinoma
- 180 patients with P1 disease (18%)—lamina propria invasion
- 90 patients with P2 disease (9%)—tumour invades superficial (inner half) muscle

● 91 patients with P3a disease (9%)—tumour invade deep (outer half) muscle

● 126 patients with P3b disease (13%)—tumour extends into the perivesical tissue

● 76 patients with P4 disease (7%)—tumour invades contiguous structures or the pelvic side-wall

● 238 patients with lymph node involvement with tumour (24%)

The 5- and 10-year recurrence-free survival for the 58 patients with P0 (lymph node negative) disease was found to be 92% and 86%, respectively (Table 11.1). The estimated overall probability of survival for these patients with P0 disease is 85% at 5 years, and 71% at 10 years. These results are similar to patients with Pis (lymph node negative) disease. The 5- and 10-year recurrence-free survival for patients with Pis is 91% and 87%, respectively, with an estimated overall probability of survival of 91% and 74% at 5 and 10 years respectively. A total of 38 patients demonstrated Pa (lymph node negative) disease; 27 (71%) with and 11 without associated carcinoma *in situ*. The association of carcinoma *in situ* did not significantly affect the 5- and 10-year recurrence or overall survival in these small groups of patients ($P = 0.1$). The 5- and 10-year recurrence-free survival for the entire 38 patients with Pa (lymph node negative) disease is 78% and 71%, respectively, with

Table 11.1

THE REPORTED 5- AND 10-YEAR RECURRENCE-FREE SURVIVAL AND OVERALL SURVIVAL RATES FOR PATIENTS UNDERGOING RADICAL CYSTECTOMY FOR BLADDER CANCER ACCORDING TO PATHOLOGICAL STAGE

Pathological stage*	No. of patients	Recurrence-free survival (%)		Overall survival (%)	
		5 years	10 years	5 years	10 years
P0	58	92	86	85	71
Pis	96	91	87	91	74
Pa	38	78	71	79	66
P1	179	80	76	76	57
P2	90	90	87	77	56
P3a	91	77	74	67	50
P3b	125	62	61	51	32
P4	72	53	47	43	31
LN† +	227	35	33	32	26
All	976	68	65	62	47

* Based on T-N-M pathologic staging system.
† Lymph node involvement

an estimated overall probability of survival of 79% and 66% at 5 and 10 years, respectively. Furthermore, of the 180 patients with P1 (lymph node negative) disease; 142 (80%) specimens were found to have associated carcinoma *in situ*, while 38 demonstrated no evidence of associated carcinoma *in situ*. The presence of carcinoma *in situ* in this group of patients also did not significantly affect the 5- and 10-year recurrence or overall probability of survival (*P* = 0.12). The 5- and 10-year recurrence-free survival for the entire 180 patients with P1 (lymph node negative) disease is 80% and 76%, respectively, with an estimated overall probability of survival of 76% and 57% at 5 and 10 years respectively. When collectively evaluating the 371 patients (38%) with superficial tumours (P0, Pis, Pa, P1), the 5- and 10-year recurrence-free survival was 85% and 80%, respectively. The overall probability of survival in this group was 82% at 5 years and 64% at 10 years.

The 5- and 10-year recurrence-free survival for patients with superficial muscle invasive (P2) lymph node negative disease is 90% and 87%, respectively, with an overall probability of survival of 77% at 5 years, and 56% at 10 years. The 5- and 10-year recurrence-free survival for patients with deep muscle invasive (P3a) lymph node negative disease is 77% and 74%, respectively, with an overall probability of survival of 77% at 5 years and 74% at 10 years.

Patients with extravesical tumour extension (P3b) lymph node negative disease demonstrated a 5- and 10-year recurrence-free survival of 62% and 61%, respectively, and an overall probability of survival of 51% at 5 years and 32% at 10 years. The 5- and 10-year recurrence-free survival for patients with locally extensive P4 lymph node negative disease was 53% and 47%, respectively, with an overall probability of survival of 43% at 5 years and 31% at 10 years.

The overall 5- and 10-year recurrence rates for all patients with organ confined (P0, Pis, Pa, P1, P2, P3a) bladder tumours is 84% and 80%, respectively, with an overall probability of survival of 78% at 5 years and 60% at 10 years (Table 11.2). This suggest that patients with pathologically organ confined bladder cancer have a good prognosis. Patients with superficial and muscle invasive bladder tumours that are confined to the bladder have low recurrence rates and excellent survival following radical cystectomy. The overall 5- and 10-year recurrence-free survival rates for patients with extravesical or locally extensive bladder tumours (P3b, P4) without evidence of lymph node involvement is 59% and 56%, respectively, with an overall probability of survival of 48% at 5 years and 31% at 10 years. These data demonstrate that the pathological stage of the primary bladder tumour is an important prognostic factor; patients with higher pathological stages have increased recurrence rates and poorer overall survival rates.

Table 11.2

THE REPORTED 5- AND 10-YEAR RECURRENCE-FREE SURVIVAL AND OVERALL SURVIVAL RATES FOR PATIENTS UNDERGOING RADICAL CYSTECTOMY FOR BLADDER CANCER ACCORDING TO PATHOLOGICAL GROUPS					
		Recurrence-free survival (%)		Overall survival (%)	
Pathological group	No. of patients	5 years	10 years	5 years	10 years
Organ confined*	552	84	80	78	60
Extravesical†	197	59	56	48	31
Lymph node positive	227	35	33	32	26

* Lymph node negative tumours (P0, Pis, Pa, P1, P2, P3a).
† Lymph node negative tumours (P3b, P4).

A total of 227 (23%) patients demonstrated tumour involvement of their regional or pelvic lymph nodes. The overall 5- and 10-year recurrence-free survival in this group of patients was 35% and 33%, respectively, with a 32% overall probability of survival at 5 years and 26% probability of survival at 10 years (Table 11.1). These patients could be stratified by their extent of lymph node involvement (Table 11.3). The 5-year recurrence-free survival for

Table 11.3

THE REPORTED 5- AND 10-YEAR RECURRENCE-FREE SURVIVAL AND OVERALL SURVIVAL RATES FOR PATIENTS UNDERGOING RADICAL CYSTECTOMY FOR BLADDER CANCER ACCORDING TO LYMPH NODE INVOLVEMENT					
		Recurrence-free survival (%)		Overall survival (%)	
	No. of patients	5 years	10 years	5 years	10 years
No. of lymph nodes involved					
1 lymph node	85	43	39	43	33
2–4 lymph nodes	67	38	36	37	29
>5 lymph nodes	75	23	23	17	15
Subgroup by p-stage*					
(P0, Pis, Pa, P1)	18	55	55	53	52
(P2, P3a)	54	45	43	51	39
(P3b, P4)	155	29	25	23	18

* All patients with lymph node involvement stratified by their p-stage.

patients with one ($n = 85$), two to four ($n = 67$), and five ($n = 75$) or more lymph nodes was 43%, 38%, and 23%; with a 10-year recurrence-free survival of 39%, 36%, and 23%, respectively, in the same groups of patients. The overall probability of survival in those patients with one, two to four, and five or more lymph nodes was 44%, 37%, and 17% at 5 years, and 33%, 29%, and 15% at 10 years, respectively.

Patients with lymph node involvement could also be stratified according to their primary bladder tumour (Table 11.3). Of the 227 patients with lymph node involvement, a total of 18 (8%) had superficial bladder tumours (P0, Pa, Pis, P1), 54 (27%) had muscle invasive, organ confined tumours (P2, P3a), and 155 (65%) had extravesical extension (P3b, P4) of their bladder tumour. The 5- and 10-year recurrence-free survival for those patients with lymph node involvement whose primary bladder tumour was superficial, muscle invasive, and extending extravesical was 55% and 55%, 45% and 43%, and 29% and 23%, respectively. The 5- and 10-year overall probability of survival in these same groups of patients with lymph node involvement was 53% and 52%, 51% and 39%, and 23% and 18%, respectively. Although these data demonstrate that lymph node involvement is an adverse prognostic factor, this group of patients could be stratified according to the number of lymph nodes involved and the primary characteristics of the primary bladder tumour (p-stage).

These data from a large group of patients, uniformly treated, over a long period of time, with long-term follow-up clearly define that pathological evaluation of the primary bladder tumour and the status of the lymph nodes is an important prognostic factor in patients undergoing radical cystectomy. Pathological evaluation of the cystectomy specimen, including assessment of the primary bladder tumour and the status of the lymph nodes, currently provides the most reliable and accurate determination of a patients' prognosis regarding recurrence-free and overall survival.

BLADDER CANCER MARKERS

At the present, conventional histopathological evaluation of bladder cancer (tumour grade and stage) is most commonly performed to provide information regarding prognosis and treatment. However, there is clearly a need to identify additional tumour markers which may better define the tumour characteristics than tumour grade or stage. With a better understanding of the cell cycle, cell-to-cell interactions, and cell-to-extracellular matrix interactions, along with improved diagnostic techniques, progress is being made to identify and characterize additional potential prognostic markers for patients with transitional cell carcinoma of the bladder. The ultimate goal is to develop reliable prognostic markers which will accurately predict not only the course of an individual bladder tumour but also the response of that tumour to therapy. This information may then be employed to dictate more aggressive treatment regimens for those patients with tumours that are likely to progress, and less aggressive treatment regimens for those patients with tumours that are unlikely to progress.

TUMOUR-ASSOCIATED ANTIGENS

Although a number of monoclonal antibodies have been generated that are specific to transitional cell carcinoma of the bladder (18), only three antigens (M344, 19A211, and T138) appear to posses any proven prognostic clinical application (19). The monoclonal antibodies M344 and 19A211 are reactive to superficial bladder tumours antigens which are absent in normal transitional epithelium. The M344 antigen is a cytoplasmic mucin-like antigen that is expressed in 70% of superficial (Ta, T1) bladder tumours, 25% of carcinoma *in situ* (TIS) tumours, and approximately 15% of invasive bladder tumours. In general, M344 expression decreases with increasing tumour grade and is rarely positive in poorly differentiated, aneuploid bladder tumours (19). The 19A211 antigen is a sialoglycoprotein cell–surface antigen that is expressed in 70% of Ta and T1 tumours, 60% of TIS tumours, and approximately 50% of invasive tumours (19). In a prospective study evaluating M344 and 19A211 expression, 260 bladder irrigations from 140 patients with a history of bladder cancer were analysed (20). Overall, 95% of Ta and T1 tumours with positive urinary cytology, and 85% of those with negative urine cytology were positive for these antibodies. In addition, 30% of patients with a normal cystoscopic examination and a previous history of a bladder tumour demonstrated a positive antibody test. Those patients with a positive test had a 75% recurrence rate compared with only a 20% recurrence rate for those without M344 or 19A211 expression. These data suggest a potential role for these antibodies in evaluating for and monitoring superficial bladder cancer.

The T138 antigen is a surface glycoprotein that is expressed in approximately 15% of superficial Ta and T1 bladder tumours and 60% of muscle invasive bladder cancers (19). This antigen is not expressed in normal transitional epithelium. However, reactive urothelium may be positive for this antigen. The expression of

T138 in patients with bladder cancer was found to be associated with the development of metastatic disease in two independent studies (21,22). Fradet and associates evaluated 68 patients with bladder cancer and found that cancer-specific death occurred in 35% of patients with diploid, T138 positive tumours, in no patient with diploid, T138 negative tumours, and in 65% of patients with aneuploid, T138 positive tumours (22). Furthermore, 80% of patients with Ta or T1, T138 positive tumours demonstrated disease progression in this study. The T138 antigen appears to be a promising bladder cancer marker, but will require further evaluation to define its true clinical role as a prognostic marker.

Recently, several additional tests have been developed that can be performed on voided urinary specimens in an attempt to provide predictive information for the presence of bladder cancer in patients with a history of bladder cancer. These urinary tests include the BTA test (Bard Urological, Covington, GA, USA), the BTA Stat test (Bard Diagnostic Sciences, Inc., Redmond, WA, USA), the BTA TRAK assay (Bard Diagnostic Sciences, Inc.), and the determination of urinary nuclear matrix protein (NMP22, Matritech Inc., Newton, MA, USA).

The BTA test is a latex agglutination assay which detects the presence of basement membrane antigens that have been isolated and characterized in the urine of patients with bladder cancer (19). Early studies with the BTA test suggested that it may be more sensitive than voided urine cytology in the detection of newly diagnosed and recurrent superficial bladder cancer (23,24). However, the sensitivities of voided urine cytology reported in these studies were considerably lower than what had previously been reported in the literature, and the BTA test did not perform much better than cytology in the detection of low-grade/low-stage disease. More recent studies have demonstrated that the sensitivity of the BTA test may be no better than that of voided urine cytology, and that the BTA test may be limited by false positive reactions in patients with inflammatory bladder conditions or other genitourinary malignancies (25,26). Consequently, two newer assays, the BTA Stat and BTA TRAK assays, have been introduced which may prove to be more sensitive than the original BTA test in the detection of bladder cancer (27–31). These assays detect a human complement factor H-related protein that is produced *in vitro* by several human bladder cancer cell lines but not by other epithelial cell lines (27,30). However, both the BTA Stat and BTA TRAK assays continue to be limited by false positive reactions in those patients with a recent history of genitourinary trauma, stone disease, urinary tract inflammation, and other genitourinary malignancies (27,30).

Nuclear matrix proteins (NMPs) make up the non-chromatin structure of the nucleus. Certain NMPs have been identified as specific markers for particular tumours including bladder cancer (NMP22) (32). Recent studies have examined the ability of the urinary NMP22 assay to detect newly diagnosed and recurrent bladder tumours (32–35). Although results have been promising, these studies are preliminary and further investigation will be required to determine the appropriate use of the urinary NMP22 assay in the evaluation and detection of bladder cancer.

PROLIFERATING ANTIGENS

The fraction of proliferating cells (the growth fraction) of a tumour is an important prognostic feature of many malignancies and may help better to define the biological potential of a tumour. Markers used to assess cellular proliferation have included mitotic count, silver-stained nucleolar organizer regions (AgNORs), Ki-67, and the proliferating cell nuclear antigen (PCNA). The two most promising markers of cellular proliferation appear to be Ki-67 and PCNA. Increased expression of these antigens indicates a higher level of proliferative activity in tumour cells and in general is associated with tumours of more aggressive biological potential with an increased propensity for tumour progression and metastasis (19).

Ki-67

Ki-67 is a murine monoclonal antibody which reacts with a nuclear antigen expressed in proliferating cells (36). Although the exact nature of this antigen has not been well characterized, it is thought that Ki-67 recognizes a nuclear protein involved in the DNA replicase complex (37). Since the discovery of this antibody in 1983, it has been extensively evaluated in a variety of human malignancies (38). Okamura and associates evaluated 55 bladder cancers with Ki-67 immunostaining and found a correlation between increased expression of this antigen and increased tumour grade and stage (39). Several other studies have confirmed this relationship and have also found a significantly higher recurrence rate in bladder cancer patients whose tumours demonstrated a higher proliferative index as determined by increased Ki-67 immunoreactivity (40–45). Overall, there appears to be some evidence to suggest that the cellular proliferative index of a tumour as determined by Ki-67 labelling index, may supplement the routine use of histological grade and stage in assessing a bladder tumour's aggressiveness and metastatic potential.

Proliferating cell nuclear antigen

PCNA is a well-characterized antigen critical to DNA polymerase delta activity (47,48). This antigen is present in all proliferating eukaryotic cells and plays an important part in the cell cycle. Recently developed techniques allow for the immunohistochemical evaluation of PCNA expression in formalin-fixed tissues. Cohen and associates evaluated 25 transitional cell carcinomas of the bladder for PCNA expression and found a strong correlation between tumour grade and stage and PCNA expression by immunohistochemistry (41). With further investigation PCNA may become a more widely employed prognostic tumour marker for bladder cancer. None the less, before any marker of proliferative activity can be applied in clinical practice, its prognostic ability must be evaluated prospectively in larger groups of patients.

ONCOGENES

Oncogenes are normal cellular genes that can become altered by mutations or gene amplification which can result in deregulation of cellular growth-control mechanisms. Oncogenes believed to be important in human malignancies include: c-H-ras, c-myc, mdm2, and c-erbB2.

c-H-ras

The c-H-ras gene is an active oncogene thought to be involved in the development and progression of human bladder cancer (48). Mutational studies of the ras gene family have demonstrated that alterations in codons 12 and 61 of the H-ras gene occur in up to 20% of bladder cancers (49–52). One study employing polymerase chain reaction (PCR) amplification followed by oligonucleotide-specific hybridization reported that 36% of bladder tumours had the same mutation on codon 12 of the H-ras gene (53). In general, the activation of H-ras occurs by a single point mutation (G→A) in codon 12. However, three other mutations have been described in bladder cancer including: c-H-ras point mutation at codon 13 (G→T), codon 61 (A→T), and amplification of the c-K-ras oncogene (49,54). Nagata and associates have shown that mutations of the c-ras genes in bladder cancer can occur in any member of the c-ras gene family, although mutations of the c-H-ras gene is reportedly the most common (51). Clinically, Fontana and colleagues have demonstrated a statistically significant relationship between the overexpression of the c-ras oncogene and early recurrence in patients with superficial bladder cancer (55). These preliminary data suggest a potential prognostic role for the c-ras oncogene in patients with superficial bladder cancer, but currently these techniques apply only in a research setting.

c-myc

The myc gene family is an important regulator of cellular proliferation and encodes for nuclear phosphoproteins containing DNA-binding activity (56–59). The c-myc oncogene has been shown to be overexpressed in several human tumours (60,61), including bladder cancer (62). Deregulation of the myc gene family occurs with chromosomal translocation and gene amplification (57,60,61) and studies have demonstrated that myc overexpression promotes cellular proliferation (56,57).

Although the genetic mechanism causing overexpression of the c-*myc* gene in bladder cancer is unknown, overexpression of c-*myc* has been shown to be associated with high-grade bladder cancer (62). Kotake and associates have demonstrated that expression of the c-*myc* gene product correlates with the nuclear grade of bladder cancer. However, in a conflicting study Lipponen found no independent prognostic value for myc proteins with respect to prognosis for patients with transitional cell carcinoma of the bladder (63). Currently, the prognostic significance of c-*myc* gene expression is unknown and will require further evaluation to determine accurately the prognostic role for the c-myc oncogene in bladder cancer.

mdm2

The mdm2 gene resides on chromosome 12 and encodes a nuclear protein that can bind to, and negatively regulate or suppress the normal cell function of the p53 protein (64). The overexpression of mdm2 may be considered an alternate pathway for p53 inactivation. Amplification of the mdm2 gene is infrequently seen in bladder cancer (65). However, some studies have reported overexpression of the mdm2 protein in 20–30% of bladder cancers suggesting a potential role in tumour development (66). Further evaluation will be required to determine the true prognostic value of this oncoprotein in bladder cancer.

c-erbB-2

The proto-oncogene c-erbB-2 (also known as HER-2/neu) has been extensively studied and implicated in a number of tumours including breast, prostate, and bladder cancer (67). The c-erbB-2 oncogene encodes a transmembrane glycoprotein similar to the epidermal growth factor (EGF) receptor. Accumulating evidence suggests that the c-erbB-2 protein is a growth factor receptor possessing structural homology to the EGF receptor (68,69), with similar tyrosine kinase activity (70,71), and the ability to stimulate cellular growth (72).

The initial studies of c-erbB-2 were performed in breast carcinoma which demonstrated a significant relationship between gene expression, tumour progression and overall survival (73,74). Subsequently, several studies have reported that c-erbB-2 expression in patients with bladder cancer is associated with higher stage tumours (75–78), increased tumour progression (79), increased incidence of metastasis (77,78), and decreased overall survival (76). Although these studies suggest a prognostic value of c-erbB-2 expression in human bladder cancer, other studies have reported conflicting results concluding that evaluation of c-erbB-2 provides no additional prognostic value over previously established predictors (grade and stage) for transitional cell carcinoma of the bladder (79–81). In view of these discrepant results further evaluation will be required to determine accurately the prognostic value of c-erbB-2 in bladder cancer.

EPIDERMAL GROWTH FACTOR RECEPTOR

Epidermal growth factor receptor (EGFR) is a 175 000 Dalton transmembrane glycoprotein which is the product of the c-erb-1 gene and is structurally similar to the c-erbB2 and v-erbB1 oncogenes. EGFR is activated by the binding of EGF (82), and transforming growth factor alpha (TGF-α) (83) to its external domain. This results in phosphorylation of intracellular tyrosine kinases by the cytoplasmic portion of EGFR and subsequent cellular proliferation, transformation and division (84). The primary ligand (EGF or TGF-α) responsible for EGFR activation has yet to be determined (85,86).

EGFR is found in many cell types, including transitional epithelium and is normally confined to the basal cell layer of the bladder (87,88). However, EGFR distribution may be altered in patients with transitional cell carcinoma of the bladder and, in fact has been identified throughout the entire urothelium in the involved mucosa (89–93) This 'malignant distribution' is also seen in the normal appearing mucosa of bladder cancer patients. This information supports the notion of a 'field defect' of the transitional mucosa in patients with bladder cancer, and implicates a possible premalignant lesion involving an otherwise histologically normal appearing urothelium (identified by the presence of increased levels of EGFR expression).

EGFR may be identified immunohistochemically (93), with the use of radiolabelled ligand binding studies (94), and with the use of the PCR of bladder washings (92). Ligand binding studies appear to be more sensitive in tumours with low levels of receptor; otherwise, investigators have found a strong correlation between immunohistochemistry and radioassays and have therefore relied primarily on immunohistochemistry to evaluate EGFR. PCR has not been shown to be as accurate as either of the other two methods in the evaluation of EGFR.

The immunohistochemical expression of EGFR has proven to be a potential prognostic marker for TCC of the bladder. A strong correlation exists between EGFR overexpression and higher tumour grade, stage, and ploidy status (81,87–91). The correlation between EGFR expression and clinical outcome has been evaluated in two large study populations with bladder cancer (92,93). Overexpression of EGFR correlates with an increase in cancer-specific death, a significantly shorter interval to recurrence, a higher rate of recurrence, and an increased rate of progression in patients with superficial bladder tumours. Interestingly, a significant difference in survival between EGFR-positive and EGFR-negative tumours has not been observed when evaluating patients with muscle invasive bladder cancer alone. This finding, coupled with the fact that high levels of EGFR are found in normal transitional epithelium distant from the tumour site (94), suggests that increased EGFR expression may be an early event in bladder cancer tumorigenesis.

Finally, investigators have evaluated the potential of using EGFR overexpression as a target for treatment purposes. Conjugating the receptor ligand EGF or TGF-α to a cytotoxic agent has been attempted. A recent interesting report found a hybrid protein of TGF-α and *Pseudomonas* exotoxin-A protein to bind selectively tissues expressing EGFR, with a resultant growth-inhibitory effect on several bladder cancer cell lines (95). Although the clinical application of EGFR as a prognostic factor in bladder cancer is yet to be determined there appears to be some potential usefulness.

PEPTIDE GROWTH FACTORS

Peptide growth factors are the paracrine mediators of cell-to-cell interactions within the microenvironment. In the non-malignant state, peptide growth factors mediate cellular response to injury or infection and regulate the events of embryogenesis. In addition, these factors are intimately involved in cellular growth, differentiation, and death. Alterations in expression of peptide growth factors may contribute to uncontrolled cell growth and malignant transformation. Three major families of peptide growth factors have been studied in bladder cancer: EGF, fibroblast growth factor (FGF), and transforming growth factor (TGF).

Epidermal growth factor

EGF is found in high concentrations in a biologically active form in the urine. Indirect evidence that EGF may play a part in the development of bladder cancer comes from animal studies demonstrating that EGF from normal rat urine can promote the formation of transitional cell tumours in the bladder (96). In addition, EGF isolated from human urine has been shown to stimulate the growth of cultured human bladder cancer cell lines *in vitro* (97). Several studies have evaluated urinary levels of EGF in patients with bladder cancer. Matilla *et al.* found no significant difference between EGF excretion in the urine of patients with bladder cancer and controls (98). However, several other studies have shown significantly lower levels of EGF in the urine of patients with bladder cancer as compared with controls (99–101). Lower levels of EGF in the urine of bladder cancer patients may reflect binding of EGF to abnormally expressed EGFRs. However, an association between the stage or grade of a bladder tumour and EGF levels in the urine have not been identified (100,101). Urinary EGF measurements were found to increase after transurethral resection of a bladder tumour, leading to speculation that the appropriate use of EGF in patients with bladder cancer may be in following urinary concentrations of the protein over time to predict tumour persistence or recurrence (100).

A recent study evaluated immunohistochemical expression of EGF in 43 patients with invasive bladder cancer; EGF was detected in 45% of the tumours and did not correlate with survival from bladder cancer (102).

Fibroblast growth factor

FGF expression has also been studied in bladder cancer. An FGF-like angiogenic factor capable of stimulating capillary endothelial cell migration has been identified in the urine of patients with bladder cancer (103). It has been shown that exposure of bladder cancer cell lines to FGF *in vitro* results in increased cellular motility, higher metastatic potential, and changes in cellular morphology, all of which are properties of tumorigenesis (104,105).

Chopin *et al.* demonstrated a 10-fold increase in tissue acidic FGF in transitional cell carcinoma compared with normal transitional epithelium (106). This increased expression was found to correlate with tumour stage (107). Basic FGF excretion in the urine has also been shown to be associated with bladder tumour stage, with one study suggesting that basic FGF may be more sensitive, but less specific, than urinary cytology for diagnosing bladder cancer (107). O'Brien *et al.* also demonstrated significantly higher urinary levels of basic FGF in patients with bladder cancer compared with controls (108). However, no difference was found between urinary basic FGF levels in patients with high- versus low-stage bladder cancer. Furthermore, increased levels of basic FGF were found in patients about to undergo transurethral resection of the prostate for benign prostatic hypertrophy (108). The lack of specificity of urinary basic FGF as a marker for bladder cancer is probably related to its association with other disease processes such as benign prostatic hypertrophy as well as a wide spectrum of other tumours (109). Therefore, the ability of FGF to serve as an indicator for prognosis or survival of patients with bladder cancer may be limited.

Transforming growth factor-beta

TGF-β has a wide range of activities including enhancing the proliferative rate of cells such as fibroblasts and lymphoblasts, and inhibiting the proliferation of lymphocytes, vascular endothelial cells, and most epithelial cells. TGF-β also has demonstrated potent angiogenic activity in a dose-dependent manner *in vitro* (110). Increased levels of TGF-β have been identified in the serum of patients with bladder cancer (111), while levels of TGF-β extracted from tumour specimens were found to be highest in patients with low-grade and low-stage tumours (112,113). To date, no correlation has been found between TGF-β levels in the serum and in the tumour tissue of patients with bladder cancer. Urinary levels of TGF-β have not been shown to be significantly related to bladder tumour stage or grade (111).

The ability of TGF-β to serve as an indicator for prognosis or survival of patients with bladder cancer has not been demonstrated. Coombs *et al.* suggest that the loss of TGF-β (at the tissue level) could potentially serve as a marker of progression in transitional cell carcinoma (114). Further studies are warranted to confirm this observation.

Transforming growth factor-alpha

It has been shown that TGF-α transfection into rat bladder carcinoma cells results in changes at the cellular level that cause these cells to possess a more aggressive and/or less differentiated appearance (115). TGF-α levels, as measured by radioimmunoassay, are significantly higher in bladder cancer tissue as compared with normal bladder controls (86). In addition, levels of TGF-α correlate with EGFR levels as assessed by immunohistochemical techniques, suggesting that TGF-α is the ligand for EGFR in bladder tumours (86). An immunohistochemical evaluation in 43 specimens with invasive bladder cancer demonstrated expression of TGF-α in 60% of the tumours, and a strong association between TGF-α levels and death from bladder cancer (102). This has not been confirmed by other studies. Currently, the use of TGF-α as a prognostic indicator for bladder cancer is not presently recommended without further investigation.

ANGIOGENESIS AND ANGIOGENESIS INHIBITORS

Tumour angiogenesis

There is considerable direct evidence to support the notion that tumour growth and metastases require a neovascular response (116–120). The process by which this neovascularization occurs is known as tumour angiogenesis. New vessel growth is tightly regulated by the combination of angiogenic stimulators, such as the FGFs and vascular endothelial growth factor, as well as by angiogenic inhibitors such as thrombospondin-1 (TSP) and angiostatin (121). These factors may be produced by the tumour cells themselves, or they may be released from the surrounding extracellular matrix, the tumour-associated stromal cells or they may be products of inflammatory cells that infiltrate the tumour (121–124). As both tumour growth and tumour invasion depend on this angiogenic response, the ability to quantitate the degree of angiogenesis within or around a given tumour may provide important prognostic information for that particular tumour. To this end, methods have been developed that are capable of quantitating the neovascular response induced by a given tumour. This has been accomplished by determining the 'microvessel density' via immunohistochemical methods within and around a given tumour using antibodies that recognize vascular endothelial cells, such as antibodies to factor VIII and CD34.

Microvessel density has been demonstrated to be a useful prognostic indicator in a variety of malignancies including melanoma (125,126), breast cancer (127–128), and prostate cancer (129,130). In general, increased microvessel density counts have been associated with tumour progression and decreased overall survival

(125–130). The relationship between microvessel density count and tumour progression has recently been examined in patients with bladder cancer (131–134). Jaeger and associates demonstrated a significant correlation between tumour angiogenesis (as determined by microvessel density) and lymph node metastases in 41 patients with invasive bladder cancer (132). Dickinson *et al.* evaluated a series of 45 patients with invasive bladder tumours with a median follow-up of 37 months (132). They found microvessel density count to be an independent prognostic indicator of disease progression. Patients with an elevated microvessel density count demonstrated a 2.5-fold greater risk of dying than those patients with a lower microvessel count.

Bochner and associates recently evaluated the relationship between the immunohistochemical determination of tumour angiogenesis and tumour progression in 164 patients with invasive bladder cancer (131). In this study, we found that microvessel density was significantly associated with both disease recurrence and overall survival in patients with invasive bladder cancer. Patients with elevated microvessel density counts demonstrated a significantly increased risk of disease recurrence and a significantly decreased overall survival when compared with patients with low microvessel density counts. Furthermore, microvessel density count was found to be an independent prognostic indicator of both disease progression and overall survival in patients with invasive bladder cancer when evaluated in the presence of histological grade, pathological stage, and regional lymph node involvement.

The above data indicate that the immunohistochemical determination of tumour angiogenesis is an important prognostic indicator in patients with invasive bladder cancer. Although further studies are warranted, tumours exhibiting an angiogenic phenotype may benefit from an aggressive treatment regimen including adjuvant chemotherapy following cystectomy. In the future, determination of microvessel density in transurethral bladder biopsies may prove to be useful in helping clinicians to decide which patients with minimally invasive (T1) disease should undergo early aggressive treatment of their bladder cancer. Furthermore, the significance of tumour angiogenesis in superficial bladder tumours should be studied in order to determine the potential role of this marker in superficial bladder cancer. If microvessel density is able to predict which superficial tumours are likely to recur or progress, this information could help the clinician to decide which patients with superficial tumours are most likely to benefit from intravesical treatment following transurethral resection.

Angiogenesis inhibitors

As tumour angiogenesis and the evaluation of microvessel density have proven to be important predictors of bladder cancer progression, interest has been focused on the isolation and evaluation of inhibitors of this angiogenic process. Many inhibitors of angiogenesis exist including thalidomide (135), interleukin-12 (136), angiostatin (120,137,138), and TSP (139,140). While angiostatin has been shown to inhibit the growth of Lewis lung carcinoma (138,139), human breast cancer, human colon cancer, and human prostate cancer in animal models, only TSP has been examined in human bladder cancer.

TSP is an extracellular matrix glycoprotein that has been shown to be a potent inhibitor of angiogenesis both *in vitro* and *in vivo* (140,141). Our group has recently reported that TSP expression can be determined using antigen retrieval immunohistochemistry in routinely processed formalin-fixed, paraffin-embedded tissue (142). Employing this technique, we then evaluated 163 patients with invasive bladder cancer for TSP expression, and found a highly significant association between TSP expression and both tumour recurrence and overall survival in this group of patients (143). Patients with low TSP expression exhibited higher recurrence rates and decreased overall survival when compared with patients with moderate or high TSP expression. This association was strongest in those patients with organ-confined disease. Furthermore, TSP expression remained an independent predictor of both disease recurrence and overall survival in the presence of tumour stage, histological grade, and lymph node status.

Given previous studies establishing a link between TSP expression, tumour angiogenesis, and the p53 tumour suppressor gene in cultured fibroblasts, we sought to examine the relationship between TSP expression, microvessel density count and p53 expression in this cohort of 163 patients with invasive bladder cancer (143). Using immunohistochemical techniques, we demonstrated that TSP expression was significantly associated with both microvessel density count and p53 nuclear reactivity in patients with invasive bladder cancer. Tumours with p53 alterations were significantly more likely to demonstrate low TSP expression, while tumours with low TSP expression were significantly more likely to demonstrate high microvessel density counts. Results of an analysis of variance were compatible with the hypothesis that p53 affects tumour angiogenesis by regulating the level of TSP expression. These data were in agreement with the findings of Dameron *et al.* (144), and provided strong support for one possible mechanism by which both p53 and TSP exert their tumour inhibitory effects in patients with invasive bladder cancer.

Further studies will be required to evaluate the relationship between the various angiogenesis inhibitors and bladder tumour progression. Nevertheless, inhibitors of angiogenesis, such as TSP, hold promise as prognostic markers for patients with invasive bladder cancer. The utility of these angiogenesis inhibitors for bladder cancer patients, however, may not be limited to that of prognostic marker. If an angiogenesis inhibitor, such as TSP or angiostatin, can be delivered directly to the extracellular matrix surrounding a tumour cell, it may function to inhibit tumour neovascularity and thereby decrease the likelihood of tumour invasion and metastasis. Angiogenesis inhibitors may also be combined with traditional chemotherapeutic agents to enhance anticancer therapy and induce 'dormancy' in the tumour cells remaining after chemotherapy. Given that several angiogenesis inhibitors are currently being studied in phase 1 or 2 clinical trials as treatment for a wide spectrum of solid tumours (145), the possibility of anti-angiogenic therapy for solid tumours, including bladder cancer, is no longer a far-fetched idea.

CELL CYCLE REGULATORY PROTEINS

Malignant diseases are characterized by uncontrolled cell growth. Normal cellular proliferation occurs by an orderly progression through the cell cycle which is regulated by cell-cycle-associated protein complexes composed of cyclins and cyclin-dependent kinases (146). These complexes exert their control mechanism by phosphorylating key proteins involved in cell cycle transition points, including the protein encoded by the retinoblastoma gene (pRB) or the p53 protein. Loss of this cell cycle control appears to be an early step in the development of carcinogenesis and ultimately cancer progression. Recent investigative efforts have examined several genes and their protein products that are involved in cell cycle regulation, to determine their prognostic significance in bladder cancer progression.

Retinoblastoma tumour suppressor gene

The retinoblastoma (Rb) tumour suppressor gene was the first tumour suppressor gene identified. The Rb gene is located on chromosome 13q14 and encodes for a 110 kDa nuclear phosphoprotein (147). Although initially discovered to be mutated in patients with inherited retinoblastoma, altered Rb gene expression has been reported in various human tumours including transitional cell carcinoma of the bladder (148–151). In its physiological active hypophosphorylated form, pRb acts by inhibiting cell-cycle progression at the G_1–S check-point by binding to a number of cellular proteins including the transcription factor E2F (152,153). pRb is phosphorylated in a cell-cycle-dependent manner, with under-phosphorylated pRb being the predominant form in G_1 resulting in a tumour suppressor effect. With entry into the S phase, pRb becomes phosphorylated.

Inactivation of the Rb gene is thought to be an important step in bladder cancer progression. Several monoclonal and polyclonal antibodies have been discovered which allow the reliable evaluation of pRb expression through immunohistochemical methods (154). With a combination of immunohistochemical techniques and molecular analysis, several groups have demonstrated that the proportion of tumours demonstrating Rb alterations increases with higher grade and stage bladder cancers (155,156). The results of these studies suggest that loss of pRb expression may be an important prognostic factor in transitional cell carcinoma of the bladder. Cordon-Cardo and associates reported that patients with muscle invasive bladder tumours who have lost Rb immuno-expression had a statistically significant shorter 5-year survival ($P = 0.001$) than those patients with normal Rb protein expression (149). Similarly, Logothetis and associates studied 43 patients with invasive bladder cancer and demonstrated that Rb alterations were more common in advanced tumours, and that those patients who had lost pRb expression had a shorter overall survival compared with those patients who maintained Rb expression (152). Based on the aforementioned data, it appears that pRb expression is an important prognostic factor in patients with invasive bladder cancer.

p53 tumour suppressor gene

Mutations in the p53 gene are the most common genetic defect in human tumours (157). The p53 gene is located on chromosome 17p13 and encodes for a 53-kDa protein. The p53 gene functions as a tumour suppressor gene. Specifically, the p53 protein plays a vital part in the regulation of the cell cycle (158). When DNA damage occurs, the level of p53 protein increases causing cell cycle arrest. This allows for the repair of DNA and prevents propagation of the DNA defect. Mutations in the p53 gene result in the production of an abnormal and usually dysfunctional protein product with a prolonged half-life compared with the wild-type protein. Consequently, this abnormal protein accumulates in the cell nucleus and can be detected by immunohistochemical staining. It has been shown that nuclear accumulation of p53 protein as determined by immunohistochemical staining correlates with gene mutations as detected by DNA sequence analysis (159).

It has been shown that p53 alteration, as determined by immunohistochemical techniques, is an important prognostic indicator for bladder cancer progression (160–163). Increased p53 immunoreactivity has been found in higher grade and stage bladder cancers and is associated with disease progression and decreased overall and disease-specific survival. Our group evaluated p53 nuclear reactivity in 243 patients with invasive bladder cancer who were uniformly treated by radical cystectomy (160). We found that immunohistochemical detection of the p53 protein in tumour nuclei provided important prognostic information in this group of patients with bladder cancer. Patients with an increased p53 expression (altered p53) were found to have a significantly increased risk of disease recurrence and a significantly decreased overall survival when compared with those patients without altered p53. This association was independent of tumour grade, pathological stage, and lymph node status and was strongest in patients with organ confined tumours (P1, P2, P3a). Furthermore, nuclear accumulation of p53 was found to be the only independent predictor of disease progression in a multivariable analysis of p53 status, histological grade, and pathological stage.

Lipponen and associates reported their findings in 212 patients with primary bladder cancer who were evaluated for p53 immunoreactivity (162). Increased p53 nuclear reactivity was found to be a significant adverse prognostic factor in patients with muscle invasive bladder cancers. Increased tumour grade, as well as tumour progression were associated with increased p53 expression. In another study, Sarkis and associates evaluated p53 expression in 11 patients with muscle invasive bladder tumour treated with neoadjuvant chemotherapy (163). They found that increased p53 nuclear reactivity was significantly associated with disease progression and cancer specific death when compared with those patients without increased p53 nuclear reactivity.

Based on an accumulating amount of evidence supported by a number of independent studies, p53 immunoreactivity appears to be a reliable and consistent prognostic marker for bladder cancer progression. Increased expression of p53 as determined by immunohistochemical methods is generally seen in high-grade and high-stage bladder tumours. In addition, increased p53 immunoreactivity is associated with a higher likelihood of disease progression and cancer-specific death.

Combination of Rb and p53 tumour suppressor genes

Two independent studies have evaluated the prognostic significance of combining the Rb and p53 status of bladder cancers as determined by immunohistochemical techniques (164,165). Preliminary data from these studies support the concept that bladder tumours with alterations in both p53 and Rb have a poorer prognosis and decreased overall survival when compared with tumours with wild-type p53 and wild-type Rb. Tumours with an alteration of only one of these genes (as determined by immunohistochemistry) behave in an intermediate fashion. These data suggest that the status of both p53 and Rb are important, and that these two proteins act in an independent yet synergistic manner in patients with bladder cancer.

p21 tumour suppressor gene

Although p53 nuclear accumulation, as detected by immunohisto-chemical methods, is a significant predictor of bladder cancer progression, not all p53-altered bladder tumours recur or progress (159,163). One of the primary functions of p53 is as a cell cycle regulatory protein (145,159). p53 mediates its effects on the cell cycle through the regulation of p21 (WAF1/CIP1) expression (146). Alterations in p53 result in loss of p21 expression, which leads to unregulated cell growth. This is thought to be one of the mechanisms through which p53 alterations may influence tumour progression. However, it has recently been demonstrated that p21 expression may also be mediated through p53-independent pathways (165–168). This important finding suggests that despite the presence of a p53 alteration, p21 expression (and therefore cell cycle control) can be maintained.

With a better understanding of cell-cycle regulation, including the interactions of p53 and p21, we sought to determine whether the presence or absence of p21 expression in bladder tumours that demonstrated p53 alterations might be an important factor in predicting clinical behaviour. We reasoned that the expression of p21 through p53-independent pathways might abrogate the dele-terious effects of p53 alterations by resulting in the maintenance of cell cycle control.

We evaluated bladder tumours from 101 patients who under-went radical cystectomy for invasive bladder cancer for p21 expression using immunohistochemical techniques (169). All patients had been previously determined to have p53 altered tumours (160). We found that immunohistochemical detection of p21 protein in the nuclei of bladder cancers which show p53 alterations (p53-altered) provides important additional prognostic information for patients with bladder cancer. Patients with p53-altered transitional cell carcinomas of the bladder that were p21-negative demonstrated a significantly increased probability of recurrence and a significantly decreased probability of overall survival when compared with patients with p53-altered tumours that maintained expression of p21 (p21-positive). The association between p21 status and prognosis in p53-altered bladder tumours was independent of tumour grade, pathological stage, and lymph node status. The strongest association between p21 status and tumour progression was observed in patients with organ-confined disease (Pis, P1, P2, P3a) and extravesical disease (P3b, P4) without evidence of lymph node metastases. Loss of p21 expression was strongly associated with an increased probability of recurrence and decreased probability of survival in patients with lymph node negative organ confined disease and lymph node negative extravesical disease. In fact, p21 was the only independent predictor of disease progression in p53-altered bladder tumours in a multivariate analysis of p21 status, histological grade, and pathological stage. These findings suggest that p21 expression through p53 independent pathways exist, and that cell-cycle control may be maintained through these pathways. Those patients with p53 altered tumours that lose p21 expression have a poor prognosis and should be considered for adjuvant treatment.

CONCLUSIONS

It is clear that conventional histopathological evaluation of bladder cancer, including determination of tumour grade and stage, is now inadequate to predict accurately the behaviour of most bladder cancers. Tumour heterogeneity, even within the same clinical subgroups of patients, prevents the reliable determination of a bladder cancer's biological potential. Consequently, dedicated efforts have been made to identify other potential prognostic markers that may better stratify and identify a tumour's true malignant potential. With a better understanding of the cell-cycle and cell-to-cell interactions, along with improved diagnostic techniques (immunohistochemistry), progress is being made to characterize other potential prognostic markers. It is hoped that it will soon be possible to use these techniques to help dictate more aggressive treatment schemes for those patients with a tumour that demonstrates a biologically aggressive phenotype, and less aggressive therapeutic regimens for those patients with a tumour demonstrating a less aggressive biological phenotype.

The development of uncontrolled cellular proliferation leads to invasive and metastatic capabilities is a complex process that remains poorly understood. The measurable determinants of these properties will unlikely involve a single marker. A considerable amount of redundancy is inherent in all biological systems, and the evaluation of one particular marker will not logically guarantee the behaviour of the tissue. It is becoming more apparent that tumour progression may occur through several different mechanisms including alterations in cell-cycle regulation, cellular adhesion and signal transduction, and the expression of certain growth factors. In the future, evaluation of multiple markers may be more logical and provide more information than a single marker. The ultimate application of tumour markers may therefore involve the evaluation of multiple tumour markers for an individual tumour or specimen; a so-called 'test-battery' of markers. Simultaneous evaluation of these multiple tumour markers using a 'test -battery' approach may therefore better evaluate a tumour's individual growth capability, help to dictate adjuvant treatment strategies, and more accurately predict a tumour's responsiveness to various forms of adjuvant therapy.

Despite the significant progress made in the development and evaluation of various tumour markers, currently there is an inability to make solid recommendations about most studied markers in the management of bladder cancer. This relates to the present maturity of methodological principles seen in prognostic factor studies. Furthermore, although prognostic factor studies are receiving greater critical attention, there is still a need for well designed, randomized, prospective, phase 3 trials evaluating the strongest candidate markers. These studies are only beginning to be performed. Currently, although great enthusiasm exists with the application of various tumour makers in the management of bladder cancer, concrete clinical recommendations must be tempered at this time.

Key Points

1. Conventional tumour grade and stage remain the primary prognostic determinants in patients with invasive bladder cancer
2. Although a number of monoclonal antibodies have been generated that are specific to transitional cell carcinoma of the bladder, only the antigens M344, 19A211, and T138 appear to posses any proven prognostic clinical application.
3. There appears to be some evidence to suggest that the tumour suppressor genes Rb and p53, as determined by immunohistochemical techniques, may supplement the routine use of histological grade and stage in assessing a bladder tumour's aggressiveness and metastatic potential.
4. Bladder tumour heterogeneity, even within the same clinical subgroups of patients, prevents the reliable determination of a bladder cancer's biological potential and currently there is an inability to make solid recommendations about most studied markers. There is a need for well designed, randomized, prospective, phase 3 trials evaluating the strongest candidate markers.

References

1 Malkowicz BS. Superficial bladder cancer: the role of molecular markers in the treatment of high-risk superficial disease. *Semin Urol Oncol* 1997, **15**, 169–78.
2 Skinner DG, Lieskovsky G. Management of invasive and high-grade bladder cancer. In: *Diagnosis and management of genitourinary cancer* (ed. Skinner DG, Lieskovsky G), Vol. 1. WB Saunders, Philadelphia 1988, 295–312.
3 Droller MJ. Individualizing the approach to invasive bladder cancer. *Contemp Urol* 1990, **July/August**, 54–61.
4 Skinner DG, Lieskovsky G. Contemporary cystectomy with pelvic node dissection compared to preoperative radiation therapy plus cystectomy in management of invasive bladder cancer. *J Urol* 1984, **131**, 1069–72.
5 Montie JE, Strafton RA, Stewart BH. Radical cystectomy without radiation therapy for carcinoma of the bladder. *J Urol* 1984, **131**, 477–82.
6 Frazier HA, Robertson JE, Dodge RK, Paulson DF. The value of pathologic factors in predicting cancer-specific survival among patients treated with radical cystectomy for transitional cell carcinoma of the bladder and prostate. *Cancer* 1993, **71**, 3993–4001.
7 Skinner DG, Tift JP, Kaufman JJ. High dose, short course preoperative radiation therapy and immediate single stage radical cystectomy with pelvic node dissection in the management of bladder cancer. *J Urol* 1982, **127**, 671–4.

8 Lerner SP, Skinner DG, Lieskovsky G *et al.* The rationale for en bloc pelvic lymph node dissection for bladder cancer patients with nodal metastases: long-term results. *J Urol* 1993, **149**, 758–65.

9 Soloway MS, Lopez AE, Patel J, Lu Y. Result of radical cystectomy for transitional cell carcinoma of the bladder and the effect of chemotherapy. *Cancer* 1994, **73**, 1926–31.

10 Voges GE, Tauschke E, Stockle M *et al.* Computerized tomography: an unreliable method for accurate staging of bladder tumors in patients who are candidates for radical cystectomy. *J Urol* 1989, **142**, 972–4.

11 Malkowicz SB, Nichols P, Lieskovsky G *et al.* The role of radical cystectomy in the management of high grade superficial bladder cancer (Pa, P1, Pis, P2). *J Urol* 1990, **144**, 641–5.

12 Freeman JA, Esrig D, Stein JP *et al.* Radical cystectomy for high risk patients with superficial bladder cancer in the era of orthotopic urinary reconstruction. *Cancer* 1995, **76**, 833–9.

13 Lerner SP, Skinner E, Skinner DG. Radical cystectomy in regionally advanced bladder cancer. *Urol Clin N Am* 1992, **19**, 713–23.

14 Esrig D, Freeman JA, Elmajian DA *et al.* Transitional cell carcinoma involving the prostate with a proposed staging classification for stromal invasion. *J Urol* 1996, **156**, 1071–6.

15 American Joint Committe on Cancer (AJCC). *Cancer staging manual.* Lippincott-Raven JB, Philadelphia 1997.

16 Stein JP, Freeman JA, Boyd SD *et al.* Radical cystectomy in the treatment of invasive bladder cancer: long-term results in a large group of patients. *J Urol*

17 Skinner DG, Daniels JR, Russell CA *et al.* The role of adjuvant chemotherapy following cystectomy for invasive bladder cancer: a prospective comparative trial. *J Urol* 1991, **145**, 459–64.

18 Dalbagni G, Reuter VE, Sheinfeld J *et al.* Cell surface differentiation antigens of normal urothelium and bladder tumors. *Semin Surg Oncol* 1992, **8**, 293–9.

19 Fradet Y, Cordon-Cardo C. Critical appraisal of tumor markers in bladder cancer. *Semin Urol* 1993, **11**, 145–9.

20 Fradet Y, Gauthier J, Bedard G *et al.* Monitoring and prognostic determination of bladder tumors by flow cytometry with monoclonal antibodies on bladder irrigations. *J Urol* 1991, **145**, 250A (abstract 149).

21 Fradet Y, Tardif M, Bourget L, Robert J, the Laval University Urology Group. Clinical cancer progression in urinary bladder tumors evaluated by multiparameter flow cytometry with monoclonal antibodies. *Cancer Res* 1990, **50**, 432–7.

22 Bretton P, Cordon-Cardo C, Wartinger D *et al.* Expression of the T-138 antigen and survival of patients with bladder cancer. *Proc Am Assoc Cancer Res* 1990, **31**, 186 (abstract 1105).

23 Sarosdy MF, De Vere White RW, Soloway MS *et al.* Results of a multicenter trial sing the BTA test to monitor for and diagnose recurrent bladder cancer. *J Urol* 1995, **154**, 379–83.

24 D'Hallewin MA, Baert L. Initial evaluation of the bladder tumor antigen test in superficial bladder cancer. *J Urol* 1996, **155**, 475–6.

25 Johnston B, Morales A, Emerson L, Lundie M. Rapid detection of bladder cancer: a comparative study of point of care tests. *J Urol* 1997, **158**, 2098.

26 Murphy WM, Rivera-Ramirez I, Medina CA *et al.* The bladder tumor antigen (BTA) test compared to voided urine cytology in the detection of bladder neoplasms. *J Urol* 1997, **158**, 2102–6.

27 Ellis WJ, Blumenstein BA, Ishak LM, Enfield DL. Clinical evaluation of the BTA TRAK assay and comparison to voided urine cytology and the Bard BTA test in patients with recurrent bladder tumors. *Urology* 1997, **50**, 882–7.

28 Ishak LM, Enfield DL, Sarosdy MF. Detection of recurrent bladder cancer using a new quantitative assay for bladder tumor antigen. *J Urol* 1997, part 2, **157**, 337 (abstract 1317).

29 Leyh H, Marberger M, Pagano F *et al.* Results of a European multicenter trial comparing the BTA stat test to urine cytology in patients suspected of having bladder cancer. *J Urol* 1997, part 2, **157**, 337 (abstract 1316).

30 Sarosdy MF, Hudson MA, Ellis WJ *et al.* Improved detection of recurrent bladder cancer using the Bard BTA stat Test. *Urology* 1997, **50**, 349–53.

31 Sarosdy MF, Hudson MA, Ellis WJ *et al.* Detection of recurrent bladder cancer using a new one-step test for bladder tumor antigen. *J Urol* 1997, part 2, **157**, 337 (abstract 1317).

32 Soloway MS, Briggman JV, Carpinito GA *et al*. Use of a new tumor marker, urinary NMP22, in the detection of occult or rapidly recurring transitional cell carcinoma of the urinary tract following surgical treatment. *J Urol* 1996, **156**, 363–7.

33 Akaza H, Miyanaga N, Tsukamoto T *et al*. Evaluation of nuclear matrix protein 22 (NMP22) as a diagnostic marker for bladder cancer: a multicenter trial in Japan. *J Urol* 1997, part 2, **157**, 337 (abstract 1315).

34 Carpinito GA, Stadler WM, Briggman JV *et al*. Urinary nuclear matrix protein as a marker for transitional cell carcinoma of the urinary tract. *J Urol* 1996, **156**, 1280–4.

35 Rodriguez-Villanueva JR, Dinney CPN, Grossman HB, Fritsche HA. Evaluation of the NMP22 immunoassay in the detection of transitional cell carcinoma (TCC) of the urinary tract. *J Urol* 1997, part 2, **157**, 336 (abstract 1314).

36 Gerdes J, Schwab U, Lemke H, Stein H. Production of a mouse monoclonal antibody reactive with a human nuclear antigen associated with cell prolfieration. *Int J Cancer* 1983, **31**, 13–7.

37 Loke SL, Jaffe ES, Neckers LM. Inhibition of in vitro DNA synthesis by the monoclonal antibody Ki-67. *Blood* 1987, **70** (Suppl.), 1579–83.

38 Brown DC, Gatter KC. Monoclonal antibody Ki-67: its use in histopathology. *Histopathology* 1990, **17**, 489–503.

39 Okamura K, Miyake K, Koshikawa T, Asai J. Growth fractions of transitional cell carcinomas of the bladder defined by the monoclonal antibody Ki-67. *J Urol* 1990, **144**, 875–8.

40 Fontana D, Bellina M, Gubetta L *et al*. Monoclonal antibody Ki-67 in the study of the proliferative activity of bladder carcinoma. *J Urol* 1992, **148**, 1149–51.

41 Cohen MB, Waldman FM, Carroll PR *et al*. Comparison of five histopathologic methods to assess cellular proliferation in transitional cell carcinoma of the urinary bladder. *Hum Pathol* 1993, **24**, 772–8.

42 Tsujihashi H, Nakanishi A, Matsuda H *et al*. Cell proliferation of human bladder tumors determined by BrdUrd and Ki-67 immunostaining. *J Urol* 1991, **145**, 846–9.

43 Mulder AH, Van Hootegem JCSP, Sylvester R *et al*. Prognostic factors in bladder carcinoma: histologic parameters and expression of a cell cycle-related nuclear antigen (Ki-67). *J Pathol* 1992, **166**, 37–43.

44 Bush C, Price P, Norten J, Parkins CS *et al*. Proliferation in human bladder carcinoma measured by Ki-67 antibody labelling: its potential clinical importance. *Br J Cancer* 1991, **64**, 357–60.

45 King ED, Matteson J, Jacobs SC, Kyprianou N. Incidence of apoptosis, cell proliferation and bcl-2 expression in transitional cell carcinoma of the bladder: association with tumor progression. *J Urol* 1996, **155**, 316–20.

46 Ogata K, Celis JE, Tan EM. Proliferating cell nuclear antigen: cyclin. *Methods Enzymol* 1987, **150**, 147–9.

47 Robbins BA, De la Vega D, Ogata K *et al*. Immunohistochemical detection of proliferating cell nuclear antigen in solid human malignancies. *Arch Path Lab Med* 1987, **111**, 841–5.

48 Kroft SH, Oyasu R. Urinary bladder cancer: mechanisms of development and progression. *Lab Invest* 1994, **71**, 158–74.

49 Strohmeyer TG, Slamon DJ. Proto-oncogenes and tumor suppressor genes in human urological malignancies. *J Urol* 1994, **151**, 1479–86.

50 Moriyama N, Umeda T, Akaza H *et al*. Expression of ras p21 oncogene product on human bladder tumors. *Urol Int* 1989, **44**, 260–3.

51 Nagata Y, Abe M, Kobayashi K *et al*. Point mutation of C-ras gene in human bladder cancer and kidney cancer. *Jpn J Cancer Res* 1990, **81**, 22–7.

52 Fradet Y. Markers of prognosis in superficial bladder cancer. *Semin Urol* 1992, **10**, 28–38.

53 Czerniak B, Deitch D, Simmons H *et al*. Ha-ras gene condon 12 mutation and DNA ploidy in urinary bladder carcinoma. *Br J Cancer* 1990, **62**, 762–3.

54 Stanley LA. Molecular aspects of chemical carcinogenesis: the roles of oncogenes and tumor suppressor genes. *Toxicology* 1995, **96**, 173–81.

55 Fontana D, Bellina M, Scoffone C *et al*. Evaluation of c-ras oncogene product (p21) in superficial bladder cancer. *Eur Urol* 1996, **29**, 470–6.

56 Evan GI, Littlewood TD. The role of c-myc in cell growth. *Curr Opin Gene Dev* 1993, **3**, 44–62.

57 Koskinen PJ, Alitalo K. Role of myc amplification and overexpression in cell growth, differentiation and death. *Semin Cancer Biol* 1993, **4**, 3–11.

58 Cole MD. The myc oncogene: its role in transformation and differentiation. *Ann Dev Gene* 1986, **20**, 361–8.

59 Watt RA, Shatzman AR, Rosenberg M. Expression and characterization of the human c-myc DNA binding protein. *Mol Cell Biol* 1985, **5**, 448–56.

60 Roux-Dossetto M, Romain S, Dussault N *et al*. C-myc gene amplification in selected node-negative breast cancer patients correlates with high rate of relapse. *Eur J Cancer* 1992, **28A**, 1600–4.

61 Berns EM, Klijn JG, Van Putten WL *et al*. C-myc amplification is a better prognostic factor then Her2/neu amplification in primary breast cancer. *Cancer Res* 1990, **52**, 1107–9.

62 Kotake T, Saiki S, Kinouchi T *et al*. Detection of c-myc gene product in urinary bladder cancer. *Jpn J Cancer Res* 1990, **81**, 1198–201.

63 Lipponen PK. Expression of c-myc protein is related to cell proliferation and expression of growth factor receptors in transitional cell bladder cancer. *J Pathol* 1995, **175**, 203–9.

64 Momand J, Zambetti GP, Olson DC *et al*. The mdm-2 oncogene product forms a complex with the p53 protein and inhibits p53 mediated transactivation. *Cell* 1992, **69**, 1237–45.

65 Habuchi T, Kinoshita H, Yamada H *et al*. Oncogene amplification in urothelial cancers with p53 gene mutation or mdm2 amplification. *J Natl Cancer Inst* 1994, **86**, 1331–4.

66 Lianes P, Orlow I, Zhang ZF *et al*. Altered patterns of MDM2 and Tp53 expression in human bladder cancer. *J Natl Cancer Inst* 1994, **86**, 1325–30.

67 Underwood M, Bartlett J, Reeves J *et al*. C-erbB-2 gene amplification: a molecular marker in recurrent bladder tumors? *Cancer Res* 1995, **55**, 2422–5.

68 Bargmann CI, Hung MC, Weinberg RA. The neu oncogene encodes an epidermal growth factor receptor-related protein. *Nature* 1986, **319**, 226–30.

69 Yamamoto T, Ikawa S, Akiyama T *et al*. Similarity of protein encoded by the human c-erbB-2 gene to epidermal growth factor receptor. *Nature* 1986, **319**, 230–4.

70 Stern DF, Heffernan PA, Weinberg RA. P185, a product of the neu proto-onogene, is a receptor like protein associated with tyrosine kinase activity. *Mol Cell Biol* 1986, **6**, 1729–40.

71 Akiyama T, Sudo C, Ogawara H *et al*. The product of the human c-erbB-2 gene: a 185-kilodalton glycoprotein with tyrosine kinase activity. *Science* 1986, **232**, 1644–6.

72 Lee J, Dull TJ, Lax I *et al*. HER2 cytoplasmic domain generates normal mitogenic and transforming signals in a chimeric receptor. *EMBO J* 1989, **8**, 167–73.

73 Slamon DJ, Godolphin W, Jones LA *et al*. Studies of the HER-2/neu proto-oncogene in human breast and ovarian cancer. *Science* 1989, **244**, 707–12.

74 Borg A, Baldetorp B, Ferno M *et al*. ERBB-2 amplification in breast cancer with a high rate of proliferation. *Oncogene* 1991, **6**, 137–43.

75 Gorgoulis VG, Barbatis C, Poulias I, Karameris AM. Molecular and immunohistochemical evaluation of epidermal growth factor receptor and c-erbB-2 gene product in transitional cell carcinomas of the urinary bladder. A study in Greek patients. *Mod Pathol* 1995, **8**, 758–64.

76 Sato K, Moriyama M, Mori S *et al*. An immunohistologic evaluation of c-erbB-2 gene product in patients with urinary bladder carcinoma. *Cancer* 1992, **70**, 2493–8.

77 Moch H, Sauter G, Moore D *et al*. P53 and erbB-2 protein overexpression are associated with early invasion and metastasis in bladder cancer. *Virchows Arch A Pathol Anat Histopathol* 1993, **423**, 329–34.

78 Moriyama M, Akiyama T, Yamamoto T *et al*. Expression of c-erbB-2 gene product in urinary bladder cancer. *J Urol* 1991, **145**, 423–7.

79 Lipponen P. Expression of c-erbB-2 oncoprotein in transitional cell bladder cancer. *Eur J Cancer* 1993, **29A**, 749–52.

80 Mellon JK, Lunec J, Wright C *et al*. C-erbB-2 in bladder cancer: molecular biology, correlation with epidermal growth factor receptors and prognostic value. *J Urol* 1996, **155**, 321–6.

81 Lipponen P, Eskelinen M. Expression of epidermal growth factor receptor in bladder cancer as related to established prognostic factors, onocprotein (c-erbB-2, p53) expression and long-term prognosis. *Br J Cancer* 1994, **69**, 1120–4.

82 Adamson E, Rees A. Epidermal growth factor receptors. *Mol Cell Biochem* 1981, **34**, 129–52.

83 Massague J. EGF-like TGF. *J Biol Chem* 1983, **258**, 13614–8.

84 Partanen AM. Epidermal growth factor and transforming growth factor-A in the development of epithelial-mesenchymal organs of the mouse. *Curr Top Dev Biol* 1990, **24**, 31–7.

85 Mellon JK, Cook S, Chambers P, Neal DE. Tranforming growth factor alpha and epidermal growth factor in bladder cancer and their relationship to epidermal growth factor receptor. *Br J Cancer* 1996, **73**, 654–8.

86 Messing EM, Reznikoff CA. Epidermal growth factor and its receptor: markers of—and targets for—chemoprevention of bladder cancer. *J Cell Biochem* 1992, **161** (Suppl.), 56–68.

87 Liebert M. Growth factors in bladder cancer. *World J Urol* 1995, **13**, 349–55.

88 Messing EM. Clinical implications of the expression of epidermal growth factor receptors in human transitional cell carcinoma. *Cancer Res* 1990, **50**, 2530–7.

89 Neal DE, Sharples L, Smith K *et al.* The epidermal growth factor receptor and the prognosis of bladder cancer. *Cancer* 1990, **65**, 1619–25.

90 Sauter G, Haley J, Chew K *et al.* Epidermal growth factor receptor expression is associated with rapid tumor proliferation in bladder cancer. *Int J Cancer* 1994, **57**, 508–14.

91 Berger MS, Greenfield C, Gullick WJ *et al.* Evaluation of epidermal growth factor receptors in bladder tumours. *Br J Cancer* 1987, **56**, 533–7.

92 Neal DE, Marsh C, Bennett MK *et al.* Epidermal-growth-factor receptors in human bladder cancer: comparison of invasive and superficial tumours. *Lancet* 1985, **i**, 366–8.

93 Messing EM, Hanson P, Ulrich P, Erturk E. Epidermal growth factor-interactions with normal and malignant urothelium: in vivo and in situ studies. *J Urol* 1987, **138**, 1329–35.

94 Neal DE, Smith K, Fennelly J *et al.* The epidermal growth factor receptor in human bladder cancer: a comparison of immunohistochemistry and radioligand binding. *J Urol* 1989, **141**, 517–21.

95 Lonn U, Lonn S, Nylen U *et al.* Gene amplification detected in carcinoma cells from human urinary bladder washings by the polymerase chain reaction method. *Cancer* 1993, **71**, 3605–10.

96 Yura Y, Hayashi O, Kelly M, Oyasu R. Identification of epidermal growth factor as a component of rat urinary bladder tumor-enhancing urinary fractions. *Cancer Res* 1989, **49**, 1548–53.

97 Kuranami M, Yamaguchi K, Fuchigami M *et al.* Effect of urine of clonal growth of human bladder cancer cell lines. *Cancer Res* 1991, **51**, 4631–5.

98 Matilla AL, Saario I, Viinikka L *et al.* Urinary epidermal growth factor concentrations in various human malignancies. *Br J Cancer* 1988, **57**, 139–42.

99 Kristensen JK, Lose G, Lund F, Nexo E. Epidermal growth factor in urine from patients with urinary bladder tumors. *Eur Urol* 1988, **14**, 313–4.

100 Fuse H, Mizuno I, Sakamoto M, Karayama T. Epidermal growth factor in urine from the patients with urothelial tumors. *Urol Int* 1992, **48**, 261–4.

101 Messing EM, Murphy-Brooks N. Recovery of epidermal growth factor in voided urine of patients with bladder cancer. *Urology* 1994, **44**, 502–4.

102 Ravery V, Grignon D, Angulo J *et al.* Evaluation of epidermal growth factor receptor, transforming growth factor alpha, epidermal growth factor and c-erbB2 in the progression of invasive bladder cancer. *Urol Res* 1997, **25**, 9–17.

103 Chodak GW, Hospelhorn V, Judge SM *et al.* Increased levels of fibroblast growth factor-like activity in urine from patients with bladder cancer. *Cancer Res* 1988, **48**, 2083–8.

104 Valles AM, Boyer B, Badet J *et al.* Acidic fibroblast growth factor is a modulator of epithelial plasticity in a rat bladder carcinoma cell line. *Proc Natl Acad Sci USA* 1990, **87**, 1124–8.

105 Jouanneau J, Gavrilovic J, Caruelle D *et al.* Secreted or nonsecreted forms of acidic fibroblast growth factor produced by transfected epithelial cells influence cell morphology, motility, and invasive potential. *Proc Natl Acad Sci USA* 1991, **88**, 2893–7.

106 Chopin DK, Caruelle JP, Colombel M *et al.* Increased immunodetection of acidic fibroblast growth factor in bladder cancer, detectable in urine. *J Urol* 1993, **150**, 1126–30.

107 Nguyen M, Watanabe H, Budson AE *et al.* Elevated levels of the angiogenic peptide basic fibroblast growth factor in urine of bladder cancer patients. *J Natl Cancer Inst* 1993, **85**, 241–2.

108 O'Brien TS, Smith K, Cranston D *et al*. Urinary basic fibroblast growth factor in patients with bladder cancer and benign prostatic hypertrophy. *Br J Urol* 1995, **76**, 311–4.

109 Nguyen M, Watanabe H, Budson AE *et al*. Elevated levels of an angiogenic peptide, basic fibroblast growth factor, in the urine of patients with a wide spectrum of cancers. *J Natl Cancer Inst* 1994, **86**, 356–61.

110 Kehrl JH. Transforming growth factor-beta: an important mediator of immunoregulation. *Int J Cell Cloning* 1991, **9**, 438–50.

111 Eder IE, Stenzl A, Hobisch A *et al*. Transforming growth factors beta-1 and beta-2 in serum and urine from patients with bladder cancer. *J Urol* 1996, **156**, 953–7.

112 Miyamoto H, Kubota Y, Shuin T *et al*. Expression of transforming growth factor beta-1 in human bladder cancer. *Cancer* 1995, **75**, 2565–70.

113 Eder IE, Stenzl A, Hobisch A *et al*. Expression of transforming growth factors beta-1, beta- 2 and beta -3 in human bladder carcinomas. *Br J Cancer* 1997, **75**, 1753–60.

114 Coombs LM, Pigott DA, Eydmann ME, Proctor AJ, Knowles MA. Reduced expression of TGF beta is associated with advanced disease in transitional cell carcinoma. *Br J Cancer* 1993, **67**, 578–84.

115 Gavriloc J, Moens J, Thiery JP, Jouanneau J. Expression of transfected transforming growth factor alpha induces a motile fibroblast-like phenotype with extracellular matrix-degrading potential in a rat bladder carcinoma cell line. *Cell Regulation* 1990, **1**, 1003–14.

116 Folkman J, Cole P, Zimmerman S. Tumor behavior in isolated perfused organs: in vitro growth and metastases of biopsy material in rabbit thyroid and canine intestinal segment. *Ann Surg* 1966, **164**, 491–502.

117 Sutherland RM, McCredie JA, Inch WR. Growth of multicell spheroids in tissue culture as a model of nodular carcinomas. *J Natl Cancer Inst* 1971, **46**, 113–20.

118 Gimbrone MA Jr, Leapman SB, Coltran RS, Folkman J. Tumor dormancy in vivo by prevention of neovascularization. *J Exp Med* 1972, **136**, 261–76.

119 Gimbrone MA Jr, Cotran RS, Leapman SB, Folkman J. Tumor growth neovascularization: an experimental model using the rabbit cornea. *J Natl Cancer Inst* 1974, **52**, 413–27.

120 O'Reilly MS, Holmgren L, Chen C, Folkman J. Angiostatin induces and sustains dormancy of human primary tumors in mice. *Nature Med* 1996, **2**, 689–92.

121 LeQuerrec A, Duval D, Tobelem G. Tumour angiogenesis. *Baillières Clin Haematol* 1993, **6**, 711–30.

122 Blood CH, Zetter BR. Tumor interactions with the vasculature: angiogenesis and tumor metastasis. *Biochim Biophys Acta* 1990, **1032**, 89–91.

123 Polverini PJ, Leibovich SJ. Induction of neovascularization in vivo and endothelial proliferation in vitro by tumor-associated macrophages. *Lab Invest* 1984, **51**, 635–42.

124 Folkman J, Klagsbrun M. Angiogenic factors. *Science* 1997, **235**, 442–6.

125 Srivastava A, Laidler P, Davies RP *et al*. The prognostic significance of tumor vascularity in intermediate-thickness (0.76–4.0 mm thick) skin melanoma. *Am J Pathol* 1988, **133**, 419–23.

126 Barnhill RL, Levy MA. Regressing thin cutaneous malignant melanomas (< 1.0mm) are associated with angiogenesis. *Am J Pathol* 1992, **143**, 99–104.

127 Weidner N, Folkman J, Pozza F *et al*. Tumor angiogenesis: a new significant and independent prognositic indicator in early-stage breast carcinoma. *J Natl Cancer Inst* 1992, **84**, 1875–87.

128 Horak ER, Leek R, Klenk N *et al*. Angiogenesis, assessed by platelet/endothelial cell adhesion molecule antibodies, as indicator of node metastases and survival in breast cancer. *Lancet* 1992, **340**, 1120–4.

129 Weidner N, Carrol PR, Flax J, Blumenfeld W, Folkman J. Tumor angiogenesis correlates with metastasis in invasive prostate carcinoma. *Am J Pathol*, 1993, **143**, 401–3.

130 Brawer MK, Deering RE, Brown M *et al*. Predictors of pathologic stage in prostatic carcinoma. The role of neovascularity. *Cancer* 1994, **73**, 678–87.

131 Bochner BH, Cote RJ, Weidner N *et al*. Angiogenesis in bladder cancer: relationship between microvessel density and tumor prognosis. *J Natl Cancer Inst* 1995, **87**, 1603–12.

132 Jaeger TM, Weidner N, Chew K *et al*. Tumor angiogenesis correlates with lymph node metastases in invasive bladder cancer. *J Urol* 1995, **154**, 69–71.

133 Dickinson AJ, Fox SB, Persad RA *et al.* Quantification of angiogenesis as an independent predictor of prognosis in invasive bladder carcinomas. *Br J Urol* 1994, **74**, 762–6.

134 O'Brien T, Cranston D, Fuggle S *et al.* Different angiogenic pathways characterize superficial and invasive bladder cancer. *Cancer Res* 1995, **55**, 510–3.

135 Cambell SC, Bouck N. Harnessing the tumor-fighting power of angiogenesis. *Contemp Urol* 1996, **June**, 27–40.

136 D'Amato RJ, Loughnan MS, Flynn E, Folkman J. Thalidomide is an inhibitor of angiogenesis. *Proc Natl Acad Sci USA* 1994, **91**, 4082–5.

137 Voest EE, Kenyon BM, O'Reilly MS *et al.* Inhibition of angiogenesis in vivo by interleukin 12. *J Natl Cancer Inst* 1995, **87**, 581–6.

138 O'Reilly MS, Holmgren L, Shing Y *et al.* Angiostatin: a novel angiogenesis inhibitor that mediates the suppression of metastases by a Lewis Lung carcinoma. *Cell* 1994, **79**, 315–28.

139 O'Reilly MS, Holmgren L, Shing Y *et al.* Angiostatin: a circulating endothelial cell inhibitor that suppresses angiogenesis and tumor growth. *Cold Spring Harbor Symp* 1994, 471–7.

140 Iruela-Arispe ML, Bornstein P, Sage H. Thrombospondin exerts an antiangiogenic effect on cord formation by endothelial cells in vitro. *Proc Natl Acad Sci USA* 1991, **88**, 5026–30.

141 Good DJ, Polverini PJ, Rastinejad F *et al.* A tumor suppressor-dependent inhibitor of angiogenesis is immunologically and functionally indistinguishable from a fragment of thrombospondin. *Proc Natl Acad Sci USA* 1990, **87**, 6624–8.

142 Grossfeld GD, Shi SR, Ginsberg DA *et al.* Immunohistochemical detection of thrombospondin-1 in formalin-fixed, paraffin-embedder tissue. *J Histochem Cytochem* 1996, **44**, 761–6.

143 Grossfeld GD, Ginsberg DA, Stein JP *et al.* Thrombospondin-1 expression in bladder cancer: association with p53 alterations, tumor angiogenesis and tumor progression. *J Natl Cancer Inst* 1997, **89**, 219–27.

144 Dameron KM, Volpert OV, Tainsky MA, Bouck N. Control of angiogenesis in fibroblasts by p53 regulation of thrombospondin-1. *Science* 1994, **265**, 1582–4.

145 Folkman J. Clinical applications of research on angiogenesis. *N Engl J Med* 1995, **333**, 1757–9.

146 Cordon-Cardo C. Mutation of cell cycle regulators. Biological and clinical implicaitons of human neoplasia. *Am J Pathol* 1995, **147**, 545–8.

147 Fung YKT, Murphree AL, T' Ang A *et al.* Structural evidence for the authenticity of the human retinoblastoma gene. *Science* 1987, **236**, 1657–61.

148 Cairns P, Proctor AJ, Knowles MA. Loss of heterozygosity at the Rb locus is frequent and correlates with muscle invasion in bladder carcinoma. *Oncogene* 1991, **6**, 2305–9.

149 Cordon-Cardo C, Wartinger D, Petrylak D *et al.* Altered expression of the retinoblastoma gene product: prognostic indicator in bladder cancer. *J Natl Cancer Inst* 1992, **84**, 1251–6.

150 Logothetis CJ, Xu HJ, Ro JY *et al.* Altered expression of retinoblastoma protein and known prognostic variables in locally advanced bladder cancer. *J Natl Cancer Inst* 1992, **84**, 1256–61.

151 Presti JC Jr, Reuter VE, Galan T *et al.* Molecular genetic alterations in superficial and locally advanced human bladder cancer. *Cancer Res* 1991, **51**, 5405–9.

152 Bagchi S, Weinman R, Raychaudhuri P. The retinoblastoma protein copurifies with E2F-1, and E1A-regulated inhibitor of the transcription factor E2F. *Cell* 1991, **65**, 1063–72.

153 Wang JY, Knudsen ES, Welch PJ. The retinoblastoma tumor suppressor protein. *Adv Cancer Res* 1994, **64**, 25–85.

154 Geradts J, Hu SX, Lincoln C *et al.* Aberrant Rb gene expression in routinely processed, archival tumor tissues determined by three different anti-Rb antibodies. *Int J Cancer* 1994, **58**, 161–7.

155 Xu HJ, Cairns P, Hu SX *et al.* Loss of Rb protein expression in primary bladder cancer correlates with loss of heterozygosity at the Rb locus and tumor progression. *Int J Cancer* 1993, **53**, 781–4.

156 Ishikawa J, Xu HJ, Hu SX *et al.* Inactivation of the retinoblastoma gene in human bladder and renal cell carcinomas. *Cancer Res* 1991, **51**, 5736.

157 Hollstein M, Sidransky D, Volgelstein B, Harris CC. P53 mutations in human cancers. *Science* 1991, **253**, 49–53.

158 Lane DP. Cancer: p53, guardian of the genome. *Nature* 1992, **358**, 15–6.

159 Esrig D, Spruck CH III, Nichols PW *et al.* P53 nuclear protein accumulation correlates with mutations in the p53 gene, tumor grade, and stage in bladder cancer. *Am J Pathol* 1993, **143**, 1389–97.

160 Esrig D, Elmajian D, Groshen S *et al.* Accumulation of nuclear p53 and tumor progression in bladder cancer. *N Engl J Med* 1994, **331**, 1259–64.

161 Cordon-Cardo C, Dalbagni G, Saez GT *et al.* P53 mutations in human bladder cancer: genotypic versus phenotypic patterns. *Int J Cancer* 1994, **56**, 347–53.

162 Lipponen PK. Over-expression of the p53 nuclear onocprotein in transitional cell carcinoma of the bladder and its prognostic value. *Int J Cancer* 1993, **53**, 365–9.

163 Sarkis AS, Dalbagni G, Cordon-Cardo C *et al.* Nuclear over-expression of p53 protein in transitional cell bladder carcinoma: a marker for disease progression. *J Natl Cancer Inst* 1993, **85**, 53–9.

164 Esrig D, Shi SR, Bochner B *et al.* Prognostic importance of p53 and Rb alterations in transitional cell carcinoma of the bladder. *J Urol* 1995, **153**, 362A (abstract 536).

165 Lerner S, Linn D, Chakraborty S *et al.* Correlation of p53 and retinoblastoma protein expression with established pathologic prognostic features in radical cystoprostatectomy specimens. *J Urol* 1995, **153**, 363A (abstract 537).

166 Michieli P, Chedid M, Lin D *et al.* Induction of WAF1/CIP1 by a p53-independent pathway. *Cancer Res* 1994, **54**, 3391–5.

167 Bond JA, Blaydes JP, Rowson J *et al.* Mutant p53 rescues human diploid cells from senescence without inhibiting the induction of SDI1/WAF1. *Cancer Res* 1995, **55**, 2404–9.

168 Parker SB, Eichele G, Zhang P *et al.* p53-independent expression of p21 in muscle and other terminal differentiating cells. *Science* 1995, **267**, 1024–7.

169 Stein JP, Ginsberg DA, Grossfeld GD *et al.* The effect of p21 expression on tumor progression in p53 altered bladder cancer. *J Urol* 1996, **155**, 628A (abstract 1270).

12. STAGING OF BLADDER CANCER

David Farrugia and R. Timothy Oliver

The last five decades have seen a gradual evolution of systems used for the staging of bladder cancer. These systems are still undergoing changes as it is increasingly realized that close correlation between pathological and clinical staging is required, and that staging should distinguish between patients requiring different approaches to therapy. Additionally, the desire to have one internationally acceptable and universally applicable staging system continues to gain momentum.

TUMOUR–NODE–METASTASES (TNM) SYSTEM

The TNM system adopted by the 'Union Internationale Contre le Cancer' (UICC) in 1963 (1) was based on the original concepts of Denoix, who devised his system between 1943 and 1952. The TNM system classifies tumours by the anatomical extent of disease, and has a pretreatment clinical system designated TNM, and a postoperative histopathological system designated pTNM. For bladder tumours, the pretreatment classification is nowadays based on findings of clinical examination, examination under anaesthesia (EUA), radiological imaging, and cystoscopic biopsies, whereas the postsurgical classification includes evidence from definitive surgery, which may be transurethral resection (TUR) or a cystectomy specimen. Clinical staging of the depth of invasion has been notoriously unreliable with discordance rates of up to 44% reported in the literature (2). The role of novel imaging modalities in the preoperative staging of bladder cancer is discussed below.

The 1st edition of the UICC TNM system was published in 1968, followed by the 2nd edition in 1974. This system was well received and was seen as a concise, descriptive method of recording staging data relevant to prognosis and treatment. The 3rd edition, published in 1978 (1), rapidly gained acceptance worldwide, and was recognized for the staging of urological tumours by the World Health Organization (WHO) and the European Organization for Research on Treatment of Cancer (EORTC). A

4th edition was published in 1987 (3), and was revised in 1990 (Table 12.1a and 12.1b). Among the changes made in the 1990 revision were the subdivision of T3b tumours (invading perivesical fat) into (I) microscopic and (II) macroscopic invasion, and T4 tumours into T4a if involving prostate, uterus, or vagina, and T4b if involving pelvic or abdominal walls (4).

Table 12.1a

COMPARISON OF THE 1987, 1990, AND THE 1997 REVISED TNM SYSTEMS[3-5]

Definition	1987	1990	1997
Primary tumour			
Primary tumour cannot be assessed		TX	TX
No evidence of primary tumour		T0	T0
Non-invasive papillary carcinoma	Ta	Ta	Ta
Carcinoma *in situ*: flat tumour	Tis	Tis	Tis
Invades subepithelial connective tissue	T1	T1	T1
Superficial (inner half) muscle invasion	T2	T2	T2a
Deep (outer half) muscle invasion	T3a	T3a	T2b
Invades perivesical fat	T3b	T3b	T3
microscopic			T3a
macroscopic			T3b
Invades prostate, uterus, or vagina	T4	T4a	T4a
Invades pelvic or abdominal wall	T4	T4b	T4b
Lymph nodes			
Regional lymph nodes cannot be assessed		NX	NX
No regional node involvement	N0	N0	N0
Single node, <2 cm largest diameter	N1	N1	N1
Single node 2–5 cm or multiple nodes < 5 cm	N2	N2	N2
Nodal involvement > 5 cm	N3	N3	N3
Distant metastasis			
No distant metastases	M0	M0	M0
Distant metastases	M1	M1	M1

Table 12.1b

STAGE GROUPING[3]

Stage group	TNM stages		
Stage 0	Tis	N0	M0
	Ta	N0	M0
Stage I	T1	N0	M0
Stage II	T2	N0	M0
Stage III	T3a	N0	M0
	T3b	N0	M0
Stage IV	T4	N0	M0
	Any T	N 1–3	M0
	Any T	Any N	M1

The latest modification to the TNM staging of bladder cancer was published in 1997 (5). This modification has re-classified invasion of the outer half of the muscle wall as T2b, thus grouping all muscle invasive but not penetrant tumours under stage T2. Any tumour penetrating through to the perivesical fat was re-classified as stage T3, with T3a denoting microscopic as opposed to macroscopic (T3b) disease (Table 12.1). Support for this re-definition of stages T2 and T3 came from observations such as those of Pearse (6) and Blandy *et al.* (7), who reported little difference in survival between superficial (previously T2) and deep (previously T3a) muscle invasive tumours. More emphasis in staging is therefore being placed on whether or not the tumour is organ confined (T2b or less according to the 1997 revision) or non-organ confined (T3 or greater) (8). Additionally, the accuracy of clinical determination of the degree of muscle infiltration remains at best modest, and even in experienced hands, the correlation between depth of invasion, based on the cystoscopic evaluation, and the findings after cystectomy is only 50–60% (9). In most centres, it is the presence of muscle invasion, rather than its depth, which dictates therapy and significantly influences prognosis.

Another issue that requires further clarification is that regarding prostatic involvement and its correlation with prognosis. A distinction must be made between tumour growing into the prostate from the urethra along the prostatic ducts, i.e. a non-invasive lesion, and that directly invading the prostatic stroma (i.e. a true T4a tumour). Pugh (10) in 1981 was among the first to draw attention to this deficiency in the UICC TNM system, and to the differences in outcome associated with these two distinct pathological entities. He suggested that non-invasive tumour in the prostatic ducts should be labelled P4aa, while stromal invasive disease should be designated P4ab, and showed that the former was associated with superior survival in a series of 33 patients. Wood *et al.* (11) identified transitional cell carcinoma of the prostatic epithelium in 40% of 25 men undergoing radical cystectomy. In 24 of these, preoperative cystoscopy had shown a normal urethra, but transurethral resection had revealed the presence of carcinoma with 90% accuracy, compared with 20 and 40% accuracy for prostate needle biopsy and fine needle aspiration respectively. Pagano *et al.* (2), showed that the 5-year survival for non-invasive transitional cell carcinoma (TCC) in the prostate coincidental with bladder tumour was 37% compared with 6% for transmural prostatic invasion. These findings were similar to those of Esrig *et al.* (12), who recently correlated pathological staging of cystectomy specimens with survival in 143 cystectomy specimens collected between 1971 and 1989, in which prostatic involvement was present. They concluded that prostatic urethral or ductal TCC without prostatic stromal involvement did not alter the survival determined by bladder staging alone. Prostatic stromal involvement adversely affected prognosis, reducing the 5-year survival from 71% where no stromal involvement was present, to 36% in cases of stromal invasion (whether transurethral or transmural). Within the subgroup with prostatic stromal involvement, transurethral spread had superior 5-year survival (55%) than transmural prostatic infiltration (21%).

The classification of nodal status has also been successively revised. The 1978 UICC staging system defined N1 as involvement of a single homolateral regional node; N2 as involvement of contralateral, or bilateral, or multiple regional nodes; N3 for regional nodes which were fixed to the pelvic wall; and N4 for involved juxtaregional (inguinal, common iliac, and para-aortic nodes. In line with staging systems for other solid tumours, size of involved nodes is now the main distinguishing feature between nodal stages rather than multiplicity or fixity of involved nodes. Thus in 1987, N1 was defined as a single regional node <2 cm in greatest dimension; N2 as a single regional node 2–5 cm in greatest dimension or multiple nodes all <5cm; and N3 as one or more regional nodes >5 cm in greatest dimension. This annotation has remained unchanged in all subsequent revisions of the TNM staging system (Table 12.1).

Further information can be added to the TNM staging by the use of additional descriptors that are denoted by the prefixes or suffixes listed in Table 12.2. Additionally, the degree of certainty with which each TNM category was allocated can be denoted by the 'C-factor' following each category (Table 12.3 and see example below). The C-factor may be reviewed and upgraded as information becomes available from additional staging modalities.

Table 12.2

USE OF ADDITIONAL DESCRIPTORS IN TNM STAGING[3]	
Descriptor	**Definition**
Suffix 'm'	Synchronous multiple tumours within the bladder. Alternatively, the number of primaries in parenthesis may be used.
Suffix 'is'	Associated carcinoma *in situ*.
Prefix 'y'	Classification was made during or following other treatment, e.g. surgery preceded by intravesical instillation therapy.
Prefix 'r'	Tumour is a recurrence within a previously treated area.
Prefix 'R'	Residual tumour after treatment; RX: not assessable, R0: not present, R1: microscopic, R2: microscopic.

Table 12.3

C-FACTOR CATEGORY(3)	
C-factor	**Definition**
C1	Evidence from standard diagnostic means, e.g. clinical examination, and standard radiography.
C2	Evidence from special diagnostic means, e.g. CT and MRI imaging, and cystoscopy.
C3	Evidence from surgery exploration.
C4	Evidence from pathological examination of therapeutically resected specimen.
C5	Evidence from autopsy.

The use of the system is illustrated in the following clinical case. A patient presented with macroscopic haematuria and a filling defect in the bladder on urography. Examination under anaesthesia was negative, but cystoscopy revealed two papillary tumours which were biopsied and found not to infiltrate the lamina propria (Ta(m)C2), while computed tomography (CT) scanning did not show evidence of nodal or metastatic disease (N0C2M0C2). A TUR was performed revealing invasion of the lamina propria (pT1(m)C4N0C2M0C2). The patient returned a year later with pain and haematuria and was found to have a palpable recurrence at the original site (rT2C1). A TUR shows infiltration of superficial muscle but no evidence of nodal or metastatic spread on imaging (rT2aC3N0C2M0C2). He received neo-adjuvant chemotherapy and proceeded to radical cystectomy, which revealed deep muscle infiltration and involvement of multiple pelvic nodes all less than 5 cm in greatest dimension (yrpT2bC4N2C4M0C2).

As will be appreciated, the addition of further information leads to increased complexity and may limit the more widespread use of this system. However, the advantages of adopting a detailed, universally accepted system are clearly evident.

THE JEWETT AND STRONG (AMERICAN) STAGING SYSTEM

This system was developed following the examination of autopsy specimens from 107 patients, and was intended to correlate the depth of bladder wall invasion with the probability of metastasis (13). Depth of invasion was also correlated with 5-year survival (14), emphasizing the importance of proper preoperative staging with adequate biopsy and EUA. This classification, further modified by Marshall (15), became standard in the United States and

Table 12.4

COMPARISON OF JEWITT/STRONG/MARSHALL AND AJCC (2ND EDITION) CLASSIFICATIONS		
Jewitt/Strong/Marshall[12-14]	**AJCC**	**TNM[15]**
0 Limited to mucosal surface	TX	Minimum staging requirements not met
	T0	No evidence of primary tumour
	Tis	Carcinoma *in situ*
	Ta	Papillary non-invasive carcinoma
A Invasion of lamina propria	T1	Invasion of lamina propria
B1 Muscle invasion <50%	T2	Muscle invasion <50%
B2 Muscle invasion >50%	T3a	Muscle invasion >50%
C Invasion of perivesical fat or	T3b	Invasion of perivesical fat
adjacent organs (prostate	T4a	Invasion of prostate, uterus or vagina
uterus, vagina, bowel) or		
fixed to pelvic wall.	T4b	Fixed to pelvic or abdominal wall
D1 Nodal metastases	N0	No regional node involvement
	N1	Single homolateral regional node
	N2	Contralateral, bilateral, or multiple regional nodes
	N3	Fixed pelvic wall mass separate from primary tumour
D2 Distant metastases	M0	No evidence of distant metastases
	M1	Distant metastases present

is shown in Table 12.4 compared with the AJCC TNM system. Although this system was useful as it correlated pathological findings with prognosis, the use of the same terms to describe pre-operative and pathological findings led to some confusion. Additionally, as can be appreciated particularly from the description of stage C and D disease, it lacked the detail present in the TNM system.

The American Joint Committee on Cancer Staging and End Results Reporting (AJCC) recommended a modified version of the TNM system which has gradually gained popularity. The 2nd edition of the AJCC classification, published in 1983, is shown in Table 12.4, and the similarities with the UICC TNM system are clearly evident (16). As well as being a more detailed system, this classification was one major step towards having an internationally comparable system for reporting treatment results.

IMAGING MODALITIES IN THE STAGING OF BLADDER CANCER

Ultrasonography

Bladder ultrasonography has developed from transabdominal, to transrectal (TRUS), to transurethral, with progressive miniaturization of transducers. Transabdominal ultrasonography suffers from poor definition of bladder wall invasion, and has largely been superseded by CT and magnetic resonance (MR) imaging. TRUS was compared by Yaman *et al.* (17) with CT and TUR, and the findings correlated with pathological staging of the cystectomy specimen. In their hands the staging accuracy of TRUS, CT, and TUR was 40, 35, and 46%, respectively, and they concluded that the two imaging techniques did not complement TUR and failed to contribute additional information. TRUS led to overstaging of superficial tumours in 49% of cases, and to understaging of invasive tumours in 11% of cases.

Transurethral ultrasound has the potential to identify individual layers of bladder muscle and may be particularly useful for the staging of superficial lesions. Schuller *et al.* (18), reported 82% staging accuracy with this technique. Koraitim *et al.* (19), correlated preoperative transurethral ultrasound staging with pathological staging of cystectomy specimens and reported 100% correlation in non-invasive tumours (Ta and T1). This dropped off with increasing depth of invasion to about 96% for T2a and b, and 70% for T3 tumours. The main disadvantage of transurethral ultrasonography is the need to undertake the investigation under general or spinal anaesthesia at the time of cystoscopy, and this has limited its use to centres with a special interest in bladder cancer.

Computerized tomography

CT has been among the mainstay of bladder cancer staging modalities for some time. Kellett *et al.* (20), who reported an 80% concordance between CT and pathological staging, noted that whereas clinical staging tended to underestimate muscle invasive disease, CT scanning tended to overstage tumours. Numerous other studies have evaluated the role of CT in this setting, and among the larger ones in which correlation with pathological staging was sought, accuracy rates ranging from 64 to 81% were reported for assessment of depth of invasion (21–23). MacVicar and Husband (24) in a review of CT staging of bladder cancer observed that CT, like ultrasound, was unable to show accurately the depth of muscle invasion due to its inability to distinguish between individual layers of muscle wall. However, CT was useful in discriminating between disease confined to the bladder wall and tumour that had penetrated perivesical fat (T3). They concluded that with increasing expertise, the accuracy rate of this technique should nowadays exceed 80%. Oedema or thickening of the bladder wall secondary to biopsy or irradiation can mimic recurrent tumour on CT images and result in overstaging. Conversely, T3 disease may be understaged as microscopic infiltration of perivesical tissue was not recognized by this technique.

The ability of CT to detect affected lymph nodes depends on enlargement of involved nodes and sensitivity rates of between 50 and 85% have been reported. Nodal enlargement from other causes can give false positives so that specificity rates of between 67 and 100% have been reported (21,23,25,26). One application for CT imaging not shared by MR is its use in guided biopsy of the bladder wall. Malmstrom *et al.* (27) evaluated CT-guided transmural core biopsy of the bladder wall in 17 patients, and found this more useful at identifying transmural infiltration than transurethral biopsies.

Magnetic resonance imaging

MR is well suited for the imaging of pelvic organs, with better contrast resolution compared with CT. T1-weighted sequences produce low signal (dark) from tumours and generate contrast with high signal perivesical fat (light). T2-weighted sequences generate low signal from bladder wall, intermediate signal from tumour, and high signal from urine within the bladder. However, individual layers of bladder wall are still poorly visualized making it difficult to distinguish T2a from T2b tumours, while accuracy is improved for higher tumour stages (T3 and T4) (28).

The use of gadolinium-DTPA enhancement may improve the assessment of bladder wall invasion, and early reports suggested that this technique was superior to CT or conventional unenhanced MR at delineating bladder wall anatomy and depth of tumour invasion (29). However, this technique is also affected by late tissue changes which may occur up to several years following previous radiotherapy (30). Thus, in a comparison of CT with unenhanced and dynamic gadolinium-enhanced MR, Kim *et al.* (28) found that with all techniques, overstaging was the most common error and occurred in about a third of cases across all imaging modalities. A trend towards greater sensitivity and accuracy was seen with dynamic gadolinium-enhanced MR, but this was not significant in this small series. These findings supported those of Persad *et al.* (31), and Narumi *et al.* (32) who encountered both over- and understaging, as well as difficulties in visualizing the depth of muscle wall penetration. The latter study used oblique enhanced T1-weighted and unenhanced T2-weighted MR and found the former to be more accurate at assessing depth of muscle invasion (78% accuracy) compared with the latter (60% accuracy, $P < 0.05$). Scattoni *et al.* (33), also found dynamic contrast-enhanced T1 imaging to be superior to unenhanced T1- and

T2-weighted and late enhanced MR imaging in the assessment of superficial (T1) disease, with 84% accuracy of the former compared with 44–68% for the other modalities.

Recent advances in MR imaging resulting in improved image quality in the pelvis may yet translate into more accurate preoperative staging of bladder cancer. Barentz *et al.* (34), recently reported on the use of a fast dynamic first-pass MR technique with contrast enhancement. This is based on an earlier enhancement of tumour compared with normal tissues, which can be detected by serial turbo FLASH (fast low angle shots) images at 2 s intervals. Compared with unenhanced T1- and T2-weighted images, dynamic contrast enhancement improved the accuracy of staging of both bladder wall disease and nodal spread in 61 patients staged 1–4 weeks after TUR or biopsy.

Positron emission tomography (PET)

Initial impressions from studies of PET scanning in the staging of bladder cancer have been somewhat disappointing. In a small series of 23 primary tumours reported by Ahlstrom *et al.* (35), PET was able to detect 18 of 23 primary tumours, but its accuracy at staging was probably inferior to that of MR or CT. The presence of large amounts of 18F-fluoro-deoxy-glucose tracer in urine was found to impair the visualization of the primary tumour. Thus PET may be more useful in defining nodal or metastatic spread, but this remains to be tested.

CORRELATION OF TUMOUR STAGING WITH BEHAVIOUR AND PROGNOSIS

Ta lesions tend to grow as exophytic lesions, have a tendency to bleed and recur, but generally do not invade and have an excellent prognosis. A tumour invading the lamina propria (T1), also has a good prognosis with a 5-year survival of about 75% in most series (Table 12.5). Once invasion into the muscle layer is documented, the risk of nodal and subsequent distant metastases increases. Thus only 5–13% of patients with bladder muscle confined disease (T1–T2) have positive nodes, but this proportion increases to 18–44% for patients with extravesical invasion (>T3) (36). Once nodal disease is documented, outcomes without systemic therapy are poor, with overall survival ranging from 4% to 36% at 5 years (Table 12.5). Similarly, patients with metastatic disease also exhibit a bleak prognosis, with median survival ranging from 6 to 9 months and few patients surviving at 5 years.

Table 12.5

CORRELATION OF STAGING WITH % 5-YEAR SURVIVAL							
Series	No. of patients	Definitive treatment	T1	T2	T3*	T4	N+
Blandy[7] 1980	704	RT + salvage cystectomy	70	27	38	9	
Smith[36] 1981	134	cystectomy	—	—	—	—	7
Skinner[37] 1984	197	Cystectomyn ± RT	75	64	44	36	36
Pagano[2] 1991	261	cystectomy	75	63	31	21	4

* Refers to the older classification and includes deep muscle invasion as well as extramural penetration. RT = radiotherapy.

CONCLUSIONS

The TNM system appears to provide an accurate method for the documentation of bladder cancer stage, and has been shown to correlate with prognosis. Its strongest point, however, is that it has become the most widely accepted and used bladder staging system to date, thereby enabling world-wide comparisons of treatment results. Although MR is rapidly overtaking CT as the pelvic imaging modality of choice in many centres (24), patients found to have superficial tumours may benefit in terms of increased staging accuracy if this were to be supplemented by transurethral ultrasonography. Both CT and MR appear equally effective at visualizing nodal and metastatic disease, although the efficacy of PET scanning in detecting small tumour deposits in normal sized nodes is still under evaluation.

Key Points

1. The TNM system provides an accurate method for the documentation of bladder cancer stage and has been shown to correlate with prognosis.
2. MRI is rapidly overtaking CT as the pelvic imaging modality of choice.
3. Patients with superficial tumours may benefit in terms of increased staging accuracy if MRI were to be supplemented by transurethral ultrasonography.

References

1 UICC. *TNM classification of malignant tumours* (ed. Harmer MH). Union Internationale Contre Le Cancer, Geneva, 1978.
2 Pagano F, Bassi F, Prayer-Galetti T *et al*. Results of contemporary radical cystectomy for invasive bladder cancer: a clinicopathological study with an emphasis on the inadequacy of the tumor, nodes and metastases classification. *J Urol* 1991, **145**, 45–50.
3 UICC. Staging of urinary bladder cancer. In: *TNM classification of malignant tumours* (ed. Hermanek P, Sobin LH), Springer-Verlag, Berlin, 1987, pp. 118–123
4 UICC. Staging of urinary bladder cancer. In: *TNM atlas: illustrated guide to the TNM/pTNM classification of malignant tumours* (ed. Spiessel B, Beahrs OH, Hermanek P, Hutter RVP, Scheibe O, Sobin LH, Wagner G). Springer-Verlag, Berlin, 1992, pp. 174–179
5 UICC. (1997): Staging of urinary bladder cancer. In: *TNM classification of malignant tumours* (ed. Sobin LH, Wittekind C). John Wiley and Sons, New York, 1997, pp. 201–213
6 Pearse HD, Reed RR, Hodges CV. Radical cystectomy for bladder cancer. *J Urol* 1978, **119**, 216–18.
7 Blandy JP, England HR, Evans JW *et al*. T3 bladder cancer—the case for salvage cystectomy. *Br J Urol* 1980, **52**, 506–10.

8   Hall RR, Prout GR. Staging of bladder cancer. Is tumor, node, metastases system adequate? *Semin Oncol*, 1990, **17**, 517–23.

9   Whitmore WF. Management of invasive bladder neoplasms. *Semin Urol* 1983, **1**, 34–41.

10 Pugh RCB. Bladder cancer. In: *Principles of combination therapy* (ed. Oliver RTD, Hendry WF, Bloom HJG). Butterworths, London, 1981, pp. 3–8.

11 Wood DP, Montie JE, Pontes JE, Levin HS. Identification of transitional cell carcinoma of the prostate in bladder cancer patients: a prospective study. *J Urol* 1989, **141**, 83–5.

12 Esrig DFJ, Elmajian DA, Stein JP *et al.* Transitional cell carcinoma involving the prostate with a proposed staging classification for stromal invasion. *J Urol* 1996, **156**, 1071–6.

13 Jewett HJ, Strong GH. Infiltrating carcinoma of the bladder: relation of depth of penetration of the bladder wall to incidence of local extension and metastases. *J Urol* 1946, **55**, 366–72.

14 Jewett HJ. Carcinoma of the bladder: influence of the depth of infiltration on the 5-year results following complete extirpation of the primary growth. *J Urol* 1952, **67**, 672–80.

15 Marshall VF. The relation of the preoperative estimate to the pathologic demonstration of the extent of vesical neoplasms. *J Urol* 1952, **68**, 714–23.

16 American Joint Committee on Cancer. *Manual for staging of cancer*. Lippincott, Philadelphia, 1983.

17 Yaman O, Baltaci S, Arikan N *et al.* Staging with computed tomography, transrectal ultrasonography and transurethral resection of bladder tumour: comparison with final pathological stage in invasive bladder carcinoma. *Br J Urol* 1996, **78**, 197–200.

18 Schuller J, Walther V, Schmiedt E *et al.* Intravesical ultrasound tomography in staging bladder carcinoma. *J Urol* 1982, **128**, 264–6.

19 Koraitim M, Kamal B, Metwalli N, Zaky Y. Transurethral ultrasonographic assessment of bladder carcinoma: its value and limitation. *J Urol* 1995, **154**, 375–8.

20 Kellett MJ, Oliver RTD, Husband JE, Kelsey Fry I. Computed tomography as an adjunct to bimanual examination for staging bladder tumours. *Br J Urol* 1980, **52**, 101–6.

21 Koss JC, Arger PH, Coleman BG *et al.* CT Staging of bladder carcinoma. *Am J Roentgenol*, 1981, **137**, 359–62.

22 Vock P, Haertel M, Fuchs WA *et al.* Computed tomography in staging of carcinoma of the urinary bladder. *Br J Urol* 1982, **54**, 158–63.

23 Weinerman PM, Arger PH, Pollack HM. CT evaluation of bladder and prostate neoplasms. *Urol Radiol*, 1982, **4**, 105–14.

24 MacVicar D, Husband J. Radiology in the staging of bladder cancer. *Br J Hosp Med* 1994, **51**, 454–8.

25 Walsh JW, Amendola MA, Konerding KF *et al.* Computed tomographic detection of pelvic and inguinal lymph-node metastases from primary and recurrent pelvic malignant disease. *Radiology* 1980, **137**, 157–66.

26 Morgan CL, Calkins RF, Cavalcanti EJ. Computed tomography in the evaluation, staging, and therapy of carcinoma of the bladder and prostate. *Radiology* 1981, **140**, 751–61.

27 Malmstrom PU, Lonnemark M, Busch C, Magnusson A. Staging of bladder carcinoma by computer tomography-guided transmural core biopsy. *Scand J Urol Nephrol* 1993, **27**, 193–8.

28 Kim B, Semelka RC, Ascher SM *et al.* Bladder tumor staging: comparison of contrast enhanced CT, T1- and T2-weighted MR imaging, dynamic gadolinium-enhanced imaging, and late gadolinium-enhanced imaging. *Radiology* 1994, **193**, 239–45.

29 Tanimoto A, Yuasa Y, Imai Y *et al.* Bladder tumor staging: comparison of conventional and gadolinium-enhanced dynamic MR imaging and CT. *Radiology* 1992, **185**, 741–7.

30 Hawnaur JM, Johnson RJ, Read G, Isherwood I. Magnetic resonance imaging with gadolinium-DTPA for assessment of bladder carcinoma and its response to treatment. *Clin Radiol* 1993, **47**, 302–10.

31 Persad R, Kabala J, Gillatt D *et al.* Magnetic resonance imaging in the staging of bladder cancer. *Br J Urol* 1993, **71**, 566–73.

32 Narumi Y, Kadota T, Inoue E *et al.* Bladder tumours: staging with gadolinium-enhanced oblique MR imaging. *Radiology* 1993, **187**, 145–50.

33 Scattoni V, Da Pozzo LF, Colombo R *et al.* Dynamic gadolinium-enhanced magnetic resonance imaging in staging of superficial bladder cancer. *J Urol* 1996, **155**, 1594–9.

34 Barentsz JO, Jager GJ, Van Vierzen PB *et al.* Staging urinary bladder cancer after transurethral biopsy: value of fast dynamic contrast-enhanced MR imaging. *Radiology* 1996, **201**, 185–93.

35 Ahlstrom H, Malmstrom PU, Letocha H *et al.* Positron emission tomography in the diagnosis and staging of urinary bladder cancer. *Acta Radiol* 1996, **37**, 180–5.

36 Smith JA, Whitmore WF. Regional lymph node metastases from bladder cancer. *J Urol* 1981, **126**, 591–3.

37 Skinner D, Lieskovsky G. Contemporary cystectomy with pelvic node dissection compared to preoperative radiation therapy plus cystectomy in management of invasive bladder cancer. *J Urol* 1984, **131**, 1069–72.

13. THE MANAGEMENT OF SUPERFICIAL BLADDER CANCER

P. Van Erps and L.J. Denis

INTRODUCTION

Seventy to 80% of patients with transitional cell carcinoma of the bladder have superficial tumours without invasion of the detrusor muscle at initial presentation. The standard primary treatment of superficial bladder cancer is a wide transurethral resection (TUR) of all visible tumours. This surgical therapy has a high success rate in eradicating the existing lesions: the persistence of incompletely resected tumours and regrowth is low. Despite this complete resection, most patients will develop new bladder tumours in remote areas of the bladder. This phenomenon called tumour recurrence is in fact a new occurrence and pre-existing areas of dysplasia or carcinoma *in situ* (CIS) account for the high frequency of tumour recurrence. The majority of these recurrent tumours are also superficial; however, about 15% of those patients with superficial bladder carcinoma will develop tumour progression with bladder muscle invasion (1). Once the tumour has invaded the detrusor muscle, the prognosis is grim, with a high risk for the development of metastases and death from bladder cancer.

As superficial bladder cancer represents a heterogeneous group with differing natural histories, it may be difficult to predict which patients will develop a recurrence or not and which patients will develop tumour progression. With the help of prognostic factors such as histological stage and grade, tumour size, number of previous bladder tumours, the presence or absence of CIS, and other predictors of the biological potential such as p53 expression, it is possible to identify subgroups of patients with a different risk of recurrence and progression.

A minority of patients present with a primary small, solitary, well-differentiated superficial bladder tumour, that does not recur after TUR. Adjuvant therapy seems to be unnecessary in this low risk patient. However, the majority of patients with superficial bladder cancer will develop superficial recurrences and have a low risk of tumour progression ultimately. As TUR alone may not control all tumours and cannot prevent tumour recurrences, adjuvant therapy such as intravesical instillations of chemotherapy or bacille Calmette–Guérin (BCG), may be administered to these patients in order to decrease the recurrence rate and prevent or delay tumour progression. Another small group of patients present initially with a relatively aggressive superficial tumour and is at high risk for the development of infiltrating bladder cancer. It is important to select these high-risk patients as early as possible and to make every effort to improve the outcome with maximal intravesical treatment in order to avoid cystectomy. Patients with primary or concomitant CIS form a separate group. CIS is an anaplastic, preinvasive form of bladder cancer that does not respond to radiotherapy. The only effective treatment for CIS apart from cystectomy is intravesical chemotherapy or BCG.

STAGING AND NATURAL HISTORY

The tumour stages discussed in this section include Ta, T1, and TIS (Table 13.1). These tumour stages are all superficial to the deep muscle layer of the bladder. The basement membrane plays a major part in the staging of superficial bladder cancer. There is an important prognostic difference between tumours confined by this basement membrane and tumours invading the lamina propria, that consists of loose connective tissue and is rich with vascular and lymphatic channels. Within the lamina propria lies the muscularis mucosa, an attenuated layer of smooth muscle. Some authors have suggested that invasion of this muscular layer has prognostic significance: patients with lamina propria invasion into the muscularis mucosa had a significantly higher incidence of tumour recurrence and progression, than patients with superficial tumours not invading the muscularis mucosa (2). Unfortunately, the muscularis mucosa is variably present, making it an unreliable landmark, with less than half of pathologists agreeing on a given case (3).

The most commonly used grading systems employ three grades: low, intermediate, and high grade. Low-grade bladder tumours

Table 13.1

T CLASSIFICATION OF SUPERFICIAL BLADDER TUMOURS	
Stage	**Definition**
Ta	Non-invasive papillary tumour (above the basement membrane)
T1	Tumour invades subepithelial connective tissue
TIS	Carcinoma *in situ*: 'flat tumour'

usually have a benign natural history, while high-grade tumours behave aggressively. However, as most tumours are classified in the intermediate grade group, these grading systems fail to discriminate tumours with varying biological potential, and it also has been shown that they lack reproducibility (4). At diagnosis about 70% of superficial bladder tumours are pTa and 30% are pT1 (5). Only 10–20% of patients with muscle invasive bladder cancer have ever started as superficial bladder cancer (6), indicating that superficial and invasive bladder carcinoma are probably biologically completely different entities.

Ta tumours are usually low or intermediate grade (G1 and G2), whereas the majority of T1 tumours are high grade (G2–G3). TIS is always a high-grade neoplasm. The natural history of superficial bladder carcinoma has been studied by the National Bladder Cancer Collaborative Group prospectively following 249 patients after TUR alone without any adjuvant treatment (7). Both tumour stage and grade significantly influenced the likelihood of recurrence and progression to invasive disease (Table 13.2). Only 30% of the patients with pT1 bladder tumours remain free of tumour for 3 years, compared with about 50% for patients with stage Ta tumours. Progression to deeply invasive bladder cancer occurred in more than a third of patients with stage T1 tumours, while progression was absent in more than 90% of patients with stage Ta tumours. Fifty to 60% of patients with grades 1 and 2 tumours have tumour recurrences, which are mostly also low stage and low grade, and only 2–11% will progress to invasive disease. On the contrary, 80% of patients with grade 3 bladder tumours have tumour recurrence and more than half of them develop invasive bladder cancer within 3 years after diagnosis. The initial stage and grade remain important with long-term follow-up: in patients with grade 1 disease 10- and 20-year survival have been reported to be 98% and 93%, respectively, whereas with grade 3 disease 10- and 20-year survival decrease to 35% and 28%, respectively.

Table 13.2

IMPORTANCE OF TUMOUR STAGE AND GRADE ON RECURRENCE AND PROGRESSION RATE AFTER 3 YEARS (7)		
Stage	Recurrence	Progression
Ta	50%	<10%
T1	>70%	>30%
G1–2	50–60%	<10%
G3	80%	>50%

Table 13.3

PROGNOSTIC FACTORS OF SUPERFICIAL BLADDER CARCINOMA	
1. Number of tumours	1, 2–3, >4
2. Prior recurrence rate	Primary, Rec < 1/year, Rec > 1/year
3. T category	Ta, T1
4. G grade	G1, G2, G3
5. Tumour diameter	<3 cm, >3 cm
6. Tumour configuration	Papillary versus sessile
7. Urine cytology	Positive versus negative
8. Carcinoma *in situ*	Present or absent

The factor most predictive of tumour recurrence is the number of tumours at first presentation (8), and other factors affecting tumour recurrence or progression (Table 13.3) are tumour size, prior recurrence rate, tumour configuration (papillary versus sessile), positive or negative cytology, and the presence or absence of CIS. Tumour recurrence rate after initial therapy varies from 30% in patients with a solitary papillary tumour to more than 90% in patients with multiple tumours (9). Multiple tumours are also predictive of a short disease-free interval. Disease recurrence at the time of the first follow-up cystoscopy is highly predictive of future recurrences, and the probability of developing future recurrences decreases with each negative cystoscopy, reaching 8% at 5 years and 0% at 10 years (10). CIS can be focal but is mostly diffuse, can be symptomatic or clinically silent, and may or may not be associated with superficial bladder tumours. Diffuse CIS, particularly when associated with symptoms and/or papillary tumours, is a negative prognostic factor. A compilation of the urological literature on CIS indicates an average incidence of progression to muscle invasive disease of 54% (11). Another highly deleterious aspect of CIS is its multicentricity, with possible lesions in the urethra, the ureters, or the prostatic ducts. Therefore, CIS possesses a great biological threat to the patient in terms of both disease progression and the development of tumours elsewhere in the urinary tract.

URINARY CYTOLOGY

The most prominent symptom of bladder cancer is haematuria, occurring in about half of the patients, and cystoscopic evaluation with biopsy and routine cytology are the main tools for bladder cancer diagnosis.

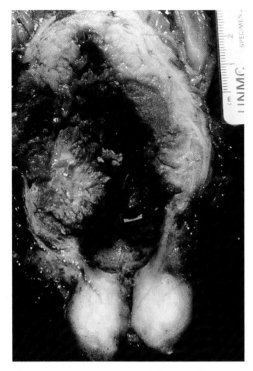

Plate 1 Cystectomy specimen with large papillary urothelial carcinoma. (*See page 100*)

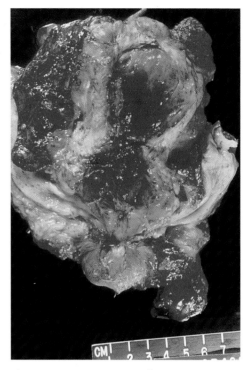

Plate 2 Cystectomy specimen with carcinoma in situ. Note the reddish velvety mucosal surface. (*See page 105*)

Plate 3 Gross appearance of a squamous cell carcinoma which developed in a quadriplegic woman with an indwelling catheter for 24 years. (*See page 113*)

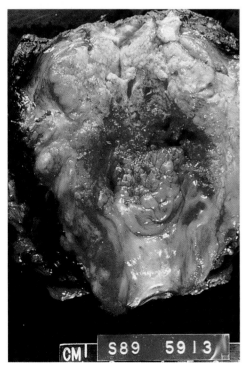

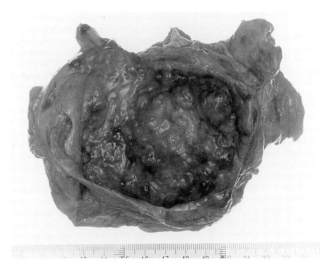

Plate 4 Gross appearance of urinary bladder showing metastatic melanoma. (*See page 118*)

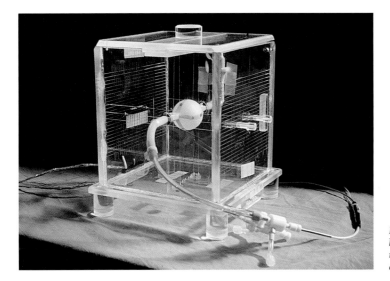

Plate 5 Phantom simulating treatment including ballon catheter for the heat deposition measurement at different distances from the microwaves applicator. (*See page 395*)

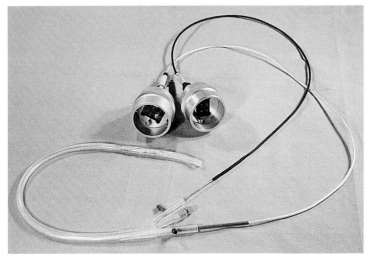

Plate 6 Ultimate version of the Synergo® *System operative catheter ready for treatment. The lure cone connections for closed loop circulation of cytotoxic solution and the connections of microwaves applicator to central unit are shown.* (*See page 397*)

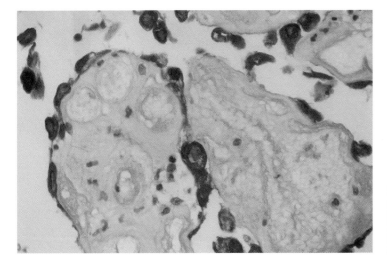

Plate 7 Massive calcification and sclerohyaline necrosis extended to lamina propria in T1 tumours after chemothermotherapy treatment. Thrombosis of vascular structure at the tumoral basis are also evident. Haematoxylin and eosin, ×400. (*See page 401*)

Urothelial cells are continuously sloughed in the urine as they enter apoptosis (programmed cell death). These exfoliated cells provide a rich resource for cytological analysis. The majority of the morphological features of malignancy are associated with the nucleus: hyperchromasia or hypochromasia, irregular coarse chromatin clumping, irregular nuclear membranes, and increased nuclear/cytoplasme ratio. The accuracy of urinary cytology is primarily affected by the grade of the tumour. The reported sensitivity of cytology for grade 3 carcinoma and CIS varies between 65% and 100% (25). Cells exfoliated from grade 1 carcinoma are so closely similar to normal cells that only about 30% are detected by Papanicolau cytology, while the sensitivity of the test for grade 2 carcinomas achieves about 50% (25).

Urinary cytology is not invasive and an important tool in the diagnosis of bladder cancer. The cells for cytological analysis are obtained either in voided urine or during cystoscopy from bladder washing. Cytology can be used for diagnosis of high urinary tract or bladder cancer, for monitoring during and after treatment of urothelial cancer for the detection of recurrences, for screening a high risk population exposed to environmental carcinogens and for predicting the biological potential of cancer or premalignant lesions. False-positive cytology is caused by a number of morphological pitfalls including inflammatory lesions, post-radiation changes, and changes of the bladder epithelium by intravesical therapy with chemo- or immunotherapeutic agents.

Tumour markers

As the clinical behaviour of superficial tumours is unpredictable by stage and grade alone, efforts have been directed to the development of other measures to increase prognostic capabilities (Table 13.4). One of the most commonly used modalities is probably the measurement of the DNA content by flow cytometry on voided urine or on paraffin-embedded tissue. Normal cells are diploid, and aneuploidy is indicative of malignancy. It has been shown that aneuploidy is more common in high-grade tumours and that patients with aneuploid tumours are more prone to disease recurrence, progression, and cancer death (12,13). In one study no progression occurred in 175 patients with diploid DNA tumours whereas 35% of 54 patients with aneuploid tumours had disease progression (12).

Another predictor of biological potential in superficial bladder cancer is the loss or gain of antigen expression. All cells express a variety of antigens on their surface, associated with a variety of

Table 13.4

TUMOUR MARKERS FOR SUPERFICIAL BLADDER CARCINOMA
DNA content by flow cytometry
ABO blood group antigens
Tumour-associated antigens
Lewis X
M344 antigen
DD23 antigen
T138 antigen
BTA
NMP22
Tumour suppressor genes
P53
RB protein

normal cell activities such as cell recognition, cell signalling, and cellular adhesion. Malignant change is associated with the loss of differentiation, leading to the loss of antigenic expression and the expression of new antigens unique to malignant cells. ABO blood group antigens are expressed not only on erythrocytes but also on urothelial cells and numerous reports have suggested an association between the absence of ABO antigens on the tumour cell surface and tumour progression, recurrence and failure of intravesical BCG (14,15). However, this test has not been accepted widely because of methodological difficulties and it has been shown that not every normal person expresses these antigens on their urothelial cells: the absence of ABO expression occurs in 20% of the population and is called 'negative secretor status' (16).

A large number of tumour-associated antigens have been identified, which can be detected on exfoliated urothelial cells by monoclonal antibody staining. The Lewis X (LeX) blood-group-related antigen is one example of an immunocytologically detectable tumour marker. LeX antigen is not normally expressed on benign urothelial cells except for occasional umbrella cells (superficial urothelial cells). Immunocytological detection of LeX antigen on two voided urine specimens has a reported sensitivity of 97%, specificity of 85%, positive predictive value of 76% and negative predictive value of 98% in predicting the presence of transitional cell carcinoma of the bladder (17). If the high sensitivity and specificity of this technique are confirmed in large prospective studies, LeX antigen detection may prove useful in early detection regimens and post-treatment monitoring. Other bladder tumour antigens are the M344 antigen, which is expressed on roughly 70% of superficial bladder tumour specimens (18), the DD23 antigen, which is found in 80% of bladder tumours (19) and the T138 antigen detectable in advanced stage lesions as well as aggressive Ta/T1 lesions (20). To date these tumour-associated antigens are primarily of research interest. Two bladder tumour antigens with commercially available tests are potentially promising: the Bard Bladder Tumour Antigen test (BTA-Bard) and the Nuclear Matrix Protein 22 test (NMP22 Matritech). The BTA-Bard measures the urinary complexes formed by the aggregation of proteolytically fragmented basement membranes. In a recent study 65% of 60 patients with Ta, grades 1–3 and CIS lesions were detected with the BTA-Bard test on voided urine as compared with a 32% detection rate for conventional bladder wash cytology (21). Neither the BTA test nor urinary cytology are effective in identifying grade 1 tumours. The specificity of the test was shown to be 95.9% in healthy volunteers and decreased to 82% in patients with urinary tract disease. The high levels of nuclear matrix protein 22 in the urine of persons with active TCC compared with normal subjects forms the basis for the NMP22 Matritech-test. This test appears promising for both detection and postresection surveillance (22).

Finally, the overexpression of the suppressor gene p53 was found to be associated with tumour progression to muscle invasion and metastases (23). p53 protein positivity in more than 20% of cells was associated with a relative risk of tumour progression of 11 : 1. The Rb protein is believed to inhibit the cell cycle and decreased pRb expression has been associated with disease progression and decreased disease-free survival (24).

TREATMENT OF SUPERFICIAL BLADDER TUMOURS

Surgery

Nearly all bladder tumours can be treated by TUR (Table 13.5). Resection begins with a careful cystoscopic examination of the entire urethra, the prostate, and all surfaces of the bladder. Several findings of prognostic significance are noted and mapped on a bladder diagram: number and size of tumours, the exact location of the tumours in reference to bladder neck and ureteric orifices, and the configuration of the tumour: whether they are papillary or sessile, broad based or peduncular. When the bladder is carefully inspected the risk to overlook a tumour is small. In one study only two of 242 (0.8%) of presumed single tumours were missed at the time of TUR, discovered by endoscopy done less than 35 days after TUR (26). The mucosa remote from the tumour is inspected for changes suggestive for CIS, i.e. red velvety patches.

Table 13.5

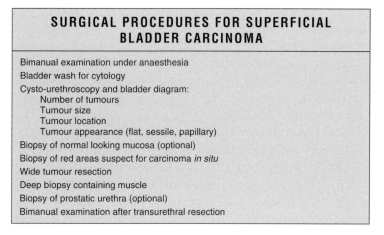

SURGICAL PROCEDURES FOR SUPERFICIAL BLADDER CARCINOMA
Bimanual examination under anaesthesia
Bladder wash for cytology
Cysto-urethroscopy and bladder diagram:
Number of tumours
Tumour size
Tumour location
Tumour appearance (flat, sessile, papillary)
Biopsy of normal looking mucosa (optional)
Biopsy of red areas suspect for carcinoma *in situ*
Wide tumour resection
Deep biopsy containing muscle
Biopsy of prostatic urethra (optional)
Bimanual examination after transurethral resection

Selected-site or random mucosal biopsies will confirm the presence of CIS when suspected. Very recently it has been reported that multiple biopsies of normal looking urothelium in Ta, T1 bladder cancer do not show abnormalities in about 90% of the cases and that performing such biopsies does not attribute to the staging nor to the choice of adjuvant therapy in a group of 995 patients with Ta, T1 bladder cancer (27). In patients with a positive cytology, no visible bladder tumour and normal upper tracts, bladder biopsies and biopsies of the prostatic urethra are mandatory. Once the cystoscopic findings are noted and biopsies if necessary are taken, tumour resection can begin. The tumour resection should be deep enough to obtain muscle as part of the evaluation of the T-category. The resected tissue samples are potted separately with ample information for the pathologist. The pathology report should indicate grade and depth of the tumour invasion, and it should mention the presence or absence of bladder muscle in the specimen. In special situations such as studies to evaluate the efficacy of intravesical chemotherapy a single bladder tumour can be left on purpose: this is the concept of the marker lesion to study the marker tumour response.

Laser treatment

Tumours that are papillary and low grade in appearance in a patient with a documented previous history of low-grade, low-stage tumours can be coagulated with a neodymium/YAG (Nd/YAG) laser. When multiple tumours are present, a tumour should be biopsied and sent for pathology. Nd/YAG laser treatment produces thermal coagulation with a penetration depth of 3–5 mm. However, the depth of penetration can be variable and transmural coagulation of the bladder wall has been observed in some situations when the total energy output was only 30 J, whereas in other circumstances, penetration depth was less than 2 mm when 200 J of energy was applied to the bladder wall (28). But even after a transmural coagulation the bladder mostly maintains its structural integrity, hence bladder perforation with extravasation into the perivesical tissues or laser injury to adjacent organs is uncommon (29). Other lasers such as the argon lasers (30) and KTP lasers (31) have been used to treat superficial bladder cancer. More recently there have been reports of holmium/YAG laser treatment of bladder cancer (32). A decreased incidence of overall recurrence within the bladder for laser-treated patients as compared with electrocautery resection has been reported (33); however, in a randomized, prospective study no difference was found in overall recurrence rate between laser-treated patients and those undergoing electrocautery resection (34). Laser treatment can be considered a safe and effective treatment for tumours that are papillary and low grade in appearance. If there is a question of a high-grade tumour or invasion suggested by a more sessile appearance, electrocautery resection is preferred over laser treatment so that an adequate histological examination of the resection specimen containing detrusor muscle can be performed.

Intravesical therapy

Intravesical therapy can be divided into prophylactic (or adjuvant) therapy, to prevent recurrences after endoscopic resection of all visible tumours, and therapeutic or definitive intravesical therapy (also called chemoresection) designed to treat established papillary tumours that cannot be resected (e.g. tumours that are too numerous or too large, inaccessible tumours) or CIS.

Advantages of the intravesical route of administration are the high concentrations of drugs in contact with tumour-bearing mucosa or bladder epithelium at risk, and little or no systemic uptake of the drug; disadvantages are the local side-effects in the bladder because of the high local drug concentration and the need for transurethral manipulation (44). The earliest attempts to reduce recurrences utilizing intravesical chemotherapy are reported in 1961 using thiotepa (35) and more than three decades later this drug is still frequently used, along with a number of other chemotherapeutic agents. The use of BCG for superficial bladder cancer was first reported in 1976 (36) and BCG has become the mainstay in the treatment of CIS of the bladder and has been shown to be very effective in the prevention of recurrence of superficial tumours as well (37,38).

Effect of intravesical adjuvant therapy on the incidence of recurrent superficial tumours

Many agents have been used for intravesical therapy and a number of these agents have been shown to be effective in randomized, prospective trials with sufficient numbers of patients including thiotepa, epodyl, doxorubicin, mitomycin C (MMC), epirubicin, and BCG . During the past two decades the European Organization for Research and Treatment of Cancer (EORTC) Genitourinary Tract Cancer Co-operative Group (GU-Group) has performed a series of randomized phase 3 studies investigating the prophylactic treatment of stage Ta, T1 bladder cancer (39–43) (Table 13.6). Many of these studies have demonstrated the advantage of adjuvant prophylactic treatment after TUR compared with TUR alone in decreasing the recurrence rate or in prolonging the disease-free interval. Very recently long-term results of an EORTC trial comparing doxorubicin, ethoglucid, and TUR alone in a total of 443 patients were published (42). Time to first recurrence was significantly prolonged by both drugs compared with TUR alone. Recurrence rate per year was 0.30 for both adjuvant treatment arms and 0.68 for the resection alone group. For all patients the absolute benefit according to the formula, % recurrence in resection only arm minus % recurrence in the adjuvant treatment arms, is approximately 20% for doxorubicin and 27% for ethoglucid at 3 years.

Table 13.6

EORTC TRIALS FOR SUPERFICIAL BLADDER CARCINOMA

30751	Thiotepa versus VM26 (epipodophyllotoxin) versus TUR only
30781	Oral pyridoxine versus placebo
30782	Thiotepa versus adriamycin versus cisplatin
30790	Adriamycin versus Epodyl (ethoglucid) versus TUR only
30831	Mitomycin C early versus delayed maintenance versus no further tmt
30832	Adriamycin early versus delayed maintenance versus no further tmt
30845	BCG versus mitomycin C (CIS)
30861	BCG (CIS)
30863	Epirubicin (single) versus sterile water
30864	Mitomycin C phase II marker lesion phase III maintenance versus no further tmt
30869	Epirubicin: phase II marker lesion phase III maintenance versus no further treatment
30897	Mitomycin C and BCG sequential
30901	TUR only versus biopsy + laser
30906	BCG versus Epirubicin (CIS)
30911	Epirubicin versus BCG versus BCG + INH
30952	Quarter dose BCG (marker lesion)
30962	BCG standard dose versus 1/3 dose long-term versus short-term maintenance

TUR, transurethral resection; CIS, carcinoma *in situ*; BCG, bacille Calmette–Guérin.

Impact of intravesical adjuvant therapy on progression to muscle-invasive bladder cancer and survival

The long-term benefit compared with TUR alone with regard to progression to muscle invasive disease and duration of survival cannot be assessed in individual trials because while only 10–15% of patients entered in these trials are expected to progress to invasive disease, the studies have insufficient statistical power to detect differences with respect to time to progression and survival (43). Hence a combined analysis of completed trials using meta-analysis techniques has been performed recently by the EORTC GU group and the British Medical Research Council (MRC) working party on superficial bladder cancer (45) (Table 13.7). This meta-analysis included six randomized trials comprising 2535 patients. The results confirm the favourable impact of adjuvant prophylactic treatment on the disease-free interval of patients with stage Ta, T1 bladder cancer. The hazard ratio of treatment versus no treatment for all trials was 0.8, which is equivalent to a mean plus or minus standard deviation 20 ± 6% decrease in the risk of recurrence in the treated group compared with the no treatment group. For example, the estimate of the average absolute benefit in the percentage of patients disease-free at 8 years for those randomized to receive adjuvant treatment was 8.2% (44.9 versus 36.7%) with a 95% confidence interval of 3.8%–12.5%. However, no long-term benefit could be shown for prophylactic treatment compared with TUR alone in terms of time to invasive disease, or duration of survival or progression-free survival. No differences were observed in the incidence of second malignant tumours in the treatment groups refuting the suggestion by some of a possible carcinogenic effect locally on the epithelium or systematically of intravesical chemotherapy (46–48).

Table 13.7

EUROPEAN ORGANIZATION FOR RESEARCH AND TREATMENT OF CANCER (EORTC) AND MEDICAL RESEARCH COUNCIL (MRC) TRIALS INCLUDED IN THE COMBINED ANALYSIS (45)			
Trial number	Drugs used	Total no. patients	No. controls
EORTC			
30751	Thiotepa (VM-26)	370	124
30791	Doxorubicin Epodyl	443	73
30863	Epirubicin	512	255
30781	Pyridoxine (oral)	291	144
MRC			
BSO1	Thiotepa	417	139
BSO3	Mitomycin C	502	171
Total no. patients		2535	906

Bacille Calmette–Guérin or cytotoxic intravesical adjuvant therapy

In this combined analysis intravesical BCG was not addressed, as no trials were conducted in the EORTC or the MRC in which TUR alone was compared with TUR plus BCG. However, some investigators would consider intravesical BCG and not chemotherapy to be the first-line treatment of choice in the adjuvant therapy of stage Ta, Tl bladder cancer, particularly in high risk cases (recurrent, multifocal stage T1G3 disease and/or CIS) (49–56). In most of these trials BCG is superior over chemotherapeutic agents with respect to the recurrence rate (49,53,56) (Table 13.8). A Dutch trial comparing MMC with BCG as intravesical adjuvant therapy has shown that both agents are equieffective in patients with low and intermediate risk for recurrence (57).

Early or delayed and short versus long-term intravesical adjuvant therapy

The effects of a single early (within 6 h after TUR) instillation of 80 mg Epirubicin was investigated in 399 patients with low-risk prognostic factors by the EORTC-GU group (23). This early single instillation significantly prolonged the time to first recurrence: the recurrence rate for patients treated with epirubicin was 0.16 compared with 0.40 for patients in the control group treated with sterile water only ($P = 0.02$). Probably the early instillation of chemotherapy immediately after TUR may destroy viable floating tumour cells, which otherwise may lead to implantation. Two other randomized EORTC trials with MMC and doxorubicin comparing early versus delayed and short-term versus long-term treatment have shown that for patients treated within 6–24 h after TUR a 6-month course of therapy is sufficient, whereas a 12-month course provides better results for patients in whom such early intravesical instillation is not feasible (58).

Table 13.8

INTRAVESICAL AGENTS FOR SUPERFICIAL BLADDER CANCER

Drug	Recommended dose	Chemoresection (CR rate)	Prophylactic treatment (RR)	Advantage to control	Carcinoma *in situ* (CR rate)
Thiotepa	30 mg	38%,	45%	17%	—
Adriamycin	50 mg	28–56%	38%	18%	34%
Mitomycin	40–60 mg	43%	37%	15%	58%
Epirubicin	80 mg	56%			
BCG	depends on strain	50–66%	31 %	44%	70%

Thiotepa

Thiotepa is an alkylating agent that interferes with protein synthesis of the cancer cell by inhibiting the synthesis of RNA. It has a low molecular weight of 189, resulting in absorption and possible systemic toxicity. Initial reports claimed that approximately 25% of the patients treated with intravesical thiotepa were suffering from leucopenia and thrombocytopenia (59), but in a review of 670 instillations in 1983 thiotepa-induced myelosuppression was considered to be rare, usually mild, and transient (60). The incidence of chemical cystitis, which is characterized by dysuria, frequency, and pain in the bladder region, ranges from 12 to 69% depending on the dose and instillation schedules (interval between first instillation and TUR, number of instillations and time between instillations) (61). Six fatal cases of acute non-lymphocytic myelodysplastic syndrome have been reported, with a mean interval of 57 months (range 27–84 months) between thiotepa instillation and the diagnosis (61). Thiotepa has been used as definitive therapy for superficial bladder tumours with a success rate of approximately 38% in 10 small series (62). Adjuvant therapy with intravesical instillations with thiotepa after a complete TUR has been studied with differing results. Lamm compared the recurrence rate of thiotepa (45%) with the recurrence rate in control groups (62%) in a series of 10 controlled studies with 1009 patients, an advantage of thiotepa of 17% (63). These results depended highly on the follow-up period and half of the included series failed to reach statistical significance, including one of the largest, the MRC study (64). Another large series, EORTC study 30751 failed to show a statistical difference in disease-free interval between patients treated with thiotepa, epipodophyllotoxin (VM 26), and controls, although the recurrence rate of the treated patients was significantly lower than that of the control group (65).

Doxorubicin

Doxorubicin or Adriamycin is an anthracycline antibiotic that binds to pairs of DNA. It has a relatively high molecular weight of 580, resulting in a very low absorption and rare systemic toxicity. Chemical cystitis occurs in about 20–30% of treated patients (66,67). The response rates for doxorubicin used as definitive treatment for papillary tumours varies between 28% and 56% (mean 38%) depending on the dose (62). For CIS only 34% of patients treated with doxorubicin had a complete response in a multicentre trial (49), and the median time to treatment failure was only 5 months with only 18% of patients remaining free of CIS. There is a large experience with doxorubicin as prophylactic intravesical therapy in the Japanese Urological Cancer Research Group, who conducted a series of large randomized trials with different agents and different schedules. The disease-free rates were significantly better for adjuvant therapy with doxorubicin and MMC compared with controls, but no differences were found between short term schedules and a 2-year maintenance schedule (42). Also pre-TUR treatment with six instillations of doxorubicin in the 2 weeks before TUR has been shown to be significantly less effective than adjuvant instillations (68).

Mitomycin C

The mode of action of mitomycin C (MMC) is still not fully clear, but it has an intracellular effect resulting in the production of a cytotoxic alkylating agent. With a molecular weight of 329 MMC is barely absorbed, so myelosuppression is rare. The most frequent side-effects are chemical cystitis with an incidence ranging between 6% and 41% and a mean of 15% (61), and allergic reactions. Allergic reactions are mainly cutaneous, such as palmar rash. Up to 9% of patients treated with intravesical MMC experienced cutaneous side-effects, due to a delayed-type hypersensitivity reaction (69,70). These symptoms usually occur after the second instillation, and disappear after cessation of therapy. A contracted bladder was seen in three of 538 (0.5%) patients in one study (61) and bladder wall calcifications have been reported after instillation (71). In a large Dutch trial comparing MMC (30 mg in 50 ml) with two BCG strains in 469 patients, MMC had significantly fewer side-effects than BCG in regard to drug-induced cystitis and systemic side-effects (72).

Intravesical MMC as definitive therapy for superficial bladder tumours gives a complete response of 43% in papillary lesions and 58% in CIS (62). In EORTC study 30864 the effect of eight instillations with 80 mg MMC were studied on a marker lesion left after TUR. After 10 weeks the marker lesion was resected if still present. The complete response rate for the marker lesion was 50% (48 of 96 patients), no change was observed in 29 patients and increase in size was seen in 19 (62). The prophylactic value of intravesical MMC has been reviewed in five controlled trials with 859 patients giving an advantage of 15% for MMC (52% recurrences in the control groups versus 37% in the MMC group) (63). Huland *et al.* compared long-term MMC instillation therapy (42 instillations of 20 mg in 3 years) with no intravesical therapy in a randomized trial after complete TUR (73). The percentage of recurrences was 10.4% in the MMC group compared with 51% in the control group. This was confirmed by a later prospective multicentre trial, although the recurrence rate was slightly higher

(15.3%) with the same long-term prophylaxis (74). Short-term prophylaxis (20 instillations of 20mg MMC in 20 weeks) was shown to give similar results, indicating the lack of advantage of maintenance therapy (74).

Epirubicin

Epirubicin has an antitumour effect similar to that of doxorubicin, but less side-effects. In a large series of 911 patients receiving 8-weekly instillations of 50 mg epirubicin only 14% of patients experienced chemical cystitis, without treatment delay (75). Systemic toxicity was absent. In the EORTC study 30863 a single instillation of 80 mg epirubicin immediately after TUR was compared with an instillation of sterile water (76). Local irritative symptoms were seen in 11.7% of the patients receiving epirubicin versus 2 % in the patients treated with sterile water. The recurrence rate was significantly less in the epirubicin group ($P < 0.0001$). Epirubicin was of no benefit for solitary pTa grade I tumours. In EORTC study 30869 the effect of epirubicin on a marker lesion was studied (62). Only 36 patients were recruited, and a complete response with disappearance of the marker lesion was observed in 20 (56%), but no definitive conclusions could be drawn due to the small number of patients.

Bacille Calmette–Guérin

Used for more than 20 years now as adjuvant therapy for superficial bladder cancer, BCG is currently the most active intravesical immunotherapy and is considered as the first-line treatment for CIS of the bladder and T1G3 tumours. The precise way through which BCG exerts its antitumour activity is still not well understood, but two premises seem absolutely certain: direct contact between tumour cells and BCG is necessary and T lymphocytes are required for BCG-mediated antitumour activity (77). Direct contact allows fibronectin-mediated attachment of the bacteria to the normal urothelial cells as well as to the tumoral cells. After active phagocytosis these cells present the bacterial antigen to T lymphocytes which in turn initiate a cascade of local and systemic immunological events.

Intravesical therapy with BCG has proven to be very effective in the prophylaxis and treatment of superficial bladder cancer and CIS. In most series BCG seems to be more effective than intravesical chemotherapy, but BCG is clearly more toxic. The risk benefit for the individual patient has to be considered and it is obvious that BCG is not the first choice for every patient with superficial TCC. There is a clear indication to treat prophylactically patients with bad prognostic factors, such as G3 tumours and all T1 tumours irrespective of the grade. The adverse impact of Tl stage and G3 grade in the final outcome of the patients is well known and in this category of patients the benefit of the therapy exceeds the risk of possible side-effects and the disadvantage of long-term treatment. CIS is the optimal indication for intravesical BCG.

As BCG as first-line treatment produces very high and durable response rates in CIS, radical cystectomy is no longer the initial choice for this disease (78). Unfortunately, about 30% of the patients with CIS do not respond to a first BCG treatment and about 30 % of the initial responders have a relapse at 5 years after an initial complete response, and at 10 years only 31% of patients treated with BCG instillations for CIS remain tumour-free (79). BCG is contraindicated in immunocompromised subjects such as HIV-positive patients or patients undergoing immunosuppressive treatment, in patients with other progressing malignancies, leukaemia or Hodgkin's disease, and in pregnant or lactating women.

A significant reduction in tumour recurrence is noted in most of prospective controlled studies comparing BCG with TUR alone for superficial bladder cancer (63). Overall, the rates of tumour recurrence were 75% for the control arm patients, versus 31% for the BCG-treated patients, a net benefit of 44% in 402 patients. Studies comparing BCG with intravesical chemotherapy have demonstrated superiority of BCG over thiotepa and adriamycin (49,53), while a Dutch study did not find any difference between two strains of BCG and MMC (72). Complete remission rates of about 70% have been reported in patients with CIS treated with BCG, at 5 years about 50% of these patients remain tumour-free while at 10 years only 30% of patients experience a durable remission (49,80). In comparison a review of intravesical chemotherapy in CIS revealed that the long-term tumour-free response rates were 15% for thiotepa and 18% for adriamycin, although the initial response rates were 38 and 48%, respectively (11). A considerable proportion of failures is due to extravesical progression of the disease, either to the lower ureters or to the prostatic urethra and prostatic ducts. In the literature, reports of prostatic urethral involvement after BCG therapy ranges from 1.5 to 6.3%, which is much lower than those for chemotherapy (33–37%) (81). Some urologists advocate prompt cystectomy after failure of BCG treatment in CIS. Although patients with residual CIS after intravesical treatment are at increased risk for tumour progression, this progression usually occurs after 2 years and second-line intravesical therapies may be attempted with reasonable safety (82). The ablative effect of BCG on papillary tumours present in the bladder at the time of instillation was evaluated in a prospective phase 2 study done by the Tokyo BCG Study Group. Sixty-six per cent of patients with a Ta T1 tumour showed complete disappearance of the tumour after 8-weekly instillations of 80 mg of Tokyo BCG (83). In EORTC study 30897 the ablative effect of intravesical BCG in combination with MMC was studied. After complete resection of all tumours except the marker tumour, 4-weekly instillations of MMC 40 mg were followed by 6-weekly instillations of BCG. Complete response (no tumour in a biopsy at the site of the marker lesion and negative cytology) was observed in 50% of the patients.

BCG produces more intense local effects than does chemotherapy. It produces an intense local inflammatory reaction in most patients. Symptoms of this local reaction are dysuria, frequency, urgency, painful micturition, and haematuria. Local symptoms generally do not require dose reduction or cessation of therapy. Serious systemic complications are uncommon but can occur. As many as 25% of patients have an influenza-like syndrome lasting from 12 to 24 h after instillation. Those patients suspected of having systemic BCG infection or allergic reactions are treated successfully in most cases with antituberculous medication. At least seven deaths have been attributed to BCG instillations, where BCG was given immediately after TURB was performed, or after a traumatic catheterization, leading to high systemic absorption. In order to reduce the side-effects of BCG some investigators administer short-term isoniazid prophylactically at each instillation. Additionally, the administration of isoniazid might impair the growth of urothelial tumours, as has been shown in an animal study (84). The precise role of isoniazid used prophylactically is currently being investigated in EORTC protocol 30911. One hundred and ninety-five patients were treated with BCG only, while 188 patients have received BCG plus isoniazid. An interim analysis of the toxicity has been carried out which demonstrates that the incidence of local side-effects did not significantly differ between patients treated with BCG and those treated with BCG plus isoniazid (85–87). Also no statistically significant differences in the incidence of the systemic side-effects, such as fever, influenza-like symptoms, and allergic reactions were shown in the same EORTC study. However, isoniazid given in a dose of 300 mg daily for only 3 days during a maximum of 6 consecutive weeks, induced transient liver function disturbances, therefore it does not seem advisable to use isoniazid as a prophylactic agent to diminish the adverse effects of BCG intravesical therapy (85).

The optimal length of BCG therapy is still under debate. A prospective randomized trial comparing non-maintenance with maintenance BCG therapy once per month for 2 years after the standard induction 6-week intravesical BCG regimen in both groups demonstrated no reduction in tumour recurrences or progression, and long-term BCG increased cumulative local toxicity. In CIS patients it has been shown that 3-week BCG treatments at 3 months increased the complete response rate at 6 months from 73% to 87% and 3-week BCG treatments every 6 months for 3 years resulted in an increase in long-term disease-free status from 65% in the group receiving only the 6-week induction therapy to 83% in patients receiving regular retreatment.

Other immunotherapeutic agents

Many other agents have been investigated or are currently investigated in superficial bladder cancer, as definitive treatment of residual tumours or prophylactically to prevent recurrences. These include interferon, interleukin-2, keyhole limpet haemocyanin, lactobacillus casei, bropirimin, levamisole, transfer factor, and many more. Today none has proved more effective than BCG.

CARCINOMA IN SITU OF THE BLADDER

This form of superficial bladder cancer was first described by Melicow in 1952 as areas of hyperplasia and anaplasia in grossly normal-appearing mucosa of a tumour-bearing bladder (86). CIS can be focal but is mostly diffuse. About 90% of cases of CIS are found in association with visible bladder tumours. The likelihood of the development of a muscle-invasive cancer in such patients is 42–83% (87). Only 10% of all cases of CIS are an isolated pathological finding and microinvasive carcinoma is found in 20–34% of these patients at cystectomy (11). Classically, patients with CIS present with lower urinary tract symptoms including dysuria, frequency, nocturia, perineal pain, and haematuria, but up to 25% of patients with CIS may be asymptomatic (88). On cystoscopy the bladder mucosa may look normal, but more often erythema and increased vascularity are noticed, and raised velvety patches or ulcerations can be present. Histologically, CIS appears as flattened areas of epithelium composed of anaplastic cells with an anarchical pattern of growth without extension into the bladder lumen, nor penetration of the basement membrane. CIS has been found in all areas of the urothelium, including the renal pelvis, ureters, bladder, prostatic, and anterior urethra. Cytological examination of the urine has proved highly accurate in the diagnosis and monitoring of response to treatment in patients with CIS of the bladder. More than 95% of the patients with biopsy proved CIS have been reported to have a positive urine cytology result (89).

Treatment of carcinoma *in situ*

Because CIS may not be visible endoscopically and because the visible lesions are often too extensive to resect and have ill-defined margins, TUR and fulguration is not considered a definitive treatment for this disease. In the series by Herr *et al.* none of the patients with CIS undergoing TUR alone was cured of the disease and 65% of patients required cystectomy for muscle invasive tumours or intractable CIS (90). As CIS is associated with invasive disease in the majority of patients radical cystectomy was deemed the most appropriate treatment for CIS by urologists from the 1960s to the mid-1980s. But the results of immediate cystectomy have never proved superior to cystectomy performed promptly after failure of intravesical therapy (49). CIS is the optimal target for intravesical therapy, as close contact between agent and tumour cells occurs and the tumour burden is low. A review of intravesical chemotherapy in CIS reveals that initial response rates are 38% for thiotepa and 48% for adriamycin, but long-term tumour-free response rates are only 15% and 18%, respectively (11). Approximately 42% of CIS patients treated with MMC have a long-term tumour-free response (91,92). In studies comparing MMC and BCG, initial tumour-free response rates are comparable for the two agents, with some studies suggesting an advantage for BCG therapy (93). The highest tumour-free success rates have been reported after intravesical BCG therapy. Results of multiple studies suggest an overall complete response rate of 70% in patients with CIS treated by intravesical BCG; about 50% have a durable remission of 5 years or longer while at 10 years 30% are still tumour free (79,80). Primary CIS (no previous transitional cell carcinoma), secondary CIS (occurring after previous transitional cell carcinoma), and concurrent CIS (associated with superficial transitional cell carcinoma) respond similarly to BCG treatment (94). Today BCG is recommended as first-line treatment for CIS.

The treatment of CIS refractory to initial intravesical BCG therapy is still under debate. As patients with persistent CIS are at high risk for tumour progression, prompt cystectomy is often recommended for patients with BCG-resistant CIS. But many patients with a relatively asymptomatic form of CIS prefer to maintain normal bladder function. Alternative therapies have proved effective for some patients failing initial intravesical BCG therapy. Sarosdy reported six complete remissions in 17 cases (35%) of BCG-resistant CIS with the oral interferon-inducer bropirimine (95). No significant difference in survival was noted in patients with CIS undergoing prompt cystectomy after failure of one course of BCG compared with patients undergoing delayed cystectomy after additional intravesical therapy (96). Although the number of patients with refractory CIS treated by alternative agents is small, there are patients who appear to respond to second lines of treatment and avoid cystectomy. However, consideration of early, aggressive surgery should not be abandoned in all patients with CIS. The association of CIS and high-grade, lamina propria invasive disease (T1G3) has a substantial risk for disease progression and may be an indication for early cystectomy after failed initial intravesical therapy (97).

CURRENT GUIDELINES FOR INTRAVESICAL THERAPY

Low-risk patients

Appropriate therapy is based on risk versus benefit. Many patients will derive little benefit from intravesical therapy. An ideal intravesical drug which is inexpensive, highly effective and non-toxic has not been discovered yet, so not all patients should be treated. Primary, small, solitary, and low-grade Ta tumours are at such a low risk of tumour progression that intravesical therapy is not required. They can be managed with TURB alone followed by standard surveillance.

Low progression risk, high recurrence risk

Recurrent low-grade superficial tumours may benefit from a single early instillation of chemotherapy after TURB (23). In this EORTC trial epirubicin 80 mg was instilled within 6 h after TURB. A variety of other chemotherapeutic agents and regimens have been used successfully in a multiplicity of trials and it has been demonstrated that they prolong the disease-free interval with statistical significance (45). A small percentage of patients will develop chemical cystitis. The use of BCG may not be indicated in these low progression risk patients because of its increased morbidity.

High progression risk patients

Patients with high-grade (G3) and/or high-stage (T1) tumours and patients with diffuse CIS are at substantial risk for disease progression and death from bladder cancer. They require a complete TURB followed by adjuvant intravesical therapy. The treatment of choice is BCG, as response rates to BCG appear to be higher and more durable than to chemotherapy. The optimal

length of therapy with BCG (maintenance or not) is still controversial. A complete response is indicated by repeated negative
biopsy specimens and negative urine cytology. Six months after
the start of the therapy a complete response to the continued use
of an active agent should be expected. A positive biopsy specimen
for persistent bladder cancer or a positive urine cytology at
6 months after the start strongly indicates that an alternative
therapy should be tried. An alternative intravesical therapy is
reasonable for persistent non-invasive disease, but should not be
continued beyond 1 year in non-responding patients. Persistent or
recurrent high-grade Tl tumours or CIS have a bad prognosis and
cystectomy is currently the safest approach in these cases.

References

1 Althausen AF, Prout GRJr, Daly JJ. Non-invasive papillary carcinoma of the
bladder associated with carcinoma in situ. *J Urol* 1976, **116**, 575–80.

2 Hasui Y, Osada Y, Kitada S, Nishi S. Significance of invasion to the muscularis
mucosae on the progression of superficial bladder cancer. *Urology*, 1994, **43**,
782–6.

3 Younes M, Sussman J, True LD. The usefulness of the level of the muscularis
mucosae in the staging of invasive transitional cell carcinoma of the urinary
bladder. *Cancer* 1990, **66**, 543–8.

4 Abel PD, Henderson D, Bennett MK *et al*. Differing interpretations by pathologists of the pT category and grade of transitional cell cancer of the bladder.
Br J Urol 1988, **62**, 339–42.

5 Ro JY, Starerkel GA, Ayala AG. Cytologic and histologic features of superficial
bladder cancer. *Urol Clin North Am*, 1992, **19** (3), 435–53.

6 Hopkins CS, Ford KS, Soloway MS. Invasive bladder cancer: support for
screening. *J Urol* 1983, **130**, 61–4.

7 Heney NM, Ahmed S, Flanagan MJ *et al*. Superficial bladder cancer: progression and recurrence. *J Urol* 1983, **130**, 1083–6.

8 Dalesio O, Schulman CC, Sylvester R *et al*. Prognostic factors in superficial
bladder tumors: a study of the European Organization for Research on
Treatment of Cancer: Genitourinary Tract Cancer Cooperative Group. *J Urol*
1983, **129**, 730–3.

9 Cutler SJ, Heney NM, Friedall GH. Longitudinal study of patients with bladder
cancer: factors associated with disease recurrence and progression. In: *Bladder
cancer* (ed. Bonney VW, Prout GR). Williams & Wilkins, Baltimore, 1982,
p. 35–47.

10 Fitzpatrick WM, West AB, Butler MR *et al*. Superficial bladder tumors (stage
pTa, grade I and II): the importance of recurrence pattern following initial
resection. *J Urol* 1986, **135**, 920–2.

11 Lamm DL. Carcinoma in situ. *Urol Clin North Am*, 1992, **19**, 499–511.

12 Gustafson H, Tribukait B, Esposti PL. DNA profile and tumour progression in
patients with superficial bladder tumours. *Urol Res*, 1982, **10**, 13–8.

13 Blomjous CEM, Schipper NW, Baak JPA *et al*. Retrospective study of prognostic importance of DNA flow cytometry of urinary bladder carcinoma. *J Clin
Pathol*, 1988, **41**, 21–5.

14 Newman AJ Jr, Carlton CE Jr, Johnson S. Cell surface A, B, or O (H) blood
group antigens as an indicator of malignant potential in stage A bladder carcinoma. *J Urol* 1980, **124**, 27–9.

15 Sanders H, McCue P, Graham SD JrABO, (H.) antigens and beta-2 microglob-
ulin in transitional cell carcinoma.Predictors of response to intravesical bacillus CalmetteGuerin. *Cancer* 1991, **67**, 3024–8.

16 Aprikan AG, Sarkis AS, Reuter VE *et al*. Biological markers of prognosis in
transitional cell carcinoma of the bladder: current concepts. *Semin Urol* 1993,
11, 137–44.

17 Golijanin D, Sherman Y, Shapiro A, Pode D. Detection of bladder tumours by immunostaining of the Lewis X antigen in cells from voided urine. *Urol* 1995, **46**, 173–7.

18 Bonner RB, Hemstreet IIIGP, Fradet Y *et al.* Bladder cancer risk assessment with quantitative fluorescence image analysis of tumor markers in exfoliated bladder cells. *Cancer* 1993, **72**, 2461–9.

19 Grossman HB, Washington RW Jr, Carey TE, Liebert HB. Alternations in antigen expression in superficial bladder cancer. (Review.) *J Cell Biochem*, 1992, **161**, 63–8.

20 Fradet Y, Tardif M, Bourget L *et al.* Clinical cancer progression in urinary bladder tumors evaluated by multiparameter flow cytometry with monoclonal antibodies. *Cancer Res*, 1990, **50**, 432–7.

21 D'Hallewin MA, Baert L. Initial evaluation of the bladder tumor antigen test in superficial bladder cancer. *J Urol* 1996, **155**, 475–6.

22 Soloway MS, Briggman JV, Carpinito GA *et al.* Use of a new tumor marker, urinary NMP22, in the detection of occult or rapidly recurring transitional cell carcinoma of the urinary tract following surgical treatment. *J Urol* 1996, **156**, 363–7.

23 Sarkis AS, Dalbagni G, Cordon-Corda C *et al.* P53 nuclear overexpression in T1 bladder carcinoma: a marker for disease progression. *J Natl Cancer Inst*, 1993, **85**, 53–9.

24 Logothetis CJ, Xu H, Ro JY *et al.* Altered expression of retinoblastoma protein and known prognostic variables in locally advanced bladder cancer. *J Natl Cancer Inst*, 1992, **84**, 1256–61.

25 Koss LG. Tumors of the urinary tract and prostate in urinary sediment. In: *Diagnostic cytology and its histologic basis* (ed: Koss LG). JB Lippincott, Philadelphia, 1992.

26 Oosterlinck W, Kurth KH, Schroder F, Bultinck J, Hammond B, Sylvester R, and Members of the European Organization for Research and Treatment of Cancer Genitourinary Group: A prospective EORTC GU group randomized trial comparing transurethral resection followed by a single intravesical instillation of epirubicin or water in single stage Ta,TI papillary carcinoma of the bladder. *J Urol* 1993, **149**, 749–52.

27 Van der Meijden A, Oosterlinck W, Members of the EORTC-GU, group Superficial Bladder Committee. The significance of bladder biopsies in TA, Tl bladder tumors.Report from the EORTC-GU GROUP. *J Urol* 1997, 157 (abstract 215).

28 Smith JA Jr, Landau ST. Nd:YAG laser specifications for safe intravesical use. *J Urol* 1989, **141**, 1238–9.

29 Hofstetter A, Frank F, Keiditsch E. Endoscopic Nd:YAG laser application for destroying bladder tumors. *Eur Urol* 1981, 7, 278–82.

30 Smith JA Jr, Dixon JA. Argon laser phototherapy of superficial transitional cell carcinoma of the bladder. *J Urol* 1984, **131**, 655–6.

31. Benson RC. Laser treatment. In: High tech urology: technologic innovations and their clinical applications (ed: Smith JA Jr), Saunders WB, Philadelphia, 1992, 47.

32 Johnson DE. Use of the holmium:YAG laser for treatment of superficial bladder carcinoma. *Lasers Surg Med*, 1994, **14**, 213–5.

33 Hofstetter A, Kriegman M, Baumgartner R. Evaluation of laser treatment of bladder cancer. In: *Lasers in urologic surgery* (ed: Smith JA). Mosby YearBook, Chicago, 1994, p. 114.

34 Beisland HO, Seland O. A prospective randomized study on Nd:YAG laser irradiation versus TUR in the treatment of urinary bladder cancer. *Scand J Urol Nephrol*, 1986, **20**, 209–12.

35 Jones HC, Swinney J. Thiotepa in the treatment of tumours of the bladder. *Lancet*, 1961, **ii**, 615.

36 Morales A, Eidinger D, Bruce AW. Intracavitary Bacillus Calmette-Guerin in the treatment of superficial bladder tumors. *J Urol* 1976, **116**, 180–3.

37 Sarosdy MF, Lamm DL. Long-term results of intravesical Bacillus Calmette-Guérin therapy for superficial bladder carcinoma. *J Urol* 1989, **142**, 719–22.

38 Morales A, Nickel JC, Wilson JWL. Dose–response of Bacillus Calmette-Guérin in the treatment of superficial bladder cancer. *J Urol* 1992, **147**, 1256–59.

39 Schulman CC, Robinson M, Denis L *et al.* Prophylactic chemotherapy of superficial transitional cell bladder carcinoma: an EORTC randomized trial

comparing thiotepa, an epipodophyllotoxin (VM-26) and TUR alone. *Eur Urol* 1982, **8**, 207–12.

40 Bouffioux C, Denis L, Oosterlinck W *et al.* Adjuvant chemotherapy of recurrent superficial transitional cell carcinoma: results of a European Organization for Research and Treatment of Cancer randomized trial comparing intravesical instillation of thiotepa, doxorubicin and cisplatin. *J Urol* 1992, **148**, 297–301.

41 Kurth KH, Denis L, Bouffioux C *et al.* Factors affecting recurrence and progression in superficial bladder tumours. *Eur J Cancer* 1995, **11**, 1840–6.

42 Kurth KH, Tunn U, Ay R *et al.* Adjuvant chemotherapy for superficial transitional cell bladder carcinoma: long-term results of a European Organization for research and treatment of cancer randomized trial comparing doxorubicin, ethoglucid and transurethral resection alone. *J Urol* 1997, **158**, 378–84.

43 Van der Meijden APM. Ta,T1 Bladder cancer: What can we learn from EORTC trials. *Urol Int*, 1997, **4**, 15–19.

44 Witjes JA, Oosterhof GON, Debruyne FMJ. Management of superficial bladder cancer Ta/T1/TIS Intravesical chemotherapy. In: *Comprehensive textbook of genitourinary oncology* (ed. Vogelzang NJ, Sardino PT). Williams and Wilkins, Baltimore, 1996, p. 416.

45 Pawinski A, Sylvester R, Kurth KH *et al.* for the members of the European Organization for Research and Treatment of Cancer Genitourinary Tract Cancer Cooperative Group and the Medical Research Council Working Party on Superficial Bladder Cancer. A combined analysis of European Organization for Research and treatment of Cancer and Medical Research Council randomized clinical trials for the prophylactic treatment of stage Ta,T1 bladder cancer. *J Urol* 1996, **156**, 1934–40.

46 Sonneveld P, Kurth KH, Hagemeyer A, Abels J. Secondary haematologic neoplasm after intravesical chemotherapy for superficial bladder carcinoma. *Cancer* 1990, **65**, 23–5.

47 Friedman D, Moopan UMM, Rosen Y, Kim H. The effect of intravesical instillations of thiotepa, mitomycin C, and Adriamycin on normal urothelium: an experimental study in rats. *J Urol* 1991, **145**, 1060–3.

48 Soloway MS, Murphy WM, de Furia MD *et al.* The effect of mitomycin C on superficial bladder cancer. *J Urol* 1981, **125**, 646–8.

49 Lamm DL, Blumstein BA, Crawford ED *et al.* A randomized trial of intravesical doxorubicin and immunotherapy with bacille Calmette-Guérin for transitional cell carcinoma of the bladder. *N Engl J Med*, 1991, **325**, 1205–9.

50 Herr HW, Schwalb DM, Zhang ZF *et al.* Intravesical Bacillus Calmette-Guérin therapy prevents tumor progression and death from superficial bladder cancer: ten year follow-up of a prospective randomized trial. *J Clin Oncol* 1995, **13**, 1404–8.

51 Lamm DL, Griffith G. Intravesical therapy: does it affect the natural history of superficial bladder cancer? *Sem Urol* 1992, **10**, 39–44.

52 Pagano F, Bassi P, Milani C *et al.* A low dose bacillus Calmette-Guérin regimen in superficial bladder cancer therapy: is it effective? *J Urol* 1991, **146**, 32–5.

53 Martinez-Pineiro JA, Leon JJ, Martinez-Pineiro L Jr *et al.* Bacillus Calmette-Guérin versus doxorubicin versus thiotepa: a randomized prospective study in 202 patients with superficial bladder cancer. *J Urol* 1990, **143**, 502–4.

54 Rintala E, Jauhiainen K, Alfthan O, the Finnbladder Research Group. MMC, BCG. In: *Intravesical chemotherapy, immunotherapy of superficial bladder cancer*. EORTCGU Group Monograph 6. Alan R, Liss Inc., New York, 19894, pp. 271–74.

55 Soloway MS, Perry A. Bacillus Calmette-Guérin for treatment of superficial transitional cell carcinoma of the bladder in patients who have failed thiotepa and/or mithomycin C. *J Urol* 1987, **137**, 871–3.

56 Lamm DL, Blumenstein BA, Crawford ED *et al.* Randomized intergroup comparison of bacillus Calmette-Guérin immunotherapy and mitomycin C chemotherapy prophylaxis in superficial transitional cell carcinoma of the bladder. *Urol Oncol* 1995, **1**, 119–21.

57 Witjes WPJ, Witjes JA, Oosterhof GON, Debruyne FMJ. on behalf of the Dutch South-East Cooperative Urological Group: Update on the Dutch Cooperative Trial: Mitomycin versus Bacillus Calmette-Guérin-Tice versus Bacillus Calmette-Guérin RIVM in the treatment of patients with pTa-pT1 papillary carcinoma and carcinoma in situ of the urinary bladder. *Semin Urol Oncol* 1996, **14**, 10–14.

58 Bouffioux CH, Kurth KH, Bono A *et al.* Intravesical adjuvant chemotherapy for superficial transitional cell bladder carcinoma: Results of two EORTC

randomized trials with mitomycin C and doxorubicin comparing early versus delayed and short-term versus, long-term treatment. *J Urol* 1995, **153**, 934–41.

59 Hollister D, Coleman M. Hematologic effects of intravesical thiotepa therapy for bladder carcinoma. *JAMA*, 1980, **244**, 2065–7.

60 Soloway MS, Ford KS. Thiotepa-induced myelosuppression: review of 670 bladder instillations. *J Urol* 1983, **130**, 889–91.

61 Trasher JB, Crawford ED. Complications of intravesical chemotherapy. *Urol Clin North Am*, 1992, **19**, 529–37.

62 Bouffioux C, Meijden AD, Kurth KH *et al.* Objective response of superficial bladder tumors to intravesical treatment (including review of response of marker lesions). *Prog Clin Biol Res*, 1992, **378**, 29–32.

63 Lamm DL. Long-term results of intravesical therapy for superficial bladder cancer. *Urol Clin North Am*, 1992, **19**, 573–84.

64 Medical Research Council. The effect of intravesical thiotepa on the recurrence rate of newly diagnosed superficial bladder cancer. An MRC study. *Br J Urol* 1985, **57**, 680–1.

65 Schulman CC, Robinson M, Denis L *et al.* Prophylactic chemotherapy of superficial transitional cell bladder carcinoma: an EORTC randomized trial comparing thiotepa, an epipodophyllotoxin (VM 26) and TUR alone. *Eur Urol* 1982, **8**, 207–12.

66 Crawford ED, McKenzie D, Mannson W *et al.* Adverse reactions to the intravesical administration of doxorubicin hydrochloride: a report of six cases. *J Urol* 1986, **136**, 668–9.

67 Akaza H, Isaka S, Koiso K *et al.* Comparative analysis of short-term and long-term prophylactic intravesical chemotherapy of superficial bladder cancer. *Cancer Chemother Pharmacol*, 1987, **20**, 91–6.

68 Matsumura Y, Akaza H, Isaka S *et al.* The 4th study of prophylactic intravesical chemotherapy with adriamycin in the treatment of superficial bladder cancer: the experience of the Japanese urological cancer research group for adriamycin. *Cancer Chemother Pharmacol*, 1992, **30**, 10–14.

69 De Groot AC, Meijden APM, Conemans JMH, Maibach HI. Frequency and nature of cutaneous reactions to intravesical instillation of mitomycin for superficial bladder cancer. *Urology*, 1992, **40**, 16–9.

70 Colver GB, Inglis JA, McVittie E *et al.* Dermatitis due to intravesical Mitomycin-C: a delayed type hypersensitivity reaction? *Br J Dermatol*, 1990, **122**, 217–24.

71 Drago PC, Badalament RA, Lucas J, Drago JR. Bladder wall calcifications after intravesical Mitomycin-C treatment of superficial bladder cancer. *J Urol* 1989, **142**, 1071–2.

72 Witjes JA, Meijden APM, Witjes WPJ *et al.* A randomized prospective study comparing intravesical instillations of Mitomycin-C, BCG-Tice and BCG-RIVM in pTa-pT1 tumors and primary carcinoma in situ of the urinary bladder. Intravesical instillations in superficial bladder cancer. *Eur J Cancer* 1993, **29A**, 1672–5.

73 Huland H, Otto U, Droese M, Kloeppel G. Long-term mitomycin-C instillation after resection of superficial bladder carcinoma: influence on recurrence, progression and survival. *J Urol* 1984, **132**, 27–9.

74 Huland H, Kloeppel G, Feddersen I *et al.* Comparison of different schedules of cytostatic intravesical instillations in patients with superficial bladder carcinoma: final evaluation of a prospective multicenter study with 419 patients. *J Urol* 1990, **144**, 68–71.

75 Burk K, Kurth HK, Newling D. Epirubicin in treatment and recurrence prophylaxis of patients with superficial bladder cancer. *Prog Clin Biol Res*, 1989, **303**, 423–34.

76 Oosterlinck W, Kurth KH, Schroder F *et al.* A prospective European Organization for Research and Treatment of Cancer Genitourinary group randomized trial comparing transurethral resection followed by a single intravesical instillation of epirubicin or water in single Ta,T1 papillary carcinoma of the bladder. *J Urol* 1993, **149**, 749–52.

77 Martinez-Pineiro JA, Martinez-Pineiro L. BCG Update: Intravesical therapy. *Eur Urol* 1997, **31**, 31–8.

78 Reitsma DJ, Guinan P, Lamm DL et al. Long-term effects of intravesical bacillus Calmette-Guérin-TICE strain in flat carcinoma in situ of the bladder. In: *BCG in superficial bladder cancer* (ed. Debruyne FMJ, Denis L, Van der Meijden APM). Alan R. Liss, New York, 1989, p. 171–6.

79 Herr HW, Wartinger DD, Fair WR, Oetgen HF. Bacillus Calmette-Guérin therapy for superficial bladder cancer: A 10-year follow-up. *J Urol* 1992, **147**, 1020–3.

80 Hudson MA, Herr HW. Carcinoma in situ of the bladder. *J Urol* 1995, **153**, 564–72.

81 Schellhammer PF. Intravesical BCG treatment for superficial transitional cell carcinoma of the bladder and prostatic urethra. In: *BCG immunotherapy in superficial bladder cancer* (ed. Pagano F, Bassi P), Cleup, Padova, 1994, p. 63–7.

82 Herr HW, Badalement RA, Amato DA *et al.* Superficial bladder cancer treated with bacillus Calmette-Guérin: a multivariate analysis of factors affecting tumor progression. *J Urol* 1989, **141**, 22–9.

83 Akaza H, Kameyana S, Koiso K, Aso Y, Tokyo BCG. Study Group: Ablative and prophylactic effects of BCG Tokyo 172 strain for intravesical treatment in patients with superficial bladder cancer. *J Urol* 1991, **145**, 427–31.

84 De Boer LC, Steerenberg PA, Van der Meijden APM *et al.* Impaired immune response by isoniazid treatment during intravesical BCG administration in the guinea pig. *J Urol* 1992, **148**, 1577–9.

85 Lamm DL, Van der Meijden A, Morales A *et al.* Incidence and treatment of complications of BCG intravesical therapy in superficial bladder tumors. *J Urol* 1992, **147**, 596–9.

86 Melicow MM. Histological study of vesical urothelium intervening between gross neoplasms intotal cystectomy. *J Urol* 1952, **68**, 261.

87 Althausen AF, Prout GR Jr, Daly JJ. Non-invasive papillary carcinoma of the bladder associated with carcinoma in situ. *J Urol* 1976, **116**, 575–80.

88 Skinner DG, Richie JP, Cooper PH *et al.* The clinical significance of carcinoma in situ of the bladder and its association with overt carcinoma. *J Urol* 1974, **112**, 68–71.

89 Zein TA, Milad MF. Urine cytology in bladder tumors. *Int Surg*, 1991, **76**, 52–4.

90 Herr HW, Pinsky CM, Whitmore WF Jr *et al.* Long-term effect of intravesical bacillus Calmette-Guérin on flat carcinoma in situ of the bladder. *J Urol* 1986, **135**, 265–7.

91 Cant JD, Murphy WM, Soloway MS. Prognostic significance of urine cytology on initial followup after intravesical mitomycin C for superficial bladder cancer. *Cancer* 1986, **57**, 2119–22.

92 Stricker P, Grant ABF, Hosken BM, Taylor JS. Topical mitomycin C therapy for carcinoma in situ of the bladder: a follow up. *J Urol* 1990, **143**, 34–6.

93 Pagano F, Bassi P, Milani C *et al.* BCG in superficial bladder cancer: a review of phase III European trials. *Eur Urol* 1992, **21**, 7–11.

94 Steg A, Belas M, Lenen C, Boccon-Gibod L. Intravesical BCG therapy in patients with superficial bladder tumors. In: *BCG in superficial bladder cancer* (ed. Debruyne FMJ, Denis L, Van der Meijden APM), EORTC Genitourinary Group Monograph 6. Alan R. Liss Inc, New York, 1989, 153.

95 Sarosdy M, Lowe B, Schellhammer P. Bropirimine immunotherapy of bladder cancer CIS. Positive phase II results of an oral interferon inducer. *J Urol* 1994, **151**, 304–7.

96 Klein EA, Rogatko A, Herr HW. Management of local bacillus Calmette-Guérin failures in superficial bladder cancer. *J Urol* 1992, **147**, 601–5.

97 Mohamed SR, Mishriki SF, Persad RA *et al.* Urological audit: the role for an aggressive approach to high grade superficial bladder tumours. *Br J Urol* 1992, **70**, 156–60.

14. SURGICAL TREATMENT OF MUSCLE-INVASIVE BLADDER CANCER

Aria F. Olumi and Jerome P. Richie

Mortality related to bladder cancer is usually due to the invasive and/or metastatic disease. The greatest improvement in death rates from bladder cancer can be made from appropriate management of the invasive bladder cancer, or those superficial bladder cancers with greatest risk of progression. This chapter will focus on the surgical treatment of invasive bladder cancer. In particular, surgical technique of radical cystectomy, various options of urinary diversion and some recent molecular biology findings with clinical applications will be discussed.

RATIONALE FOR CYSTECTOMY IN LOCALLY INVASIVE TRANSITIONAL CELL CARCINOMA

Transitional cell carcinoma (TCC) is highly resistant to radiation even at high doses of 7000 cGy. Although radiation was used as definitive therapy prior to 1970, with improvements of surgical technique and anaesthesia, very few centres recommend irradiation as primary treatment for advanced TCC. The natural history of high-grade bladder cancer is to invade progressively through lamina propria, muscularis, perivesical fat, and adjacent pelvic structures (1). The wide-*en bloc* resection of the bladder is designed to provide clear surgical margins with intent to cure.

The curability of bladder cancer after cystectomy is directly correlated with the extent of muscle invasion. In 1946 Jewett and Strong correlated the incidence of pelvic node metastasis with the pathological stage of the tumour (2). Subsequently, Richie *et al.* observed that any degree of TCC muscle invasion adversely affected the 5-year survival (3). Similarly, Pagano and coworkers showed in 1991 that muscle invasion to any extent decreased the 5-year survival, even without pelvic lymph node metastasis (4). Table 14.1 summarizes the 5-year survival after radical cystectomy in various series (3–9).

Table 14.1

PERCENTAGE 5-YEAR SURVIVAL AFTER RADICAL CYSTECTOMY ACCORDING TO STAGE IN EACH SERIES					
Refs	pT0–pT1 (O–A) with or without CIS	pT2 (B1)	pT3a (B2)	pTeb (C)	pT4 (D)
3	67–75	40	40	19.7	6.2
5*		64	50	20	18
6	61	54	48	25	18
7	67–73	88	57	40	29
8**	75	64	44	—	36
9	83	83	69	29	22
4***	68–76	68	67	22	27

* Combined scoring of stages A and B1.
** pT1/pT2 and pT2/pT3a combined.
*** Patients without pelvic lymph node metastasis.

SURGICAL TECHNIQUE

Radical cystectomy

The overview of the surgical technique of radical cystectomy in this chapter is based on Skinner and Lieskovsky's description (10). Radical cystectomy refers to the removal of the anterior pelvic organs. In males it includes the resection of the prostate, seminal vesicles, bladder with its peritoneum, and perivesical fat. In females it includes the urethra, bladder, cervix, vaginal cuff, uterus, ovaries, and anterior pelvic peritoneum. One day prior to surgery, bowel preparation and cleansing is begun with oral neomycin, erythromycin, and various available laxatives and enemas.

Intraoperatively, the patient is placed in a hyperextended supine position. Operation begins with a long mid-line incision. Once the peritoneum has been opened, the intra-abdominal organs are explored to determine any intrahepatic metastasis or any unrelated pathological abnormality. The ascending colon and peritoneal attachments to the small bowel mesentery are dissected toward the ligament of Treitz. Next, the left colon and sigmoid mesentery are mobilized along the avascular line of Toldt.

After retraction of the small bowel and right colon with the aid of moist gauze pads, proper exposure of the pelvic viscera is obtained. Both ureters are transected in the deep pelvis, several centimetres after crossing the common iliac arteries. Samples of the distal ureters are sent to the pathology laboratory for frozen section to assure tumour-free margins.

Pelvic lymphadenectomy is begun, extending lateral to the genitofemoral nerve. The fibroareolar/lymphatic tissue is swept off the distal aorta, vena cava, common iliac vessels, and the sacral promontory. The pelvic peritoneum is dissected over the external iliac artery and incised medial to the spermatic vessel in the male and lateral to the ovarian vessel in the female. Vas deferens and the round ligaments are clipped in the male and female, respectively. The node of Cloquet, medial to the external iliac artery at the femoral canal, represents the distal limit of lymphatic dissection. Deep in the pelvis, the obturator fossa represents the posterior limit of the lymphatic dissection. Great care should be taken to protect the obturator nerve in this region. It is important to note that meticulous *en-bloc* pelvic node dissection in patients with microscopic pelvic lymph node metastases has been shown to improve survival when combined with adjuvant chemotherapy (11).

Mobilization of the bladder is begun by skeletonizing and ligating the hypogastric vessels. The lateral fascial pedicles, extending from the anterior pelvic organs to the rectum are resected. The posterior fascial pedicle, the peritoneal reflection between the rectum and the anterior visceral organs, is resected after anterior retraction of the urachal remnant in the male and the uterus in the female.

After complete resection of the lateral and posterior pedicles, attention is turned anteriorly. In the male, attachments between the anterior bladder wall and prostate to the pubis are freed. The urethra, distal to the prostate is clamped and resected. The prostate, seminal vesicle, and the posterior bladder wall are carefully dissected off the rectum. Better definition of the neurovascular structures that supply the pelvic viscera, has led to development of nerve sparing radical cystoprostatectomy in order to preserve sexual potency (12). This technique has not compromised resection of tumour, and has had moderate impact in improving quality of life after surgery by preservation of sexual potency (13).

To complete the pelvic exenteration in the female, urethropubic ligaments are divided, the urethra is resected along with the anterior vaginal wall. When feasible, the anterior vaginal wall is preserved and closed to give a functional vagina.

Urethrectomy

If the urethra is retained after radical cystectomy, the patient has the option of obtaining a continent urinary diversion with urethral anastamosis. This is more socially acceptable because of the near normal pattern of voiding after cystectomy. Indications for urethrectomy are based on the probability of urethral tumour involvement at time of cystectomy or subsequent risk of urethral recurrence. The incidence of urethral tumour recurrence after cystectomy is 8–12% (14–16). However, those with multiple bladder cancers or foci of carcinoma *in situ* (CIS) have a two- to threefold increased risk of urethral tumour recurrence (17,18).

Traditionally, urethrectomy has been routine in women with invasive TCC because of inability to maintain continence after creation of an orthotopic neobladder with urethral anastamosis secondary to poor urethral sphincter mechanism. However, better neuroanatomical and histological studies of the female pelvis and urethra have shown that women are able to maintain continence if the distal two-thirds of the urethra are preserved (19). Also, better patient selection with careful biopsies of the bladder, trigone, and bladder neck preoperatively with careful pathological review have shown that women who undergo orthotopic diversion with urethral anastamosis are capable of maintaining continence without compromising resection of cancer (20–23).

URINARY DIVERSION

There are three classes of urinary diversion which can be offered to the patient. Cutaneous urinary diversions using a segment of ileum, jejunum, or sigmoid colon have been used in the past. This requires the patient to wear a urinary appliance over the abdomen for collection of urine at all times. Bricker popularized the ileal conduit for urinary diversion in 1950 (24). Prior to surgery the stoma site is marked on the abdomen. It should be as far lateral of the mid-line as possible, but should always lead the bowel for urinary diversion through the split rectus muscle to avoid a high incidence of parastomal hernias. In brief, intraoperatively a suitable segment of small bowel is chosen and divided proximally and distally along the avascular parts of the mesentery. The ureters are mobilized, with special care not to damage its collateral blood supply from the spermatic cord or infundibulopelvic ligament. The ureter is partially transected in an oblique fashion, and the spatulated ureter is anastamosed to the isolated small bowel.

Continent catheterizing pouches are the second form of cutaneous urinary diversion. This form of cutaneous stoma gives the patient the added advantage of intermittent catheterization, without need of wearing an abdominal urinary collection appliance. The pioneering work of Gilchrist (25), Ashken (26), Mansson (27),

and Benchckroun (28) were used to develop our current understanding of continent cutaneous urinary diversion. After 20 years of
animal experimentation and human studies, Kock and colleagues
found that if the ileum is detubularized and reconstructed in a
spherical shape, a reservoir with lower filling pressures, higher
volumes, and improved continence is created (Fig. 14.1) (29). The
Indiana pouch (30), the Mainz pouch (31), and the Penn pouch
(32) are other forms of continent cutaneous urinary reservoir that
have been developed, all of which use segments of ileum and/or
colon. They all use the same principle of the Kock pouch, providing a high volume, low pressure system. [See Benson and Olsson
for a detailed review (33).]

Orthotopic voiding diversion is the third possible option for
the patient facing radical cystectomy. It refers to creation of a collecting urinary reservoir followed by anastamosis to the retained
urethra. This is more socially accepted by the patient, as there is
no need for an abdominal urinary appliance or catheterization of
the urinary stoma as mentioned above. Generally, this option has
been available only to men after cystectomy. However, recent
work at the University of Southern California by Stein et al. (34)
and others (20–22) have shown favourable results in providing orthotopic diversion to women. A method favoured at our

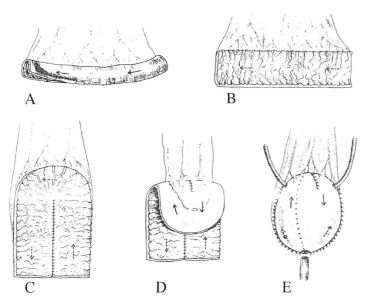

A   B

C   D   E

Fig. 14.1 Creation of a high capacity low pressure ileal urinary reservoir. (A,B)
Detubularization of a segment of small bowel along its anti-mesenteric border. (C) The
segment of bowel is folded into a U. (D) The loop is closed in a craniocaudal fashion,
(E) followed by ureteral and urethral anastamoses

institution is the orthotopic neobladder developed by Hautmann and colleagues at the University of Ulm (35). A spherical pouch utilizing 60–80 cm of the ileum in the shape of an M or W (Fig. 14.2) achieves a low pressure, high capacity system that is anastamosed to the urethra (35). This pouch is well tolerated by patients with minimal complications (36) and minimal metabolic derangements (37).

Patient selection is a key component of choosing the appropriate urinary diversion. Continent diversions are inappropriate for the patient with compromised renal function, because of the increased risk of metabolic abnormalities associated with these reservoirs. Similarly, the patient who is not motivated or is physically handicapped to care for his urinary reservoir is considered a poor candidate for continent diversion.

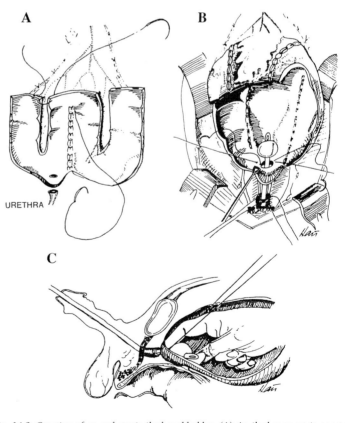

Fig. 14.2 Creation of an orthotopic ileal neobladder. (A) An ileal segment is anastamosed side by side in the shape of an **M** or **W**. (B) Ileo-urethral anastamosis, and subsequent closure of the urinary reservoir in a cranio-caudal direction. (C) Sagittal view of the ileo-urethral anastamosis

CONSERVATIVE THERAPY

Muscle invasive TCC can also be treated with bladder preservation techniques. Only a portion of the bladder is removed with the intention of full resection of cancer, retaining physiological bladder function, continence, potency, and ability to sample regional pelvic lymph nodes (38). Indicators for partial cystectomy include solitary, primary, and muscle invasive or high-grade lesions in a region of the bladder that allows complete excision with adequate margins, and a biopsy proven absence of cellular atypia or CIS in the remaining bladder. The biggest drawback of partial cystectomy is the high rate of tumour recurrence ranging from 38% to 78% (38). Because partial cystectomy has been used for highly selected patients who are poor surgical candidates, it is difficult to make direct comparisons in studies utilizing radical cystectomy for treatment of invasive TCC. As expected, patients with higher histological grade, treated with partial cystectomy, have a higher mortality rate at 5- and 10-year follow up (38). Another conservative approach to preserve the bladder is to combine local transurethral resection, radiotherapy, and systemic chemotherapy (39). In select patients this combination of treatments may be beneficial; however, randomized clinical trials for direct comparison with other treatments remains to be done.

NEOADJUVANT AND ADJUVANT CHEMOTHERAPY

Metastasis to local pelvic lymph nodes is treated by combination of surgery and chemotherapy. Cisplatin and methotrexate are the most active single chemotherapeutic agents used in urothelial carcinoma (40). Combination chemotherapy with methotrexate, vinblastine, doxorubicin, and cisplatin is most effective in invasive TCC (41). Both adjuvant chemotherapy (chemotherapy after surgery) and neoadjuvant chemotherapy (chemotherapy prior to surgery) have been used. Beneficial results have been found with adjuvant chemotherapy after cystectomy in multiple randomized trials (42–46). In neoadjuvant chemotherapy trials, median survival for invasive TCC may be improved (47,48); however, no benefit in survival has been found in treating patients with neoadjuvant chemotherapy who have lamina propria (pT1) or early muscle (pT2) invasion of TCC (47,48). The issue of neoadjuvant or adjuvant chemotherapy is further discussed in another chapter of this volume (Chapter 17).

Key Points

1. Radical cystectomy in males includes the resection of the prostate, seminal vesicles, bladder with its peritoneum, and perivesical fat. In females it includes the urethra, bladder, cervix, vaginal cuff, uterus, ovaries, and anterior pelvic peritoneum.
2. There are three classes of urinary diversion which can be offered to the patient: (i) use of a segment of ileum, jejunum, or sigmoid colon; (ii) continent catheterizing pouches; and (iii) orthotopic voiding diversion.
3. Patient selection is a key component of choosing the appropriate urinary diversion.

Points of controversy

1. Creation of orthotopic neobladder with urethral anastamosis in women.
2. Radical cystectomy versus conservative partial cystectomy combined with radiation and chemotherapy.
3. Use of adjuvant or/and neoadjuvant chemotherapy.

CONCLUSIONS

In appropriately selected patients, the best chance for cure of invasive bladder cancer is radical cystectomy with pelvic lymphadenectomy, as the primary treatment. Probably, the greatest progress in management of the surgical candidate is development of various forms of urinary diversion. Patient satisfaction has improved with creation of orthotopic bladders, which enables the patient to lead a near normal life after treatment for invasive bladder cancer. Neoadjuvant and adjuvant chemotherapy improve the long-term survival of this patient population. Many areas remain to be explored in the laboratory to better understand the molecular biology of bladder carcinogenesis. The efforts from the laboratory will hopefully lead to better drug designs and new modes of therapy, which will work more effectively in synergy with surgical treatment.

References

1 Lieskovsky G, Ahlering T, Skinner DG. *Diagnosis and staging of bladder cancer* (ed. Skinner DG, Lieskovsky G). WB Saunders, Philadelphia, 1988.

2 Jewett HJ, Strong GH. Infiltrating carcinoma of the bladder: Relation of depth of penetration of the bladder wall to incidence of local extension and metastases. *J Urol* 1946, **55**, 366–72.

3 Richie JP, Skinner DG, Kaufman JJ. Radical cystectomy for carcinoma of the bladder: 16 years of experience. *J Urol* 1975, **113**, 186–9.

4 Pagano F, Bassi P, Milani C *et al.* A low dose bacillus Calmette-Guerin regimen in superficial bladder cancer therapy: is it effective? *J Urol* 1991, **146**, 32–5.

5 Pearse HD, Reed RR, Hodges CV. Radical cystectomy for bladder cancer. *J Urol* 1978, **119**, 216–18.

6 Bredael JJ, Croker BP, Glenn JF. The curability if invasive bladder cancer treated by radical cystectomy. *Eur Urol* 1980, **6**, 206–10.

7 Mathur VK, Krahn HP, Ramsey EW. Total cystectomy for bladder cancer. *J Urol* 1981, **125**, 784–6.

8 Skinner DG, Lieskovsky G. Contemporary cystectomy with pelvic node dissection compared to preoperative radiation therapy plus cystectomy in management of invasive bladder cancer. *J Urol* 1984, **131**, 1069–72.

9 Skinner DG, Lieskovsky G. Management of invasive and high-grade bladder cancer. In: *Diagnosis and management of genitourinary cancer* (ed. Skinner DG, Lieskovsky G). WB Saunders, Philadelphia, 1988, pp. 295–312.

10 Skinner DG, Lieskovsky G. Technique of radical cystectomy. In: *Diagnosis and management of genitourinary cancer* (ed. Skinner DG, Lieskovsky G). WB Saunders, Philadelphia, 1988, pp. 607–21.

11 Lerner SP, Skinner DG, Lieskovsky G *et al.* The rationale for en bloc pelvic lymph node dissection for bladder cancer patients with nodal metastases: long-term results. *J Urol* 1993, **149**, 758–64.

12 Walsh PC, Mostwin JL. Radical prostatectomy and cystoprostatectomy with preservation of potency. Results using a new nerve-sparing technique. *Br J Urol* 1984, **56**, 694–7.

13 Schoenberg MP, Walsh PC, Breazeale DR *et al.* Local recurrence and survival following nerve sparing radical cystoprostatectomy for bladder cancer: 10-year followup. *J Urol* 1996, **155**, 490–4.

14 Ahlering TE, Lieskovsky G, Skinner DG. Indications for urethrectomy in men undergoing single stage radical cystectomy for bladder cancer. *J Urol* 1984, **131**, 657–9.

15 Faysal MH. Urethrectomy in men with transitional cell carcinoma of bladder. *Urology* 1980, **16**, 23–6.

16 Schellhammer PF, Whitmore WF Jr. Transitional cell carcinoma of the urethra in men having cystectomy for bladder cancer. *J Urol* 1976, **115**, 56–60.

17 Hendry WF, Gowing NF, Wallace DM. Surgical treatment of urethral tumours associated with bladder cancer. *Proc R Soc Med* 1974, **67**, 304–7.

18 Zincke H, Patterson DE, Utz DC, Benson RC Jr. Pelvic lymphadenectomy and radical cystectomy for transitional cell carcinoma of the bladder with pelvic nodal disease. *Br J Urol* 1985, **57**, 156–9.

19 Colleselli K, Strasser H, Moriggl B *et al*. Hemi-Kock to the female urethra: anatomical approach to the continence mechanism to the female urethra. *J Urol* 1994, **151**, 500A (abstract).

20 Stenzl A, Colleselli K, Poisel S *et al*. The use of neobladders in women undergoing cystectomy for transitional-cell cancer. *World J Urol* 1996, **14**, 15–21.

21 Stenzl A, Draxl H, Posch B *et al*. The risk of urethral tumors in female bladder cancer: can the urethra be used for orthotopic reconstruction of the lower urinary tract? *J Urol*, 1995, **153**, 950–5.

22 Stenzl A, Colleselli K, Poisel S *et al*. Rationale and technique of nerve sparing radical cystectomy before an orthotopic neobladder procedure in women. *J Urol* 1995, **154**, 2044–9.

23 Stein JP, Stenzl A, Esrig D *et al*. Lower urinary tract reconstruction following cystectomy in women using the Kock ileal reservoir with bilateral ureteroileal urethrostomy: initial clinical experience. *J Urol* 1994, **152**, 1404–8.

24 Bricker EM. Symposium on clinical surgery: bladder substitution after pelvic evisceration. *Surg Clin North Am* 1950, **30**, 1511–21.

25 Gilchrist RK, Merricks JW, Hamlin HH, Rieger IT. Construction of substitute bladder and urethra. *Surg Gynecol Obstet* 1950, **90**, 752–60.

26 Ashken MH. Urinary cecal reservoir. In: *Bladder reconstruction and continent diversion* (ed. King LR, Stone AR, Webster GD). YearBook Medical Publishers, Chicago, 1987, pp. 238–51.

27 Mansson W, Colleen S, Forsberg L *et al*. Renal function after urinary diversion. A study of continent caecal reservoir, ileal conduit and colonic conduit. *Scand J Urol Nephrol* 1984, **18**, 307–15.

28 Benchekroun A. The ileocecal continent bladder. In: *Bladder reconstruction and continent diversion* (ed. King LR, Stone AR, Webster GD). YearBook Medical Publishers, Chicago, 1987, pp. 224–37.

29 Kock NG, Nilson AE, Nilsson LO *et al*. Urinary diversion via a continent ileal reservoir: clinical results in 12 patients. *J Urol* 1982, **128**, 469–75.

30 Rowland RG, Mitchell ME, Bihrle R *et al*. Indiana continent urinary reservoir. *J Urol* 1987, **137**, 1136–9.

31 Thuroff JW, Alken P, Riedmiller H *et al*. 100 cases of Mainz pouch: continuing experience and evolution. *J Urol* 1988, **140**, 283–8.

32 Duckett JW, Snyder H, Md. Use of the Mitrofanoff principle in urinary reconstruction. *Urol Clin North Am* 1986, **13**, 271–4.

33 Benson MC, Olsson CA. Urinary diversion. *Urol Clin North Am* 1992, **19**, 779–95.

34 Stein JP, Cote RJ, Freeman JA *et al*. Indications for lower urinary tract reconstruction in women after cystectomy for bladder cancer: a pathological review of female cystectomy specimens. *J Urol* 1995, **154**, 1329–33.

35 Hautmann RE, Egghart G, Frohneberg D, Miller K. The ileal neobladder. *J Urol* 1988, **139**, 39–42.

36 Hautmann RE, Miller K, Steiner U, Wenderoth U. The ileal neobladder: 6 years of experience with more than 200 patients. *J Urol* 1993, **150**, 40–5.

37 Matsui U, Topoll B, Miller K, Hautmann RE. Metabolic long-term follow-up of the ileal neobladder. *Eur Urol* 1993, **24**, 197–200.

38 Sweeney P, Kursh ED, Resnick MI. Partial cystectomy. *Urol Clin North Am* 1992, **19**, 701–11.

39 Kaufman DS, Shipley WU, Griffin PP. *et al*. Selective bladder preservation by combination treatment of invasive bladder cancer. *N Engl J Med* 1993, **329**, 1377–82.

40 Scher HI. Systemic chemotherapy in regionally advanced bladder cancer. Theoretical considerations and results. *Urol Clin North Am* 1992, **19**, 747–59.

41 Sternberg CN, Yagoda A, Scher HI *et al*. Methotrexate, vinblastine, doxorubicin, and cisplatin for advanced transitional cell carcinoma of the urothelium. Efficacy patterns response relapse. *Cancer* 1989, **64**, 2448–58.

42 Richards B, Bastable JR, Freedman L *et al*. Adjuvant chemotherapy with doxorubicin (Adriamycin) and 5-fluorouracil in T3, NX, MO bladder cancer treated with radiotherapy. *Br J Urol* 1983, **55**, 386–91.

43　Skinner DG, Daniels JR, Russell CA *et al.* The role of adjuvant chemotherapy following cystectomy for invasive bladder cancer: a prospective comparative trial. *J Urol* 1991, **145**, 459–64.

44　Stockle M, Meyenburg W, Wellek S *et al.* Advanced bladder cancer (stages pT3b, pT4a, pN1 and pN2): improved survival after radical cystectomy and 3 adjuvant cycles of chemotherapy. Results of a controlled prospective study. *J Urol* 1992, **148**, 302–6.

45　Studer UE, Bacchi M, Biedermann C *et al.* Adjuvant cisplatin chemotherapy following cystectomy for bladder cancer: results of a prospective randomized trial. *J Urol* 1994, **152**, 81–4.

46　Freiha F, Reese J, Torti FM. A randomized trial of radical cystectomy versus radical cystectomy plus cisplatin, vinblastine and methotrexate chemotherapy for muscle invasive bladder cancer. *J Urol* 1996, **155**, 495–9.

47　Schultz PK, Herr HW, Zhang ZF *et al.* Neoadjuvant chemotherapy for invasive bladder cancer: prognostic factors for survival of patients treated with M-VAC with 5-year follow-up. *J Clin Oncol* 1994, **12**, 1394–401.

48　Malmstrom PU, Rintala E, Wahlqvist R, Hellstrom P, Hellsten S, Hannisdal E. Five-year followup of a prospective trial of radical cystectomy and neoadjuvant chemotherapy: Nordic Cystectomy Trial I. *The Nordic Cooperative Bladder Cancer Study Group J Urol* 1996, **155**, 1903–6.

15. Radiotherapy in the Management of Muscle-Invasive Bladder Cancer

K.J. Harrington and K. Sikora

Introduction

The patient population that presents with bladder cancer offers a number of specific challenges. These patients are frequently elderly, with a poor performance status and a number of concurrent medical conditions, often related to prior or ongoing tobacco smoking. Such patients are often unfit for radical surgery, either by virtue of the extent of the disease or the risk posed by the anaesthesia, and may not tolerate combined bladder-conserving therapeutic approaches using radiotherapy and chemotherapy. Careful selection of the most appropriate treatment strategy can result in effective palliation of symptoms and even complete resolution of the disease process before death due to an intercurrent illness intervenes (1–3).

The management of muscle-invasive bladder cancer remains an area of great controversy. A wide variety of treatment strategies are supported by clinicians practising in different countries, different specialties, and even within the same specialty in different units. In general terms, there is a dichotomy in which one camp strongly supports radical surgery as the treatment of choice and the other believes that bladder conservation by means of a combination of different treatment modalities represents the way forward. This split is exemplified by the titles of two recent editorials, 'Is there a role for radiation treatment in the treatment of bladder cancer' and 'Organ-sparing treatment for bladder cancer: Time to beat the drum' (4,5). As in many arenas where uncertainty persists, this controversy is fuelled by the paucity of available data from large-scale, prospective, randomized clinical trials. As a consequence, the fundamental questions regarding treatment selection for individual patients have not received definitive answers. Instead, there is a large body of literature addressing the various issues in this field, careful review of which allows a number of recommendations to be made. Nevertheless, the need for further large randomized studies cannot be overemphasized, as it is only by conducting such investigations that clear answers will eventually emerge.

THE ROLE OF RADIOTHERAPY

Modalities of radiotherapy

Radiotherapy is the therapeutic use of ionizing radiation. It can be divided into three broad classes of treatment: teletherapy, brachytherapy, and the use of unsealed sources. Teletherapy or external beam radiotherapy involves the use of treatment machines at a distance (usually about 1 m) from the patient. Production of radiation is by means of X-ray tubes for energies less than 1 MeV and by linear accelerators or high activity radioisotope sources for energies greater than 1 MeV. Other forms of high energy radiation, such as neutrons, protons and π-mesons, can also be produced in specialist units. Brachytherapy describes treatment with sealed radioactive sources, which are placed in very close proximity to the treated tissue. This can involve sources placed on the surface of tumours (moulds), within the substance of the tumour (interstitial), within the lumen of a hollow viscus (intraluminal), and within a cavity (intracavitary). Unsealed sources are radioactive materials which are not confined within a container and that come into direct contact with the patient. Each of these different types of treatment may be used in the treatment of bladder cancer. However, in general, radiotherapy for bladder cancer is largely restricted to the use of external beam therapy using high energy photons from a linear accelerator. Brachytherapy is under investigation as a means of delivering a very high local tumour boost after external beam radiotherapy (see below). The use of unsealed sources, including radiolabelled monoclonal antibodies and colloidal solutions, is an interesting avenue for research, but, as yet, remains experimental.

THE RADIOBIOLOGICAL BASIS OF RADIOTHERAPY

Radiobiology is the study of the effect of radiation on living matter. Although a detailed account of the science of radiobiology is beyond the scope of this chapter, a brief description of five of its central themes (the five Rs of radiobiology) will serve to highlight the important areas of interest and their clinical relevance. The five Rs of radiobiology are repair, repopulation, reoxygenation, redistribution, and radiosensitivity.

Repair

The damage caused by radiation to the DNA of both normal and malignant cells takes a number of different forms. Single- and double-strand DNA breaks are the most important phenomena and double-stranded breaks, in particular, have been found to correlate with cell kill over a wide range of doses. However, once damage has occurred, complex cellular repair mechanisms come into effect to attempt to restore the integrity of the DNA sequence. It is thought that all reparable damage is completely repaired within 6 h of irradiation. Although repair is a highly desirable property of normal cells, its occurrence in cancer cells will tend to reduce the efficacy of therapeutic radiation. The ability of normal and tumour cells to repair radiation-induced DNA damage varies and lies at the heart of the design of fractionated courses of radiotherapy. In general, normal tissues are said to repair damage more efficiently. Therefore, dividing a course of radiation into a number of fractions with an interval between them to allow normal tissue repair allows differential killing of normal and tumour cell populations. The therapeutic ratio is the term used to describe the ratio between the cell kill in the tumour compared with that in normal tissue. Changes in the pattern of fractionation alter the differential cell killing between tumours and late-responding normal tissues, in effect modifying the therapeutic ratio. Increasing the dose per fraction may be hazardous as this causes relatively more damage in normal tissues than in the tumour and reduces the therapeutic ratio. On the other hand, reducing the dose per fraction may be advantageous as there will be differential sparing of normal tissues relative to the tumour, increasing the therapeutic ratio. Balanced against this is the need to increase the total dose and the number of radiation fractions to achieve equal total tumour cell kill. If this requires undue prolongation of treatment, the beneficial effects of fractionation may be lost by the occurrence of tumour cell repopulation (see below) and a decreased chance of cure. In the case of low dose rate interstitial brachytherapy, the treatment can be viewed as a large number of very small radiation fractions given one after another. Repair occurs throughout the treatment and this gives rise to differential sparing of normal tissues while allowing high curative doses to be delivered to the tumour. Part of this advantage is lost if high dose rate brachytherapy is used. Such treatment must be delivered in fractions with sufficient time between them to allow for repair of damage in normal tissues.

Repopulation

During a course of fractionated radiotherapy, viable tumour cells continue to divide. As some cells are destroyed by a dose of radiotherapy, new cells replace them. Some studies have suggested that after approximately 3 weeks of fractionated radiotherapy viable clonogenic tumour cells are able to enter a phase of accelerated repopulation. Therefore, in order to eradicate a tumour completely, the radiotherapy must destroy not only all of the original tumour cells but also any formed by repopulation during the treatment period. This has led to the concept of 'wasted' radiation dose (i.e. some of the next fraction of radiotherapy is used up in killing cells born in the interval between fractions). Therefore, prolongation of the overall treatment time would be expected to have an adverse effect on local control and patient survival. Clinical studies have confirmed this prediction for a number of different tumour types, including bladder cancer (6,7). Changes in conventional fractionation regimens, classically 2 Gy fractions once daily for 5 days per week, are under investigation. These include: hyperfractionation, in which an increased number of small fractions is given more than once daily within the same overall treatment time as conventional radiotherapy; and accelerated hyperfractionation, where the treatment is given more than once a day within a shorter total period of time than conventional radiotherapy, either continuously (CHART) or with a gap to allow resolution of the acute radiation reaction.

Re-oxygenation

Well-oxygenated (euoxic) cells are more susceptible to the effects of ionizing radiation than hypoxic cells. The euoxic zone around tumour blood vessels tends to contain healthy, dividing cells, whereas the areas distant from the blood vessels often show areas of necrosis thought to be due to anoxic cell death. Radiotherapy is generally effective at killing the euoxic cells and those that have already died from profound anoxia no longer pose a threat. However, in the intervening territory between the euoxic and anoxic cell populations, there exists a population of hypoxic cells that is able to remain viable in a quiescent, non-cycling phase. There is evidence to suggest that this group of cells is relatively radioresistant and is a major determinant of the outcome of radiotherapy. Fractionation of radiotherapy provides a mechanism to circumvent this problem. As euoxic cells are killed by radiation, they no longer absorb and metabolize oxygen allowing it to diffuse further from the blood vessels into previously hypoxic areas. This effect of tumour reoxygenation tends to reverse the relative radioresistance of the hypoxic cell population.

Redistribution

Cellular radiosensitivity varies at different phases of the cell cycle. Cells in G_1, early S and G_2/M phases are highly sensitive, whereas cells in late S phase are highly resistant to the effects of ionizing radiation. Fractionated courses of radiotherapy aim to exploit the tendency for tumour cells to redistribute into different phases of the cell cycle throughout the course of treatment. Therefore, it is hoped that cells in a relatively radioresistant phase at the time of one treatment fraction will be in a more sensitive phase at the time of the next fraction.

Radiosensitivity

Different types of tumours have differing inherent sensitivities to ionizing radiation. Therefore, radiotherapy is more effective in treating some tumours than others (e.g. lymphomas and seminomas are extremely radiosensitive and gliomas and melanomas are relatively radioresistant). However, within a given tumour type, such as bladder cancer, it is impossible to predict in advance what the inherent radiosensitivity of any individual tumour will be. If it were possible to assay radiosensitivity on a biopsy specimen before therapeutic radiation started, it might be possible to select the most appropriate radiotherapy regimen or even to identify tumours which would be unlikely to be cured by radiotherapy. As yet, such assays have proved to be little more than a research tool and have not found their way into routine radiotherapy treatment strategies.

ACUTE AND LATE RADIATION REACTIONS

During radiotherapy normal tissues unavoidably receive some of the radiation dose. The effect of this absorbed dose in normal tissues is of considerable importance and limits the amount of treatment that can be delivered safely. Normal tissue reactions are conventionally divided into acute and late reactions, depending on the cellular populations at risk and the timing of onset of the reactions. Acute reactions occur in rapidly proliferating tissues, such as the bone marrow, skin, and the mucosae of the gastrointestinal and respiratory tracts due to cell death in the stem cell population. Typical acute radiation reactions include skin desquamation, radiation-induced diarrhoea, and mucosal ulceration. They tend to be self-limiting and, if the dose delivered has not been excessive, resolve promptly without long-term sequelae. In contrast, late reactions occur in slowly proliferating tissues and manifest themselves many weeks or months after the irradiation. They are irreversible and tend to be progressive. They are thought to be due to vascular damage, most probably at the level of the endothelial cells. Late radiation reactions include such severe complications as bowel stenosis, fistula formation, bladder fibrosis, and radiation-induced myelopathy. In general, it is the risk of late normal tissue reactions which dominates clinical practice. Every course of radical radiotherapy involves balancing the chance of curing the disease against the risk of causing unacceptable late normal tissue damage. Figure 15.1 illustrates the dilemma and the relatively narrow therapeutic window within which curative treatment is given. In this hypothetical example, at a dose of 60 Gy very few tumours are cured but there are no serious adverse reactions. By increasing the dose to 65 Gy, the cure rate increases dramatically to about 35% but this is achieved at the expense of 5% of patients suffering a serious adverse reaction. This equates to a complication-free cure rate of 30%. If attempts are made to increase the cure rate further by increasing the radiation dose to 75 Gy, the cure rate may increase to 70% but the complication rate has leapt to 40%, a complication-free survival, which has remained unchanged at 30%. Therefore, for conventionally fractionated radiotherapy, the incidence of normal tissue damage effectively imposes a dose ceiling on treatment which limits the total dose that can be delivered.

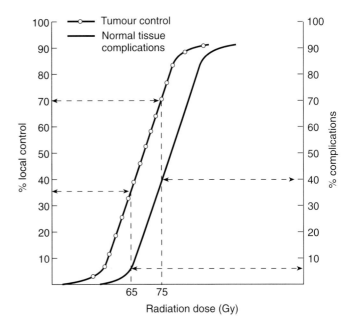

Fig. 15.1 Local tumour control and normal tissue complications as a function of radiation dose. The occurence of severe late normal tissue damage effectively imposes a therapeutic ceiling on the dose of radiation that can be administered safely. Strategies aimed at circumventing this problem include the use of altered fractionation schedules, radiation sensitizers, and conformal planning techniques

RADIOTHERAPY PLANNING

Definition of treatment volumes

The purpose of radiotherapy planning is to define the volumes of tissues which need to be treated to a therapeutic dose and to avoid important uninvolved normal structures. Figure 15.2 shows a schematic illustration of the different volumes that must be considered during this process (8). The gross tumour volume (GTV) represents the palpable or visible extent of the tumour, as assessed by clinical examination and standard imaging techniques. This volume of tissue corresponds to that part of the disease in which the malignant cells are at their greatest concentration. The GTV may include the primary tumour, metastatic lymph node disease and/or other metastatic foci. However, the GTV does not accurately represent the entire local tumour burden, as clinical and radiological examination will only demonstrate areas of macroscopic disease involvement. Therefore, it is necessary to consider a larger volume of tissue which may contain microscopic amounts of disease. The clinical target volume (CTV) comprises the GTV with an added margin to take account of direct, local subclinical spread. In practice, the definition of a CTV requires consideration of factors such as the tendency for the tumour type to invade local structures and its likely pattern of spread to loco-regional lymph nodes. In addition, when delineating this volume, it is necessary to consider adjacent critical normal structures and the general health of the patient. The CTV, therefore, can be considered to be

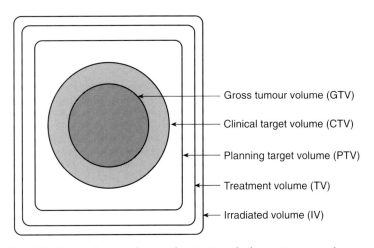

Gross tumour volume (GTV)

Clinical target volume (CTV)

Planning target volume (PTV)

Treatment volume (TV)

Irradiated volume (IV)

Fig. 15.2 Tissue volumes under consideration in radiotherapy treatment planning. ICRU 50 has defined a number of tissue volumes that must be considered during the planning of radical radiotherapy

the volume of tissue which must be treated to a predetermined dose in order to achieve the goal of therapy, whether radical or palliative.

In order that all the tissues within the CTV receive the prescribed radiation dose, it is necessary to plan to deliver irradiation to a geometrically larger volume of tissue than the CTV. This is a consequence of a number of factors: (i) movement of tissues which contain the CTV, e.g. patient movement during treatment and physiological respiratory and bowel movements; (ii) day to day variations in the size and shape of the tissues that contain the CTV, e.g. different filling states of the bladder and bowel; and (iii) day to day variations in the radiotherapy beam geometry characteristics. Therefore, another volume, the planning target volume (PTV) must be recognized. The PTV is a geometrical concept which allows selection of appropriate beam sizes and arrangements to ensure that the prescribed radiation dose is actually delivered to the CTV. In clinical practice, the CTV and the PTV should be very similar in shape and size. When radiotherapy is delivered, technical limitations dictate that some tissues beyond the PTV will also receive the full therapeutic radiation dose. The volume of tissue that receives a radiation dose which is considered important for local cure or palliation is known as the treated volume. Finally, there will be a larger volume of tissue beyond the treated volume that will receive a radiation dose below the full therapeutic dose which may, none the less, represent a clinically significant dose in terms of normal tissue tolerance. This volume of tissue is the irradiated volume.

Radiotherapy planning techniques in bladder cancer

There are a number of possible approaches to planning radiotherapy for muscle-invasive bladder cancer. Previously, the standard approach was to instil a urographic contrast agent into the bladder in order to define the target volume. This approach had the disadvantage of only being able to delineate the bladder cavity and failed to demonstrate the extent of invasion into muscle or extravesical structures. It is now standard to perform a computed tomography (CT) scan of the pelvis and abdomen to assist planning of radical radiotherapy, although contrast cystography is usually sufficient to allow planning of palliative radiotherapy.

Two-phase technique
Radiotherapy is first administered to a large volume comprising the primary tumour and its local extensions, the entire bladder, and the loco-regional pelvic lymph nodes. The margins of the

volume for phase I are as follows: the upper border is at the level of the L4/L5 junction, the lower border is at the level of the bottom of the obturator foraminae, laterally the volume extends 1 cm beyond the bony margins of the pelvis, the anterior border lies 2 cm in front of the anterior wall of the bladder and the posterior margin extends to cover the entire bladder and the internal iliac lymph nodes. This volume is treated to a dose of 40 Gy in 20 fractions over 4 weeks using a three-field (or occasionally a four-field) beam arrangement (a direct anterior and two wedged lateral fields). Thereafter, a smaller phase II volume is treated which encompasses the entire bladder, primary tumour and its local extensions with a 1.5–2 cm margin. This volume is treated to a dose of 20–26 Gy, again using a three-field arrangement as above.

Single-phase technique

Radiotherapy is directed solely at the primary bladder cancer, its local extensions, and the whole bladder with a margin of 1.5–2.0 cm. No attempt is made to treat the pelvic lymph nodes. Planning this type of radiotherapy requires the aid of CT planning scans, which allow accurate definition of the extent of disease. However, treatment is still delivered by a standard three- or four-field pelvic technique.

Conformal radiotherapy

Recent developments in physics, engineering, and computing have opened the way for the application of conformal therapy and three-dimensional treatment planning and delivery (9). Although a detailed consideration of conformal therapy is beyond the scope of this chapter, it is sufficient to state that the specific aim of this approach is to optimize the physical basis of radiotherapy in order to tailor the high-dose volume to match the PTV, sparing at-risk normal structures where possible. The natural consequence of achieving such a result is to allow a larger radiation dose to be delivered more accurately to the PTV without increasing toxicity and, therefore, potentially to increase local control of the tumour. Thames et al. (1992) (10) have estimated that the use of conformal techniques offers the prospect of increasing tumour control by up to 20%. As yet, this approach is still under development, although a number of clinical studies have been reported. Reduced acute toxicity has been reported in some studies (11,12), but not in others (13,14). Tait et al. (1988) (15) studied the potential tissue sparing effect of conformal radiotherapy in 20 patients with invasive bladder cancer suitable for radical radiotherapy. The median treatment volume for conventional radiotherapy planning was 2275 cm^3 compared with 1416 cm^3 for conformal planning. In 13 of 20 patients (65%) the percentage volume of rectum irradiated to 90% of the isocentric dose was reduced by more than 30%. However, conformal planning was less likely to reduce the volume of large and small bowel irradiated to a high dose. In addition, the new technology offers the possibility of monitoring the accuracy of patient set-up before delivery of each radiotherapy fraction. In a randomized trial of patients receiving pelvic radiotherapy, Gildersleve *et al.* (1994) (16) were able to show that an on-line megavoltage imaging system was able to improve the accuracy of setting the treatment field with the result that the number of treatments given with a field placement error of ≥ 5 mm decreased from 69% to 7%. Such accurate field placement may yield advantages both in terms of more accurate delivery of therapeutic radiation to the tumour and reduced irradiation of normal tissues.

CLINICAL APPLICATIONS OF RADIOTHERAPY IN BLADDER CANCER

In the last decade there has been a substantial re-evaluation of the standard therapy for muscle-invasive bladder cancer. Previously, radical cystectomy was regarded as the treatment of choice, with radiotherapy reserved for either preoperative use or for the treatment of patients judged to have inoperable disease or to be medically unfit for surgery. This policy was perpetuated by the fact that there has never been a properly conducted large randomized trial of surgery versus radiotherapy. Instead, retrospective reviews were able to point to the relatively poor survival and high rates of recurrence in patients treated with radiotherapy alone, despite the fact that many of these poor-risk patients had been actively excluded from radical surgical series. In recent times there has been a strong move towards the development of organ-sparing therapeutic strategies in a range of common solid malignancies, including breast, head and neck, gastrointestinal, and bladder cancers. The aim of this movement is to develop combination strategies using conservative surgery, radiotherapy, and cytotoxic chemotherapy, which are at least as effective as radical surgery without the need for organ ablation (e.g. total cystectomy). Randomized trials are currently under way to determine if survival can be improved with adjuvant or neoadjuvant chemotherapy and to examine the most efficacious timing of chemotherapy administration. In addition, a new generation of studies includes detailed assessment of the patients' quality of life as well as the relatively crude measures of overall and disease-specific survival (17,18).

As part of the move towards the development of organ-sparing treatment, its proponents have often pointed to the adverse effect of cystectomy on the patients quality of life, using the presence of a urostomy and the occurrence of erectile impotence as powerful arguments against surgical treatment. During recent years, however, there have also been considerable advances in the surgical management of bladder cancer, both in terms of operative mortality and functional outcome. For example, Stockle et al. (19) reported the improvements in perioperative mortality for 246 cystectomies performed over an 18-year period in their centre. Perioperative mortality declined from 15% in the early years to 0% in 1985. In addition, modern surgical techniques of continent urinary diversion or total bladder replacement combined with sparing of the pelvic nerves (and thus preservation of potency) mean that radical cystoprostatectomy need no longer be regarded as mutilating surgery. Furthermore, if patients are well-prepared in advance for the effects of surgery, the overall quality of life achieved can be good (20).

A clear assessment of the place of radiotherapy in the treatment of bladder cancer will only be achieved by conducting well-supported, multicentre, randomized clinical trials. Unfortunately, there is a tendency for groups to conduct small, phase II studies or to embark on limited phase III studies with insufficient numbers of patients to provide statistically significant answers (21). Rigid adherence to previously accepted treatment strategies represents a significant obstacle to the evaluation of the place of new approaches. Similarly, the temptation to adopt intensive multimodality approaches should be resisted until it is clear that they improve the outcome of therapy and the quality of life achieved (22).

Definitive radiotherapy

The attraction of radiotherapy is that it offers the possibility of cure while preserving normal bladder and sexual function (23). There have been no randomized studies comparing radiotherapy alone with radical surgery. To compound the issue further, there is no firm agreement as to what constitutes standard radiotherapy. Wide variations in dose, fractionation, schedule, and energy of radiation exist. In addition, the use of interstitial brachytherapy boosts, non-photon radiation beams, radiosensitizing drugs, and physical therapies such as hyperthermia confuses the picture further. Therefore, an accurate assessment of the place of definitive radiotherapy in the management of muscle-invasive bladder cancer is difficult. In order to attempt this, it is necessary to rely on retrospective series in which radiotherapy was used as a single modality treatment.

Conventional fractionation

The definition of conventional fractionated radiotherapy is not clear. Classically, it involves the delivery of a radiation dose of 1.8–2.0 Gy daily for 5 days per week to a total dose of between 60 and 66 Gy. However, in a number of centres in the UK, a radical dose of radiotherapy delivered in 20 fractions would be considered to be conventional treatment. More recently, the advent of conformal planning techniques has offered the possibility of dose escalation beyond previously recognized safe limits. Therefore, this area represents a changing field of study.

Conventional external beam irradiation, using modern megavoltage techniques and doses that do not harm bladder function, will permanently eradicate local bladder cancer in 30–50% of patients, compared with 70–90% with cystectomy (24). A number of recent studies of conventional radiotherapy for muscle-invasive bladder cancer have reported overall 5-year survival rates of between 20 and 40 %, with the cause-specific rates being a little higher (25–30). A typical result of such a treatment policy was provided by Jenkins *et al.* (25) who reported their results in 182 patients with T2/T3 disease. The overall 5-year survival rate was 40%. Seventy-five (41.2%) patients had a complete response (CR) without subsequent local or distant relapse during follow-up. A further 20 patients had a local relapse, which was salvaged by cystectomy in 11 cases with a 5-year survival of 36%. Of the 87 patients who failed to achieve a CR after radiotherapy, 22 were able to undergo salvage cystectomy with a 5-year survival of 47%. The most important question for conventional fractionated radiotherapy, at present, is whether the opportunity afforded by conformal planning techniques to increase the absorbed dose delivered to the tumour will result in improved outcomes.

Opponents of radiotherapy have often stated that salvage cystectomy following radical radiotherapy is more difficult and associated with a prohibitively high rate of complications. This argument has often been used to argue in favour of immediate cystectomy as the treatment of choice. Abratt *et al.* (31) reported on 46 patients who underwent salvage surgery for persistent or recurrent disease after radical radiotherapy. The peri-operative mortality rate was 7% and 35% of patients suffered complications over a 5-year period. The risk of complications was significantly lower in those patients treated with conventional fractionation (2 Gy per day, 5 days per week) compared with altered fractionation regimens. The overall survival rate was 43% and, interestingly, this was found to be greater for those patients with an inCR to the initial radiotherapy. This finding can probably be explained by the fact that non-responders underwent early cystectomy, in contrast to the complete responders in whom the diagnosis of relapse and subsequent surgery was delayed.

Many studies have attempted to define factors which allow prediction of the likely outcome of treatment with radiotherapy. Well-recognized clinical prognostic factors include tumour stage, tumour grade, tumour histology, presence of ureteric obstruction, patient's age, Karnofsky performance status, pretreatment haemoglobin level, grossly complete resection at transurethral resection of the bladder tumour (TURBT) and the presence of tumour at follow-up cystoscopy at 3 months (26,27,29–34). However, many of these factors are significant only in univariate analyses. Attempts to define objective laboratory-based predictors of prognosis have met with mixed success. A number of studies have pointed out factors which seem to be associated with a poor outcome, but, as yet, none of these has found a place in the routine assessment of patients with bladder cancer. Jenkins *et al.* (35), obtained original pre-radiotherapy histological sections from 125 patients with invasive transitional cell bladder cancer. The presence of squamous metaplasia or positive staining for beta-human chorionic gonadotrophin (β-hCG) was associated with lack of a response to radiotherapy and the presence of both of those features in the same specimen was associated with failure to respond in 26 of 28 (93%) tumours. The response rate to radiotherapy in tumours without either of these features was 40 of 45 (89%). The DNA ploidy of 86 of the tumours was measured by flow cytometry. The response of diploid and aneuploid tumours was not significantly different.

Altered fractionation regimens

The results of the above retrospective analyses confirm that radical radiotherapy can cure muscle-invasive bladder cancer but the results are generally disappointing. A cure rate of only about 30% leaves a great deal of room for improvement. In recent years, there has been considerable interest in the potential of altered fractionation schedules to improve on the results of conventional radiotherapy. The most widely studied of the altered fractionation regimens is hyperfractionation, which involves the use of two to three low dose radiotherapy fractions per day with a planned break in treatment usually after half of the dose has been administered. Pure hyperfractionated radiotherapy allows a larger total dose of radiotherapy to be delivered within the same overall treatment time.

Stuschke and Thames (36) have recently conducted an overview analysis of the use of hyperfractionated radiotherapy in the treatment of bladder cancer. Their analysis included two randomized trials published since 1980 in which conventional fractionation (2 Gy per day, 5 days per week for 6–7 weeks) was compared directly with hyperfractionated radiotherapy. The two studies concerned were those of Edsmyr *et al.* (37) and Goldobenko *et al.* (38). The former reported the results of a phase III study in which 168 patients with T2–T4 disease were randomly allocated between conventional fractionation (64 Gy in 32 daily fractions over 8 weeks) and hyperfractionated radiotherapy (84 Gy in 84 thrice daily fractions over 8 weeks). The latter reported a complex four-arm randomized study in 177 patients with T2–T3 disease. In both of these designs, there was a 2-week rest period after half of the total dose had been given. The meta-analysis of the pooled data confirmed a benefit in terms of both local control and survival from the use of hyperfractionated radiotherapy with odds ratios of local failure and death of 0.44 and 0.55, respectively. Further analysis of the data confirmed that these effects were most marked for the high T stage tumours. There was no reported increase in the severe late normal tissue damage, although acute effects were intensified. These data are encouraging but must be viewed in light of the fact that the total doses employed in the conventional fractionation arms may not have been optimal and the 2-week gap in the middle of conventional radiotherapy is unnecessary and may run the risk of decreasing local control by extending treatment time and allowing accelerated repopulation to occur. In future, comparison of hyperfractionated radiotherapy with dose-escalated conformal radiotherapy may provide a more meaningful comparison.

The effect of treatment delays has been reported by a number of authors. Salminen *et al.* (39) reported a retrospective study of 119 patients with T1–T4 disease who received split course radiation to a total dose of 66 Gy, with a 3-week rest period in the middle of treatment. The actuarial 5-year survival for these patients was only 20%. Maciejewski and Majewski (6), have provided evidence that acceleration of treatment delivery may result in therapeutic advantages. They estimated that, for a dose of 63.3 Gy, protraction of overall treatment time from 40 to 55 days gave a decrease in local control rate from 50% to about 5%. Similarly, De Neve *et al.* (7), demonstrated that split course radiotherapy with a gap of 1 month and an overall duration of greater than 75 days was associated with a worse outcome than continuous fractionated radiotherapy completed in less than 75 days. No significant difference between radiotherapy completed in less than 44 days and radiotherapy completed between 44 and 75 days was detected, although the numbers of patients in each group were rather small. These findings may be explicable in terms of accelerated tumour repopulation during treatment. Analysis of the literature suggests that, on average, tumour clonogen repopulation in bladder cancer accelerates after a lag period of about 5–6 weeks from the start of treatment, with an estimated dose increment of 0.36 Gy per day required to compensate for this repopulation. It suggests that overall treatment time is an important factor in the dose fractionation and protraction of time may have a significant impact on treatment outcome.

Interstitial brachytherapy

Interstitial brachytherapy with iridium-192 has been used in selected patients in a few specialist centres with good effect. Rozan *et al.* (40), treated 205 patients with a short course of preoperative pelvic irradiation followed by surgery (partial cystectomy or tumour resection) and interstitial brachytherapy with iridium-192 wires. In most patients the tumour was early stage (164 patients had pT1 or pT2 disease) and relatively small (mean size 2.9 cm). Local failure occurred in 35 patients (17%), of whom 29% also had metastases or regional recurrence. The overall 5-year survival rates were 77%, 63%, and 47% for pT1, pT2, and pT3 disease, respectively. A quarter of the patients had acute side-effects and three patients died from surgical complications. Late bladder side-effects (haematuria, fistula, chronic cystitis) occurred in 29 patients. A functioning bladder was retained in 96% of disease-free survivors. In a smaller series, Moonen *et al.* (41) treated 40 patients with G3T1 and muscle-invasive T2–T3a disease of less than 5 cm in diameter with a combination of TURBT, external beam radiotherapy, and interstitial brachytherapy. Six patients developed local recurrence, four of whom also had systemic metastatic disease. Three other patients relapsed with distant metastatic disease alone. Acute complications of this approach included urine leakage and delayed wound healing and infections, whereas the only late reaction was that of self-limiting mucosal ulceration at the implant site. Similarly, Pernot *et al.* (42) reported 85 patients with pT1–pT4 disease treated with a combination of preoperative radiotherapy (10.5 Gy in three fractions), conservative surgery (TURBT or partial cystectomy) and iridium-192 interstitial brachytherapy to a dose of between 30 and 50 Gy. The majority of patients (68%) had pT1 or pT2 disease. Patients with advanced stage disease received pelvic radiotherapy and the lower dose of brachytherapy. The local control rate was 85%, 64%, and 70% for pT1, pT2, and pT3 disease, respectively. The complications included delayed wound healing and fistula formation. These complications were considerably reduced by delaying the afterloading of the iridium wires by 1 week. Recently, Wijnmaalen *et al.* (43) reported their results in treating 66 patients with a similar protocol consisting of external beam radiotherapy, TURBT ± pelvic lymph node dissection ± partial cystectomy, and interstitial iridium-192 brachytherapy (30 Gy at 0.58 Gy/h). The brachytherapy was started within 24 h after insertion of the loading tubes. The probability of bladder relapse-free survival at 5 years was 88%. In the surviving patients, the probability of bladder preservation was 98%.

The use of an intraoperative radiation boost has been suggested as an alternative to interstitial brachytherapy (24,44). They suggest that appropriately chosen patients can be treated with intraoperative radiotherapy delivered directly to the tumour by either a removable radium or iridium implant or a large single dose of electrons. Cure with preserved bladder function in more than 75% of patients with solitary tumours that invade into but not beyond the bladder muscle has been reported.

Non-photon irradiation

The use of forms of irradiation other than megavoltage photons has been reported in recent years. Such approaches have included neutron therapy (45–48), proton therapy (49) and π-meson therapy (50). These alternative radiotherapy approaches will be reviewed briefly but it should be remembered that they are experimental and their use should be restricted to clinical trials.

Russell et al. (45) reviewed the role of neutron therapy in bladder cancer, concluding that, although data suggest that preoperative neutron therapy may result in a greater degree of pathological downstaging than conventional photon regimens, this has not led to an improved survival rate for neutron-treated patients. Similarly, Kirkove et al. (46) reported a retrospective series of 58 patients with locally advanced bladder cancer treated with fast neutron therapy according to a number of different protocols. The overall 5-year actuarial survival was 30% (equivalent to what might have been expected with photon irradiation) and this was achieved with only modest adverse effects. Although the authors of that study placed their emphasis on the fact that neutrons are 'at least as effective as photon beam treatment', the clinical role of fast neutron therapy has been called into question as a result of recent analyses of data from the available randomized trials (47,48). Duncan (47) reviewed the data from 25 randomized trials of neutrons versus photons, including a number of patients with bladder cancer. There was no evidence of an advantage for the use of neutrons and, furthermore, the late complications were found to be unacceptably frequent and severe. Warenius (48) reviewed the recent study at the Clatterbridge Hospital, UK comparing 8 MeV photon therapy with 62.5 MeV neutron therapy. This study was stopped early because of a significantly worse survival in the neutron therapy group for reasons which are not clear. Therefore, at present, it seems unlikely that neutron therapy will have a significant role in future therapeutic strategies for bladder cancer.

The results of treatment with 250 MeV proton beam therapy in 147 patients (including 10 patients with bladder cancer) was reported by Tsujii et al. (49). Most patients were treated with proton beams alone and the total dose exceeded 80 Gy in the majority. Fraction sizes were greater than in conventional radiotherapy (>2.5 Gy) and the margins around the tumour volume were kept to a minimum (0.5–1.0 cm) in an attempt to minimize toxicity. The local control rate was 70% for the patients with bladder cancer. Further studies of this experimental radiotherapy technique are proceeding.

Studer et al. (50) reported very poor results of π-meson therapy in 41 patients with both superficial and muscle-invasive bladder tumours. An unacceptably high rate of local pelvic complications was observed and eight (21%) of the patients died as a consequence of severe late radiation reactions which occurred between 1 and 8 years after treatment. All of these patients had received high dose therapy (>33 pion Gy). Such data highlight the difficulties of introducing novel therapies with theoretical advantages into the clinic.

Radiosensitizers

A number of agents have the ability to enhance the effects of ionizing radiation on both normal and cancer cells. Such radiosensitizing agents include the hypoxic cell sensitizers (misonidazole, pimonidazole, etanidazole), the S-phase sensitizers (bromodeoxyuridine, iododeoxyuridine) and a variety of cytotoxic chemotherapeutic drugs (cisplatin, mitomycin C). This section will review the role of the hypoxic cell sensitizers and the cytotoxic agents will be considered separately below.

Bydder et al. (51) treated 89 patients in a multicentre, randomized trial with either misonidazole or placebo added to the first 40 Gy of radiotherapy. Depending on their referring clinician, patients then completed treatment with either further radiotherapy to a radical dose, or surgery 4 weeks later. No significant difference in local control, survival, or pathological downstaging of the tumour was demonstrated between the groups. There was considerable neurotoxicity in the misonidazole group with 43% of patients developing a peripheral neuropathy which persisted in 80%. Abratt et al. (52) reported their experience in treating 53 evaluable patients with G3T2 and T3 bladder cancer in a randomized study of radiation alone or radiation plus misonidazole. Patients in both groups initially received 40 Gy in 20 fractions.

Thereafter, patients either received a further 20 Gy in 10 fractions or a further 12 Gy in two fractions 1 week apart plus oral (3.0 g/m^2) and intravesical (1.0 g) misonidazole, 4 h and 2 h, respectively, before each fraction of 6 Gy. There was no significant difference in response rates, local control, or survival between the two groups, although there was some evidence of increased bowel toxicity in the group treated with misonidazole, perhaps as a result of the unconventional radiation fractionation schedule.

Hyperthermia

Hyperthermia can enhance the effect of radiation and chemotherapy against a variety of tumour types, both *in vitro* and *in vivo*. In the setting of bladder cancer, the tumour may be heated by bladder irrigation with a warmed solution of saline (53) or by external heating with radiofrequency capacitive heating devices (54). The aim of treatment is to heat the whole tumour to a temperature in excess of 41¡C for a period of up to 1 h shortly after radiotherapy. The use of hyperthermia and radiotherapy in the treatment of bladder cancer has, thus far, been restricted to small pilot studies. Matsui *et al.* (53) reported a response rate of 84% in 56 patients treated with a combination of radiotherapy (40 Gy in 4 weeks), local hyperthermia, and bleomycin. Kakehi *et al.* (54) reported a diverse group of patients treated with radiotherapy and hyperthermia or chemotherapy and hyperthermia. A CR rate of 71% was documented for the patients with bladder cancer. Further studies of local hyperthermia, with an emphasis on its integration into multimodality strategies certainly appear to be warranted.

Preoperative radiotherapy

Preoperative radiotherapy is used with the aim of treating microscopic local disease extension and nodal micrometastatic disease, downstaging the primary tumour, increasing the ease of operability of the lesion, and increasing local disease control. In recent years, the importance of securing local control has been clearly recognized. Pollack *et al.* (29) reported a significant correlation between local control and freedom from distant metastasis in 240 patients treated with radical cystectomy with or without combination chemotherapy. While this may represent an indication of the biological nature of the tumour, with more aggressive tumours which are more likely to metastasize also being more likely to recur locally, it is possible that local failure may subsequently give rise to the occurrence of distant metastases. Therefore, securing local control should be a major objective in the management of bladder cancer. In this regard, preoperative radiotherapy is an attractive therapeutic option and one which has been the subject of extensive study. Unfortunately, most of the published data are derived from non-randomized studies, although some randomized trials have been conducted in this area. As yet, a clear consensus view has not emerged because of the apparently contradictory results from the various studies.

Parsons and Million (55) conducted an exhaustive review of the published literature, including the randomized (56–60) and non-randomized studies. The authors concluded that the addition of preoperative irradiation to cystectomy for clinical T3 bladder cancer added approximately 15–20% to the 5-year survival. A study examining a different perspective of this question has been conducted by the Co-operative Urological Cancer Group (61). The results of that randomized study in which 189 patients were treated with either preoperative radiotherapy (40 Gy in 20 fractions) followed by cystectomy or radical radiotherapy (60 Gy in 30 fractions) were recently updated (62). When analysed by the intention to treat there was no significant difference in the cause specific survival at 5 and 10 years, although there was a trend in favour of the preoperative radiotherapy.

More recently, an extensive comparison of patients treated with either preoperative radiotherapy and cystectomy or cystectomy alone was conducted at the M.D. Anderson Cancer Centre (63). Of 521 patients included in the analysis, 301 received preoperative radiotherapy (mean dose 49.2 ±0.2 Gy) and cystectomy between 1960 and 1983 and 220 patients underwent cystectomy alone between 1985 and 1990. No differences were found in local control rates between the two groups for patients with T2 or T3a disease and there were insufficient patients to allow a meaningful analysis in patients with T4 disease. For the subgroup of patients with T3b disease, actuarial local control was significantly higher for those who received preoperative radiotherapy (91% versus 72%). In addition, there was a statistically non-significant improvement in metastasis-free survival (67% versus 54%), freedom from disease (59% versus 47%), and overall survival (52% versus 40%) for this subset of patients. It is also noteworthy that the two groups were treated in different eras and one can speculate that the group treated with cystectomy alone may have benefited from modern surgical techniques and the use of neoadjuvant cytotoxic chemotherapy to downstage tumours. Therefore, it has been suggested that the effect of preoperative radiotherapy may have been underestimated by this study.

In a recently reported randomized study, 140 patients with invasive bladder cancer were randomized to receive either pelvic irradiation to a dose of 20 Gy followed within 1 week by cystectomy or surgery alone (64). The 5-year survival rates of 43% and 53% were not significantly different. The same group reported their experience in a larger group of patients using preoperative radiotherapy to a dose of between 20 and 40 Gy followed by radical cystectomy, compared with radical cystectomy alone (65). They demonstrated that preoperative radiotherapy resulted in an improvement in pelvic local control, although this translated only to a modest improvement in survival because of the high rate of systemic disease relapse.

Further retrospective studies (many of them involving small numbers of patients) have reported either no benefit or a marginal benefit in favour of preoperative radiotherapy when assessed in terms of local control, freedom from metastases, and overall survival. Langemeyer et al. (66) reported the results of 160 patients treated with irradiation between 1972 and 1980. Following a radiotherapy dose of 40 Gy to the pelvis, treatment consisted of either cystectomy or completion of radical radiotherapy to the bladder region only. A full urological examination of the bladder established whether a patient was a responder or non-responder. The patients were divided into four groups according to their response to the initial radiotherapy and their subsequent treatment: group 1—27 radiotherapy responders treated with cystectomy and diversion; group 2—48 radiotherapy responders treated with radical radiotherapy up to 65 Gy; group 3—24 radiotherapy non-responders treated with cystectomy and diversion; group 4—42 radiotherapy non-responders treated with radical radiotherapy up to 65 Gy. Those patients who responded to the initial radiotherapy had a better survival rate than non-responders, regardless of further treatment. The patients who responded to the initial radiotherapy and then underwent cystectomy survived longer than those who went on to receive radical radiotherapy. Salvage cystectomy was associated with a high operative risk and short survival. Kaplan et al. (67), reviewed 58 consecutive patients who underwent cystectomy, with or without preoperative radiotherapy. Treatment selection was based solely on the physician's preference. The study showed no advantage of preoperative radiation in patients requiring cystectomy for transitional cell carcinoma of the bladder. Mameghan et al. (33), treated 205 patients with palliative radiotherapy, radical radiotherapy, or preoperative radiotherapy followed by total cystectomy. The overall actuarial 5-year survival rate (death from any cause) was 24%. The 5-year survival rates for patients treated with radical radiotherapy or preoperative radiotherapy followed by cystectomy were 25% and 38%, respectively. This difference was not statistically significant. Sell et al. (68), treated 183 patients with T2–T4a disease with either preoperative irradiation (40 Gy) followed by cystectomy or radical irradiation (60 Gy) followed by salvage cystectomy for residual tumour. There was a trend towards a higher survival rate for the combination of preoperative irradiation and cystectomy compared with radical irradiation followed by salvage cystectomy, although this did not reach the level of statistical significance and should be viewed in light of the fact that a radiation dose of 60 Gy may not be optimal. Interestingly, there was no difference in the occurrence of surgical complications in the planned and salvage cystectomy groups and there were no postoperative deaths among the cystectomized patients. The late complications experienced by the two treatment groups were different, as would be expected, but there were no major differences in the number of complications except for the inevitable occurrence of erectile impotence in male patients after cystectomy. Fossa et al. (69) reported their experience with 132 patients who underwent cystectomy after preoperative radiotherapy of either 20 Gy (65 patients) or 46 Gy (67 patients). The corrected 5-year survival rate was 60%.

Adjunctive therapies, used in addition to preoperative radiotherapy, have also been evaluated. Ono et al. (70), used the hypoxic cell radiosensitizer misonidazole in a small randomized study in 44 patients treated with preoperative irradiation of 40 Gy to the pelvic region followed by total cystectomy. The 5-year survival rate for T3 patients in the group treated by misonidazole plus radiotherapy was 59%, while that for T3 patients in the radiation only group was 43%. The differences were not statistically significant. A statistically significant effect was seen in terms of pathological downstaging of the primary tumour for patients with T3 disease treated with misonidazole plus radiotherapy. Hyperthermia plus preoperative radiotherapy has also been investigated (71). In this study, 49 patients received either 24 Gy in six fractions over 2 weeks or the same radiotherapy regimen plus twice weekly hyperthermia for 35–60 min immediately after the radiotherapy to a total of four sessions. Patients who received hyperthermia to an average intravesical temperature of more than 41.5°C achieved a significantly higher rate of tumour downstaging and degeneration than the patients treated with radiotherapy alone or those receiving hyperthermia in whom the average intravesical temperature did not exceed 41.5°C. This translated to an non-significant improvement in survival in this small group of patients.

Attempts have been made to identify factors of prognostic value in patients undergoing preoperative radiotherapy. Jacobsen et al. (72), used deoxyribonucleic acid (DNA) flow cytometry measurements in nuclear suspensions obtained from paraffin-embedded biopsies from 83 patients treated with preoperative radiotherapy and cystectomy for T2, T3, and T4a bladder carcinoma. Thirteen tumours (16%) were diploid, 18 (22%) tetraploid, and 52 (63%) aneuploid. A total of 19 tumours (23%) had two or three stemlines in addition to the diploid cells. Postradiotherapy downstaging (absence of muscle infiltration in the cystectomy specimen) occurred more often in tumours with only one non-diploid stemline than in diploid tumours or non-diploid tumours with multiple stemlines. The 5-year survival rate was significantly worse for patients with a diploid (33%) than for those with a non-diploid (66%) tumour, although this finding was true only of univariate, and not multivariate, analysis. The same group also studied DNA ploidy and S-phase fraction as a means of predicting the response to cisplatin-based chemoradiotherapy in operable bladder cancer (73). Neither DNA ploidy nor S-phase fraction was shown to be predictive for the response to neo-adjuvant treatment.

In summary, despite an extensive body of literature, the role of preoperative radiotherapy in the management of muscle-invasive bladder cancer remains unresolved. In fact, with the recent move towards more complex, intensive, combination strategies it is unlikely that this matter will be examined in detail in further studies.

Postoperative radiotherapy

The role of postoperative radiotherapy to the pelvis after cystectomy has not been clearly defined. In general, preoperative staging investigations should be able to identify in advance those patients with unresectable disease so that they can be referred for primary non-surgical management. However, there are occasions in which the margins of the resection are relatively close or in which pelvic nodal metastases have been detected unexpectedly. In these circumstances, pelvic radiotherapy may have a part to play. In general, delivery of radiotherapy to the pelvis after surgery is likely to be associated with increased morbidity as a result of disruption of the normal vascular anatomy, the presence of bowel adhesions and reductions in the motility of segments of small bowel, potentially resulting in a single segment being tethered within the high-dose volume.

The largest experience in this circumstance was reported in bilharzial bladder cancer. Zaghloul et al. (74) treated 236 patients with clinical T3 disease who survived radical surgery and were found to have pT3a or greater tumours in a randomized study of postoperative radiotherapy. Patients were divided into three groups: group 1—no further treatment (83 patients); group 2—postoperative radiotherapy using three daily fractions of 1.25 Gy each with 3 h between fractions to a total dose of 37.5 Gy in 12days (75 patients); group 3—postoperative radiotherapy using conventional fractionation to a total dose of 50 Gy in 5 weeks (78 patients). Postoperative radiotherapy was well tolerated with equal acute reactions in the hyperfractionated and conventional fractionation groups. The 5-year disease-free survival rates were 25% in group 1, 49% in group 2, and 44% in group 3. The 5-year local control rates were 50%, 87%, and 93% for groups 1, 2, and 3, respectively. Interestingly, the late complications of radiotherapy in the skin, small bowel, rectum, and the anastomotic site of the urinary division were lower with hyperfractionated than conventional radiotherapy.

Reisinger *et al.* (75) reported the results of 78 patients who were treated with combined pre- and postoperative adjuvant radiation therapy. All were given a single dose of preoperative radiation therapy of 5 Gy, either on the day of or the day before cystectomy. Forty patients with G3T2–T4a or node positive disease underwent planned high dose postoperative radiation therapy to a dose of 40–45 Gy in 1.8 Gy fractions in 5 weeks. The overall 5-year survival was 67%. Survival for patients treated with postoperative radiotherapy was approximately 50%. Late bowel complications occurred in 37% of the irradiated patients and only 8% of the unirradiated patients. There was no significant difference in the rates of genitourinary complications in both groups. These data indicate that postoperative radiotherapy is likely to be associated with unacceptably high rates of bowel toxicity. Therefore, it is unlikely that it will find a place in the routine management of bladder cancer.

Primary chemoradiotherapy

In recent years there has been enormous interest in the use of combined radiotherapy/chemotherapy treatment in a wide range of solid cancers. This approach has the twin aims of increasing local disease control and influencing the development/progression of distant metastatic disease. In many cases, the nature of the interaction of the individual modalities is not clearly understood. Indeed, it is not necessary for the radiotherapy and chemotherapy to have any interaction, so long as they each achieve a degree of cell kill in the tumour.

Tannock (76) has elegantly reviewed the inherent limitations of reports of single-arm studies of combination therapy when compared with historical controls treated with radiation alone. He described several types of bias including patient selection, stage migration, the tendency to publish positive results, or inadequate follow-up as compared with the historical series. He also pointed out that randomized controlled trials provide the only rigorous method for evaluating combined therapy, but are also subject to misinterpretation if they seek small benefits of treatment in a spectrum of patients with widely differing prognosis. Some randomized trials have demonstrated improved local control and increased toxicity from combined treatment, a result that might have been achieved by increasing the effective radiation dose. Ideally, combined treatment should be compared with radiotherapy alone at equal levels of normal tissue damage.

The majority of recent studies have focused on the use of cisplatin in combination with radiation (77–81), as this agent has significant cytotoxicity against bladder cancer and has been shown to interact with radiation in a number of tumour types. However, studies with agents such as 5-fluorouracil (5-FU), mitomycin C and vinblastine have also been reported (82–84).

Sauer et al. (77) treated 67 patients with T1–4N0–2M0 disease with radiotherapy to a dose of 50.4 Gy in 28 fractions in 6 weeks with concomitant cisplatin (25 mg/m^2 per day on 5 consecutive days in weeks 1 and 5). The CR rate was 75% and the estimated 3-year survival rates were 73%, 68%, 25% for T1, T2–3, and T4 disease, respectively. The 10-year results of a large German study of an organ preserving protocol in 245 consecutive patients treated with maximal TURBT, and definitive radiotherapy to 56 Gy in 28 fractions, with more than one-half of the patients also receiving either concomitant infusional cisplatin (25 mg/m^2 per day for 5 days, 79 patients) or infusional carboplatin (65 mg/m^2 per day for 5 days, 60 patients) confirmed the efficacy of this approach (79). The overall survival was 47% at 5 years and 26% at 10 years. Salvage cystectomies were performed in 53 patients, without severe complications and 192 patients (79%) retained a functioning bladder. The bladder preservation rate in the 5-year survivors was 83%. The use of concurrent cisplatin and radiotherapy in 109 patients with localized muscle-invasive bladder cancer was reported by Chauvet et al. (80). The patients were judged to be unfit for radical cystectomy, although one-third were able to undergo extensive TURBT. Large volume pelvic irradiation to a dose of 40–45 Gy was followed by a small volume boost to the bladder to a total dose of 55–60 Gy. Concomitant cisplatin chemotherapy (20–25 mg/m^2 per day for 5 days) was delivered during weeks 2 and 5 of treatment. The overall 4-year survival was 42% for the whole group and 51% for the complete responders. Coppin et al. (81) reported their experience with concomitant cisplatin with either preoperative or definitive radiotherapy in 99 patients with T2–T4b bladder cancer. The choice between preoperative or definitive radiotherapy was a matter of choice for the clinicians and patients, with patients randomized thereafter to receive either three cycles of cisplatin at a dose of 100 mg/m^2 per day at 2 weekly intervals or no chemotherapy. The patients treated in the cisplatin arm of the study had a significantly lower incidence of local failure in the pelvis (29.4% versus 52.1%) but there was no effect on the occurrence of distant metastases or overall survival.

Rotman et al. (82) treated 19 patients with radiotherapy and concomitant (5-FU) by intravenous infusion with or without bolus mitomycin C. Eleven of 18 evaluable patients (61%) obtained a CR and an additional five patients (28%) showed tumour regression to a superficial state controlled by local transurethral resection and intravesical chemotherapy. Russell et al. (83) treated 34 patients with radiotherapy combined with infusional 5-FU. Patients received 40 Gy of radiotherapy in 5 weeks with 1 g/m^2 per day of 5-FU administered as a 96 h infusion on days 1–4 of weeks 1 and 4. After a 3-week rest period, patients eligible for cystectomy underwent cystoscopy and biopsy. Those with residual tumour underwent cystectomy, and those without tumour received an additional cycle of chemotherapy and irradiation. Patients ineligible for cystectomy for reasons medical, surgical, or refusal received a third cycle without the 4-week delay or re-evaluation. The actuarial cancer-specific survival for the entire group of patients was 64% at 45 months, with a freedom from relapse of invasive cancer of 54%. Twenty-four of the 34 (71%) patients retained intact bladders, with 20 of 24 reporting entirely normal voiding. In 16 patients who underwent pathological restaging after two cycles of chemoradiotherapy 13 (81%) had a pathological CR. Kragelj et al. (84), treated 29 patients with concurrent radiotherapy (62–66 Gy at 1.8–2.0 Gy/day for 5 days a week with a break in the middle of treatment of 2–3 weeks and vinblastine weekly 2 mg/5–12 h intravenous infusion). The toxicity was acceptable and a clinical complete remission rate of 71% was documented.

There have also been a number of studies of intra-arterial chemotherapy plus radiotherapy. Stewart et al. (85), reported the use of cisplatin (25–120 mg/m^2 per day) injected into the internal iliac arteries of 33 patients with locally advanced bladder cancer. Of 21 patients evaluable for their response to cisplatin, three (14%) achieved complete remission, 12 (57%) achieved partial remission, two (14%) had stable disease, and four (19%) failed to respond. The same group (86) treated 25 patients with T3 and T4 disease with intra-arterial cisplatin and concurrent radical radiation (20 of 25) or intra-arterial cisplatin, concurrent preoperative radiation, and cystectomy (five of 25). One patient died from treatment-related toxicity. Other toxicities have been what one would expect from the individual treatment modalities except for a sensory sacral root neuropathy in 11 of 24 (46%) patients. Twenty-three of 24 (96%) patients achieved a CR and the projected actuarial 2-year survival is 90%. Only one of the 23 complete responders has had an invasive local recurrence. The excellent complete local response and survival rates achieved warrant further study of the combination of intra-arterial cisplatin and radiation as a bladder-preserving strategy. Kanoh *et al.* (87) used intra-arterial adriamycin (10 mg infusion twice weekly) via either the superior or inferior gluteal artery in 32 patients (eight of whom also received cisplatin) with bladder cancer prior to total cystectomy. Of the 25 patients who received inferior gluteal artery infusional chemotherapy, nine died of cancer; all nine died within 2 years due to distant metastases. There was no evidence of recurrence in any patient who survived for 2 years or more after total cystectomy. Therefore, inferior-gluteal-artery infusion chemotherapy may be effective as a preoperative adjuvant therapy with no serious side-effects. Sumiyoshi *et al.* (88) treated 60 patients with T2–T4 NX M0 disease with intra-arterial doxorubicin plus low dose radiotherapy. They reported a CR rate of 60% and all but three patients proceeded to a conservative surgical approach. The overall 5-year disease-free and cause-specific survivals were 49% and 72%, respectively.

Hug *et al.* (89) studied the tumours of 37 patients treated with a bladder preserving protocol using transurethral resection, neo-adjuvant chemotherapy and 40 Gy radiotherapy plus concomitant cisplatin. At 30 months of follow-up, patients with purely aneuploid tumours had an overall survival of 82% compared with 47% for the patients with diploid/partly diploid tumours.

Radiotherapy following neoadjuvant chemotherapy

Raghavan (21), has highlighted the attraction of using pre-emptive or neoadjuvant cytotoxic chemotherapy in patients with invasive, clinically non-metastatic bladder cancer. However, he also pointed out that the fact that the majority of eligible patients have been treated in increasingly complex phase II studies has severely retarded evaluation of these approaches in randomized clinical trials.

Updated results from the Co-operative Urological Cancer Group trial of neoadjuvant and adjuvant methotrexate chemotherapy have recently been reported (62). In that study, 397 patients were randomly allocated to receive either local therapy alone (cystectomy or radical radiotherapy) or local therapy preceded and followed by methotrexate chemotherapy. The 5-year survival rates in the two groups were 27 and 29%, respectively. Subgroup analysis confirmed increased survival for patients aged <60 years, with tumours <2.5 cm in diameter, with clinical N0 disease and no evidence of histological lymphatic involvement. Wallace *et al.* (90), reported the results of an overview of two similar, but independent, randomized studies of neoadjuvant cisplatin before radiotherapy in 255 patients with T2–T4 M0 bladder cancer. There was no difference in survival between the treated and control patients. In fact, the control groups had a marginally better outcome than the chemotherapy groups. Recently, the specific role of platinum-based neoadjuvant or concurrent chemotherapy was addressed in a meta-analysis performed by the Medical Research Council (MRC) Cancer Trials Office (91). In this study, updated patient information was available for 479 patients treated in four randomized trials comparing definitive local treatment alone with neoadjuvant or concurrent single agent platinum followed by definitive local treatment. The analysis failed to demonstrate any survival benefit for the use of platinum-based chemotherapy.

In recent years, it has become clear that combination regimens are significantly more active than single agent drugs (21). Combinations containing a platinum, a vinca alkaloid and methotrexate (with or without an anthracycline) offer the greatest chance of a response in patients with bladder cancer. Therefore, the recently closed MRC/ European Organization for Research and Treatment of Cancer trial of neoadjuvant chemotherapy used a CMV (cisplatin, methotrexate, vinblastine) combination consisting of cisplatin 100 mg/m^2, methotrexate 30 mg/m^2, vinblastine 4 mg/m^2, every 3 weeks. Preliminary findings of that study have recently been published in abstract form (92). In this study, 975 patients with T2 (G3), T3 or T4a, N0 or NX, M0 transitional cell bladder cancer were randomized to receive either three cycles of CMV chemotherapy or no chemotherapy before proceeding to radical cystectomy, full dose external beam radiotherapy or preoperative radiotherapy and cystectomy. The choice of the definitive treatment of the primary tumour was left to the policy of the institution from which the patient was referred. Equal numbers of patients were allocated to the chemotherapy and no chemotherapy arms. Cystectomy was performed in 484 patients, 414 patients received radical radiotherapy and 77 patients received preoperative radiotherapy followed by cystectomy. In those patients who underwent cystectomy, the pathological CR rate attributable to CMV chemotherapy was 21%, confirming the activity of this combination regimen. However, after a median follow-up of 22 months, there was no evidence of an overall survival advantage in patients receiving neoadjuvant CMV, with an overall 2-year survival of 62% and 60% for the treatment and no treatment arms, respectively. A much smaller randomized study of neoadjuvant cyclophosphamide, doxorubicin, and cisplatin (CAP) followed by radical radiotherapy in 60 patients was reported by Okajima et al. (93). The difference in the 5-year survival rates of the chemotherapy (96%) and control (79%) groups was not statistically significant.

Perhaps partly as a consequence of the negative findings of the studies using neoadjuvant chemotherapy alone, more aggressive multimodality bladder-preserving protocols have been developed. One approach that has been extensively evaluated is that of a combination of maximum TURBT, neoadjuvant combination chemotherapy, and induction chemoradiotherapy followed by cystoscopic and pathological evaluation of response. In patients with a CR, consolidative chemoradiotherapy offers the prospect of curing the disease and retaining the bladder, while patients with residual disease at this stage can be offered prompt salvage cystectomy (94).

Prout et al. (95) outlined a conservative therapeutic strategy using transurethral debulking surgery combined with neoadjuvant CMV chemotherapy plus two additional courses of cisplatin during the first 40 Gy of radiotherapy. If tumour was present on cystoscopic re-evaluation and biopsy after this induction therapy, immediate cystectomy was advised. If no tumour was found, consolidation by a radiotherapy boost to a total of 64.8 Gy plus an additional course of cisplatin was given. After a median follow-up of 26 months, 72% of patients were alive, 70% with bladder preservation, and 74% without distant metastases. Dose reductions were required in 39% of patients who completed the protocol but there were no treatment-related deaths. Eight patients underwent immediate radical cystectomy because of positive biopsy and/or cytology results after 40 Gy, while 34 completed full chemotherapy and radiotherapy without any significant bladder or bowel injury. Of 42 patients, 22 (52%) have retained their bladder without recurrence and, of those selected for full chemotherapy and radiotherapy, this number increased to 65%. The results of the same bladder-preserving programme of two courses of CMV, followed by induction chemoradiation to 39.6 Gy with concomitant cisplatin and assessment of response before proceeding to either a chemoradiation boost or cystectomy were reported by the Radiation Therapy Oncology Group (96). Of 91 patients with T2 M0 to T4a M0 bladder cancer, 37 required cystectomy (14 nonresponders to induction, 16 invasive recurrence, six extensive

non-invasive recurrence and one severe treatment-related complications). The 4-year actuarial survival rate of the whole group was
62% and the 4-year actuarial survival with an intact bladder was
44%. Einstein *et al.* (97) reported the results of a similar therapeutic approach in a group of 34 patients with T2–T4, NX-N2, M0
bladder cancer who were judged to be unfit for cystectomy. In this
study, there was no interval assessment of response and no option
to proceed to cystectomy. Twenty-seven patients completed the
protocol and a CR rate of 56% (19 of 34) was documented,
although 10 of the CRs were achieved by the TURBT alone. The
median overall survival was 21 months with a 5-year survival of
only 18%. These data show no evidence of an advantage when
compared with radiotherapy alone and the toxicity of the combined therapy was significant. Kachnic *et al.* (98) have reported
their experience of 106 patients with T2–T4a, NX, M0 disease
treated by maximum TURBT and two cycles of CMV chemotherapy. This was followed by pelvic irradiation to a dose of 39.6 Gy
with concomitant cisplatin. Patients were then assessed for response at cystoscopy and biopsy and those with a CR received
further chemoradiotherapy to a total dose of 64.8 Gy. Those
patients with residual disease at assessment, or those unable to
tolerate this intensive regimen, went to immediate cystectomy. The
5-year actuarial overall survival and disease-specific survival were
52% and 60%, respectively. Of the 76 patients who completed
bladder-preserving therapy, the 5-year local relapse-free survival
was 79% and the 5-year overall survival rate with a functioning
bladder was 43%. A less favourable view of this approach has been
provided by Given *et al.* (99). They reported their results in 94
patients treated with TURBT, two to three cycles of cisplatin-based
chemotherapy followed by radiotherapy, partial cystectomy, or
cystectomy. After 5 years the relapse-free survival for the entire
group was 49%. However, of the initial patient cohort, only 18%
were alive with an intact bladder. The authors of this study concluded that bladder conservation should be limited to a very select
group of patients.

   Orsatti *et al.* (100), used a slightly different approach to bladder
conservation with chemoradiotherapy in their phase II study.
Seventy-six patients with T1G3 to T4 N0 M0 bladder cancer
received alternating chemotherapy and radiotherapy. The chemotherapy used was cisplatin 20 mg/m^2 per day and 5-FU 100 mg/m^2
per day for 5 days (although the final 21 patients received
methotrexate 40 mg/m^2 per day instead of 5-FU). The radiotherapy dose schedule was two courses of 20 Gy in 10 fractions over
12 days for the first 18 patients, escalating to two courses of 25 Gy
in 10 fractions over 12 days for the remaining 58 patients. The

systemic toxicity of the chemotherapy was mild, although more than one-third of the patients experienced moderate to severe local toxicity. The clinical CR rate was 81% and the 6-year overall survival was 42%.

Palliative radiotherapy

There are many circumstances in which palliative radiotherapy can be used to treat bladder cancer. Most frequently, palliative radiotherapy is used as the primary treatment of elderly, infirm patients with symptomatic local disease who are fit for neither cystectomy nor radical radiotherapy, with or without cytotoxic chemotherapy; although age *per se* should not exclude patients from consideration of radical treatment approaches (101). Alternatively, symptomatic local disease (primary or recurrent) may be present against a background of systemic metastatic disease. Radiotherapy may also provide a useful means of palliating symptoms due to distant meastatic disease (e.g. bone and brain metastases), although these issues are considered in detail in Chapter 24 dealing with palliative therapy. Whatever the situation, the aim of palliative radiotherapy must be to produce effective palliation of disease-related symptoms without producing excessive treatment-related morbidity. In the case of pelvic disease, if a sufficient radiation dose can be delivered, it is possible to induce CRs or significant tumour growth delay which may mean that the patient remains disease-free until death from an unrelated cause occurs.

In general, palliative radiotherapy has taken the form of either hypofractionated radiotherapy (a small number of relatively high-dose radiation fractions delivered less frequently than in conventional fractionation) or split-course therapy. The potential advantage of these approaches is that the tolerability and, to some extent, the efficacy of treatment can be evaluated during the course of treatment before proceeding to the full dose. Irradiation of a small pelvic volume appears to offer the most appropriate strategy (102) and this can usually be planned with the aid of a contrast cystogram rather than with CT planning.

Hypofractionated radiotherapy has been extensively investigated. Wijkstrom *et al.* (103), reported the results and complications of palliative radiotherapy in 162 elderly or disabled patients. Improvement in tumour-associated symptoms was noted in 75 (46%) of these patients and 72 survived for more than a year. Those who responded to radiotherapy had a 5-year cancer-free survival rate of 58% compared with 4% in patients who did not respond to treatment. Survival was also affected by stage and indications for radiotherapy. In 85 patients without severe symptoms, where the tumour was judged curable but the patient was unsuitable for a full course of radiotherapy, the 5-year cancer-free survival rate was 21%, which is in accordance with what might have been achieved with full-course radiotherapy. The 5-year late complication rate was 7%. In a similar study, Salminen (104), treated 94 patients considered unsuitable for conventional radical radiotherapy for locally advanced, recurrent or metastatic urinary bladder cancer with the intention of palliating local disease. Patients received 30 Gy in six fractions given twice a week. Eighty-two patients (87%) completed the treatment as planned and 40 patients (43%) had complete palliation of their symptoms. Thirty-eight patients (40%) had initial local control of the tumour, which was lasting in 25 cases (26%). The median disease-specific survival was 13.3 months. The estimated 5-year survival was 13% and survival from bladder cancer 27%. The use of once-weekly hypofractionated radiotherapy was reported from a series of patients treated at the Royal Marsden Hospital (105). In this study, 64 patients with a median age of 81 years were treated with a weekly fractions of 6 Gy to a total dose of 36 Gy (29 patients), 30 Gy (25 patients) or less than 30 Gy (10 patients). A cystoscopic CR was seen in 62% (23 of 37) of patients evaluable for response and the median survival of the whole group was 10 months. There was moderate acute bladder toxicity and three patients experienced grade III–IV late bladder morbidity. Rostom et al. (106), conducted a preliminary dose-finding study in elderly patients or those with poor performance status. Seventy patients received once weekly irradiation; 27 to a dose of 36–39 Gy in six fractions over 35 days and 43 to a lower dose of 34.5 Gy in six fractions over 39 days. The lower dose was well tolerated with response rates and survival that were comparable with daily fractionated regimens.

Split course radiotherapy has also been the subject of a number of studies. Spanos et al. (107), used a twice-daily fractionation schedule of 3.7 Gy per fraction for 2 days (i.e. 14.8 Gy in four fractions over 2 days) with a 4-week gap between courses in 152 patients with advanced pelvic malignancies, 25% of whom had genitourinary cancers. Patients received a maximum of three courses of radiation to a total dose of 44.4 Gy. For the patients completing all three courses, the responses were as follows: complete remission (14%); partial remission (31%); no change (40%); progression (7%); and unknown (8%). There was little evidence of severe toxicity with this regimen. Vrouvas et al. (108), treated a group of 89 elderly, unfit patients with a mean dose of 45 Gy in 10–12 fractions over a mean time of 48 days. A CR was achieved in 28 of 89 patients (31%) and was highly dependent on the T stage of disease. The median survival for patients with T1/T2, T3, and T4 tumours was 22, 10, and 8 months, respectively. The treatment was well-tolerated with only 8% of patients experiencing grade II–III late toxicity. Phillips and Howard (109), reported their experience in 76 elderly patients treated with a split course radiotherapy protocol in which patients received an initial 2-week course of radiotherapy followed by a 3-week gap. Thereafter, their fitness to proceed to a second phase of radiotherapy was evaluated and 53 patients completed this course of treatment. The overall CR rate was 25%, although this figure rose to 36% of those completing the full protocol.

The ability of two different radiotherapy fractionation regimens to palliate the symptoms of bladder cancer has been evaluated in prospective study in 41 patients (110). Patients were treated in a non-randomized fashion with either 17 Gy in two fractions over 3 days or 45 Gy in 12 fractions over 26 days. Patient selection was based on the clinician's assessment of their general condition and performance status. The two fraction treatment was more effective at palliating pain and haematuria than the more protracted conventional fractionation, although the survival was shorter in this group of patients. Further evaluation of the most appropriate fractionation schedule for the palliation of bladder cancer is under way in a large, multicentre, randomized study being conducted by the MRC.

CONCLUSIONS

Radiotherapy represents an active treatment modality against muscle-invasive bladder cancer and can legitimately be applied in a number of therapeutic settings. In recent years, there has been a significant re-appraisal of its role, with a trend towards the use of more aggressive multimodality combination regimens incorporating radiotherapy as part of an organ-sparing approach. However, encouraging data from small phase II studies must not blind investigators to the fact that, as yet, none of these newer approaches has withstood the test of rigorously conducted randomized trials. Such investigations must be the priority for the next decade of study if a clearer view of the optimal therapy of this disease is to emerge.

Key Points

1. The standard treatment of muscle-invasive bladder cancer is with either radical surgery or radical radiotherapy
2. The use of altered fractionation regimens, interstitial brachytherapy, non-photon irradiation, and radiosensitizing agents should be restricted to the setting of clinical trials.
3. Preoperative and postoperative radiotherapy have not been shown to yield a clear survival advantage.
4. Organ-preserving strategies involving the use of concomitant chemotherapy and radiotherapy represents the most active field of study at present.

References

1   Keane P, Waxman J, Sikora K. Urological system. In: *Treatment of cancer* (ed. Price P, Sikora K). Chapman and Hall, London, 1995, pp. 562–568.
2   Ritchie CD, Bevan EA, Collier St J. Importance of occult haematuria found at screening. *Br Med J* 1986, **292**, 681–3.

3 Droller MJ. Bladder cancer. *Curr Probl Surg* 1981, **18**, 209–13.

4 Wajsman Z. Is there a role for radiation therapy in the treatment of invasive bladder cancer? *J Urol* 1997, **157**, 1647–8.

5 Zietman AL, Shipley WU. Organ-sparing treatment for bladder cancer: Time to beat the drum. *Int J Radiat Oncol Biol Phys* 1994, **30**, 741–2.

6 Maciejewski B, Majewski S. Dose fractionation and tumour repopulation in radiotherapy for bladder cancer. *Radiother Oncol* 1991, **21**, 163–70.

7 De Neve W, Lybeert MLM, Goor C *et al.* Radiotherapy for T2 and T3 carcinoma of the bladder: the influence of overall treatment time. *Radiother Oncol* 1995, **36**, 183–8.

8 International Commission on Radiation Units and Mesurements (ICRU) Report 50. *Prescribing, recording and reporting photon beam therapy.* ICRU, Bethesda, MD, 1993.

9 Webb S. Developments and controversies in three-dimensional treatment planning. In: *The physics of conformal radiotherapy: advances in technology* (ed. Webb S). Institute of Physics Publishing, Bristol, 1997, pp. 4–13.

10 Thames HD, Schultheiss TE, Hendry JH *et al.* Can modest escalations of dose be detected as increased tumour control? *Int J Radiat Oncol Biol Phys* 1992, **22**, 241–6.

11 Schultheiss TE, Hanks GF, Hunt MA *et al.* Factors influencing incidence of acute grade 2 morbidity in conformal and standard radiation treatment of prostate cancer: univariate and multivariate analysis. *Int J Radiat Oncol Biol Phys* 1993, **27**, 134–8.

12 Sandler H, McLaughlin PW, Ten Haken R *et al.* 3D conformal radiotherapy for the treatment of prostate cancer: low risk of chronic rectal morbidity observed in a large series of patients. *Int J Radiat Oncol Biol Phys* 1993, **27**, 135–9.

13 Tait DM, Nahum AE, Rigby L *et al.* Conformal radiotherapy of the pelvis: assessment of acute toxicity. *Radiother Oncol* 1993, **29**, 117–26.

14 Horwich A, Wynne C, Nahum A *et al.* Conformal radiotherapy at the Royal Marsden Hospital (UK). *Int J Radiat Biol* 1994, **65**, 117–22.

15 Tait D, Nahum A, Southall C *et al.* Benefits expected from simple conformal radiotherapy in the treatment of pelvic tumours. *Radiother Oncol* 1988, **13**, 23–30.

16 Gildersleve J, Dearnley DP, Evans PM *et al.* A randomised trial of patient repositioning during radiotherapy using a megavoltage imaging system. *Radiother Oncol* 1994, **31**, 161–8.

17 Fossa SD, Aaronson N, Calais Da Silva F *et al.* Quality of life in patients with muscle-infiltrating bladder cancer and hormone-resistant prostatic cancer. *Eur Urol* 1989, **16**, 335–9.

18 Caffo O, Fellin G, Graffer U, Luciani L. Assessment of quality of life after cystectomy or conservative therapy for patients with infiltrating bladder carcinoma: a survey by self-administered questionnaire. *Cancer* 1996, **78**, 1089–97.

19 Stockle M, Alken P, Engelmann U *et al.* Radical cystectomy—often too late? *Eur Urol*, 1987, **13**, 361–7.

20 Fossa SD, Reitan JB, Ous S, Kaalhus O. Life with an ileal conduit in cystectomized bladder cancer patients: Expectations and experience. *Scand J Urol Nephrol* 1987, **21**, 97–101.

21 Raghavan D. Keynote address: A critical assessment of trials of neoadjuvant (preemptive) chemotherapy for bladder cancer: Lesson for future studies of combined modality treatment. *Int J Radiat Oncol Biol Phys* 1991, **20**, 233–7.

22 Lerner SP, Skinner E, Skinner DG. Radical cystectomy in regionally advanced bladder cancer. *Urologic Clinics North Am* 1992, **19**, 713–23.

23 Gospodarowicz MK, Warde P. The role of radiation therapy in the management of transitional cell carcinoma of the bladder. *Hematologic Oncologic Clinics North Am* 1992, **6**, 147–68.

24 Shipley WU, Kaufman SD, Prout GR. Jr Intraoperative radiation therapy in patients with bladder cancer. A review of techniques allowing improved tumor doses and providing high cure rates without loss of bladder function. *Cancer* 1987, **60**, 1485–8.

25 Jenkins BJ, Caulfield MJ, Fowler CG *et al.* Reappraisal of the role of radical radiotherapy and salvage cystectomy in the treatment of invasive (T2/T3) bladder cancer. *Br J Urol* 1988, **62**, 343–6.

26 Gospodarowicz MK, Hawkins NV, Rawlings GA *et al.* Radical radiotherapy for muscle invasive transitional cell carcinoma of the bladder: Failure analysis. *J Urol* 1989, **142**, 1448–54.

27 Greven KM, Solin LJ, Hanks GE. Prognostic factors in patients with bladder carcinoma treated with definitive irradiation. *Cancer* 1990, **65**, 908–12.

28 Skolyszewski J, Reinfuss M, Weiss M. Radical external beam radiotherapy of urinary bladder carcinoma: An analysis of results in 500 patients. *Acta Oncol* 1994, **33**, 561–5.

29 Pollack A, Zagars GK, Cole CJ *et al.* The relationship of local control to distant metastasis in muscle invasive bladder cancer. *J Urol* 1995, **154**, 2059–64.

30 Whillis D, Howard CGW, Kerr GR *et al.* Radical radiotherapy with salvage surgery for invasive bladder cancer: Results following a reduction in radiation dose. *J R Coll Surg Edinburgh* 1992, **37**, 42–5.

31 Abratt RP, Wilson JA, Pontin RA, Barnes RD. Salvage cystectomy after radical irradiation for bladder cancer—prognostic factors and complications. *Br J Urol* 1993, **72**, 756–60.

32 Micheletti E, Morrica B, Bonanno I, Buffoli A. Bladder cancer prognostic indices: Analysis of 286 patients treated with radical radiation therapy. *Tumori* 1988, **74**, 85–92.

33 Mameghan H, Fisher R. Invasive bladder cancer. Prognostic factors and results of radiotherapy with and without cystectomy. *Br J Urol* 1989, **63**, 251–8.

34 Davidson SE, Symonds RP, Snee MP *et al.* Assessment of factors influencing the outcome of radiotherapy for bladder cancer. *Br J Urol* 1990, **66**, 288–93.

35 Jenkins BJ, Martin JE, Baithun SI *et al.* Prediction of response to radiotherapy in invasive bladder cancer. *Br J Urol* 1990, **65**, 345–8.

36 Stuschke M, Thames HD. Hyperfractionated radiotherapy of human tumours: overview of the randomised clinical trials. *Int J Radiat Oncol Biol Phys* 1997, **37**, 259–67.

37 Edsmyr F, Andersson L, Esposti PL *et al.* Irradiation therapy with multiple small fractions per day in urinary bladder cancer. *Radiother Oncol* 1985, **4**, 197–203.

38 Goldobenko GV, Matveev BP, Shipilov VI *et al.* Radiation treatment of bladder cancer using different radiation regimes. *Med Radiol Moskow* 1991, **36**, 14–6.

39 Salminen E. Split-course radiotherapy for urinary bladder cancer. *Radiother Oncol* 1989, **15**, 327–31.

40 Rozan R, Albuisson E, Donnarieix D *et al.* Interstitial iridium-192 for bladder cancer (a multicentric survey: 205 patients). *Int J Radiat Oncol Biol Phys* 1992, **24**, 469–77.

41 Moonen LM, Horenblas S, Van der Voet JC *et al.* Bladder conservation in selected T1G3 and muscle-invasive T2–T3a bladder carcinoma using combination therapy of surgery and iridium-192 implantation. *Br J Urol* 1994, **74**, 322–7.

42 Pernot M, Hubert J, Guillemin F *et al.* Combined surgery and brachytherapy in the treatment of some cancers of the bladder (partial cystectomy and interstitial iridium-192). *Radiother Oncol* 1996, **38**, 115–20.

43 Wijnmaalen A, Helle PA, Koper PCM *et al.* Muscle invasive bladder cancer treated by transurethral resection, followed by external beam radiation and interstitial iridium-192. *Int J Radiat Oncol Biol Phys* 1998, **39**, 1043–52.

44 Calvo FA, Henriquez I, Santos M *et al.* Intraoperative and external beam radiotherapy in invasive bladder cancer: Pathological findings following cystectomy. *Am J Clin Oncol Cancer Clin Trials* 1990, **13**, 101–6.

45 Russell KJ, Laramore GE, Griffin TW *et al.* Fast neutron radiotherapy for the treatment of carcinoma of the urinary bladder. *Am J Clin Oncol Cancer Clin Trials* 1989, **12**, 301–6.

46 Kirkove C, Richard F, Van Cangh PJ *et al.* Neutron therapy of bladder cancer: can a high rate of severe complications be avoided in neutron therapy? *Eur Urol* 1993, **24**, 52–7.

47 Duncan W. An evaluation of the results of neutron therapy trials. *Acta Oncol* 1994, **33**, 299–306.

48 Warenius HM. Fast neutron therapy. The UK experience. *Acta Oncol* 1994, **33**, 289–92.

49 Tsujii H, Tsuji H, Inada T *et al.* Clinical results of fractionated proton therapy. *Int J Radiat Oncol Biol Phys* 1993, **25**, 49–60.

50 Studer UE, Gerber E, Zimmermann A *et al.* Late results in patients treated with p-mesons for bladder cancer. *Cancer* 1993, **71**, 439–47.

51 Bydder PV, Burry AF, Gowland S *et al.* A controlled trial of misonidazole in the curative treatment of infiltrating bladder cancer. *Australas Radiol* 1989, **3**, 8–14.

52 Abratt RP, Craighead P, Reddi VB, Sarembock LA. A prospective randomised trial of radiation with or without oral and intravesical misonidazole for bladder cancer. *Br J Cancer* 1991, **64**, 968–70.

53 Matsui K, Takebayashi S, Watai K *et al.* Combination radiotherapy of urinary bladder carcinoma with chemohyperthermia. *Int J Hyperthermia* 1991, **7**, 19–26.

54 Kakehi M, Ueda K, Mukojima T *et al.* Multi-institutional clinical studies on hyperthermia combined with radiotherapy or chemotherapy in advanced cancer of deep-seated organs. *Int J Hyperthermia* 1990, **6**, 719–40.

55 Parsons JT, Million RR. Planned preoperative irradiation in the management of clinical Stage B2-C (T3) bladder carcinoma. *Int J Radiat Oncol Biol Phys* 1988, **14**, 797–810.

56 Slack NH, Bross IDJ, Prout GR Jr. Five-year follow-up results of a collaborative study of therapies for carcinoma of the bladder. *J Surg Oncol* 1977, **9**, 393–405.

57 Awwad H, Abd El-Baki H, El-Bokainy N *et al.* Preoperative irradiation of T3 carcinoma in bilharzial bladder: a comparison between hyperfractionation and conventional fractionation. *Int J Radiat Oncol Biol Phys* 1979, **5**, 787–94.

58 Ghoneim MA, Ashamallah AK, Awwad HK, Whitmore WF Jr. Randomised trial of cystectomy with or without preoperative radiotherapy for carcinoma of the bilharzial bladder. *J Urol* 1985, **134**, 266–8.

59 Anderstrom C, Johansson S, Nilsson S *et al.* A prospective randomised study of preoperative irradiation with cystectomy or cystectomy alone for invasive bladder cancer. *Eur Urol* 1983, **9**, 142–7.

60 Blackard CE, Byar DP, the Veterans Administration Co-operative Urological Research Group. Results of a clinical trial of surgery and radiation in stages II and III carcinoma of the bladder. *J Urol* 1972, **108**, 875–8.

61 Bloom HJG, Hendry WF, Wallace DM, Skeet RG. Treatment of T3 bladder cancer: Controlled trial of preoperative radiotherapy and radical cystectomy versus radical radiotherapy: Second report and review (for the Clinical Trials Group, Institute of Urology). *Br J Urol* 1982, **54**, 136–51.

62 Horwich A, Law M. on behalf of the Co-operative Urological Cancer Group (CUCG). *Br J Cancer*, 1994, **70** (22), 15.

63 Cole CJ, Pollack A, Zagars GK *et al.* Local control of muscle-invasive bladder cancer: preoperative radiotherapy and cystectomy versus cystectomy alone. *Int J Radiat Oncol Biol Phys* 1995, **32**, 331–40.

64 Smith JA Jr, Crawford ED, Paradelo JC *et al.* Treatment of advanced bladder cancer with combined preoperative irradiation and radical cystectomy versus radical cystectomy alone: a phase III intergroup study. *J Urol* 1997, **157**, 805–8.

65 Smith JA Jr, Fowler JE Jr, Ghoneim MA. Summary of preoperative irradiation and cystectomy for bladder cancer. *Semin Urologic Oncol* 1997, **15**, 86–93.

66 Langemeyer TNM, Peer PGM, Janknegt PA, Leers WH. Invasive bladder cancer. Should patients who respond to radiotherapy be treated by cystectomy? *Br J Urol* 1987, **60**, 248–51.

67 Kaplan SA, Sawczuk IS, O'Toole K, Olsson CA. Contemporary cystectomy versus preoperative radiation plus cystectomy for bladder cancer. *Urology* 1988, **32**, 485–91.

68 Sell A, Jakobsen A, Nerstrm B *et al.* Treatment of advanced bladder cancer category T2, T3 and T4a. A randomized multicenter study of preoperative irradiation and cystectomy versus radical irradiation and early salvage cystectomy for residual tumor. DAVECA protocol 8201. Danish Vesical Cancer Group. *Scand J Urol Nephrol* 1991, **138** (Suppl.), 193–201.

69 Fossa SD, Ous S, Berner A. Clinical significance of the 'palpable mass' in patients with muscle-infiltrating bladder cancer undergoing cystectomy after pre-operative radiotherapy. *Br J Urol* 1991, **67**, 54–60.

70 Ono K, Akuta K, Takahashi M *et al.* Effect of misonidazole in preoperative irradiation for bladder cancer followed by total cystectomy. *Radiat Med Med Imaging Radiat Oncol* 1989, **7**, 105–9.

71 Masunaga SI, Hiraoka M, Akuta K *et al.* Phase I/II trial of preoperative thermoradiotherapy in the treatment of urinary bladder cancer. *Int J Hyperthermia* 1994, **10**, 31–40.

72 Jacobsen AB, Pettersen EO, Amellem O *et al.* The prognostic significance of deoxyribonucleic acid flow cytometry in muscle invasive bladder carcinoma treated with preoperative irradiation and cystectomy. *J Urol* 1992, **147**, 34–7.

73 Jacobsen AB, Berner A, Juul M *et al.* DNA flow cytometry and neo-adjuvant chemotherapy/radiotherapy in operable muscle-invasive bladder carcinoma. *Eur Urol* 1992, **22**, 316–22.

74 Zaghloul MS, Awwad HK, Akoush HH *et al.* Postoperative radiotherapy of carcinoma in bilharzial bladder: Improved disease free survival through improving local control. *Int J Radiat Oncol Biol Phys* 1992, **23**, 511–7.

75 Reisinger SA, Mohiuddin M, Mulholland SG. Combined pre- and postoperative adjuvant radiation therapy for bladder cancer—A ten year experience. *Int J Radiat Oncol Biol Phys* 1992, **24**, 463–8.

76 Tannock IF. Combined modality treatment with radiotherapy and chemotherapy. *Radiother Oncol* 1989, **16**, 83–101.

77 Sauer R, Dunst J, Altendorg-Hofmann A *et al.* Radiotherapy with and without cisplatin in bladder cancer. *Int J Radiat Oncol Biol Phys* 1990, **19**, 687–91.

78 Utsunomiya M, Itoh H, Yoshioka T *et al.* (1992). Preliminary results of concurrent cisplatin and radiation therapy in locally advanced bladder cancer. *Br J Urol* 1992, **70**, 399–403.

79 Dunst J, Sauer R, Schrott KM *et al.* Organ-sparing treatment of advanced bladder cancer: A 10 year experience. *Int J Radiat Oncol Biol Phys* 1994, **30**, 261–6.

80 Chauvet B, Brewer Y, Felix-Faure C *et al.* Concurrent cisplatin and radiotherapy for patients with muscle invasive bladder cancer who are not candidates for radical cystectomy. *J Urol* 1996, **156**, 1258–62.

81 Coppin CML, Gospodarowicz MK, James K *et al.* Improved local control of invasive bladder cancer by concurrent cisplatin and preoperative or definitive radiation. *J Clin Oncol* 1996, **14**, 2901–7.

82 Rotman M, Macchia R, Silverstein M. Treatment of advanced bladder carcinoma with irradiation and concomitant 5-fluorouracil infusion. *Cancer* 1987, **59**, 710–14.

83 Russell KJ, Boileau MA, Higano C *et al.* Combined 5-fluorouracil and irradiation for transitional cell carcinoma of the urinary bladder. *Int J Radiat Oncol Biol Phys* 1990, **19**, 693–9.

84 Kragelj B, Jereb B, Kragelj L, Stanonik M. Concurrent vinblastine and radiation therapy in bladder cancer. *Cancer* 1992, **70**, 2885–90.

85 Stewart DJ, Eapen L, Hirte WE *et al.* Intra-arterial cisplatin for bladder cancer. *J Urol* 1987, **138**, 302–5.

86 Eapen L, Stewart D, Danjoux C *et al.* Intraarterial cisplatin and concurrent radiation for locally advanced bladder cancer. *J Clin Oncol* 1989, **7**, 230–5.

87 Kanoh S, Noguchi R, Ohtani M *et al.* Intra-arterial chemotherapy for bladder cancer. *Cancer Chemother Pharmacol* 1987, **20**, S6–9.

88 Sumiyoshi Y, Yokota K, Akiyama M *et al.* Neoadjuvant intra-arterial doxorubicin chemotherapy in combination with low dose radiotherapy for the treatment of locally advanced transitional cell carcinoma of the bladder. *J Urol* 1994, **152**, 362–6.

89 Hug EB, Donnelly SM, Shipley WU *et al.* Deoxyribonucleic acid flow cytometry in invasive bladder carcinoma: A possible predictor for successful bladder preservation following transurethral surgery and chemotherapy-radiotherapy. *J Urol* 1992, **148**, 47–51.

90 Wallace DMA, Raghavan D, Kelly KA *et al.* Neo-adjuvant (pre-emptive) cisplatin therapy in invasive transitional cell carcinoma of the bladder. *Br J Urol* 1991, **67**, 608–15.

91 Ghersi D, Stewart LA, Parmar MKB *et al.* Does neoadjuvant cisplatin-based chemotherapy improve the survival of patients with locally advanced bladder cancer; A meta-analysis of individual patient data from randomised clinical trials. *Br J Urol* 1995, **75**, 206–13.

92 Hall RR. Neoadjuvant CMV chemotherapy and cystectomy or radiotherapy in muscle invasive bladder cancer. First analysis of MRC/EORTC intercontinental trial. *Proceedings of the American Society of Clinical Oncology* 1996, 15, abstract 612.

93 Okajima E, Ozono S, Fujimoto K *et al.* (1992). Neoadjuvant chemoradiotherapy for locally invasive bladder cancer: Nara Urooncology Research Group prospective randomized study *Ann Oncol* 1992, 3 (5), 110–3.

94 Douglas RM, Kaufman DS, Zietman AL *et al.* Conservative surgery, patient selection and chemoradiation as organ-preserving treatment for muscle-invading bladder cancer. *Semin Oncol* 1996, **23**, 614–20.

95 Prout GR Jr, Shipley WU, Kaufman DS *et al.* Preliminary results in invasive bladder cancer with transurethral resection, neoadjuvant chemotherapy and combined pelvic irradiation plus cisplatin chemotherapy. *J Urol* 1990, **144**, 1128–34.

96 Tester W, Caplan R, Heaney J *et al.* Neoadjuvant combined modality program with selective organ preservation for invasive bladder cancer: Results of Radiation Therapy Oncology Group phase II trial 8802. *J Clin Oncol* 1996, **14**, 119–26.

97 Einstein AB Jr, Wolf M, Halliday KR *et al.* Combination transurethral resection, systemic chemotherapy and pelvic radiotherapy for invasive (T2–T4) bladder cancer unsuitable for cystectomy: A phase I/II Southwestern Oncology Group study. *Urology* 1996, **47**, 652–7.

98 Kachnic LA, Kaufman DS, Heney NM *et al.* Bladder preservation by combined modality therapy for invasive bladder cancer. *J Clin Oncol* 1997, **15**, 1022–9.

99 Given RW, Parsons JT, McCarley D, Wajsman Z. Bladder-sparing multi-modality treatment of muscle-invasive bladder cancer: a 5 year follow-up. *Urology* 1995, **46**, 499–505.

100 Orsatti M, Curotto A, Canobbio L *et al.* Alternating chemoradio-therapy in bladder cancer: A conservative approach. *Int J Radiat Oncol Biol Phys* 1995, **33**, 173–8.

101 Raghavan D, Grundy R, Greenaway TM *et al.* Pre-emptive (neo-adjuvant) chemotherapy prior to radical radiotherapy for fit septuagenarians with bladder cancer: Age itself is not a contra-indication. *Br J Urol* 1988, **62**, 154–9.

102 Heimdal K, Fossa SD. Urologic cancer in elderly patients. *Curr Opin Oncol* 1993, **5**, 568–73.

103 Wijkstrom H, Naslund I, Ekman P *et al.* (1991). Short-term radiotherapy as palliative treatment in patients with transitional cell bladder cancer. *Br J Urol* 1991, **67**, 74–8.

104 Salminen E. Unconventional fractionation for palliative radiotherapy of urinary bladder cancer. A retrospective review of 94 patients. *Acta Oncol* 1992, **31**, 449–54.

105 Price A, Jose CC, Norman A *et al.* (1994). Hypofractionated radiotherapy for patients with bladder cancer. *Br J Cancer* 1994, **70** (22), 15–17.

106 Rostom AY, Tahir S, Gershuny AR *et al.* Once weekly irradiation for carcinoma of the bladder. *Int J Radiat Oncol Biol Phys* 1996, **35**, 289–92.

107 Spanos W Jr, Guse C, Perez C *et al.* Phase II study of multiple daily fractionations in the palliation of advanced pelvic malignancies: Preliminary report of RTOG 8502. *Int J Radiat Oncol Biol Phys* 1989, **17**, 659–61.

108 Vrouvas J, Dodwell D, Ash D, Probst H. Split course radiotherapy for bladder cancer in elderly unfit patients. *Clin Oncol* 1995, **7**, 193–5.

109 Phillips HA, Howard GCW. Split course radical radiotherapy for bladder cancer in the elderly: Nonsense or commonsense? A report of 76 patients. *Clin Oncol* 1996, **8**, 35–8.

110 Srinivasan V, Brown CH, Turner AG. A comparison of two radiotherapy regimens for the treatment of symptoms from advanced bladder cancer. *Clin Oncol* 1994, **6**, 11–13.

16. Systemic chemotherapy of muscle-invasive bladder cancer

Cora N. Sternberg, Fabio Calabró, Luca Marini, and Paola Scavina

Introduction

Bladder cancer is the fifth most common cancer in men and the seventh in women, with 52 900 cases in the United States in 1996 and 11 700 deaths (1,2). The male to female occurrence is 3 : 1. It is, primarily a disease of the elderly, with 80% of cases in the 50–79 year age group, and a peak incidence in the seventh decade.

The majority of patients are diagnosed at an early, treatable stage. At initial presentation 75% of bladder tumours are superficial, limited to the mucosa, submucosa, or lamina propria. Recurrence after initial treatment for superficial tumours is discovered in 50–80% of patients. Progression to muscle-invasive disease occurs in 10–25%. For patients with muscle-invasive bladder cancers, there is a 50% risk of distant metastases. It is important to identify those tumours that are biologically aggressive and that have the potential to result in mortality. For patients with metastatic disease progress continues to be made with the development of new chemotherapeutic regimens.

Metastatic disease

With the advent of cisplatin-based combination chemotherapy regimens, long-term survival may be attainable in selected patients with metastatic or advanced transitional cell carcinoma (TCC). Response rates to single agent chemotherapy are detailed in Table 16.1. Antitumour activity has been demonstrated with several single agents, with only rare improvements in survival (3).

The most active regimens for advanced TCC may lead to a survival benefit for those patients who attain complete remission (CR) (4,5). These include M-VAC (methotrexate, vinblastine, adriamycin, cisplatin), CMV (cisplatin, methotrexate, vinblastine), CM (cisplatin, methotrexate), and CISCA/CAP (cyclophosphamide, adriamycin, cisplatin).

At Memorial Hospital, New York, USA, 121 patients with measurable disease were treated with M-VAC. One hundred had

Table 16.1

RESPONSE TO SINGLE AGENTS IN ADVANCED UROTHELIAL CANCER			
Single agent chemotherapy	n	CR + PR%	95% Confidence limits
Methotrexate	236	29	23–35
Cisplatin	578	30	26–34
Adriamycin	269	19	14–24
Vinblastine	42	14	3–25
Cyclophosphamide	26	8	0–10
Ifosfamide	47	21	9–33
Epirubicin	33	15	3–27
Carboplatin	174	13	8–18
Piritrexim	29	38	20–56
Trimetrexate	51	17	7–30
Mitomycin C	42	13	3–23
5-Fluorouracil	75	35	24–46
Gemcitabine	120	28	20–36
Gallium nitrate	66	17	8–26
Taxol	26	42	23–63
Lobaplatin	22	12	0–30
Topotecan	46	10	3–23

CR = Complete response, PR = Partial response
* Phase I study only.

metastatic (M+), and 21 advanced nodal (N+) disease. The overall response rate was 72% (95% confidence limits 64–80%). CR was achieved in 36% of whom 14% were clinically proven, 12% were proven pathologically at surgery, and 11% required further surgery to attain CR. The partial response (PR) rate was 36%; 6% had a minor response (MR), and 25% had progression (PROG). Median survival for patients who achieved CR was 41 months. Two-year survival was 68% for patients with CR versus 5% in those who failed to attain CR. In patients who underwent surgical resection of the remaining residual disease, survival was 25 months. In this group survival was 2.5 times longer than in the PR group (6).

The most responsive tumours were of renal pelvis, and ureteral origin with CR in 50–54%. Urethral tumours were less responsive with CR in 13%. The most responsive metastatic sites were abdominal nodes and pelvic masses with CR in 35%, bone with CR in 26%, and lung with CR in 24%. While 69% of hepatic and 90% of subcutaneous masses and lymph nodes regressed, only 15% and 20%, respectively, were CR.

In more than one study, chemotherapy has shown to be more effective against nodal disease than visceral metastases (4,7). Responses are 71% versus 40%, respectively (4) and survival (33 months versus 12 months) (7). The central nervous system remains a sanctuary site. Durable responses are rarely seen in the liver. Select patients with urothelial tumours and loco-regional metastases may benefit from consolidation therapy with surgery or radiation therapy (RT) after maximum response to chemotherapy (8,9), although this has not been evaluated in a prospective randomized study.

The Southeastern Cancer Study Group studied M-VAC versus single agent cisplatin (DDP). In 239 evaluable patients, 11% treated with DDP responded compared with 36% treated with M-VAC. Eighteen (15%) patients achieved CR with M-VAC. Median survival for M-VAC treated patients was 13.5 months (similar to the Memorial data) compared with 8.2 months in patients given DDP ($P = 0.04$) (10).

The question of M-VAC superiority versus CISCA was evaluated at MD Anderson (Texas, USA). M-VAC was found to be superior to CISCA with survival of 82 weeks after M-VAC versus 40 weeks with CISCA. The CR + PR rate was 65% with M-VAC and 46% with CISCA ($P < 0.05$). It was rather unusual that patients with mixed histologies responded in both arms (11).

The importance of adriamycin (ADM) in M-VAC versus its absence in the CM and CMV studies, may be bypassed as growth factors have become available. In a phase I–II trial of G-CSF and M-VAC at Memorial Hospital, days of antibiotics with fever were reduced from 35 to 1. The number of days of absolute neutrophil count <1000 was reduced by 90%. There were significantly fewer days (91%) of an absolute neutrophil count less than 1000. All patients were able to receive the full dose of chemotherapy as planned and on time. Mucositis was reduced from 44% to 11% (12).

Response to cisplatin-based therapy is rapid. Elderly patients >70 years old, particularly those with compromised performance status, may be treated by reducing all doses of chemotherapy by 20–30%.

Randomized trials in advanced disease suggest that three or four drug regimens should be considered standard therapy. M-VAC and CMV have never been compared in a prospective study. In two prospective, randomized trials, M-VAC was proven superior to cisplatin alone (10) and to CISCA (11). New active regimens will include the taxanes (taxol and taxotere) and gemcitabine.

NEW DRUGS, AND COMBINATIONS IN ADVANCED DISEASE

Combination chemotherapy results in long-term survival in only 15–20% of patients. Most patients succumb to their disease.

Effective salvage regimens are therefore needed. New drugs have historically been tested in patients who have had at least one prior chemotherapeutic regimen. Owing to this tactic, few drugs have demonstrated responses above 15%. New agents must clearly be evaluated in patients with minimal disease and a good performance status.

Following first-line chemotherapy in patients with metastatic bladder carcinoma, currently available therapeutic options include: (i) escalated doses of chemotherapy with haematopoietic growth factors; (ii) novel chemotherapeutic agents, such as the taxanes, gemcitabine, gallium nitrate; (iii) fluoropyrimidine modulation; and (iv) new antifolates, such as piritrexim (3).

Haematopoietic growth factors and dose intensity

Strategies to increase CR include augmenting the dose of chemotherapy with haematological growth factor support. In a trial of escalated dose M-VAC plus GM-CSF at the MD Anderson, the dose of vinblastine and DDP were increased and the ADM dose was doubled. Thirty (40%) previously treated patients (primarily M-VAC) responded, of whom 23% achieved CR (13).

After such initial favourable reports of responses in heavily pretreated patients with escalated M-VAC and growth factors (13), other phase II trials of escalated chemotherapy were initiated. Most were abandoned due to excessive toxicity (14). The European Organisation for Research and Treatment of Cancer (EORTC) Genitourinary Group has proposed an every 2 weeks schedule of M-VAC plus growth factors. In a preliminary phase II trial, response rates were 70% (95% CI 60–80%), with a CR of 30% and a PR of 39% (15). A subsequent randomized trial is comparing this dose escalated M-VAC schedule to classic M-VAC. With the every 2 weeks schedule plus G-CSF it was possible to deliver twice the dose of DDP and ADM in half the time, with less dose delays and toxicity (16). Whether or not this approach can lead to an improvement in survival has yet to be determined.

Growth factors provide the possibility of treating patients with higher doses of chemotherapy for longer periods, with less morbidity and perhaps improved results. Escalated M-VAC is not recommended as second-line therapy in patients who have failed initial M-VAC chemotherapy, as these patients are probably resistant to such treatment.

Gemcitabine

This an analogue of cytosine arabinoside, and is a new antimetabolite that inhibits DNA synthesis. Gemcitabine is usually given weekly for 3 weeks, every 4 weeks. As a single agent response rates of 25–29% have been obtained in studies both in pretreated patients and in those who have not had prior therapy (17–20). Gemcitabine has also been combined with cisplatin (21,22).

In a joint Scandinavian, Italian, and German study, cisplatin was given weekly to patients who had no prior chemotherapy. A 40% response rate was obtained, with a median survival of 12.1 months. Significant myelosuppression, particularly thrombocytopenia resulted, most likely due to the unusual dosage schedule of cisplatin chemotherapy (21). The dosage and schedule of cisplatin have been modified to an every 3 weeks dosage in an ongoing randomized trial compared with M-VAC. Published studies with Gemcitabine can be found in Table 16.2.

Taxoids

The taxoids are a new class of antineoplastic drugs. Paclitaxel (Taxol) and Docetaxel (Taxotere) share a similar mechanism of action: the promotion of microtubule assembly and inhibition of microtubule disassembly. Taxol is the active ingredient of the bark. Taxotere was prepared from the needles of Taxus baccata. A 42% response rate (27% CR) was first seen in previously untreated patients when a relatively high dose of Taxol (250 $\mu g/m^2$) was administered with G-CSF. Tu *et al.* combined Taxol, methotrexate and DDP and reported a 40% response rate in patients who had received prior M-VAC (23).

Other investigators have combined Taxol with either cisplatin or carboplatin, plus growth factors in untreated patients, and have revealed high response rates of 50–80% (24–27). Studies of Taxol and Taxotere-containing regimens in advanced TCC are in progress. Table 16.3 reviews some of the more recent studies with Taxol (23–26,28–31).

Table 16.2

GEMCITABINE CHEMOTHERAPY IN ADVANCED TRANSITIONAL CELL CARCINOMA						
Author	Year	*n*	Prior Rx	RR	Gemzar mg/m²	DDP mg/m²
Pollera (17)	1994	15	Yes	27%	1000	
Stadler (18)	1996	38	No	29%	1200	
Lorusso (19)	1996	36	Yes	25%	1200	
Moore (20)	1996	31	No	29%	1200	
Von der Maase (21)	1997	44	No	41%	1000	35
Stadler (22)	1997	16	No in 14	75%	1000	100, 75

Table 16.3

TAXOL AND TAXOTERE CHEMOTHERAPY IN ADVANCED TRANSITIONAL CELL CARCINOMA						
Author	Year	*n*	Prior Rx	RR	Taxol mg/m^2	Therapy
McCaffrey (27)	1997	30	Yes	30%	—	Taxotere
Roth (28)	1994	26	No	42%	250 + GCSF	Taxol
Tu (23)	1995	25	Yes	40%	200 + GCSF	Taxol/methotrexate/DDP
Vaughn (24)	1997	33	No	64%	200	Taxol/carbo
Schnack (25)	1997	15	No	67%	175	Taxol/carbo AUC 5
Redman (26)	1997	19	No	53%	200	Taxol/carbo AUC 5
Roth (29)	1997	24	Yes	25%	135 + GCSF	Taxol/IFO
McCaffrey	1997	24	No	83%	200 + GCSF	Taxol/IFO/DDP

DDP, cisplatin
IFO, ifosfamide
AUC, area under the curve
GCSF, granulocyte colony stimulating factor

Table 16.4

ONGOING COMBINATION TRIALS IN TCC OF THE BLADDER			
Investigator	Institution	Protocol	Eligibility
Sternberg	San Raffaele	gemcitabine, taxol	refractory TCC
Murphy	Vanderbilt Univ.	gemcitabine, taxol	advanced TCC, refractory TCC
Meluch	Sarah Cannon	gemcitabine, taxol	advanced TCC
Redman	Wayne State	gemcitabine, taxol	advanced TCC
Wilding	Univ. of Wisconsin	gemcitabine, taxol, piritrexim	bladder or breast cancer
Gitlitz	UCLA	gemcitabine, taxotere	advanced TCC
Glode	Univ. of Colorado	CI gemcitabine	HRPC, bladder, kidney cancer
Baselga	Barcelona	gemcitabine, taxol, DDP	Phase I advanced TCC
Logan	Univ. of Pittsburg	gemcitabine, carboplatin	bladder cancer
Pagliaro	Univ. of Texas	DDP, gemcitabine, ifosfamide	refractory TCC
Smith	Univ. of Michigan	gemcitabine, RT	bladder preservation
Bajorin	MSKCC	gemcitabine, taxol, DDP, ADM	adjuvant in locally advanced
Ebbinghaus	Univ. of Alabama	gemcitabine, taxol	advanced TCC
Edelman	Univ. of California	gemcitabine, taxol, MTX	locally advanced, metastatic TCC
Petrylak	Columbia Univ.	gemcitabine, taxotere, carboplatin	TCC
Poo	Yale	gemcitabine, DDP, MTX	advanced TCC

TCC, transitional, cell carcinoma; MTX, methotrexate
DDP, cisplatin
RT, radiotherapy
ADM, adriamycin

Much interest has been generated by these new active agents. In Tables 16.4 and 16.5 some of the ongoing, unpublished, combination trials with gemcitabine and taxol or taxotere are reviewed.

Table 16.5

RANDOMIZED TRIALS OF NEO-ADJUVANT CHEMOTHERAPY				
Study group	Investigational arm	Standard arm	Patients	Results
EORTC/MRC	CMV/RT or Cyst.	RT or Cyst.	976	No difference
USA Intergroup	MVAC/Cyst.	Cyst.	266 (298)	Ongoing
Nordic	ADM/DDP/RT/Cyst.	RT/Cyst. in T3–T4a	311	15% surv difference
Australia/UK	DDP/RT	RT	255	No difference
Canada (NCI)	DDP/RT or preoperative RT+Cyst.	RT or preoperative RT+Cyst.	99	No difference
Spain (Cueto)	DDP/Cyst.	Cyst.	121	No difference
Italy (GISTV)	MVAC/Cyst.	Cyst.	171 (240)	No difference
Italy (Genoa)	DDP/5-fluorocil/RT/Cyst.	Cyst.	104	No difference
Nordic 2	Methotrexate/DDP/Cyst.	Cyst.		Ongoing

RT, radiotherapy
Cyst, cystectomy
MVAC, methotrexate, vinblastine, adriamycin, cisplatin
ADM, adriamycin
DDP, cisplatin
CMV, cisplatin, methotrexate, vinblastine.

Fluoropyrimidine modulation

Modulation of 5-fluorouracil (5-FU) by interferon-α was evaluated in 30 previously untreated patients, with a 30% response rate. When cisplatin was then added to create the FAP regimen, 17 of 28 heavily pretreated M-VAC patients responded. The 61% response rate was impressive for this population (32). An EORTC Genitourinary Group trial is in progress to confirm these results.

Gallium nitrate

This is a heavy metal like cisplatin. A 31% response was found in patients who had failed prior DDP therapy (33). Nephrotoxicity was dose limiting, due to the intravenous bolus schedule. With a 5-day continuous infusion schedule in patients who had prior M-VAC, partial responses were observed in four of 23 patients (17%) who received more than 350 mg/m^2 per day (34). When gallium was combined with 5-FU in a pilot study, responses were seen in seven of 14 (50%) previously treated patients. However, when gallium and 5-FU were randomized against M-VAC, the response rate was disappointingly low 12% versus 94% respectively (27).

VIG (vinblastine, ifosfamide, and gallium) is another gallium-containing regimen. This regimen combines ifosfamide, which had a 20% response rate in previously treated patients with G-CSF, given every 21 days (35). Eighteen of 27 (67%) patients, who had no prior chemotherapy, responded to the VIG regimen. This included eight PR and five CR with chemotherapy alone and five CR rendered disease-free with chemotherapy and surgery. Median duration of response was 20 weeks. Toxicities were significant, and included myelosuppression, renal dysfunction, neurological toxicity, and a case of temporary blindness (36). Owing to these toxicities and the availability of newer equally effective, less toxic agents, gallium is rarely used. Another VIG study was evaluated in non-pretreated patients. Responses were observed in 17 of 27 patients (63%) (37).

Antifolates

Newer antifolates such as trimetrexate and piritrexim have been evaluated. Piritrexim is a lipid-soluble inhibitor of dihydrofolate reductase (DHFR). Bioavailability after an oral dose is 60–75%. The drug is easily administered in a 5-day low-dose oral schedule. In a phase II trial in 29 unpretreated patients, a 38% response was attained (38). The combination of piritrexim and cisplatin will be of interest. trimetrexate is effective in methotrexate-resistant cell lines. Trimetrexate has been evaluated in 31 patients who had prior treatment with MTX; 28 of whom had had M-VAC. The response rate was 15% (39).

NEO-ADJUVANT CHEMOTHERAPY

Following cystectomy for muscle invasive bladder carcinoma, up to 50% of patients may develop metastases, often within 2 years (3). Most patients have distant relapses. Only one-third reoccur in the pelvis alone. The responses in advanced disease have led investigators to an integrated strategy of chemotherapy and surgery or RT in locally invasive bladder cancer.

Neo-adjuvant chemotherapy is delivered prior to cystectomy, or definitive RT. This method has been used in the treatment of several solid tumours. Neo-adjuvant chemotherapy was conceived in order to tackle micrometastatic disease, present at diagnosis in patients with T2–T4a bladder tumours. This approach provides useful prognostic information concerning response to chemotherapy. The bladder tumour serves as an *in vivo* marker to evaluate response to chemotherapy. This may permit continuation of treatment to maximal response, or discontinuation of ineffective therapy. Response of micrometastases presumably reflects response in the primary tumour. The optimal time to treat micrometastases is when tumour volume is minimal.

The use of chemotherapy prior to RT may enable better delivery of drugs than is possible after RT, which may damage the vascular bed. In selected cases the bladder may be preserved with or without RT. Surgery may become possible after an inoperable tumour responds to chemotherapy. Partial cystectomy rather than radical cystectomy may be indicated in selected patients (40).

Toxicity after neo-adjuvant chemotherapy has been lower than toxicity in patients with metastatic disease. Patients generally have operable disease and a better performance status. The major disadvantage is in those patients who do not respond to neo-adjuvant chemotherapy, as definitive local therapy is delayed.

The overall response rate in single arm, non-randomized pilot studies to neo-adjuvant chemotherapy is between 60 and 70%, with CR rates of 30% (40). Neo-adjuvant chemotherapy can produce tumour 'downstaging', which does not necessarily implicate a survival advantage.

Table 16.5 illustrates the randomized trials of neo-adjuvant chemotherapy in the literature, and several that are in progress (41–48; Fossa SD, personal communication, 1993). Randomized studies do not reveal an important survival difference in patients treated with neo-adjuvant chemotherapy.

The Nordic cystectomy trial evaluated ADM and DDP plus RT prior to cystectomy. This trial found a 20% difference in cancer-specific survival and a 15% difference in overall survival for patients with T3a–T4 disease (43). Most of the other trials have not enrolled the large numbers of patients that may be required to detect a survival difference.

The Medical Research Council/EORTC randomized trial compared neo-adjuvant CMV versus no chemotherapy, followed by either radical cystectomy or RT. In this study, 976 patients were enrolled in order to detect a 10% survival difference (41). At a median follow-up of 29 months, no difference in overall survival was observed. Survival was 63% for CMV versus 60% for patients who did not receive chemotherapy. Relapse-free survival was somewhat better in CMV-treated patients, 58% versus 50%. Relapsing patients in the observation arm were usually given chemotherapy. The United States Intergroup and the Guone Group in Italy are comparing M-VAC plus cystectomy versus cystectomy alone.

Even if neo-adjuvant chemotherapy does not lead to a significant survival difference, patients who respond to chemotherapy have a better prognosis. At eight institutions where patients were treated with neo-adjuvant chemotherapy and radical or partial cystectomy, 5-year survival was 75% for patients who had downstaging of the primary tumour to superficial disease or pT0 versus only 20% in those who had residual muscle-infiltrating disease

(>pT2) (49). The most significant prognostic factor for survival is attainment of P0 status (50). Response to chemotherapy is a prognostic factor of extreme importance.

NEO-ADJUVANT CHEMOTHERAPY AND BLADDER PRESERVATION

Bladder preservation is a controversial topic, and is not considered to be standard therapy. Bladder preservation may be accomplished by an integrated approach of neo-adjuvant chemotherapy and conservative surgery or RT (51). For patients who attain a CR to neo-adjuvant chemotherapy, it is often difficult to accept radical surgery. Despite the increased availability of ileal neo-bladders and continent reservoirs, it is better to preserve the bladder. Neo-bladders cannot be constructed in many patients undergoing cystectomy. Sexual function is usually absent following this procedure. Nocturnal incontinence can be debilitating after surgery. If patients can avoid cystectomy, with equivalent survival results by a conservative procedure, quality of life may be improved. The main goal of bladder cancer treatment, however, is patient survival.

Partial cystectomy

Candidates for partial cystectomy after neo-adjuvant chemotherapy include those who have: (i) attained a clinical CR (cCR) or significant clinical partial response (cPR) to neo-adjuvant chemotherapy; (ii) solitary lesions in favourable anatomical locations; (iii) no history of previous or recurrent infiltrative bladder cancer; (iv) no CIS; and (v) good bladder capacity. Several investigators have shown that partial cystectomy can be performed in patients with initial monofocal lesions who respond to neo-adjuvant chemotherapy at restaging transurethral resection of the bladder (TURB) (51,52). Appropriate patients are those with small T3 tumours. Such an approach appears to offer local control equivalent to that attained by radical cystectomy. Neo-adjuvant chemotherapy and partial cystectomy requires longer follow-up prior to any definitive statements regarding its efficacy.

Transurethral resection of the bladder alone

Pilot studies indicate that selected patients with muscle-invasive bladder cancer can be cured by the combination of a thorough TURB and systemic chemotherapy, without cystectomy or RT (51,53,56). In Rome, patients are selected for bladder preservation if they have a CR or downstaging to superficial disease after neo-adjuvant M-VAC. Of 41 patients who underwent chemotherapy and TURB alone, 5-year survival was 71% (54,55).

Bladder preservation remains a controversial topic, as radical cystectomy must still be considered the gold standard in muscle-invasive bladder cancer. Bladder sparing in patients selected on the basis of response to chemotherapy is a feasible approach, which will need confirmation in prospective randomized trials.

Radiation

RT is the method of bladder preservation in some countries in Europe and in Canada. Most recent series have employed a dose of 6500 cGy at daily doses of 180–200 cGy to the tumour region, with a restricted dose of 4750–5500 cGy dose to the whole bladder and perivesical region. If treatment is delivered with fractions less than 200 cGy, toxicity is reduced (57).

Up to 40–50% of patients achieve CR with RT, with approximately a 30% cure rate with normal bladder function (58–60). In an update from the Massachusetts General Hospital in Boston, 106 patients with T2–T4a bladder tumours were treated with MCV chemotherapy followed by 39.6 Gy pelvic irradiation and concomitant DDP. Responding patients received further 64.8 Gy. Cystectomy was performed on those who did not obtain T0. Five-year survival was 52%; 43% retained an intact bladder (61). Table 16.6 details results of recent multimodality chemoradiotherapy trials. Five-year survival ranges from 42% to 63%, with organ preservation in 40% (61–66). Toxicities which may be associated with RT include: decreased bladder function, cystitis, haematuria, and adhesions. Prognostic factors for local curability are absence of ureteral obstruction, papillary histology, and visibly, complete tumour resection by TURB prior to RT.

Table 16.6

NON-RANDOMIZED TRIALS OF COMBINED CHEMOTHERAPY AND RADIOTHERAPY

Series	Year	n	Chemo	5-year survival	5-year survival with intact bladder
Radiation Therapy Oncology Group-1	1993	42	DDP	52%	42%
University of Erlangen	1994	139	DDP, or Carbo	52%	41%
Genoa	1995	76	DDP/5FU	42%	
Radiation Therapy Oncology Group-2	1996	91	MCV	62%*	44%
Massachusetts General	1997	106	MCV	52%	43%
University of Paris	1997	120	DDP/5FU	63%	

DDP, cisplatin
MCV, methotrexate, cisplatin, vinblastine
* Four-year survival data. DDP, ?; 5FU, 5-Fluorouracil; MCV, ?.

Bladder preservation is possible with a combined multimodal approach using chemotherapy and RT (59). Attempts at bladder preservation should also evaluate the toxicity of these combined modalities. The true success of bladder-preserving treatment by chemotherapy and RT will clearly require validation in prospective randomized trials.

ADJUVANT CHEMOTHERAPY

Adjuvant chemotherapy follows cystectomy in patients at high risk for relapse. This approach has led to increases in survival in patients with several solid tumours. The principal advantage is that the cystectomy specimen is available for pathological evaluation. Prognostic factors for relapse and/or metastases can be evaluated. Patients who may derive the most benefit can be selected for chemotherapy. As cystectomy is performed early, no delay in definitive treatment results. Non-compliance, which may occur when a cCR has been achieved with chemotherapy, is avoided (40).

The major disadvantage to adjuvant chemotherapy is the delay in giving systemic therapy for occult metastases while treatment for the primary tumour is emphasized. An additional disadvantage is that it is very difficult to administer chemotherapy after cystectomy in elderly, debilitated patients.

Table 16.7 reviews adjuvant chemotherapy trials in the literature (67–73). In a non-randomized trial, Logothetis *et al.* selected patients at high risk for recurrence based on vascular or lymphatic invasion, nodal metastases, extravesical tumour, or resectable extension into the pelvis viscera. Adjuvant chemotherapy benefited patients with resected nodal metastases and extravesical

Table 16.7

RANDOMIZED AND NON-RANDOMIZED TRIALS OF ADJUVANT CHEMOTHERAPY AFTER CYSTECTOMY					
Investigator	Year	Chemotherapy	Chemotherapy	No Chemotherapy	Results
Einstein (67)	1984	DDP			No benefit, single agent DDP, few patients received therapy
Logothetis (68)	1988	CISCA	62	71	Benefit, but *not* a randomized trial
Skinner (69)	1991	CAP	47	44	Benefit, but few patients received therapy
Studer (70)	1994	DDP	40	37	No benefit, single agent DDP inadequate
Stockle (75)	1995	M-VAC/M-VEC M-VEC	23	26	Benefit, small patient numbers, premature closure, no therapy at relapse
Bono (72)	1996	CM	48	35	No benefit for N0M0
Freiha (73)	1996	CMV	25	25	Benefit in relapse-free survival

tumours. No advantage was seen for patients with only vascular invasion (68).

In a landmark randomized trial, Skinner found an increase in time to progression and in survival in patients treated with adjuvant CISCA. The most important prognostic factor was the extent of lymph node involvement at cystectomy (69). This trial has been heavily criticized for failure to treat patients consistently, subset analyses, and statistical methodology.

A German study with MVAC or MVEC confirmed Skinner's results. The study was prematurely closed after an interim analysis revealed a benefit for patients randomized to chemotherapy. The progression rate was 27% for treated patients versus 82% for untreated controls. Patients in the observation arm were not offered chemotherapy at relapse (71). In an update, 5-year progression-free survival was 59% after randomization to the chemotherapy arm versus 13% after cystectomy alone (74).

Randomized adjuvant chemotherapy trials suggest that there may be a benefit for selected patients who receive adjuvant chemotherapy (69,75). Studies have not clearly proven an advantage based upon muscle infiltration alone (pT2, pT3a). For patients with minimal extravesical extension (pT3b), additional therapy may be beneficial. For patients with nodal metastases (pN+) and pT4 disease, there appears to be an advantage to adjuvant chemotherapy (40).

CONCLUSIONS

Combination cisplatin-based chemotherapy has shown to be efficacious, and to prolong survival in patients who attain CR. Chemotherapy alone or combined with RT and TURB may make less aggressive surgery and bladder preservation possible in selected patients. Improvements in perioperative care, coupled with surgical, radiotherapeutic, and diagnostic achievements continue to improve results and quality of life. Haematopoietic growth factors are more widely incorporated into our therapeutic strategies. Several new active chemotherapeutic agents, particularly gemcitabine and the taxanes, show promise in the treatment of transitional cell carcinoma.

Key Points/points of controversy

1. Combination chemotherapy results in long-term survival in only 15–20% of patients. Few drugs, in previously treated patients have demonstrated responses above 15%. New agents must be evaluated in patients with minimal disease and a good performance status.
2. Should neo-adjuvant chemotherapy be given prior to cystectomy?
3. Bladder preservation is a controversial topic, and is not considered standard therapy. Bladder preservation may be accomplished by an integrated approach of neo-adjuvant chemotherapy and conservative surgery or RT.
4. Adjuvant chemotherapy may benefit selected patients. Studies have not clearly proven an advantage based in pT2 or pT3a. For pT3b, adjuvant chemotherapy may be beneficial. For pN+ and pT4 disease, there is an advantage to adjuvant chemotherapy.

References

1 Trichopoulos D, Li FP, Hunter DJ. What causes cancer? *Sci Am* 1996, **275** (3), 50–7.
2 Fact sheet. Twelve major cancers. *Sci Am* 1996, **275** (3), 92–8.
3 Sternberg CN. The treatment of advanced bladder cancer. *Ann Oncol* 1995, **6** (2), 113–26.

4 Logothetis CJ, Samuels ML, Ogden S *et al.* Cyclophosphamide, doxorubicin and cisplatin chemotherapy for patients with locally advanced urothelial tumors with or without nodal metastases. *J Urol* 1985, **134**, 460–4.

5 Stoter G, Splinter TA, Child JA *et al.* Combination chemotherapy with cisplatin and methotrexate in advanced transitional cell cancer of the bladder. *J Urol* 1987, **137**, 663–7.

6 Sternberg C, Yagoda A, Scher HI *et al.* Methotrexate, Vinblastine, Doxorubicin and Cisplatinum for advanced transitional cell carcinoma of the urothelium: efficacy and patterns of response and relapse. *Cancer* 1989, **64**, 2448–58.

7 Sternberg CN, Yagoda A, Scher HI *et al.* M-VAC (methotrexate, vinblastine, doxorubicin and cisplatin) for advanced transitional cell carcinoma of the bladder. *J Urol* 1988, **139**, 461–9.

8 Dimopoulos C, Finn L, Logothetis CJ. Pattern of failure and survival of patients with metastatic urothelial tumors relapsing after cisplatin based chemotherapy. *J Urol* 1994, **151**, 598–601.

9 Miller RS, Freiha FS, Reese JH *et al.* Cisplatin, methotrexate, and vinblastine plus surgical restaging for patients with advanced transitional cell carcinoma of the urothelium. *J Urol* 1993, **150**, 65–9.

10 Loehrer P, Einhorn LH, Elson PJ *et al.* A randomized comparison of cisplatin alone or in combination with methotrexate, vinblastine, and doxorubicin in patients with metastatic urothelial carcinoma: a Cooperative Group Study. *J Clin Oncol* 1992, **10**, 1066–73.

11 Logothetis CJ, Dexeus F, Finn L *et al.* A prospective randomized trial comparing CISCA to MVAC chemotherapy in advanced metastastic urothelial tumors. *J Clin Oncol* 1990, **8**, 1050–5.

12 Gabrilove JL, Jakubowski A, Scher H *et al.* Effect of granulocyte colony-stimulating factor on neutropenia and associated morbidity due to chemotherapy for transitional-cell carcinoma of the urothelium. *N Engl J Med* 1988, **318**, 1414–22.

13 Logothetis CJ, Dexeus FH, Sella A *et al.* Escalated therapy for refractory urothelial tumors: methotrexate-vinblastine-doxorubicin-cisplatin plus unglycosylated recombinant human granulocyte-macrophage colony-stimulating factor. *J Natl Cancer Inst* 1990, **82**, 667–72.

14 Sternberg CN. Human granulocyte macrophage colony stimulating growth factor (GM-CSF) in patients with advanced urothelial tract tumors. In: *Manual of GM-CSF* (ed. Marty M). Blackwell Science, Oxford, 1996, pp. 96–106.

15 Sternberg C, de Mulder P, Van Oosterom A, Fossa S, Giannarelli D, Soedirman J. Escalated M-VAC. chemotherapy and recombinant human granulocyte macrophage colony stimulating factor (GM-CSF) in patients with advanced urothelial tract tumors. *Ann Oncol* 1993, **4**, 403–7.

16 Sternberg CN, De Mulder P, Fossa S *et al.* for the Genito-Urinary Tract Cancer Cooperative Group of the EORTC. Interim toxicity analysis of a randomized trial in advanced urothelial tract tumors of high dose intensity MVAC chemotherapy (HD-MVAC) and recombinant human granulocyte colony stimulating factor (G-CSF) versus classic MVAC chemotherapy (EORTC 30924). *Proc Am Soc Clin Oncol* 1997, **16**, 320a (Abstract 1140).

17 Pollera CF, Ceribelli A, Crecco M, Calabresi F. Weekly gemcitabine in advanced bladder cancer: a preliminary report from a phase I study. *Ann Oncol* 1994, **5**, 182–4.

18 Stadler WM, Kuzel TM, Raghavan D *et al.* A phase II study of gemcitabine (gem) in bladder cancer (BC). *Ann Oncol* 1996, 7 (5), 58 (abstract 272P).

19 Lorusso V, Amadori D, Antimi M *et al.* Studio di fase II sulla gemcitabine nel carcinoma vescicale. *Abstract Book Soc Ital Urol Oncol* 1996, 17–18.

20 Moore MJ, Tannock I, Ernst S *et al.* Gemcitabine demonstrates promising activity as a single agent in the treatment of metastatic transitional cell carcinoma. *Proc Am Soc Clin Oncol* 1996, 15 (Abstract, **637**), 250.

21 Von der Maase H, Andersen L, Crino L *et al.* A phase II study of gemcitabine and cisplatin in patients with transitional cell carcinoma (TCC) of the urothelium. *Proc Am Soc Clin Oncol* 1997, **16**, 324a (Abstract 1155).

22 Stadler WM, Raghavan D, Voi M. Phase II, trial of gemcitabine (GEM) plus cisplatin (CDDP) metastatic urothelial cancer. *Proc Am Soc Clin Oncol* 1997, **16**, 323a (abstract 1152).

23 Tu SM, Hossa E, Amato R *et al.* Paclitaxel, cisplatin and methotrexate combination chemotherapy is active in treatment of refractory urothelial malignancies. *J Urol* 1995, **154**, 1719–22.

24 Vaughn DJ, Malkowicz SB, Zoltick BH *et al*. Paclitaxel plus carboplatin in advanced carcinoma of the urothelium: an active outpatient regimen. *J Urol* 1997, **157** (4), 376 (Abstract 1471).

25 Schnack B, Grbovic M, Brodowicz T *et al*. High effectivity of a combination of Taxol with carboplatin in the treatment of metastatic urothelial cancer. *Proc Am Soc Clin Oncol* 1997, **16**, 325a (Abstract 1160).

26 Redman B, Hussain M, Smith D *et al*. Phase II evaluation of paclitaxel and carboplatin in advanced urothelial cancer. *Proc Am Soc Clin Oncol* 1997, **16**, 325a (Abstract 1157).

27 McCaffrey JA, Hilton S, Mazumdar M *et al*. Phase II randomized trial of gallium nitrate plus fluorouracil versus methotrexate, vinblastine, doxorubicin, and cisplatin in patients with advanced transitional cell carcinoma. *J Clin Oncol* 1997, **15** (6), 2449–55.

28 Roth BJ, Dreicer R, Einhorn LH *et al*. Significant activity of paclitaxel in advanced transitional cell carcinoma of the urothelium: A phase II trial of the Eastern Cooperative Oncology Group. *J Clin Oncol* 1994, **12** (11), 2264–70.

29 Roth BJ, Finch DE, Birhle R *et al*. A phase II trial of ifosfamide + paclitaxel (IT) in advanced transitional cell carcinoma of the urothelium. *Proc Am Soc Clin Oncol* 1997, **16**, 324a (Abstract 1156).

30 McCaffrey JA, Hilton S, Mazumdar M *et al*. Phase II trial of docetaxel in patients with advanced or metastatic transitional cell carcinoma. *J Clin Oncol* 1997, **15** (5), 1853–7.

31 McCaffrey JA, Hilton S, Mazumdar M *et al*. A phase II trial of ifosfamide, paclitaxel and cisplatin (ITP) in patients (pts) with transitional cell carcinoma (TCC). *Proc Am Soc Clin Oncol* 1997, **16**, 324a (Abstract 1154).

32 Logothetis C, Dieringer P, Ellerhorst J *et al*. A 61% response rate with 5-fluorouracil, interferon-a 2b and cisplatin in metastatic chemotherapy refractory transitional cell carcinoma. *Proc Am Assoc Cancer Res* 1992, **33**, 221 (abstract).

33 Crawford ED, Saiers JH, Baker LH. Gallium nitrate in advanced bladder cancer: A Southwest Oncology Group study. *Urology* 1991, **38**, 355–7.

34 Seidman AD, Scher HI, Bajorin DF *et al*. Gallium nitrate: An active agent in advanced refractory transitional cell carcinoma of the bladder. *Cancer* 1991, **68**, 2651–5.

35 Witte RS, Elson P, Bono B *et al*. Eastern Cooperative Oncology Group phase II trial of ifosfamide in the treatment of previously treated advanced urothelial carcinoma. *J Clin Oncol* 1997, **15** (2), 589–93.

36 Einhorn LH, Roth BJ, Ansari R *et al*. Vinblastine, ifosfamide and gallium nitrate (VIG) combination chemotherapy in urothelial carcinoma. *Proc Am Soc Clin Oncol* 1994, **13**, 229 (Abstract702).

37 Dreicer R, Roth B, Propert K *et al*. for the Eastern Cooperative Oncology Group. E5892 Vinblastine, ifosfamide and gallium nitrate (VIG) in advanced carcinoma of the urothelium: A phase II trial of the Eastern Cooperative Oncology Group (ECOG). *Proc Am Soc Clin Oncol* 1995, **14**, 246 (Abstract 659).

38 De Wit R, Kaye SB, Roberts JT *et al*. Phase II study of first-line oral piritrexim (PTX) for metastatic urothelial cancer. *Ann Oncol* 1992, **3** (Suppl. 1), 136.

39 Witte RS, Elson P, Khandekar J *et al*. An Eastern Cooperative Oncology Group phase II trial of trimetrexate in the treatment of advanced urothelial carcinoma. *Cancer* 1994, **73**, 688–92.

40 Sternberg CN, Raghavan D, Ohi Y *et al*. Neo-adjuvant and adjuvant chemotherapy in locally advanced disease: what are the effects on survival and prognosis? *Int J Urol* 1995, **2** (2), 76–88.

41 Hall RR, for the MRC, Advanced Bladder Cancer Working Party E *et al*. Neoadjuvant CMV chemotheapy and cystectomy or radiotherapy in muscle invasive bladder cancer. First analysis of MRC/EORTC intercontinenta trial. *Proceedings American Society of Clinical Oncology* 1996 (abstract).

42 Crawford ED, Natale RB, Burton H, Southwest Oncology Group Study. Trial of cystectomy alone versus neo-adjuvant M-VAC and cystectomy in patients with locally advanced bladder cancer (intergroup trial 0080). In: *Neoadjuvant chemotherapy in invasive bladder cancer* (ed. Splinter TAW, Scher HI), 353th edn. Wiley-Liss, New York, 1990, pp. 111–13.

43 Malmstrom PU, Rintala E, Wahlqvist R *et al*. Five year follow up of a prospective trial of radical cystectomy and neoadjuvant chemotherapy. *J Urol* 1996, **155**, 1903–6.

44 Wallace DM, Raghavan D, Kelly KA *et al.* Neo-adjuvant (pre-emptive) cis-platin therapy in invasive transitional cell carcinoma of the bladder. *Br J Urol* 1991, **67**, 608–15.

45 Coppin C, Gospodarowicz M, Dixon P *et al.* for the NCI-Canada Clinical Trials Group, Ontario K. Improved local control of invasive bladder cancer by concurrent cisplatin and preoperative or radical radiation. *Proc Am Soc Clin Oncol* 1992, **11**, 198 (607) (abstract).

46 Martinez-Pineiro JA, Gonzalez Martin M, Arocena F *et al.* Neoadjuvant cis-platin chemotherapy before radical cystectomy in invasive transitional cell car-cinoma of the bladder: prospective randomized phase III study. *J Urol* 1995, **153**, 964–73.

47 Pellegrini A. GISTV neoadjuvant treatment for locally advanced bladder cancer: a randomized prospective clinical trial. *Eur J Cancer* 1993, **29A** (Suppl. 6), S229 (abstract 1284).

48 Vitale V, Orsatti M, Scarapati D *et al.* Integrated chemo-radiotherapy for infiltrating bladder cancer: an alternative approach to radical surgery. *Proceedings Fourth International Symposium on Advances in Urologic Oncology* 1993, 46.

49 Splinter TA, Scher HI, Denis L *et al.* The prognostic value of the pathological response to combination chemotherapy before cystectomy in patients with invasive bladder cancer. European Organization for Research on Treatment of Cancer–Genitourinary Group. *J Urol* 1992, **147**, 606–8.

50 Schultz PK, Herr HW, Zhang Z *et al.* Neoadjuvant chemotherapy for invasive bladder cancer: prognostic factors for survival of patients treated with M-VAC with 5 years follow-up. *J Clin Oncol* 1994, **12** (7), 1394–401.

51 Sternberg CN. Bladder preservation: a prospect for patients with urinary bladder cancer. *Acta Oncol*, 1995, **34** (5), 589–97.

52 Herr H, Scher HI. Neoadjuant chemotherapy and partial cystectomy for inva-sive bladder cancer. In: *Therapy for genitourinary cancer* (ed. Lepor H, Lawson PK). Kluwer Academic Publishers, Boston, 1992, pp. 99–104.

53 Hall RR, Roberts JT, Marsh MM. Radical TUR and chemotherapy aiming at bladder preservation. *Prog Clin Biol Res* 1990, **353**, 163–8.

54 Sternberg C, Arena M, Calabresi F *et al.* Neo-adjuvant M-VAC (methotrexate, vinblastine, adriamycin and cisplatin) for infiltrating transitional cell carci-noma of the urothelium. *Cancer*, 1993, **72**, 1975–82.

55 Sternberg CN, Pansadoro V, Lauretti S *et al.* Neo-adjuvant M-VAC (methotrex-ate, vinblastine, adriamycin and cisplatin) chemotherapy and bladder preserva-tion for muscle infiltrating transitional cell carcinoma of the bladder. *Urologic Oncol* 1995, **1** (3), 127–33.

56 Sternberg CN. Adjuvant chemotherapy following radical cystectomy. *World J Urol*, 1993, **11**, 169–74.

57 Fair WR, Fuks ZY, Scher HI. Cancer of the bladder. In: *Cancer, principles and practices of oncology* (ed. DeVita VT, Hellman S, Rosenberg SA). J.B. Lippincott Co., Philadelphia, 1993, pp. 1052–1072.

58 Gospodarowicz MK, Warde P. The role of radiation therapy in the manage-ment of transitional cell carcinoma of the bladder. *Hematol Oncol Clinics North Am* 1992, **6**, 147–68.

59 Douglas RM, Kaufman DS, Zietman AL *et al.* Conservative surgery, patient selection, and chemoradiation as a organ-preserving treatment for muscle invading bladder cancer. *Semin Oncol* 1996, **23** (5), 614–20.

60 Oosten JK, Janknegt RA. Bladder saving procedure and invasive local bladder cancer. Results of 3 years follow-up in 87 responders on radiotherapy. *Eur Urol* 1990, **18** (Suppl.), 79 (Abstract 159).

61 Kachnic LA, Kaufman DS, Heney NM *et al.* Bladder preservation by combined modality therapy for invasive bladder cancer. *J Clin Oncol* 1997, **15** (3), 1022–9.

62 Tester W, Porter A, Asbell S *et al.* Combined modality program with possible organ preservation for invasive bladder carcinoma: results of RTOG protocol 85–12. *Int J Radiat Oncol Biol Phys* 1993, **25**, 783.

63 Dunst J, Sauer R, Schrott KM *et al.* Organ-sparing treatment of advanced bladder cancer: A 10 year experience. *Int J Radiat Oncol Biol Phys* 1994, **30**, 261–6.

64 Orsatti M, Curotto A, Canobbio L *et al.* Alternating chemo-radiotherapy in bladder cancer: A conservative approach. *Int J Radiat Oncol Biol Phys* 1995, **33**, 173–8.

65 Tester W, Caplan R, Heaney J *et al.* Neoadjuvant combined modality program with selective organ preservation for invasive bladder cancer: Results of Radiation Therapy Oncology Group phase II trial 8802. *J Clin Oncol* 1996, **14** (1), 119–26.

66 Housset M, Dufour B, Maulard-Durdux C *et al.* Concomitant fluorouracil (5-FU) -cisplatin (CDDP) and bifractionated split course radiation therapy (BSCRT) for invasive bladder cancer. *Proc Am Soc Clin Oncol* 1997, **16**, 319A (Abstract 139).

67 Einstein A, Shipley W, Coombs J *et al.* Randomized controlled trial of cisplatin (DDP) following preoperative radiotherapy plus radical cystectomy (RT+RCy) for invasive bladder carcinoma: a national bladder cancer collaborative group A (NBCCGA) study. *Proc Am Soc Clin Oncol* 1984, **3**, 154 (C601) (abstract).

68 Logothetis CJ, Johnson DE, Chong C *et al.* Adjuvant cyclophosphamide, doxorubicin, and cisplatin chemotherapy for bladder cancer: an update. *J Clin Oncol* 1998, **6**, 1590–6.

69 Skinner DG, Daniels JR, Russell CA *et al.* The role of adjuvant chemotherapy following cystectomy for invasive bladder cancer: a prospective comparative trial. *J Urol* 1991, **145**, 459–67.

70 Studer UE, Bacchi M, Biedermann C *et al.* Adjuvant cisplatin chemotherapy following cystectomy for bladder cancer: Results of a prospective randomized trial. *J Urol* 1994, **152**, 81–4.

71 Stockle M, Meyenburg W, Wellek S *et al.* Advanced bladder cancer (stages pT3b, pT4a, pN1 nad pN2): improved survival after radical cystectomy and 3 adjuvant cycles of chemotherapy results of a controlled prospective study. *J Urol* 1992, **148**, 302–7.

72 Bono AV, Benvenuti C, Gibba A *et al.* Adjuvant chemotherapy in locally advanced bladder cancer. Final analysis of a controlled multicentre study. *Acta Urol* 1996, **38**, 60–3.

73 Freiha F, Reese J, Torti FM. A randomized trial of radical cystectomy versus radical cystectomy and cisplatin, vinblastine and methotrexate chemotherapy for muscle invasive bladder cancer. *J Urol* 1996, **155**, 495–9.

74 Stockle M, Voges GE, Meyenburg W *et al.* Locally advanced bladder cancer: long term results of radical cystectomy with and without adjuvant polychemotherapy: prospective and retrospective data. *J Urol* 1996, **155**, 628A (abstract 1267).

75 Stockle M, Meyenburg W, Wellek S *et al.* Adjuvant polychemotherapy of nonorgan-confined bladder cancer after radical cystectomy revisited: long term results of a controlled prospective study and further clinical experience. *J Urol* 1995, **153**, 47–52.

17. Integration of cytotoxic chemotherapy into management of muscle-invasive bladder cancer

Derek Raghavan and Murthy Andavolu

Introduction

Approximately 10 000 cases of invasive bladder cancer are diagnosed in the United States each year, representing about 20% of incident cases of urothelial malignancy (1). Invasive bladder cancer is now considered to be a systemic disease as more than half of the presenting cases will eventually relapse with distant metastases (2), presumably because micrometastases are present early in the course of the disease. With this in mind, systemic chemotherapy has been added to locoregional treatment in an attempt to improve cure rates (3).

The early clinical trials of chemotherapy for bladder cancer showed that several single agents have activity, including cyclophosphamide, the vinca alkaloids, methotrexate, mitomycin C, 5-fluorouracil, doxorubicin, and cisplatin (4). Ifosfamide, gallium nitrate, paclitaxel, and gemcitabine have been shown in contemporary studies to have substantial antitumour effect against transitional cell cancer of the urothelium (2,5–7).

The first randomized trial to demonstrate a survival benefit from combination chemotherapy was reported from an international group (USA, Canada, Australia), and showed that the combination of methotrexate, vinblastine, doxorobucin, and cisplatin (MVAC regimen) yields a significantly increased response rate, progression-free and total survival, compared with single agent cisplatin (8). A study from the M.D Anderson Cancer Institute (Texas, USA) confirmed this result by demonstrating a statistically improved survival from the MVAC regimen as compared with the combination of cyclophosphamide, doxorubicin, and cisplatin (9). We have recently published a long-term follow up of the international trial, revealing only two of 122 patients alive at 6 years after treatment with cisplatin alone, compared with nine of 133 alive after MVAC (10). Although MVAC constitutes the standard treatment in 1998 for patients with metastatic disease, it is clear that with such a low cure rate and a median survival of only 1 year, new treatments are urgently required (11).

Two exciting new agents appear to have an important role in the management of advanced bladder cancer. Roth *et al.* (5) have shown that paclitaxel is active against transitional cell cancer of the bladder, reporting a total response rate of 42%, including 27% complete remissions. Of importance, no responses were recorded in the liver in this series. Paclitaxel has been incorporated into combination regimens with carboplatin (12), cisplatin (13), ifosfamide plus cisplatin (14), and methotrexate plus cisplatin (15). This latter regimen is of potential importance as a substantial objective response rate was recorded among cases previously treated with cisplatin-based regimens.

We have recently reported our experience with gemcitabine, a fluorinated analogue of cytosine arabinoside with different uptake and retention characteristics from the parent compound (7). This agent has previously been shown to have activity against previously treated bladder cancer (16), and others have confirmed its single agent response rate of about 30% (17). The combination of gemcitabine with cisplatin increases the objective response rate to nearly 70% (18).

These agents are of particular importance as they appear to be much less toxic than some of the earlier agents (e.g. the MVAC regimen), and hence may be more easily introduced into combined modality regimens. In addition, paclitaxel and gemcitabine appear to be potent radiosensitizers, and thus may have a part in improving local control in combination with radiotherapy, in addition to a potential importance for the control of systemic disease.

NEOADJUVANT CHEMOTHERAPY FOR INVASIVE DISEASE

The rationale for the use of initial (neoadjuvant) chemotherapy in this clinical context has been discussed in detail before (3). In brief, possible benefits include tumour downstaging with the increased possibility of resection, the potential for *in vivo* assessment of anticancer efficacy, improved access to tumour tissues before the onset of the vascular effects of irradiation, and possible radiosensitization. By contrast, the possible drawbacks include the use of ineffective treatment, thus delaying the onset of potentially active treatment approaches (such as radiotherapy or surgery) and the use of systemic treatment with potentially more side-effects to control a local tumour.

The initial, non-randomized single agent trials were very promising, showing substantial tumour downstaging and apparently improved tumour resection rates. However, randomized clinical trials that tested single agent chemotherapy plus local treatment versus local treatment alone did not show any benefit from this strategy (Table 17.1) (19–21). Similarly, the use of combination chemotherapy regimens as neoadjuvant treatment initially appeared attractive (22), but most late follow-up studies did not indicate any apparent long-term benefit (23). By contrast, the Nordic Cooperative Bladder Cancer Study Group have reported that two cycles of neoadjuvant cisplatin and doxorubicin confer a reduced death rate in patients with T3 and T4 bladder cancer who are treated by cystectomy, although this study had only a modest statistical power because of the patient numbers (24). A recent meta-analysis of all known randomized trials, reviewing information from 479 cases comparing local treatment versus neoadjuvant chemotherapy followed by local treatment, demonstrated an overall hazard ratio of 1.02 (favouring local treatment) and a 2% increase in relative risk of death from the use of neoadjuvant chemotherapy (25). However, it should be noted that this study was heavily dominated by single agent trials.

Support for this view has been provided from the initial results of the International Intergroup [Medical Research Council (MRC)/ European Organisation for Research and Treatment of Cancer (EORTC)] Trial, in which more than 950 patients were randomly

Table 17.1

RESULTS OF CLINICAL TRIALS OF PREEMPTIVE CHEMOTHERAPY FOR INVASIVE BLADDER CANCER

Series	Regimen	Response rate after chemorx			Response rate after all Rx			Median Survival (mo)	Actuarial Long-Term Survival
		CR (%)	PR (%)	RR (%)	CR (%)	PR (%)	RR (%)		
Raghavan	C-RT/*	60		60	85		85	32	40% 5-yr 30% true 5-yr
Kaye	CyMF-RT	0	0	0	0	0	0	27	26% 3-yr, T4 26% 3-yr
Zinke*	MVDC	50	19	69	0	0	92	?	?
Scher*	MVDC	21	39	60	30	57	87	?	?
Shearer	M-RT	–	–	–	–	–	56	23	39% 3-yr
Shearer	RT only	–	–	–	–	–	50	20	37% 3-yr
Wallace	C	–	–	–	–	–	–	~24	39% 3-yr
Wallace	RT only	–	–	–	–	–	–	~22	39% 3-yr
Hall	RT/* only	–	–	–	–	–	–	–	62% 2-yr
Hall	CMV-RT/*	–	–	–	–	–	–	–	60% 2-yr

CR, complete remission
PR, partial remission
RR, total remission rate
Rx, therapy
RT, radiotherapy

C, cisplatin
M, methotrexate,
F, fluorouracil
Cy, cyclophosphamide
D, doxorubicin

* Cystectomy as definitive treatment.

allocated to neoadjuvant cisplatin/methotrexate/vinblastine plus local treatment or local treatment alone (26). The first report of this study failed to reveal a significant survival difference between the two arms, despite significant downstaging of tumours treated by neoadjuvant chemotherapy.

One important current trial (the US Intergroup Trial) has not yet been reported, but could be of particular importance. The very rigorous trial design and execution, accompanied by central pathological review, will be of particular importance in interpreting the significance of the study if the result differs from that of the larger MRC/EORTC trial.

ADJUVANT CHEMOTHERAPY

Adjuvant systemic chemotherapy, in which cytotoxics are delivered after the removal of all known local tumour (by complete resection or by radical radiotherapy), was initially developed for breast cancer and colonic cancer, and its role validated in randomized trials. In the context of bladder cancer, several early, non-randomized phase II trials have been reported, but without useful conclusions (27–29). More recently, Skinner and colleagues (30) conducted a trial for patients with deeply invasive bladder cancer, staged-at cystectomy, half of whom were randomly allocated to receive adjuvant treatment with cyclophosphamide, doxorubicin, and cisplatin. The execution of the trial was marred by the fact that some patients received different chemotherapy, predicated on the results of soft agar clonogenic sensitivity testing, and the total number of cases was small. At best, only a small survival benefit was achieved by this strategy as the survival curves had already crossed at 4 years.

Stockle et al. (31) reported the results of a randomized trial in which patients with stages pT3b–pT4 bladder cancer (defined at cystectomy and lymph node dissection) were randomly allocated to receive adjuvant chemotherapy (methotrexate, vinblastine, epirubicin, and cisplatin) or observation. A substantial disease-free survival benefit was reported (73% versus 19%), but the statistical power of the study was limited by early closure; the investigators recognized that the trial design required patients on the observation arm not to receive salvage chemotherapy at the time of relapse, and recognized that they were depriving this cohort of potentially life prolonging salvage treatment. This study, in fact, assessed only the impact of chemotherapy *at some time* after cystectomy, rather than being a true test of adjuvant treatment. These investigators have updated their experience, adding a cohort of non-randomized cases to the cases treated in the randomized trial, and comparing outcomes between groups treated by cystectomy alone and those receiving adjuvant chemotherapy (32). However, these investigators have made basic errors of trial analysis (especially with respect to the risk of selection bias) and have not recognized the fallacy of combining data sets and grouping their randomized and non-randomized experience. As a result, the more recent report adds nothing useful to the literature on this important issue.

Of greater relevance to this hypothesis, Freiha et al. (33) conducted a similar randomized trial, comparing cystectomy plus adjuvant CMV (cisplatin, methotrexate, vinblastine) chemotherapy versus cystectomy alone (with CMV offered at the time of relapse). This study was closed when only 53 cases had been randomized after it demonstrated a statistically significant increase in disease-free survival. A non-significant trend towards improved overall survival from the use of adjuvant CMV chemotherapy was also reported, but with very broad confidence intervals. However, a Taiwanese group also assessed the results of adjuvant CMV chemotherapy for stages pT2–4 and node positive disease, and reported a median disease-free survival of only 15.5 months, with a 3-year disease-free survival probability of only 28% (34).

It is not possible to make a final definitive decision about the role of adjuvant chemotherapy for invasive bladder cancer, although it seems reasonable to consider that the experience reported above from Stanford University and Mainz supports the use of adjuvant therapy when it is not feasible to enrol a patient into a clinical trial. Furthermore, one of the most provocative current trials has been developed by Cote and colleagues at the University of Southern California and collaborating institutions to test the utility of adjuvant chemotherapy in a controlled fashion. In this randomized trial, patients with superficially invasive, node-negative bladder cancer, with immunohistochemical evidence of aberrant P53 expression, an adverse prognostic determinant (35), are either observed or treated with adjuvant MVAC chemotherapy. This trial will demonstrate whether adjuvant chemotherapy offers a survival benefit when used even earlier in the disease, in addition to testing further the hypothesis that aberrant P53 expression is an adverse prognostic determinant.

PERIOPERATIVE CHEMOTHERAPY

Chemotherapy has also been administered before and after definitive locoregional treatment for bladder cancer. Shearer et al. (19), studied the role of methotrexate in this context in a randomized trial that predominantly assessed the impact of neoadjuvant chemotherapy, but also had a component of adjuvant therapy after completion of definitive treatment. No survival gain was noted when compared with standard treatment.

In a pilot study conducted by the Eastern Cooperative Oncology Group, two cycles of MVAC were administered before cystectomy, followed by another two cycles postoperatively (36). Seventeen patients had T3 disease and one had a stage T2 tumour; nearly half the cases showed down staging in response to MVAC, but at a median follow-up time of 23 months, 5096 had died. Logothetis and colleagues (37) tested a similar hypothesis in a randomized trial: 100 patients were randomized to receive either two cycles of MVAC followed by cystectomy and then three adjuvant cycles of MVAC versus initial cystectomy followed by five cycles of adjuvant MVAC. There was no statistically significant difference between the arms, despite the significant level of downstaging after neoadjuvant chemotherapy. Both trials revealed an unexpectedly high rate of intercurrent deaths from vascular complications, further demonstrating the importance of randomized trials in the assessment of these novel strategies of management.

CONCURRENT CHEMORADIATION

Several cytotoxics, including 5-fluorouracil, mitomycin, doxorubicin, carboplatin, and cisplatin are radiosensitizers, increasing the sensitivity of neoplastic and normal tissues to the cytotoxic effects of irradiation. Clinical trials have been initiated in which these cytotoxic agents are administered during the period of radiotherapy with the intention of increasing the extent of tumour lysis, with the hope that there is a sufficient difference in the pattern of toxicity between normal and malignant tissues so that the normal tissue damage will be less than that occurring in the tumour. Several phase II trials have assessed the impact of cytotoxics given alone (5-fluorouracil, carboplatin, doxorubicin, cisplatin) and in combination regimens (5-fluorouracil plus cisplatin) in radiosensitizing protocols (38–41), and have demonstrated significant tumour reduction (Table 17.2). In most of these studies, chemotherapy has been combined with radiotherapy as the definitive local treatment, although one study assessed the use of doxorubicin-induced radiosensitization as adjuvant therapy after surgery (38).

To date, it is not known whether these approaches confer a survival benefit, notwithstanding their efficacy in achieving local

Table 17.2

TRIALS OF CHEMORADIATION FOR INVASIVE BLADDER CANCER					
Series	Number of patients	Clinical T stage	Salvage cystectomy (%)	Overall survival	Median follow-up (months)
Coppin	42	T2–T4	?	61% @ 2yr	50
Dunst	139	T1–T3	?	40% @ 7yr	minimum 12
Housset	54	T2–T4	22	59% @ 3yr	18–58
Kaufmann	53	T2–T4	15	53% @ 4yr	48
Sauer	67	T1–T4	16	66% @ 3yr	
Tester	46	T2–T4	17	66% @ 3yr	36

tumour control (42). Coppin *et al.* (43), reporting a randomized trial conducted by the National Cancer Institute of Canada, showed that a statistically significantly increased level of local tumour control could be achieved by the concurrent use of cisplatin and radiotherapy (compared with radiotherapy alone), but were unable to demonstrate a statistically significant survival benefit from the combination regimen. However, it should be noted that this trial was not powered to detect a small but important survival benefit. To the present time, no other randomized trials have assessed the potential survival benefit of this approach. Given the changes in tumour classification, staging, available cytotoxics, and support therapy, it is our view that at least one convincing randomized trial will be required to establish the place of chemoradiation as a standard of therapy. This view, however, is not universally held. For example, Shipley has expressed the view that the study from Coppin and colleagues has established the place for chemoradiation in achieving local control, and that this should be incorporated into other randomized trials that test innovations in neoadjuvant or adjuvant systemic therapy.

CONCLUSIONS

There is evidence from uncontrolled trials that the combination of systemic chemotherapy and definitive local treatment may have a useful role in the management of locally advanced bladder cancer, at least by contributing to improved local control. However, the optimal schedules and the extent of true survival benefit have not yet been demonstrated, and randomized controlled trials to the present time have mostly failed to show a significant survival benefit from combined modality regimens.

Key Points

1. The advantages for the use of neoadjuvant chemotherapy include tumour downstaging with the increased possibility of resection, the potential for *in vivo* assessment of anticancer efficacy, improved access to tumour tissues before the onset of the vascular effects of irradiation, and possible radiosensitization. By contrast, the possible drawbacks include the use of ineffective treatment, thus delaying the onset of potentially active treatment approaches (such as radiotherapy or surgery) and the use of systemic treatment with potentially more side-effects to control a local tumour.

2. In adjuvant systemic chemotherapy, cytotoxics are delivered after the removal of all known local tumour, by complete resection or by radical radiotherapy.

3. There is evidence from uncontrolled trials that the combination of systemic chemotherapy and definitive local treatment may have a useful role in the management of locally advanced bladder cancer, at least by contributing to improved local control. However, the optimal schedules and the extent of true survival benefit have not yet been demonstrated, and randomized controlled trials are needed.

At present, it appears that one of the most promising future strategies will be the incorporation of adjuvant systemic chemotherapy into programmes of treatment. However, it will require well designed and carefully executed randomized trials to prove this hypothesis. This may prove to be difficult to achieve in an era in which there appear to be less available cases for entry into randomized clinical trials than in the past two decades, and where the pragmatic considerations of governmental and private managed care initiatives regularly undermine important academic initiatives.

References

1 Parker SL, Tong T, Bolden S, Wingo PA. Cancer statistics 1996. *CA* 1996, **65**, 5–27.
2 Raghavan D, Shipley W, Garnick M *et al.* Biology and management of bladder cancer. *N Engl J Med* 1990, **322**, 1129–38.
3 Raghavan D. Pre-emptive (neo-adjuvant) intravenous chemotherapy for invasive bladder cancer. *Br J Urol* 1988, **61**, 1–8.
4 Yagoda A. Chemotherapy for metastatic bladder cancer. *Cancer*, 1980, **45**, 7 1879–83.
5 Roth BJ, Dreicer R, Einhorn LH *et al.* Signiflcant activity of paclitaxel in advanced transitional cell carcinoma of the urothelium: a phase II trial of the Eastern Cooperative Oncology Group. *J Clin Oncol* 1994, **12**, 2264–70.
6 Loehrer PJ, Sr, DeMulder PP. Management of metastatic bladder cancer. In: *Principles and practice of genitourinary oncology* (ed. Raghavan D, Scher HI, Leibel SA, Lange PH). Lippincott-Raven, Philadelphia, 1997, pp. 299–305.
7 Stadler W, Kuzel T, Raghavan D *et al.* A phase II study of gemcitabine in the treatment of patients with advanced transitional cell carcinoma *J Clin Oncol* 1997, **15**, in press.
8 Loehrer PJ, Einhorn LH, Elson PJ *et al.* A randomized comparison of cisplatin alone or in combination with methotrexate, vinblastine and doxorubicin in patients with metastatic urothelial carcinoma. *J Clin Oncol* 1992, **10**, 1066–73.
9 Logothetis CJ, Dexeus FH, Finn L *et al.* A prospective randomized trial comparing MVAC and CISCA chemotherapy for patients with metastatic urothelial tumors. *J Clin Oncol* 1990, **8**, 1050.
10 Saxnan SB, Loehrer PJ, Sr Propert K *et al.* Long term follow up of phase III Intergroup study of MVAC vs. cisplatin metastatic urothelial carcinoma. *J Clin Oncol* 1997, **15**, 2564–9.
11 Levine EG, Raghavan D. MVAC for bladder cancer: time to move forward again. *J Clin Oncol* 1993, **11**, 387–8.
12 Vaughn DJ, Malkowicz SB, Zoltick B *et al.* Paclitaxel plus carboplatin in advanced carcinoma of the urothelium: A welltolerated outpatient regimen. *Proc Am Soc Clin Oncol* 1996, **15**, 240A (abstract).
13 Murphy BA, Johnson DR, Smith J *et al.* Phase II trial of paclitaxel (P) and cisplatin (C) for metastatic or locally unresectable urothelial cancer. *Proc Am Soc Clin Oncol* 1996, **15**, 245A (abstract).
14 McCaffrey J, Hilton S, Mazumdar M *et al.* A phase II trial of ifosfamide, paclitaxel and cisplatin (ITP) in patients (pts) with advanced urothelial tract tumors. *Proc Am Soc Clin Oncol* 1996, **15**, 251A (abstract).
15 Tu SM, Hossan E, Amato R *et al.* Paclitaxel, cisplatin and methotrexate combination chemotherapy is active in treatment of refractory urothelial malignancies. *J Urol* 1995, **154**, 1719–22.
16 Pollera CF, Ceribelli A, Crecco M, Calabresi F. Weekly gemcitabine in advanced bladder cancer A preliminary report. *Ann Oncol* 1994, **5**, 132–4.
17 Moore MJ, Tannock I, Ernst S *et al.* Gemcitabine demonstrates promising activity as a single agent in the treatment of metastatic transitional cell carcinoma *J Clin Oncol* 1997, in press.

18 Stadler WM, Murphy D, Kaufman D *et al*. Phase II trial of gemcitabine (BEM) plus cisplatin (CDDP) in metastatic urothelial cancer (UC). *Proc Am Soc Clin Oncol* 1997, **16**, 323A (abstract).

19 Shearer RJ, Chilvers CED, Bloom HGJ *et al*. Adjuvant chemotherapy in T3 carcinoma of the bladder. A prospective Trial: Preliminary report. *Br J Urol* 1988, **62**, 558–64.

20 Wallace DMA, Raghavan D, Kelly KA *et al*. Neo-adjuvant (preemptive) cisplatin therapy in invasive transitional cell carcinoma of the bladder. *Br J Urol* 1991, **67**, 608–15.

21 Martinez-Pineiro JA, Martin MG, Arocena F *et al*. Neoadjuvant cisplatin chemotherapy before radical cystectomy in invasive transitional cell carcinoma of the bladder: A prospective randomized phase III study. *J Urol* 1995, **153**, 964–73.

22 Scher H, Herr H, Sternberg C *et al*. Neo-adjuvant chemotherapy for invasive bladder cancer. Experience with the M-VAC regimen. *Br J Urol* 1989, **64**, 250.

23 Schultz PK, Herr HW, Zhang ZF *et al*. Neoadjuvant chemotherapy for invasive bladder cancer prognostic factors for survival of patients treated with M-VAC with 5-year follow-up. *J Clin Oncol* 1994, **12**, 1394–401.

24 Malmstrom PU, Rintala E, Wahlqvist R *et al*. Five year followup of a prospective trial of radical cystectomy and neoadjuvant chemotherapy: Nordic Cystectomy Trial I. *J Urol* 1996, **155**, 1903–6.

25 Ghersi D, Stewart LA, Parmar MKB *et al*. Does neoadjuvant cisplatin-based chemotherapy improve the survival of patients with locally advanced bladder cancer: a meta-analysis of individual patient data from randomized clinical trials. *Br J Urol* 1995, **75**, 206–13.

26 Hall RR. Neo-adjuvant CMV chemotherapy and cystectomy or radiotherapy in muscle invasive bladder cancer. First analysis of MRC/EORTC Intercontinental trial. *Proc Am Soc Clin Oncol* 1996, **15**, 323A (abstract).

27 Clyne CAC, Jenkins JD, Smart CJ *et al*. A trial of adjuvant chemotherapy for stage T3 bladder tumors. *J Urol* 1983, **129**, 736–8.

28 Richards B, Bastable JRG, Freedman L *et al*. Adjuvant chemotherapy with doxorubicin (Adriamycin) and 5-fluorouracil in T3NxMo bladder cancer treated with radiotherapy. *Br J Urol* 1983, **55**, 386–91.

29 Logothetis CJ. Postoperative adjuvant CISCA chemotherapy for high-risk invasive bladder cancer. In: *Systemic therapy for genitourinary cancers* (ed. Johnson DE, Logothetis CJ, Von Eschenbach, AC). YearBook Publishers, Chicago, 1989, pp. 73–81.

30 Skinner DG, Daniels JR, Russell CA *et al*. The role of adjuvant chemotherapy following cystectomy for invasive bladder cancer: a prospective comparative trial. *J Urol* 1991, **145**, 459–67.

31 Stockle M, Meyenburg W, Wellek S *et al*. Advanced bladder cancer (stages pT3b, pT4a, pN1 and pN2): improved survival after radical cystectomy and 3 adjuvant cycles of chemotherapy. Results of a controlled prospective study. *J Urol* 1992, **148**, 302–7.

32 Stockle M, Wellek S, Meyenburg W *et al*. Radical cystectomy with or without adjuvant polychemotherapy for non-organ-confined transitional cell carcinoma of the urinary bladder: Prognostic impact of lymph node involvement. *Urology*, 1995, **48**, 868–75.

33 Freiha F, Reese J, Torti FM. A randomized trial of radical cystectomy plus cisplatin, vinblastine and methotrexate chemotherapy for muscle invasive bladder cancer. *J Urol* 1996, **155**, 495–500.

34 Wei CH, Hsieh RK, Chiou TJ *et al*. Adjuvant methotrexate, vinblastine and cisplatin chemotherapy for invasive transitional cell carcinoma: Taiwan experience. *J Urol* 1996, **155**, 118–21.

35 Esrig D, Elmajian D, Groshen S *et al*. Accumulation of nuclear p53 and tumor progression in bladder cancer. *N Engl J Med* 1994, **331**, 1259–64.

36 Dreicer R, Messing EM, Loehrer PJ, Trump DL. Perioperative methotrexate, vinblastine, doxorubicin and cisplatin (M-VAC) for poor risk transitional cell carcinoma of the bladder: An Eastern Cooperative Oncology Group pilot study. *J Urol* 1990, **144**, 1123–7.

37 Logothetis C, Swanson D, Amato R *et al*. Optimal delivery of perioperative chemotherapy: preliminary results of a randomized, prospective, comparative trial of preoperative and postoperative chemotherapy for invasive bladder carcinoma. *J Urol* 1996, **155**, 1241–5.

38 Schaeffer AJ, Grayhack JT, Merrill JM *et al*. Adjuvant doxorubicin hydro-chloride and radiation in stage D bladder cancer: a preliminary report. *J Urol* 1984, **131**, 1073–6.

39 Housset M, Maulard C, Chretien Y *et al*. Combined radiation and chemotherapy for invasive transitional cell carcinoma of the bladder: a prospective study. *J Clin Oncol* 1993, **11**, 2150.

40 Kaufman DS, Shipley WU, Griffin PP *et al*. Selective bladder preservation by combination treatment of invasive bladder cancer. *N Engl J Med* 1993, **329**, 1377.

41 Tester W, Porter A, Asbell S *et al*. Combined modality program with possible organ preservation for invasive bladder carcinoma results of RTOG protocol 85–12. *Int J Radiat Oncol* 1993, Biology and Physics, **25**, 783.

42 Raghavan D. Editorial: Perioperative chemotherapy for invasive bladder cancer—what should we tell our patients? *J Urol* 1996, **155**, 1246–7.

43 Coppin C, Gospodarowicz M, James K *et al*. Improved local control of invasive bladder cancer by concurrent cisplatin and preoperative or definitive radiation. *J Clin Oncol* 1996, **14**, 2901–7.

18. INTRAVESICAL CHEMOTHERAPY OF BLADDER CANCER

Ali M. Ziada and E. David Crawford

INTRODUCTION

The American Cancer Society estimates that in 1998 there will be 54 500 new cases and 11 700 bladder cancer deaths in the United States (1,2). Although we have not yet succeeded to lower the incidence of bladder cancer, we have managed to improve our approach to treatment. The survival of bladder cancer in the past decade has increased by 8% despite a rise in incidence of 36% (3,4). This suggests both stage migration towards more localized disease as well as improved treatment strategies.

At presentation, superficial bladder cancer will account for 70% and 80% of patients (5). Recurrence rates after initial successful treatment range from 30% to 85% with grade progression occurring in 10–30% and stage progression in 4–30% of cases (6).

The primary standard treatment for papillary bladder tumours that do not invade the muscular layer (stages Ta or T1 transitional cell carcinoma), is transurethral resection of the bladder tumour (TURBT). The procedure of resection or fulguration or laser coagulation of the tumours can be done with minimal morbidity, with or without anaesthesia and as an outpatient procedure. In spite of opinions that some therapies of the primary tumour notably laser are associated with less incidence of recurrence, this has not been proved in the setting of controlled studies (7). Despite complete eradication of the primary tumour, about two-thirds of patients will develop tumour recurrences within the first 5 years of follow up. The high rate of recurrence can be reduced by intravesical therapies (8).

The goal is to reduce recurrence of the disease and its progression to muscle invasive bladder cancer. Intravesical therapy whether chemotherapy or immunotherapy are hence important tools of therapy. In spite of the achievement of reducing recurrence rates, our goal should still be lowering the incidence of the disease.

TYPES OF SUPERFICIAL BLADDER TUMOURS

Bladder cancers are primarily transitional cell carcinomas. Low-grade tumours have less potential of progression to invasive cancers. Low-grade tumours have a 50–70% chance of recurrence. Grades 2 or 3 have a higher chance of about 20% of progression to muscle invasive disease (5).

T1 tumours which invade the lamina propria is an indication for aggressive treatment because patients with these tumours have a 25–30% risk of progression to muscle invasive disease (9). The degree of tumour penetration is also a very important factor in determining risk of progression. Tumour penetration of the muscularis mucosa has a 54% risk of progression compared with a 7% risk with penetration of the lamina propria (10).

Carcinoma *in situ* (CIS) appears adjacent to a visible tumour in 90% of cases (11). In 10% of cases, it is an isolated pathological finding. The potential for development of muscle invasive disease is 42–83% in the case of CIS associated with papillary tumours versus 20–34% when CIS is an isolated finding (12). The risk of invasion of CIS is increased with widespread disease.

PROGNOSTIC FACTORS

Predicting the risks involved with superficial bladder tumours is difficult because not all patients have the same risk of recurrence or progression. The behaviour of superficial tumours that share the same characteristics vary remarkably from one patient to another and hence individual characteristics are not reliable to predict tumour behaviour.

The most reliable predictive characteristics for disease recurrence and progression are grade, stage, growth pattern, size, multiplicity, vascular or lymphatic invasion, and basement membrane discontinuity. The prognostic relevance of other factors has not been definitively demonstrated (5,14,15).

Badalament and Farah in 1997 (16) divided the risk factors into two major categories: dedifferentiation and increased tumour burden. Dedifferentiation was a direct measure of grade, DNA aneuploidy, growth pattern, CIS; increased tumour burden was related to the size, number, prostatic urethral involvement, and postoperative cytology. DNA ploidy status carried a better prognosis if diploid so did postoperative cytology when negative. Failure of prior intravesical therapy was also considered a marker of aggressiveness among patients with superficial bladder cancer.

INTRAVESICAL CHEMOTHERAPY: PRINCIPLES AND INDICATIONS

The advantage of intravesical chemotherapy over systemic therapy is that it directly contacts the urothelial surface. Also, the intravesical route is associated with less systemic absorption and hence less toxicity depending on the intravesical agent used. However, this route has the disadvantages of the local side-effects as well as the need for transurethral manipulations.

Intravesical chemotherapy can be used as a therapeutic agent in case of: (i) incomplete resection of tumours due to either multifocal tumour burden or CIS (ii) when tumour location interferes with complete resection; (iii) with high-grade tumours; and (iv) when urine cytology is positive for high-grade tumour after resection of all visible tumour (14).

Prophylactic administration of intravesical chemotherapy after resection of the primary tumour will reduce and delay recurrence, but clinical studies failed to show a conclusive benefit that any of the agents commonly used prevents progression or increase survival. Intravesical treatment does not permanently affect the underlying carcinogenic process in the urothelium. Most patients will eventually experience one recurrence (17).

Intravesical instillation of mitomycin C (MMC) has been used as an adjuvant therapy for superficial bladder tumours. MMC instillation immediately following transurethral resection is proposed to prevent or reduce the tumoral dissemination and regrowth that may result from endoscopic manipulation. In contrast to immunotherapy, immediate post-transurethral resection (TUR) instillation is safe with chemotherapy (18).

PHARMACOLOGY

Studies have shown several factors which influence efficacy of intravesical chemotherapeutic agents. Proper understanding of these factors can enhance the results of treatment. Bladder, bladder cavity, tumour, and drug factors can help us better understand and utilize these agents (16).

Bladder

The penetration of intravesical agents is governed by diffusion across the urothelium then across deeper tissues. The concentration of drugs is indirectly proportional to depth. The neoplastic urothelial cells may be more permeable to intravesical chemotherapeutic agents due to dedifferentiation and impaired surface mucopolysaccharide as well as intracellular junctions. TURs and cystitis can enhance drug penetration. The role of capillary circulation which increases with depth is to level off the drug concentration to be equal to blood concentrations in the deeper tissues. Another factor to be considered is the dilution effect of urine on the chemotherapeutic agent which may impede achieving cytocidal concentrations.

Bladder cavity

Six factors can influence treatment efficacy. According to Weintjes and associates (19), these factors in relative rank of importance are dose, residual urine volume, urine production, urine pH, dose volume, and dwell time.

Chemotherapeutic agents

The penetration of chemotherapeutic agents across the urothelium is dependent on molecular weight and lipid solubility. thiotepa is lipophilic and has a lower molecular weight compared with MMC and doxorubicin, which are relatively hydrophobic and have large molecular weight. Thus, MMC and doxorubicin should be used for deeper tumours whereas thiotepa should be used for more superficial lesions. The low molecular weight of thiotepa is a disadvantage because of the higher rate of systemic absorption and myelosuppression.

Tumour

Pharmacodynamic studies proved that longer exposure and higher concentrations enhance the cytocidal effects. Loss of production of intracellular reductive enzymes as a result of dedifferentiated cells can result in failure to metabolize MMC to the active form (20). The activity of MMC was demonstrated to be lower against high-grade tumours as well as rapidly proliferating tumours.

INTRAVESICAL CHEMOTHERAPY: ADMINISTRATION AND PRECAUTIONS

As chemotherapeutic drugs are cycle specific, multiple repeated instillations are more effective than single dosage. Weekly instillations, although practical, are not ideal from the biological cell cycle standpoint. The usual course consists of 6-weekly instillations depending on the agent being used. Instillations should be delayed for a week following trauma or infection (16,21). Intravesical chemotherapy in contrast to immunotherapy is safer to use earlier after TUR in the immediate postoperative period (18).

Before instillation, the bladder is emptied and then the drug instilled via the same catheter. The drug is diluted in sterile water. The patients are instructed to limit fluid intake to avoid dilution of the drug by urine in the bladder (21). The drug is left in the bladder for an empirical time of 1 h. The cytotoxicity is directly related to the drug concentration and exposure time but longer instillations are impractical (16).

The effect of the pH of the solution is not very well understood but Tarkington and his associates (22) investigated the influence of pH on sensitivity of tumour cell lines to different chemotherapeutic agents. The colony forming ability was lowest at a pH of 5.5 for thiotepa and a pH of 7.0 for doxorubicin and mitomycin. When using MMC, urinary alkalinization will reduce degradation of the drug (16).

INTRAVESICAL CHEMOTHERAPY: DRUGS

Thiotepa

Mechanism of action
Thiotepa is the oldest of the chemotherapeutic drugs. It has been used for more than 25 years. It is an alkylating agent that acts through interfering with protein synthesis by inhibiting the synthesis of nucleic acids. Thiotepa also has a direct cytotoxic effect by inhibiting cell adherence (23).

Dosage
The usual regimen is 30–60 mg in 30 ml and 60 ml, respectively. Thiotepa is used for 6-weekly instillations followed by monthly instillations for 1-year. The prophylactic failure of thiotepa when administered only five times a year, confirms the need of regular instillation regimen (24).

Toxicity
The molecular weight of thiotepa is 189 Da. This makes systemic absorption and toxicity a possibility. Myelosuppression is a side-effect because of the significant systemic absorption. Initial reports showed that one-third of the instilled dose is absorbed after an instillation period of 3 h (25) and that 25% of patients suffered from thrombocytopenia and leucopenia (26). This side-effect,

however, is not common provided proper precautions and monitoring are taken. In a review of 670 bladder instillations in 1983,
thiotepa-induced myelosuppression was a rare event, usually mild
and transient (27). Thrasher and Crawford (28) reviewing the
toxicity of thiotepa found that a wide range of reported side-effects
was due to changes in the regimen of instillation whether variation
in dose, dwell time, and schedules. The average incidence of leucopenia, thrombocytopenia, and irritative voiding symptoms was
10.4%, 9.3%, and 25%, respectively. Treatment-related deaths were
reported to be 1%. The recommended precautions were to limit
the dose to 30 mg, discontinue treatment after 1 year, hold instillation interval to at least 4 days. Patients must have platelet
(>100 000/mm^3) and leucocyte counts (>4000/mm^3) monitored
throughout therapy. Although infrequent, aplastic anaemia and
leukaemia have been reported in patients treated with thiotepa.

Therapy

The success rates of thiotepa in definitive therapy for papillary
bladder tumours is approximately 38–47% reviewing multiple
series of treatment (21).

Single adjuvant doses were used after complete TUR of all
visible lesions. Although initial reports were supportive of the
adjuvant thiotepa therapy, the large randomized study conducted
by the Medical Research Council (MRC) showed no advantage for
adjuvant therapy (29).

To evaluate the non-maintenance regimens, the National Bladder
Cancer Group found a success rate of 66% and 54% after 12 and
20 months, respectively, versus 40% and 28% with controls (receiving pyridoxone or placebo). The longer follow-up results, however,
showed only 35% remained disease-free compared with 24% of the
placebo group. Progression was noted in 17.7% of patients treated
with thiotepa and 11% in the control group (24,30).

Conclusions

Thiotepa is an inexpensive drug with a low molecular weight.
This low molecular weight results in systemic absorption and toxicity manifestations. Myelosuppression does not appear to be a
common side-effect in patients treated with thiotepa. Thiotepa
success rate was about 40% depending on duration of follow up.

Doxorubicin

Mechanism of action

Doxorubicin is an antitumour antibiotic used mainly as systemic
treatment for a wide variety of malignancies. This antitumour

agent has achieved a response in one-third to two-thirds of patients with superficial bladder cancer (14). Doxorubicin binds and pairs to DNA. It is most toxic in the S-phase of the cell cycle, although this compound is not cell cycle specific. The mechanism of action of doxorubicin is at the cell surface (17).

Dosage

The dose of doxorubicin ranges from 30 to 100 mg in several instillation schedules. Doxorubicin can be used under an escalating dose schedule, with 60–90 mg. The schedule will entail 12 instillations, with increasing intervals in between treatments (31). With this regimen of treatment, Garnick *et al.* reported a complete response rate of 53% at 18 months of follow up (31). Doxorubicin can also be used as a course of 6-weekly instillations of 50 mg with or without additional monthly instillations for 2 years as maintenance (32). It was not demonstrated in clinical studies by Flamm (32) that doxorubicin maintenance therapy adds any benefit. The recurrence rate was similar to the control groups not receiving treatment. The efficacy results of long-term doxorubicin treatment were the same as mitomycin in different long-term schedules (33) as well as equally effective to the maintenance therapy of thiotepa (34).

Toxicity

Doxorubicin has a relatively high molecular weight of 580 Daltons. Because of this, absorption and systemic side-effects are rare; however, local side-effects are more common. The main side-effect is chemical cystitis affecting an average of 28.8% (4–56%) of patients (28). Rare side-effects were allergic reactions, gastro-intestinal side-effects, and fever. These rare side-effects affected less than 2% of the patients under treatment. Only one study reported an incidence of 16% of patients having reduced bladder capacity following treatment (35). These side-effects tend to be reversible after cessation of treatment.

In a study to compare doxorubicin with immunotherapy (BCG), more side-effects were reported (36). Irritative bladder symptoms, nausea, fever, and malaise were found in 49%, 9%, 8%, and 13%, respectively. All side-effects, however, were mild.

Therapy

The average response rate to doxorubicin as definitive treatment for papillary tumours was 38% (range from 28% to 56%) depending on the dose schedule (37). The success rate for CIS ranged between 34% and 63% (36). As a single adjuvant instillation, Zincke and associates (38) in a double randomized trial showed that 32% of the treated patients, recurrence was found within a follow-up period of 4 months compared with 71% of the control group. Longer follow up was not reported.

Conclusions

Doxorubicin is a safe intravesical agent with local side-effects but no systemic absorption and toxicity. Local side-effects tend to be mild and limited to the duration of use of the drug. Chemical cystitis affects 25% of patients but is reversible with discontinuation. The success rate is about 40%. The use of doxorubicin as adjuvant therapy is more effective than no therapy. Its use as maintenance is of no additional value.

Mitomycin C

Mechanism of action

The antitumour antibiotic mitomycin has been used in the treatment of superficial bladder cancer intravesically since the early 1960s. MMC has an intracellular effect, in contrast to doxorubicin, resulting in the production of an alkylating agent. The exact mechanism of action is not fully understood.

Dose

The dose varies between 20 and 60 mg per instillation. The usual dose schedule is 40 mg in 8-weekly instillations. The following tables show the primary and secondary response rates of intravesical mitomycin with different dose schedules.

Toxicity

Because of the high molecular weight of MMC (329 Da), it is barely absorbed. Systemic toxicity is rare and it is not associated with myelosuppression or other significant systemic toxicity. Thrasher and Crawford summarized the side-effects of 11 series involving 613 patients (28) and concluded that the incidence of leucopenia and thrombocytopenia was 0.7%. One case was reported of myelosuppression leading to death following mitomycin instillation immediately following TUR (51).

The most frequent side-effects are usually local manifestations related to the intravesical instillations. Chemical cystitis and allergic reactions are the most common of the local side-effects. Chemical cystitis is characterized by dysuria, frequency, and pain. The mean incidence is 15.8% with a range between 6% and 41% (28). Allergic reactions are mainly skin symptoms. The skin reactions commonly observed were vesicular dermatitis of the hands and feet, genital dermatitis, and widespread eruptions. The incidence of skin allergic manifestations with MMC intravesical therapy reported by Thrasher and Crawford (28) was 9.8%. These symptoms usually occur after the second instillation and most of these reactions are mediated through a delayed hypersensitivity reaction. Chemical cystitis and skin reactions usually disappear after cessation of therapy.

Two comparative studies with mitomycin and BCG using RIVM, the Dutch strain of BCG, in 338 patients (52). In the second study mitomycin was compared with two different strains of BCG (53). The frequency of side-effects (drug-induced cystitis and culture proven bacterial cystitis) was comparable in both studies between the two groups of patients. However, mitomycin had significantly lower side-effects than BCG in regard to drug-induced cystitis, local and systemic side-effects.

Therapy

Numerous trials have established the efficacy of MMC (Table 18.1) (39–46). The complete response rate ranged from 39% to 77%. The success rate for definitive mitomycin therapy for CIS is 58% (37). When used after thiotepa failure as a secondary chemotherapy, the response rates ranged from 39% to 46% (Table 18.2) (47–50).

The efficacy of mitomycin has also been established as a prophylactic agent (Table 18.3). Huland *et al.* (56) compared long-term mitomycin instillation therapy with no intravesical therapy in a randomized trial after complete TUR. The percentage of recurrences was 10.4% in the mitomycin group compared with

Table 18.1

COMPLETE RESPONSES TO INTRAVESICAL MITOMYCIN IN PATIENTS WITH PRIMARY SUPERFICIAL BLADDER CANCER			
Investigator	**No. of patients**	**Dose/schedule**	**%CR**
Mishina *et al.* (39)	50	20 mg 3×/week (20 instillations)	44
DeFuria *et al.* (40)	55	20–60 mg/week×8	45
Bracken *et al.* (41)	43	various (20–60 mg)×8	49
Harrison *et al.* (42)	23	20 mg 3◊/week×7	77
Lucero *et al.* (43)	21	40 mg/week×8	48
Hetherington *et al.* (44)	43	20 mg/week×8–12	56
Heney *et al.* (45)	76	40 mg/week×8	39
Stricker *et al.* (46)	15	30 mg/week×8	73*

* One patient died from unrelated cause. Two had recurrences and were treated with transurethral resection and bacille Calmette–Guérin.
CR, complete response.

Table 18.2

COMPLETE RESPONSES (CRS) TO SECONDARY TREATMENT WITH INTRAVESICAL MITOMYCIN IN PATIENTS WITH SUPERFICIAL BLADDER CANCER			
Investigator	No. of patients	Dose/schedule	%CR
Soloway (47)	74	40 mg/week×8*	39
Prout *et al.* (48)	23	40 mg/week×8	43
Koontz *et al.* (49)	100	40 mg/week×8	46
Issell *et al.* (50)	57	40 mg/week×8	42
* Six patients received other doses.			

51% in the control group. Short-term prophylaxis (20 instillations of 20 mg in 20 weeks) was shown to give similar results, indicating the lack of advantage of maintenance therapy (33). The majority of these patients were, however, at low risk of recurrence whether because of low-grade tumours or low previous rate of recurrence. Single instillation and non-maintenance therapy after complete TUR showed an advantage of mitomycin of 15% according to Lamm (61).

In a randomized trial to compare the efficacy of mitomycin and thiotepa conducted by the National Bladder Cancer Group, patients with residual tumour were given either thiotepa 30 mg or mitomycin 40 mg weekly for 8 weeks. Mitomycin was superior to thiotepa in this trial, with a complete response rate of 39% compared with 26% for thiotepa (45).

Conclusions

MMC has few systemic side-effects. The frequency of drug-induced cystitis is similar to other agents. Reversible allergic reactions occur in up to 10% of patients. The response rate of

Table 18.3

RECURRENCE OF SUPERFICIAL BLADDER CANCER AFTER MITOMYCIN PROPHYLAXIS				
Investigator	No. of patients	Dose/schedule	%rec	follow up
Fluchter *et al.* (54)	105	20 mg/d ×10; repeat after 6 weeks	12	22.3
Niijima *et al.* (55)	139	20 mg 2× / week×4	57*	18
Huland *et al.* (56,57)	54	20 mg q2week×12 months, then 20mg/months×24 months	11	33.5
DeBruyne *et al.* (52)	167	30 mg/week×4, then 30 mg/months ×6	36	21
Tolley *et al.* (58)	138	40 mg post-TUR then 40mg×4 during 12 months	42	24
Doccardo *et al.* (59)	141	40 mg/week×8	37	15.5
* The recurrence rate for patients with a newly diagnosed tumour was 16% at 12 months (62).				

mitomycin is better than the other chemotherapeutic agents. The advantage of mitomycin maintenance therapy is, however, controversial.

OTHER INTRAVESICAL CHEMOTHERAPIES

Ethoglucid (Epodyl)

The mechanism of action of ethoglucid is poorly understood and the experience with this agent in superficial bladder cancer is limited. The molecular weight is 262 Da, and hence it is not absorbed and the systemic side-effects are rare. The most important side-effects are drug-induced cystitis ranging from 13% to 59% of patients (62,63).

The use of ethoglucid as definitive therapy was associated with 42% complete response accumulating data from three studies (37). The recurrence rates for doxorubicin and ethoglucid were found to be the exact same but both were better than no treatment in the European Organization for Research and Treatment of Cancer (EORTC)–Genitourinary Tract Cancer Co-operative (GU) group study (64). In summary, ethoglucid appears to be as effective as thiotepa and doxorubicin. The side-effects are usually mild and infrequent.

Cisplatin

Intravesical cisplatin was demonstrated not to be significantly different from doxorubicin and thiotepa as regards recurrence and progression in an EORTC trial (65). The serious side-effect in this study was anaphylaxis in 10% of patients leading to hypotension. Cisplatin is considered risky and not of benefit to these patients.

Epirubicin

The antitumour effect is similar to doxorubicin but with less incidence of side-effects (66). Burk et al. (67) reported on toxicity in a large series of 911 patients treated with epirubicin. The dose used in the majority of patients was 50 mg in 8-weekly instillations. Systemic toxicity was absent and chemical cystitis was reported in 14% of patients. The frequency of drug-induced cystitis can be reduced with a smaller dose as demonstrated by the EORTC study using a single instillation of 80 mg, the incidence of chemical cystitis was reduced to 6.8% (68). The same study demonstrated a recurrence rate with epirubicin that is significantly lower than the control group.

The main side-effect of epirubicin seem to be drug-induced cystitis. The incidence is lower than with other drugs. The studies to demonstrate the efficacy of epirubicin were underpowered to draw solid conclusions on the efficacy. Also, the use of epirubicin as a maintenance was not shown to be significantly different.

EFFICACY AND COMPARISON WITH IMMUNOTHERAPY

Multiple studies as shown in Table 18.4 have tried to compare intravesical chemotherapy with immunotherapy using BCG. In the majority of the studies, BCG provides superior protection from tumour recurrence when compared with thiotepa and doxorubicin. In the study by Witjes et al. (70), the recurrence rates with BCG were comparable with those with MMC using two different BCG strains.

The Southwest Oncology Group study comparing BCG (Connaught strain) and doxorubicin demonstrated the long-term response as well as the higher response rates attainable with BCG than chemotherapy in cases of CIS. Complete responses were achieved in 34% and 70% of patients receiving doxorubicin and BCG, respectively. Sixty-four per cent of the patients treated with BCG maintained their complete response at 5 years. At 5 years follow up, 18% versus 45% from the doxorubicin and BCG arms, respectively, remained disease free (72).

The argument against intravesical chemotherapy has been the failure to produce recurrence-free rates that lasted more than 5 years. Meta-analysis of four EORTC and two MRC trials,

Table 18.4

RECURRENCE IN CONTROLLED STUDIES COMPARING BACILLE CALMETTE–GUÉRIN (BCG) AGAINST CHEMOTHERAPEUTIC AGENTS IN THE INTRAVESICAL TREATMENT OF SUPERFICIAL TRANSITIONAL CELL CANCER OF THE BLADDER

| Investigator | Recurrence (%) | | | |
	BCG	Thiotepa	Doxorubicin	Mitomycin C
Lamm et al., 1991 (36)	63		83	
DeBruyne et al., 1988 (70)	30			25
Witjes et al., 1995 (71)	29 (RIVM) 34 (Tice)			26
Lamm et al., 1993 (72)	20			33
Martinez et al., 1990 (34)	13	36	43	

however, showed long-term median follow up of 7.7 years reduction of recurrence after intravesical chemotherapy. An advantage in reducing tumour progression, which is a higher goal, could not be demonstrated (73). However, these results should be taken with caution because of the multiple variables in these studies.

In five clinical trials comparing the intravesical MMC versus BCG, two significantly favoured BCG and three were not significantly different. The average data from these five studies show the recurrence rate of MMC to be 36% versus 29% for BCG (3).

It remains obscure why obvious reduction in recurrence does not necessarily result in decreased tumour progression. The possible explanation is that intravesical chemotherapy does not influence the deeper layers of the urothelium where potentially invasive tumours originate.

COMBINATION THERAPY

The combination of MMC (20 mg/20 ml saline) and doxorubicin (40 mg/20 ml saline) given on alternate days on days 1 and 2 of each week for 5 consecutive weeks (74). Sixty-one per cent of patients showed a complete response and were randomized to non-maintenance versus monthly instillations for a period of 1 year. The non-recurrence rates at 2 years for patients with CIS and papillary tumours were almost significant.

Rintala et al. (75) in a study of 188 patients with superficial bladder cancer used intravesical mitomycin in the first 48 h following resection of the tumour. Patients then received four additional MMC weekly treatments. The patients were randomized after that to receive MMC or alternating courses of MMC and BCG. Time to recurrence was 12 months for the MMC arm versus 7 months for the combination therapy arm.

CONCLUSIONS

Superficial transitional cell carcinoma of the bladder is a heterogeneous group of tumours, with a high tendency to recur (up to 80% in 10 years). Recurrences might be due to implantation at the time of resection. Tumour progression accounts for 10–20% of cases. Principles of intravesical therapy should be considered for maximal efficacy. These include factors related to the bladder, bladder cavity, drug, and tumour. Care should be taken to avoid injury of the bladder mucosa to prevent systemic drug absorption.

Intravesical therapy can be used in the majority of patients with superficial bladder tumours. It is safe in regard to systemic side-effects. All chemotherapeutic agents tend to cause local side-effects. Chemical cystitis is the most common. Local side-effects tend to be reversible. Differences in dosage and instillation should be considered for better results.

All chemotherapeutic agents have been shown to reduce recurrence rate. None is able to prevent progression. There is no demonstrated advantage for maintenance regimens. Use of intravesical chemotherapy should be limited to intermediate risk patients following resection of the tumour. Low risk lesions are followed up with no intravesical therapy. Immunotherapy is used in case of high risk tumours, failed chemotherapy, and CIS.

References

1 Wingo PA, Tong T, Bolden S. Cancer statistics. *CA Cancer J Clin* 1995, 45, 8–11.
2 Parker SL, Tong T, Bolden S, Wingo PA. Cancer statistics. *CA Cancer J Clin* 1997, **47**, 5–9.
3 Lamm DL, Torti FM. Bladder cancer. *CA Cancer J Clin* 1996, 46, 93–7.
4 Devesa SS, Blot WJ, Stone BJ *et al.* Recent cancer trends in the United States. *J Natl Cancer Inst* 1995, **87**, 175.
5 Abel PD. Prognostic indices in transitional cell carcinoma of the bladder. *Br J Urol* 1998, **62**, 103–5.
6 Fair WR, Fukus ZY, Scher HI. Cancer of the bladder. In: *Principles and practice of oncology* (ed. DeVita VT Jr, Hellman S, Rosenberg SA). JB Lippincott, Philadelphia, 1993, pp. 1052–1072.
7 Smith JA. Laser surgery for transitional cell carcinoma: technique, advantages and limitations. *Urol Clin North Am* 1992, **19**, 473–83.
8 Lamm DL, Griffith JG. Intravesical therapy: Does it affect the natural history of surperficial bladder cancer? *Semin Urol* 1992, **10**, 39–44.
9 Soloway MS. Introduction and overview of intravesical therapy for superficial bladder cancer. *Urology* 1988, **31**, 5–11.
10 Hasui Y, Osada Y, Kitada S *et al.* Significance of invasion to the muscularis mucosae on the progression of superficial bladder cancer. *Urology* 1994, **43**, 782–6.
11 Farrow GM. Pathology of carcinoma in situ of the urinary bladder and related lesions. *J Cell Biochem*, 1992, **161**, 39–43.
12 Hudson MA, Herr HW. Carcinoma in situ of the bladder. *J Urol* 1995, **153**, 564–72.
13 American Joint Committee on Cancer. *Manual for staging of cancer*, Lippincott, Philadelphia, 1988, pp. 193–207.
14 Crawford ED. Diagnosis and treatment of superficial bladder cancer: an update. *Semin Urol Oncol* 1996, **14**, 1–9.
15 Bostwick DG. Natural history of early bladder cancer. *J Cell Biochem*, 1992, **161**, 31–8.
16 Badalament RA, Farah RN. Treatment of superficial bladder cancer with intravesical chemotherapy. *Semin Surg Oncol* 1997, **13**, 335–41.
17 Soloway MS. Managing superficial bladder cancer: An overview. *Urology* 1992, **40**, 5–17.
18 Abderrazak M, Pentue F, Ziadé J *et al.* Pharmacokinetics of plasma mitomycin C (MMC) when instilled immediately following transurethral resection for bladder tumor. *J Urol* 1997, **157** (4), 50 (abstract 188).
19 Wientjes MG, Badalament RA, Au JL. Use of pharmacologic data and computer simulations to design an efficacy trial of intravesical mitomycin C therapy for superficial bladder cancer. *Cancer Chemother Pharmacol* 1995, **32**, 255–62.
20 Schmittgen TD, Wientjes MG, Badalament RA, Au JL. Pharmacodynamics of mitomycin C in cultured human bladder tumors. *Cancer Res* 1991, **51**, 3849–56.

21 Witjes JA, Oosterhof GO, Debruyne FM. Management of superficial bladder cancer Ta/T1/Tis: Intravesical chemotherapy. In: *Comprehensive textbook of genitourinary oncology* (ed. Vogelzang NJ, Scardino PT, Shipley WU, Coffey DS). Williams and Wilkins, New York, 1996, p. 416–29.

22 Tarkington M, Sommers CL, Gelmann EP *et al.* The effect of pH on the in vitro conlony forming ability of transitional cell carcinoma cells treated with various chemotherapeutic agents: implications for in vivo therapy. *J Urol* 1992, **147**, 511–3.

23 Weaver D, Khare N, Haigh J *et al.* The effect of chemotherapeutic agents on the ultrasturcture of transitional cell carcinoma in tissue culture. *Invest Urol* 1980, **17**, 288–92.

24 Koontz WW Jr, Prout GR, Smith W *et al.* The use of intravesical thiotepa in the management of noninvasive carcinoma of the bladder. *J Urol* 1981, **125**, 307–12.

25 Jones HC, Swinney J. Thiotepa in the treatment of tumors of the bladder. *Lancet*, 1961, **ii**, 615–6.

26 Hollister D, Coleman M. Hematologic effects of intravesical thiotepa thearpy for bladder carcinoma. *JAMA*, 1980, **244**, 2065–7.

27 Soloway MS, Ford KS. Thiotepa induced myelosuppression: review of 670 bladder instillations. *J Urol* 1983, **130**, 889–91.

28 Thrasher JB, Crawford ED. Complications of intravesical chemotherapy. *Urol Clin North Am* 1992, **19**, 529–39.

29 Medical Research Council. The effect of intravesical thotepa on the recurrence rate of newly diagnosed superficial bladder cancer. An MRC study. *Br J Urol* 1985, **57**, 680–8.

30 Prout GR, Koontz WW Jr, Coombs LJ *et al.* Long term fate of 90 patients with superficial bladder cancer randomly assigned to receive or not to receive thiotepa. *J Urol* 1983, **130**, 677–80.

31 Garnick MB, Schade D, Israel M *et al.* Intravesical doxorubicin for prophylaxis in the management of recurrent superficial bladder cancer. *J Urol* 1984, **131**, 43–8.

32 Flamm J. Long term versus short term doxorubicin hydrochloride instillation after transurethral resection of superficial bladder cancer. *Eur Urol* 1990, **17**, 119–22.

33 Huland H, Kloeppel G, Feddersen I *et al.* Comparison of different schedules of cytostatic intravesical instillations in patients with superficial bladder carcinoma: final evaluation of a prospective multicenter study with 419 patients. *J Urol* 1990, **144**, 68–71.

34 Martinez-Pineiro JA, Jimenez Leon J, Martinez-Pineiro L Jr *et al.* Bacillus Calmette Guérin versus doxorubicin versus thiotepa: a randomized retrospective study in 202 patients with superficial bladder cancer. *J Urol* 1990, **143**, 502–6.

35 Lundbeck F, Mogensen P, Jeppeson N. Intravesical therapy of noninvasive bladder tumors (stage Ta) with doxorubicin and urokinase. *J Urol* 1983, **130**, 1087–91.

36 Lamm DL, Blumenstein BA, Crawford ED *et al.* A randomized trial of intravesical doxorubicin and immunotherapy with Bacillus Calmette Guérin for transitional cell carcinoma of the bladder. *N Engl J Med*, 1991, **325**, 1205–9.

37 Bouffioux C, Meijden APM, Kurth KH *et al.* Objective response of superficial bladder tumors to intravesical treatment. *Prog Clin Biol Res* 1992, **378**, 29–42.

38 Zincke H, Utz DC, Taylor WF *et al.* Influence of thiotepa and doxoruicin instillation at the time of transurethral surgical treatment of bladder cancer on tumor recurrence: a prospective, randomized double-blind controlled trial. *J Urol* 1983, **129**, 505–9.

39 Mishina T, Oda K, Murata S *et al.* Mitomycin C bladder instillation therapy for bladder tumors. *J Urol* 1975, **130**, 217–9.

40 DeFuria MD, Bracken RB, Johnson DE *et al.* Phase I-II study of mitomycin-C topical therapy for low-grade, low stage transitional cell carcinoma of the bladder: An interim report. *Cancer Treat Rep*, 1980, **64**, 225–30.

41 Bracken RB, Swanson DA, Johnson DE *et al.* Role of intravesical mitomycin C in management of superficial bladder tumors. *Urology* 1980, **16**, 11–5.

42 Harrison GSM, Green DF, Newling DWW *et al.* A phase II study of intravesical mitomycin C in the treatment of superficial bladder cancer. *Br J Urol* 1983, **55**, 676–9.

43 Lucero SP, Wise HAII. Intravesical therapy of low stage bladder carcinoma with mitomycin C. *J Urol* 1986, **135**, 186A (abstract 39).

44   Hetherington JW, Newling DWW, Robinson MRG *et al.* Intravesical mito-
     mycin C for the treatment of recurrent superficial bladder tumors. *Br J Urol*
     1987, **59**, 239–41.

45   Heney NM, Koontz WW, Barton B *et al.* Intravesical thiotepa versus mito-
     mycin C in patients with TA, T1, TIS transitional cell carcinoma of the
     bladder: A phase III prospective randomized trial. *J Urol* 1988, **140**, 1390–3.

46   Stricker PD, Grant ABF, Hosken BM *et al.* Topical mitomycin C therapy for
     carcinoma in situ of the bladder: A follow up. *J Urol* 1990, **143**, 34–5.

47   Soloway MS. Evaluation and management of patients with superficial bladder
     cancer. *Urol Clin North Am* 1987, **114**, 771–83.

48   Prout GR Jr, Griffin PP, Nocks BN *et al.* Intravesical therapy of low stage
     bladder carcinoma with mitomycin C. Comparison of results of untreated and
     previously treated patients. *J Urol* 1982, **127**, 1096–8.

49   Koontz WW Jr, Heney N, Soloway M *et al.* The ablative effect of mitomycin C
     in patients with superficial bladder carcinoma who have previously failed
     therapy with intravesical thiotepa. *J Urol* 1984, **131**, 238A (abstr 537).

50   Issell BF, Prout GR Jr, Soloway MS *et al.* Mitomycin C intravesical therapy in
     noninvasive bladder cancer after failure on thiotepa. *Cancer*, 1984, **53**, 1025–8.

51   Zein TA, Freidberg N, Kim H. Bone marrow suppression after intravesical
     mitomycin C treatment. *J Urol* 1986, **136**, 459–62.

52   Debruyne FMJ, Meijden AVD, Witjes JA *et al.* Bacillus Calmette Guérin versus
     mitomycin C intravesical therapy in superficial bladder cancer. Results of a
     randomized trial after 21 months of follow up. *Urology* 1992, **40**, 11–7.

53   Witjes JA, Meijden AVD, Witjes WPJ *et al.* A randomized prospective study
     comparing intravesical instillations of Mitomycin C, BCG-Tice, BCG-RIVM
     in pTa-pT1 tumors and primary carcinoma in situ of the urinary bladder.
     Intravesical instillations in superficial bladder cancer. *Eur J Cancer*, 1993, **29A**,
     1672–4.

54   Fluchter SH, Harzmann R, Bichler K-H. Local mitomycin C therapy of transi-
     tional cell carcinoma of the bladder—serum resorption study and clinical
     results. In: *Mitomycin C, current impact on cancer chemotherapy* (ed. Ogawa M,
     Rozencweig M, Staquet MJ). Excerpta Medica, Amsterdam, 1982, pp. 143–52.

55   Niijima T, Koiso K, Akaza H *et al.* Randomized clinical trial on chemopro-
     phylaxis of recurrence in cases of superficial bladder cancer. *Cancer Chemother
     Pharmacol* 1983, **11**, 79–82.

56   Huland H, Otto U, Drose M *et al.* Long term Mitomycin C instillation after
     transurethral resection of superficial bladder carcinoma: Influence on recur-
     rence, progression and survival. *J Urol* 1984, **132**, 27–9.

57   Huland H, Otto U. Use of mitomycin as prophylaxis following endoscopic
     resection of superficial bladder cancer. *Urology* 1985, **26**, 32–5.

58   Tolley DA, Hargreave TB, Smith PH *et al.* Effect of intravesical mitomycin C
     on recurrence of newly diagnosed superficial bladder cancer: interim report
     from the Medical Research Council Subgroup on Superficial Bladder Cancer
     (Urological Cancer Working Party). *Br Med J*, 1998, **296**, 1759–61.

59   Boccardo F, Cannata D, Rubagotti A *et al.* Prophylaxis of superficial bladder
     cancer with mitomycin or interferon alfa-2b: Results of a multicentric Italian
     study. *J Clin Oncol* 1994, **12**, 7–13.

60   Akaza H, Isaka S, Koiso K *et al.* Comparative analysis of short term and long
     term prophylactic intravesical chemotherapy of superficial bladder cancer:
     Prospective, randomized, controlled studies of the Japanese Urological Cancer
     Research Group. *Cancer Chemother Pharmacol* 1987, **20**, S91–S96.

61   Lamm DL. Long term results of intravesical therapy for superficial bladder
     cancer. *Urol Clin North Am* 1992, **19**, 573–84.

62   Robinson MRG, Shelty MB, Richards B *et al.* Intravesical epodyl in the man-
     agement of bladder tumors: combined experience of the Yorkshire Urological
     Cancer Research Group. *J Urol* 1977, **118**, 972–3.

63   Flamm J, Bucher A. Adjuvant topical chemotherapy versus immunotherapy in
     primary superficial transitional cell carcinoma of the bladder. *Br J Urol* 1991,
     67, 70–3.

64   Meijden AVD, Kurth KH, Oosterlink W *et al.* Intravesical therapy with adri-
     amycin and 4-epirubicin for superficial bladder cancer: the experience of the
     EORTC-GU group. *Cancer Chemother Pharmacol* 1992, **30**, S95–8.

65   Bouffioux C, Denis L, Oosterlinck W *et al.* Adjuvant chemotherapy of recur-
     rent superficial transitional cell carcinoma: results of an European
     Organisation for Research on Treatment of Cancer randomized trial compar-

ing intravesical instillations of thiotepa, doxorubicin and cisplatin. *J Urol* 1992, **148**, 297–301.

66 Cersosimo RJ, Hong WK. Epirubicin: a review of the pharmacology, clinical activity and adverse effects of an adriamycin analogue. *J Clin Oncol* 1986, **4**, 425–39.

67 Burk K, Kurth KH, Newling D. Epirubicin in treatment and recurrence prophylaxis of patients with superficial bladder cancer. *Prog Clin Biol Res* 1989, **303**, 423–34.

68 Oosterlinck W, Kurth KH, Schroder F *et al.* A prospective European Organisation for Research on Treatment of Cancer randomized trial comparing transurethral resection followed by a single intravesical instillation of epirubicin or water in single Ta, T1 papillary carcinoma of the bladder. *J Urol* 1993, **149**, 749–52.

69 DeBruyne FM, Van der Meijden AP, Geboers AD *et al.* BCG (RIVM) versus mitomycin intravesical therapy in superficial bladder cancer: First results of a randomized prospective trial. *Urology* 1998, **31**, 20–6.

70 Vegt PD, Witjes JA, Witjes WP *et al.* A randomized study of intravesical mitomycin C, Bacillus Calmette Guérin Tice and Bacillus Calmette Guérin RIVM treatment in pTa-pT1 papillary carcinoma and carcinoma in situ of the bladder. *J Urol* 1995, **153**, 929–33.

71 Lamm DL, Crawford ED, Blumenstein B *et al.* A randomized comparison of Bacillus Calmette Guérin and mitomycin C prophylaxis in stage Ta and T1 transitional cell carcinoma of the bladder. *J Urol* 1993, **149**, 282A.

72 Lamm DL. Carcinoma in situ. *Urol Clin North Am* 1992, **19**, 499–514.

73 Pawinski A, Bouffioux C, Sylvester R *et al.* Meta-analysis of EORTC/MRC randomised clinical trials for the prophylactic treatment of Ta, T1 bladder cancer. *J Urol* 1996, **155**, 492A.

74 Fukui I, Kihara K, Sekine H *et al.* Intravesical combination therapy with mitomycin C and doxorubicin for superficial bladder cancer: a randomized trial of maintenance versus no maintenance following a complete response. *Cancer Chemother Pharmacol* 1992, **30**, S37–40.

75 Rintala E, Jauhiainen K, Kassinen E *et al.* Alternating mitomycin C and Bacillus Calmette Guérin instillation prophylaxis for recurrent papillary (stages Ta to T1) superficial bladder cancer. *Finnbladder Group J Urol* 1996, **156**, 56–9.

19. IMMUNOTHERAPY OF BLADDER CANCER

David Hall, John Battin, Unyime O. Nseyo, and Donald L. Lamm

INTRODUCTION

In the United States the incidence of bladder cancer increased 26% from 1956 to 1990, nevertheless mortality has declined by 8% following the introduction, of bacille Calmette–Guérin (BCG) immunotherapy and effective cisplatinum-based combination chemotherapy. Intravesical immunotherapy has reduced disease progression and may have contributed to observed decline in mortality. The antineoplastic effect of the live attenuated tuberculosis vaccine, BCG, was reported by Pearl in 1929. However, Morales, in 1976 was the first to report the results of intravesical BCG in the management of early stage bladder cancer. Many clinical investigations have demonstrated the superior benefit of intravesical BCG in the management of superficial bladder cancer, and currently BCG remains the gold standard by which treatments of aggressive superficial bladder cancer must be compared. This chapter contains highlights of the recent advances in intravesical immunotherapy of bladder cancer, summarizes the mechanisms of action of BCG, and reviews the important role of intravesical BCG immunotherapy as well as other immunotherapeutic agents in the therapy and prophylaxis of superficial transitional cell carcinoma (TCC) of the urinary bladder.

INDICATIONS FOR INTRAVESICAL IMMUNOTHERAPY

Since its introduction in the 1950s, intravesical therapy has been employed in the management of superficial bladder cancer with three specific goals: ablating existing/residual tumour, preventing recurrence of tumour after complete bladder tumour resection, and preventing progression of disease. The objectives of intravesical therapy should be tailored to the individual patient. Intravesical therapy is most effective when tumour burden is reduced by transurethral resection (TUR) of papillary disease. The inherent biological characteristics of the patient's tumour are important determinant factors in the decision for intravesical therapy. For example, an advanced grade tumour, which is at a high risk for recurrence and progression, constitutes an accepted indication for intravesical therapy. In the absence of other risk factors for progression, intravesical therapy is not required for grade I/Ta lesions which have a progression rate of only 2%. T1 disease, irrespective of grade, has the biological propensity to invade, and has a reported progression rate of 29% (1). Intravesical therapy is therefore justified in patients with T1 disease to prevent progression to muscle invasion. Carcinoma *in situ* (CIS) has a high risk of disease progression with an average of 52% of patients developing invasive disease within 4 years in the absence of intravesical therapy (2). Therefore, the presence of even small foci of CIS should be considered as a definite indication for intravesical therapy. Multifocal superficial disease irrespective of grade or stage is also associated with increased risk of tumour recurrence and progression and constitutes an indication for adjuvant intravesical therapy. Prostatic urethral involvement with CIS carries an especially high risk of progression and poor prognosis, and should be treated aggressively. The use of intravesical BCG immunotherapy has effectively spared cystectomy in many of these patients (2), and multiple reports indicate that BCG is effective in the treatment of TCC in the prostatic urethra. TUR is recommended to stage the disease and widen the bladder neck in order to facilitate BCG to bathe the prostatic urethra. Other relative indications for intravesical therapy include low-grade Ta disease recurring within 2 years, persistent positive urine cytology without associated upper tract lesions, and urothelial dysplasia or severe atypia.

Muscle-invasive disease does not generally respond to intravesical therapy and therefore such patients are offered radical cystectomy as the treatment of choice, and radiation with or without adjunctive chemotherapy as an alternative management option.

MECHANISMS OF BACILLE CALMETTE–GUÉRIN ACTION

BCG is recognized as a non-specific immune stimulant. Intravesical BCG induces inflammation of the bladder with infiltration of a broad range of cell types. BCG may activate macrophages, T lymphocytes, B lymphocytes, natural killer cells and killer cells. Intravesical BCG immunotherapy results in cytokine production, including interleukins (IL) 1, 2, and 6, interferon (IFN) gamma and tumour necrosis factor (TNF) alpha, which can be measured in the urine for many hours after instillation. McAveray reported that BCG induces a local type II immunological response mediated by

IL-4, IL-1, and IL-10, which suppress cell-mediated responses These cytokines cause a shift to type I response with the subsequent development of a protective antitumour response. Ratliff investigated the role of CD4 and CD8 lymphokines in the antitumour response of BCG and was unable to find evidence of induction of protective immunity after intravesical BCG. However, they reported a requirement of T lymphocytes, and CD4 and CD8 subsets in BCG-mediated antitumour activity. They concluded that BCG-mediated antitumour activity is a localized phenomenon, and does not involve specific immunity. BCG stimulates cytokine production, and this in turn enhances natural killer cell activity, which increases after BCG immunotherapy. Conti reported that immunotherapeutic effects of BCG in bladder cancer patients are related to its capacity to prime macrophages which enhance the release of TNF alpha and IL-1 alpha, but not IL-6, involved in tumour killing. BCG produces a T-cell-mediated immune response that has been linked to antitumour activity in both humans and mice. The antineoplastic effect of BCG is mostly likely the result of a combination of enhanced activity of various arms of the immune system. After intravesical instillation live mycobacteria attach to the urothelial lining, facilitated by fibronectin, a component of the extracellular matrix. BCG can also be internalized into bladder tumour cells by attachment to integrins. This process leaves bacterial cell surface glycoproteins attached to epithelial cell membranes, and this antigen is thought to mediate the immune response. Tumour cell motility is also thought to be inhibited by BCG through a mechanism involving the BCG fibronectin–tumour cell interaction. Bladder biopsies following BCG administration show increased expression of human leucocyte antigen DR antigens on tumour cells and infiltration of tumour and stroma with lymphocytes, predominantly T-helper cells, and macrophages The helper/suppressor ratio in infiltrating lymphocytes is increased. Changes in peripheral blood are also seen, including heightened immunoproliferative response of BCG antigen and production of BCG-specific antibody.

PRINCIPLES OF BACILLE CALMETTE–GUÉRIN IMMUNOTHERAPY

To use immunotherapy effectively in the management of bladder cancer or other malignancy it is important to consider basic principles and understand what makes BCG immunotherapy different from chemotherapy. Immunotherapy may be either non-specific or specific. More often than not, optimal responses to immunotherapy are seen at less than the maximum tolerated dose because high dose treatment invokes complex immune regulatory mechanisms. The typical dose–response curve with biological response modifiers such as BCG is therefore bell shaped, with optimal responses occurring at intermediate doses (3). Immune stimulation usually peaks with the sixth instillation in patients who have not been previously treated. In patients who receive a subsequent course of BCG, immune stimulation generally peaks at the third instillation. With continued treatment or excessively high doses of BCG, the immune response is suppressed (3). The resultant BCG-induced immune stimulation persists for many months and results in tumour destruction.

The failure of BCG immunotherapy in many previous trials in other malignancies is probably in part a result of ignoring the principles of optimal BCG immunotherapy previously defined in animal studies. These principles include juxtaposition of BCG and tumour cells, minimization of tumour burden, and use of an adequate number of viable bacteria. Clinically, ensuring direct contact of BCG with the tumour may require resection of the prostate or instillation of BCG in the upper tract for disease outside the bladder. BCG has a complete response rate of 60% or more when used to treat residual stage Ta or Tl bladder cancer, but based on the animal studies, it is generally preferable to resect all visible tumours when possible prior to beginning treatment. The optimal dose of BCG remains to be defined, and may, like the optimal treatment schedule, vary from patient to patient. Current data suggest an intravesical dose between 100 million (1×10^8) and 1 billion (1×10^{10}). Colony forming units (CFU) are effective, but responses have been reported with doses as low as 10 million CFU or 1 mg BCG. The wide variation in effective clinical doses probably relates to the mode of administration. With intravesical instillation, only those organisms that attach to the bladder wall stimulate an immune response. Consideration must therefore also be given to avoid administration of medications that can limit the effectiveness of the dose given. Agents that inhibit clot formation reduce fibronectin expression and can reduce BCG attachment, immune stimulation, and antitumour activity. Similarly, concern has been raised that administration of antitubercular antibiotics such as isoniazid (INH), which inhibit intravesical BCG attachment and immune stimulation in the guinea-pig model. Until additional data become available caution should be exercised when isoniazid, trimethoprim/sulphamethoxazole, and quinolone are used in patients receiving BCG. However, these antibiotics should be used without hesitation to treat the side-effects of BCG or infection when indicated.

Tumour biomarkers in intravesical therapy of bladder cancer

Traditionally, bladder tumour response to intravesical chemo/immunotherapy is assessed with cystoscopy and cytopathological analysis. The development of valid tumour biomarkers as intermediate end-points would be clinically useful in assessing treatment outcome in patients with superficial bladder cancer. Genomic markers which include expression and amplification of various oncogenes such as P53, ras, and epidermal growth factor (EGF) receptor could be correlated with the bladder tumour response to intravesical chemo/immunotherapy. Measurement of DNA aneuploidy has been found not to be a useful biomarker in monitoring therapy for superficial bladder cancer. However, the use of DNA ploidy and cell cycle analysis in conjunction with urinary cytology could enhance prognostication of response to intravesical therapy. Also DNA ploidy and S-phase fraction measured by flow cytometry could provide useful prognostic information for treated patients with superficial TCC. Quantitative fluorescence image analysis (QFIA) cytology can be applied to quantitate DNA changes in bladder cancer following intravesical therapy. QFIA sensitivity is tumour grade dependent, the higher the grade, the greater its sensitivity. However, its prognostic utility in monitoring response therapy in patients with superficial TCC has not yet been adequately studied.

Proliferation markers such as S-fraction and the monoclonal antibody Ki-67 are candidates as biomarkers for monitoring therapy. The percentage of cells in S-phase correlates with tumour progression and survival as well as disease stage and grade. The Ki-67 monoclonal antibody detects a nuclear antigen present in all phases of the cell cycle except G_O, and increased levels of Ki-67 have prognostic significance in bladder cancer. The proliferation markers S-fraction, DNA ploidy, and Ki-67 monoclonal antibody should be assessed for their usefulness in monitoring intravesical chemo/immunotherapy for superficial TCC.

Finally, the differentiation markers, ABO blood group family of cell surface antigens, have prognostic significance in bladder cancer. ABO antigen deletion or weak expression in bladder cancer is an early event in tumour progression and often precedes the development of DNA aneuploidy. However, application of assays of these surface antigens to monitor intravesical therapy should be studied. As we strive to improve disease survival significantly in superficial bladder cancer, incorporation of biomarker assays in monitoring intravesical therapy could enhance identification of patients harbouring resistant bladder cancer and aid in the selection of optimal treatment.

BACILLE CALMETTE–GUÉRIN USE IN CARCINOMA *IN SITU*

Immunotherapy, in the form of BCG is the only approved intravesical treatment for CIS. In a unique prospective randomized trial, Herr showed BCG therapy to be superior to TUR alone in eradicating multifocal diffuse CIS (4). Currently, more than 1500 patients with CIS of the bladder have been treated with BCG with an average complete response rate of 72% (Table 19.1). By comparison, complete response rates for chemotherapy average less than 50%. Specifically, in the treatment of CIS, the reported overall complete response is 48% in 448 patients treated with chemotherapy: 38% in 89 patients treated with thiotepa, 48% in 212 patients treated with doxorubicin, and 53% in 147 patients treated with mitomycin (MMC) (5). Controlled chemotherapy trials provide no evidence that any of the newer chemotherapies provide superior protection from tumour recurrence; however, the above studies show a statistically significant increased complete response to MMC compared with thiotepa. There is no statistically significant advantage to MMC treatment compared with doxorubicin. In most series, fewer than 20% of patients treated with chemotherapy remain disease-free for more than 5 years, whereas 64% of patients with complete response to BCG remain disease-free when treated with suboptimal treatment schedules (6). Complete response can be improved even more with maintenance BCG schedules using instillations each week

Table 19.1

COMPARISON OF BACILLE CALMETTE–GUÉRIN (BCG) STRAINS IN THE TREATMENT OF CARCINOMA *IN SITU* OF THE BLADDER			
Strain/series	**Total no. of patients**	**Complete responses (%)**	**Range of response rates (%)**
Connaught	450	357 (79%)	70–92%
Tokyo	111	86 (77%)	63–84%
Pasteur	230	171 (74%)	40–80%
Tice	277	197 (71%)	56–82%
Evans	180	117 (65%)	53–88%
A. Frappier	145	87 (60%)	39–100%
S African	13	9 (69%)	—
Danish	42	28 (67%)	—
Romanian	33	21 (64%)	—
RIVM	15	9 (60%)	—
Total	1496	1082 (72%)	39–100%

for 3 weeks at 3 months, 6 months, and every 6 months for 3 years Estimated 5-year disease-free rates can be increased to 75% using this method (7).

BACILLE CALMETTE–GUÉRIN USE IN PAPILLARY TRANSITIONAL CELL CARCINOMA

Use of BCG in superficial TCC of the bladder is a matter quite different from CIS. Patients who present with a single, low-grade, stage Ta tumour do not need BCG treatment, because the risk for recurrence and progression are low. However, T1 disease has the biological ability to invade and has a reported progression rate of 29% at 1 year (1). BCG remains the most effective intravesical agent for the therapy and prophylaxis of superficial bladder. Multiple studies confirm that BCG reduces bladder tumour recurrence and progression, increasing the disease-free interval and prolonging survival (8). Controlled comparisons of BCG immunotherapy versus surgery alone have demonstrated a statistically significant reduction in tumour recurrence in each of the six studies. The use of BCG reduced the recurrence rate from 67% to 29% on average, a 38% improvement (Table 19.2). Comparison studies of BCG and intravesical chemotherapy also demonstrate the superiority of BCG to thiotepa, doxorubicin, and MMC. The Southwest Oncology Group (7) performed a randomized study on 453 high risk patients with stage Ta or T1 disease. Patients were either given BCG (50 mg) or MMC (20 mg). Both treatments were given weekly for 6 weeks and then monthly for 1 year.

Table 19.2

EFFECT OF INTRAVESICAL BACILLE CALMETTE–GUÉRIN (BCG) ON RECURRENCE IN CONTROLLED STUDIES

| Control group (TURBT) | | BCG treatment | | | | |
Total no. patients	Control group	Recurred (no., %)	Treatment	Recurred (no., %) group	Differ. (%) recurred	P-value
57	27	14 (52%)	30	6 (20%)	32	<0.001
86	43	41 (95%)	43	18 (42%)	53	<0.001
49	26	26 (100%)	23	8 (35%)	65	<0.001
133	63	52 (83%)	70	18 (26%)	57	<0.001
94	32	19 (59%)	62	20 (32%)	27	<0.02
224	122	56 (46%)	102	26 (26%)	20	0.003
643	313	208 (67%)	330	96 (29%)	38	—

Thirty-three per cent of patients treated with MMC had tumour recurrence compared with 20% of BCG-treated patients. The median time to recurrence was prolonged up to 36 months for the BCG-treated group compared with 20 months for the MMC-treated group. In a recent series of 161 patients enrolled in a three-arm study of intravesical prophylaxis of epirubicin versus BCG versus TUR alone, Melekos *et al.* (9) reported that 60% of epirubicin-treated patients, 68% of BCG treated, and 41% of control subjects remained free of recurrences at a median follow up of 33 months. Epirubicin and BCG were superior to TUR alone; however, with regards to prophylaxis of T1 and high-grade tumours, BCG demonstrated a remarkable advantage. Cookson (10) also demonstrated this enhance effectiveness of BCG against high-grade Tl tumours. In their study, 91% of patients treated with intravesical BCG immunotherapy were free of disease at a mean follow up of 59 months. The effect of BCG on tumour progression has been investigated in three randomized studies each of which found a statistically significant reduction in progression to muscle invasion or metastasis (2). Overall progression was reduced from 28% in controls to 14% with BCG intravesical therapy. This positive impact on progression has resulted in improved survival. In another study with a median follow-up of 8 months, Herr reported that the mortality rate was reduced from 32% in patients treated with TUR alone to 14% in patients treated with BCG (11). With long-term follow up, cancer deaths were decreased from 37% to 12% and cystectomy rates were decreased from 42% to 20% with BCG (12). The current recommended maintenance BCG regimen employs 3 weekly instillations of $10^5 \times 10^8$ CFU of Connaught BCG, 3 months after initiation of treatment (8). Three weekly instillations are repeated at 6-monthly intervals for 3 years. The second or third weekly maintenance treatment is given only if the preceding instillation was without increased side-effects. In order to improve further the efficacy of BCG, Lamm reported that daily megadose vitamins A, B_6, C, and E (Oncovite, Mission Pharmacal) versus recommended daily allowances (RDA) produced protection from recurrence (13). The 5-year estimates of tumour recurrence are 91% in the RDA and 41% in the megadose. Overall recurrence was 24 of 30 (80%) patients in the RDA group and 14 of 35 (40%) in the high dose arm. These results suggest that high doses of vitamins A, B_6, C, and E may have a role in chemoprevention of bladder tumour recurrence (13). Further research will be required to confirm this study and subsequently to identify which of these vitamins protect from tumour recurrence.

TOXICITY OF BACILLE CALMETTE–GUÉRIN

Many of the adverse reactions caused from BCG therapy are a direct extension of the desired immunological response that is so important in its efficacy. Mild dysuria and urinary frequency are expected as a consequence of the inflammatory response and immune stimulation which are essential components of the mechanism of action of BCG. Most patients experience these symptoms to some degree, and up to 90% of patients are reported to have symptoms of cystitis. Symptoms typically begin after the third instillation (2,5). These mild symptoms can usually be managed with acetaminophen, diphenhydramine, and pyridium. Haematuria may occur in one-third of patients as a result of cystitis. Mild fever is common and is associated with immune stimulation and a favourable response to BCG treatment. The risk for increased absorption and major systemic BCG toxicity appears to be increased if given to patients having gross haematuria. Because of this, it is advisable to hold further BCG therapy until the haematuria has resolved. Patients with symptoms lasting more than 48 h may be treated with 300 mg isoniazid orally daily while the symptoms of cystitis and haematuria persist. Subsequently, it may be given 1 day prior to subsequent BCG instillation and continued for the 3 days following therapy. BCG treatments are postponed until all side-effects from previous instillations have resolved.

Major adverse reactions are relatively uncommon. More than 95% of patients receiving BCG therapy tolerate the treatment well. In a review of over 2600 patients, fever occurred in 3.0% and, in most instances, it resolved within 1 or 2 days. However, it is difficult to distinguish between those patients with simple BCG fever versus those who may have BCG sepsis. Because of this, it is recommended that these patients be admitted and placed on oral isoniazid 300 mg per day and rifampicin 600 mg per day. Once fever has resolved, most patients can resume BCG intravesical therapy at a half dose after receiving isoniazid for at least 1 day prior to treatment.

Other serious complications are as follows: granulomatous prostatitis 0.9%, ureteral obstruction 0.3%, epididymitis 0.4%, contracted bladder 0.2%, arthralgia 0.5%, rash 0.3%, pneumonitis/hepatitis 0.7%, and sepsis 0.4%. The most serious complication of BCG therapy is sepsis. It is believed that traumatic catheterization with bleeding is a source of BCG sepsis in most cases. BCG can also gain intravascular access in patients with severe cystitis or at the time of bladder biopsy or TUR of bladder tumour. The current recommendation is to wait at least 1 week after TUR or biopsy before starting BCG therapy. The diagnosis of BCG sepsis is generally not difficult, but unfortunately the misconception that BCG is an innocuous organism is commonly held and can delay treatment. Patients typically, but not invariably, develop high fever, shaking chills, and then hypotension. Mental confusion, disseminated intravascular coagulopathy, respiratory failure, jaundice, and leucopenia may occur. While these reactions cannot be differentiated from Gram-negative sepsis which occurs following instrumentation of the genitourinary tract, the temporal association with BCG administration makes treatment for BCG sepsis mandatory. Cultures of blood, urine, and bone marrow are typically negative in face of BCG sepsis, so treatment must be initiated on the basis of clinical suspicion. When BCG sepsis does occur, the current recommendation is isoniazid 300 mg, rifampicin 600 mg, and prednisone 40 mg daily. Prednisone is continued until signs and symptoms of sepsis persist and is then tapered gradually for an additional 2–4 weeks. Symptoms often recur if prednisone is tapered rapidly. Isoniazid and rifampicin are continued for 3–6 months, depending on the severity and duration of the reaction. Studies have confirmed that this regimen significantly improves survival and no patient receiving this regimen has died of BCG sepsis (14). It is important to proceed with antibiotic treatment when systemic BCG infection is suspected without waiting for culture results. Cultures are typically negative even in the face of progressive infection. Molecular techniques to identify BCG DNA may prove useful in the future (15).

ALTERNATIVE IMMUNOTHERAPIES

Interferons

Interferons (IFNs) are host-produced glycoproteins that are known to possess antiviral, direct antiproliferative, and immunoregulatory activities, including activation of immune effector cells, induction of cytokine production, and enhancement of tumour-associated antigen (16). They are reported also to inhibit angiogenesis and regulate differentiation (16). Clinical studies of single-agent intravesical recombinant IFN alfa-2b in patients with superficial bladder cancer suggest that IFN alfa-2b increased the cytotoxicity of both T lymphocytes and natural killer (NK) cells by increasing infiltration of these cells into the bladder wall (17).

Eradication of residual bladder tumour

Several clinical investigations have examined the ability of intravesical interferon to eradicate residual vesical papillary tumours and CIS (18,19). Torti reported 25% complete response (CR), with a mean duration exceeding 17 months in patients with recurrent papillary TCC who were treated with escalating doses(50 to 1000 MU) of rIFN alfa-2b for 8 weeks. They observed also 32% CR and 26% partial response (PR) (with persistent positive cytology) in 19 patients with CIS, approximately half of these having failed prior intravesical therapies. These responses were dose dependent. In a multicentre randomized study, Glashan found that tumour response to rIFN alfa-2b was also dose dependent, with a 5% CR and 32% PR observed with a dose of 10×10^6 units and a 43% CR and 19% PR observed with a dose of 100×10^6 units in patients treated for CIS (19). In our recent evaluation of intravesical rIFN alfa-2b high-risk patients with superficial bladder cancer were treated with 50×10^6 weekly for 6 weeks and then every 3 months for 1 year. Thirty three per cent of patients were without recurrence at 12 months. Progression occurred in 18% of the patients at a mean follow up of 28 months. None of the 28 evaluable patients were taken off the study due to side-effects. Adverse reactions following intravesical rIFN alfa-2b therapy are dose-dependent and are relatively mild and include flu-like symptoms of fever, chills, fatigue, and myalgias which occur in up to 27% of patients.

Prophylaxis

The efficacy of adjuvant intravesical rIFN alfa-2b in preventing tumour recurrence and progression of superficial vesical TCC following complete TUR has been evaluated in several studies (20–22). Recurrence rates with rIFN alfa-2b therapy ranged from 21% to 60%. In a large, multicentre, randomized study 287 patients with grade 2 primary Ta or Tl papillary TCC were treated prophylactically with either rIFN alfa-2b (50 MU) or MMC (40 mg) weekly for 8 weeks following TUR. Overall, MMC was superior to rIFN alfa-2b in terms of tumour recurrence rates (37% versus 48%) and median time to recurrence (36 versus 21 months). Hoeltl and colleagues compared 10 weekly intravesical treatments of rIFN alfa-2b (10 or 100 MU) with ethoglucid (1.13 g) and reported that the recurrence rate was substantially higher with ethoglucid than with rIFN alfa-2b (60% versus 46%). Studies comparing intravesical rIFN alfa-2b with BCG immunotherapy indicate that rIFN alfa-2b is less effective in reducing the risk of recurrence or improving the time to recurrence (22). Two induction therapies with rIFN alfa-2b (60 MU) had failed to elicit a response in 45% of treated patients compared with 8% of patients receiving BCG (6-week induction followed by six additional treatment cycles of 2 weeks).

Keyhole limpet haemocyanin

Keyhole limpet haemocyanin (KLH), a highly antigenic respiratory pigment of the mollusc *Megathura cranulata*, is a non-specific immune stimulant, that has been also investigated as an intravesical agent. In one study, Lamm demonstrated a complete response in 25 of 51 (45%) patients and partial response in 12 of 51 (21%) patients with 2, 10 mg or 50 mg of intravesical KLH for 6 weeks (24). The best responders were patients with CIS. Of 19 CIS patients, 11 (58%) had a complete response. Ten (50%) of 20 patients with papillary TCC demonstrated a response, and four (33%) of the 12 patients with both forms of bladder cancer showed response. To date, our experience includes a total of 50 patients. Overall complete response is 48% and mainly in patients who have had prior intravesical therapy (25). One group reported that KLH reduced tumour recurrence by 60% in bilharzial bladders with papillary TCC (26). In one study KLH was better than MMC in preventing recurrence of superficial bladder cancer (27). Another study compared KLH with ethoglucid for prophylaxis in patients who failed intravesical chemotherapeutic agents, and reported no difference in efficacy (28). The advantage of KLH is its apparent lack of toxicity. Lamm reported that crude preparation of KLH (i.e. C-KLH) offered greater antitumour activity than the purified KLH compound, although this has not been investigated in a clinical trial (24).

Bropirimine

Bropirimine (2-amino-5-bromo-6-phenyl-4-(3H)-pyrimidone) is a low molecular weight immunomodulator with broad-spectrum immunostimulatory activity, that can be given orally. This aryl pyrimidinone is reported to stimulate production of endogenous cytokines, including IFN alfa-2b, IL-1, TNF, and to stimulate cellular immune responses (29). It has shown efficacy in the therapy of CIS of the bladder and upper tract papillary TCC. Bropirimine also stimulates B-cell proliferation, NK, LAK, and macrophage activity. Sarosdy reported that bropirimine induced a complete response in 27 of 52 (52%) patients treated for residual disease. The best responders were among those with no prior intravesical therapy. Of those 10 patients, seven (70%) had a complete response. The median follow-up for the series was 12 months; and toxicity was dose related (30). In a separate investigation, 25 patients were treated for unilateral or bilateral positive cytology with negative retrograde pyelography. Ten of 19 (53%) evaluable patients, showed negative cytology following oral bropirimine therapy. Four patients showed the cytological conversion within

3 months, and the remaining six at 6 months. The duration of response ranged from 3 months to 30 months; the duration of therapy was 6 months in most cases. Two of the responders relapsed within the follow-up period (31).

CONCLUSIONS

Intravesical BCG remains the most effective therapy in the management and prophylaxis of superficial TCC of the urinary bladder. BCG intravesical immunotherapy has reduced tumour recurrence and progression and has prolonged survival of patients with this disease. Intravesical chemotherapy also reduces tumour recurrence but has had no positive impact on disease progression or survival. Results from newer intravesical therapies such as IFN, KLH, and bropirimine are encouraging, and have revealed significant therapeutic benefit. However, the results in prophylaxis of superficial TCC and long-term efficacy in the prevention of recurrence, disease progression, and mortality remain unknown.

> **Key Points**
>
> 1. The optimal dose and treatment schedule of BCG remains to be defined and may vary from patient to patient. The typical dose–response curve of BCG immunotherapy is bell shaped, with optimal responses occurring at less than the maximum tolerated doses.
> 2. BCG has a complete response rate of 60% or more when used to treat residual stage Ta or Tl bladder cancer, but it is generally preferable to resect all visible tumours, when possible, prior to beginning treatment. Direct contact of BCG with the tumour may require resection of the prostate or instillation of BCG in the upper tract for disease outside the bladder.
> 3. BCG remains the most effective intravesical agent for the therapy and prophylaxis of superficial bladder and is the only approved intravesical treatment for CIS, with an average complete response rate of 72%
> 4. High doses of vitamins A, B_6, C, and E may improve further the efficacy of BCG.
> 5. Results from newer intravesical therapies such as IFN, KLH, and bropirimine are encouraging, with significant therapeutic benefit.

References

1 Bostwick DG. Natural history of bladder cancer. *J Cell Biochem* 1992, **161**, 3138–43.
2 Lamm DL. Long-term results of intravesical therapy for superficial bladder cancer. *Urol Clin North Am* 1992, **19**, 573–80.
3 Lamm DL. Bacillus Calmette-Guérin immunotherapy for bladder cancer. *J Urol* 1985, **134**, 40–7.
4 Herr HW. Carcinoma in situ of the bladder. *Semin Urol* 1983, **1**, 15–22.
5 Lamm DL. Carcinoma in situ. *Urol Clin North Am* 1992, **19**, 573.
6 Lamm DL, Blumenstein BA, Crawford ED. A randomized trial of intravesical doxorubicin and immunotherapy with bacillus Calmette-Guérin for transitional-cell carcinoma of the bladder. *N Engl J Med* 1991, **325**, 1205–7.
7 Lamm DL, Crawford ED, Blumenstein B. SWOG 8795: A randomized comparison of bacillus Calmette-Guérin and mitomycin C prophylaxis in stage Ta and Tl transitional cell carcinoma of the bladder. *J Urol* 1993, **149**, 275–9.
8 Lamm DL. BCG in prospective: Advances in the treatment of superficial bladder cancer. *Eur Urol* 1995, **27**, 2–8.
9 Melekos MD, Chionis H, Pantazakos A. Intravesical bacillus Calmette-Guérin immunoprophylaxis of superficial bladder cancer: Results of a controlled prospective trial with modified treatment schedule. *J Urol* 1993, **149**, 744–8.
10 Cookson MS, Sarosdy MF. Management of stage Tl superficial bladder cancer with intravesical bacillus Calmette-Guérin therapy. *J Urol* 1992, **148**, 797–801.
11 Herr HW, Laudone VP, Badalament RA. Bacillus Calmette-Guérin therapy alters the progression of superficial cancer. *J Clin Oncol* 1988, **6**, 1450–3.
12 Herr HW. Transurethral resection and intravesical therapy of superficial bladder tumors. *Urol Clin North Am* 1991, **18**, 525–8.
13 Lamm DL, Riggs D, Shriver J. Megadose vitamins in bladder cancer: A double-blind clinical trial. *J Urol* 1994, **151**, 21–6.
14 Koukol SC, DeHaven JI, Riggs DR, Lamm DL. Drug therapy of Bacillus Calmette-Guérin sepsis. *Urol Res* 1995, **22**, 373–6.
15 Kritstjansson M, Green P, Manning HL. Molecular confirmation of bacillus Calmette-Guérin as the cause of pulmonary infection following urinary tract instillation. *Clin Infect Dis*, 1993, **17**, 228–30.

16 Baron S, Tyring SK, Fleischmann WR Jr. The interferons. Mechanisms of action and clinical applications. *JAMA*, 1991, **266**, 1375–8.

17 Alvarez-Mon M, Molto LM, Manzano L. Immunomodulatory effect of interferon-alpha 2b on natural killer cells and T lymphocytes from patients with transitional cell carcinoma of the bladder. *Anticancer Drug* 1992, **1**, 5–11.

18 Torti FM, Shortliffe LD, Williams RD. Alpha-interferon in superficial bladder cancer: a Northern California Oncology Group Study. *J Clin Oncol* 1988, **6**, 476–83.

19 Glashan R. A randomized controlled study of intravesical a-2b-interferon in carcinoma in situ of the bladder. *J Urol* 1990, **144**, 658–61.

20 Portillo J, Martin B, Hernandez R. Results at 43 months' follow-up of a double-blind, randomized, prospective clinical trial using intravesical interferon alpha-2b in the prophylaxis of stage pT1 transitional cell carcinoma of the bladder. *Urol* 1997, **49**, 187–92.

21 Hoeltl W, Hasun R, Albrecht W, Marberger M. How effective is topical alpha-2b interferon in preventing recurrence of superficial bladder cancer? *Br J Urol* 1991, **68**, 495–8.

22 Zerbib M, Botto H, Mandel E. Intravesical (IV) IFN compared to BCG therapy in 'high risk' superficial bladder cancer results of a prospective multicentric randomized study. *J Urol* 1997, **157**, A213.

23 Boccardo F, Cannata D, Rubagotti A. Prophylaxis of superficial bladder cancer with mitomycin or interferon alfa-2b: results of a multicentric Italian study. *J Clin Oncol* 1994, **12**, 7–11.

24 Lamm DL, Haven JI, Riggs DR. Keyhole limpet hemocyanin immunotherapy of murine bladder cancer. *Urol Res* 1993, **21**, 33–7.

25 Lamm DL, Morales A, Grossman HB. Keyhole Limpet Hemocyanin (KLH) immunotherapy of papillary and ln situ transitional cell carcinoma of the bladder. A multicenter phase I–II clinical trial (Meeting Abstract). *J Urol* 1996, **155**, A1405.

26 Wishahi MM, Ismail IM, Reubben H. Keyhole Limpet hemocyanin immunotherapy in bilharzial bladder: a new treatment modality? Phase II trial: superficial bladder cancer. *J Urol* 1995, **153**, 6–8.

27 Jurincic CD, Engelmann U, Gasch J. Immunotherapy in bladder cancer with keyhole-limpet hemocyanin: A randomized study. *J Urol* 1988, **139**, 723–6.

28 Flamm J, Bucher A, Holt W, Albrecht W. Recurrent superficial transition cell carcinoma of the bladder: Adjuvant topical chemotherapy versus immunotherapy: A prospective randomized trial. *J Urol* 1990, **144**, 260–3.

29 Lotzova E, Savary CA, Stringfellow DA. 5-halo-6-phenyl pyrimidinones: new molecules with cancer therapeutic potential and interferon-inducing capacity are strong inducers of murine natural killer cells. *J Immunol*, 1983, **130**, 965–9.

30 Sarosdy MF, Lowe BA, Schellhammer PF. Bropirimine immunotherapy of bladder CIS. positive Phase II results of an oral interferon inducer (Meeting Abstract). *Proc Annu Meeting ASCO*, 1994, **13**, A719.

31 Sarosdy MF, Lowe BA, Schellhammer PF. Oral bropirimine immunotherapy of carcinoma in situ of the bladder: results of a phase II trial. *Urology*, 1996, **48**, 21–7.

20. NOVEL THERAPEUTIC STRATEGIES FOR BLADDER CANCER

D.M. Papamichael and K.N. Syrigos

CONVENTIONAL CYTOTOXIC DRUGS

The most widely employed chemotherapy programmes in the advanced as well as adjuvant disease setting are the M-VAC (methotrexate, vinblastine, adriamycin, cisplatin) (1) and CMV (cisplatin, methotrexate, vinblastine) (2) regimens. Their toxicities are predictable, with neutropenic fever and mucositis being the most serious (3). However, peripheral neuropathy, renal function impairment as well as diminished auditory acuity are also observed. In a number of trials the treatment-related mortality had been of the order of 3–4% (2,3). Although overall response rates achieved with combination chemotherapy regimens range from 50% to 70%, long-term survival figures are very disappointing; 10% of patients with metastatic disease and 20–30% of patients with nodal involvement at presentation, are expected to live long term (3–6). Patients with a poor performance status and visceral or bony metastatic disease tend to fare worse, with a median survival of 6 months. Co-morbid conditions such as impaired cardiac or renal function, quite often coexisting in this group of patients, make the use of commonly employed chemotherapeutic agents very limited. Although advanced bladder cancer is a relatively chemosensitive disease, established regimens have reached a therapeutic plateau. While attempts are still being made to 'fine tune' these regimens, it is clear that new strategies, as well as more effective and less toxic agents are required to provide any hope for improving the therapeutic results in patients with advanced disease. Only after a clinical improvement in this setting, and the application of the new agents to earlier stages of the disease can we hope ultimately to affect the natural history of this malignancy. The activity of investigational chemotherapeutic as well as biological agents will be reviewed.

Platinum derivatives and other metals

Cisplatin is one of the most extensively tested single agents in advanced bladder cancer, and is the cornerstone of the most popular existing combination regimens used for the disease. The frequent presence of mild to moderate renal insufficiency in this group of patients, as well as the short duration of the responses achieved, made investigators search for alternative platinum derivatives with a better side-effect profile and higher efficacy.

So far *carboplatin* has not demonstrated significantly different results from those expected with cisplatin, either in single agent phase II studies (7), or in combination with 5-fluorouracil (5-FU) (8), methotrexate (9), or methotrexate plus vinblastine plus an anthracycline (10,11).

Oxaliplatin, a new 1,2 diaminocyclohexane (DACH) platinum complex, has exhibited an interesting spectrum of activity against a wide range of murine and human cell lines (12,13), as well as non-cross-resistance with cisplatin in others (14,15). Other *in vitro* data have suggested synergy when oxaliplatin is combined with cisplatin (16,17). In the setting of phase II and III clinical trials it has shown impressive activity in patients with advanced colorectal cancer, when used in combination with 5-FU (18,19). It has a different side-effect profile than cisplatin, with less emetogenicity, less nephrotoxicity—making pre- and posthydration unnecessary—as well as a different pattern than cisplatin for peripheral sensory neuropathy, this being its dose-limiting toxicity. Work in bladder cancer cell lines, however, has been less promising. In both RT4 and TCCSUP cell lines, oxaliplatin was shown to be more resistant than either cisplatin or carboplatin (14). Clearly, further *in vitro* as well as clinical studies are required in order to define better the future role of this interesting drug in the treatment of bladder cancer.

Gallium nitrate is a naturally occurring group IIIa metal, originally used for diagnostic scanning (20). Interest in its use as a possible antineoplastic agent was generated by the fact that it exhibited distinct intracellular uptake by certain non-osseous malignancies (21–23), as well as the observation by Rosenberg that platinum salts have potent antitumour activity (24). It was originally screened for preclinical antitumour activity against a number of rat and mouse tumour types (25,26). It has been studied in a series of phase II studies in previously treated patients with bladder cancer, with overall responses ranging from 10 to 50% (27–29). However, toxicity can be significant and can include hypocalcaemia, hypomagnesaemia, nephrotoxicity, hearing loss, and optic neuritis. Nephrotoxicity is dose limiting for this agent. A randomized phase II study in previously untreated patients, where a combination of 5-FU and gallium nitrate was used, showed only two partial responses (PRs) (12%) in 17 evaluable patients, thus calling into question the true activity of gallium nitrate (30). It was suggested though, that the dose of gallium nitrate made necessary by the combination with 5-FU in that study, was perhaps not adequate.

Taxanes

Preclinical studies have shown antiproliferative activity of taxanes against human bladder cancer cell lines (31), and superiority of these agents against classic microtubular inhibitors (32).

Single agent *paclitaxel* has the distinct advantage of not being dependent upon renal excretion for its elimination when used in a group of patients who frequently have low creatinine clearance (33,34). In a phase II study in 26 previously untreated patients, single agent paclitaxel showed an overall response of 42% with an impressive 27% complete response (CR) rate (35). When paclitaxel was tried in previously treated patients in a small phase II study, the results were disappointing, with an overall response of 7% (36). Phase II combination studies with paclitaxel, so far published only in abstract form, have reported response rates ranging from 50% to 80% (37,38). Although these results are promising, there are currently no phase III data randomizing these regimens against 'standard' ones.

The role of *docetaxel*, a semi-synthetic taxane, in bladder cancer is even less well defined. Phase II studies have shown response rates of between 20 and 40% (39,40). Additional studies especially in combination, thus increasing the numbers of patients treated, will help determine the relative efficacy of docetaxel compared with paclitaxel.

New antifolates

A number of second-generation antifolates have been synthesized in an attempt to overcome several of the mechanisms of *de novo* and acquired resistance to methotrexate. Because of the significant activity of methotrexate in bladder cancer, two agents—trimetrexate and piritrexim—have been tested in phase I and II studies.

Trimetrexate is a non-classical antifolate with previously shown *in vitro* activity in methotrexate-resistant leukaemia cells (41). In a phase II study of 48 previously treated patients with bladder cancer, the overall response rate was 17%, including one Complete Response (CR) (42). Interestingly, all eight patients who responded had received prior methotrexate, and five of them had documented Progressed Disease (PD) while on methotrexate. This would suggest that the theoretical non-cross-resistance of these agents may be clinically realized.

Piritrexim is another lipid soluble dihydrofolate reductase inhibitor. Because of a short half-life, lack of polyglutamation and 75% bioavailability after oral administration, most clinical trials have used a prolonged, oral low-dose schedule. A response seen in a previously treated patient with bladder cancer during a phase I trial (43), prompted a phase II trial in this disease. In a multi-institutional European study in 29 previously untreated bladder cancer patients, there were 10 PRs and one CR, giving an overall response rate of 38%; median duration of response was 22 weeks (44). A further study, in patients previously progressing on methotrexate based therapy, showed all three evaluable patients treated with piritrexim, to have achieved a PR, again suggesting a degree of lack of cross-resistance.

Nucleoside analogues

Gemcitabine is a novel pyrimidine antimetabolite, an analogue of cytosine arabinoside. It exerts its antitumour activity via multiple mechanisms of action: (i) incorporation into replicating DNA hence inhibiting cell growth; (ii) masked DNA chain termination; and (iii) several self-potentiation mechanisms that serve to increase intracellular levels of the active compound. Preclinical experiments in various cell lines and animal models demonstrated a broad range of cytotoxic activity (45). Responses with gemcitabine in advanced or metastatic bladder cancer were first observed in a phase I study (46) and were further confirmed in single agent and combination phase II studies (47,48). Objective responses were seen in patients with hepatic, lung, and bony metastases. A randomized trial comparing a combination of gemcitabine/cisplatin to 'standard' M-VAC is currently ongoing. This was prompted by the interesting phase I–II data , as well as encouraging activity and a good toxicity profile in combination studies in other malignancies (49,50).

Vinca alkaloids

Although vinblastine is a frequent and established component of modern combination regimens in advanced bladder cancer, there is very little phase I data available in this setting.

Vinorelbine is another vinca alkaloid closely related to vinblastine but with a different side-effect profile. It has interesting activity in breast and non-small cell lung cancer patients (51,52). Although it has not undergone single agent testing in advanced bladder cancer, because of the activity demonstrated in other malignancies, it has been incorporated into a combination regimen with 5-FU and ifosfamide, with one CR and two PRs in 10 evaluable patients (53). Vinorelbine was also used in combination with paclitaxel in previously treated patients, in the context of a phase II study; the regimen was thought to be relatively ineffective in that setting (54). It is therefore as yet unclear as to whether vinorelbine will play a significant part in the future management of the disease.

Topoisomerase-1 inhibitors

Irinotecan (CPT-11) is a semi-synthetic analogue of camptothecin with a novel mechanism of action and encouraging activity in patients with previously treated colorectal cancer (55). In preclinical studies it has exhibited cytotoxic activity against cisplatin resistant transitional cell carcinoma cell lines. It has also exhibited synergistic activity with cisplatin *in vivo* against certain lung cancer xenografts as well as TCC DU4184 (a nude mouse supported human xenograft) (56). The role of irinotecan in the clinical setting is currently being evaluated in ongoing studies.

Topotecan is another S-phase specific topoisomerase-1 inhibitor with well established activity in ovarian cancer. In a single agent phase II study in previously treated patients with advanced bladder cancer, however, it exhibited only minimal activity with an overall response rate of 10% (57).

Biological response modifiers

Interferons are host-produced glycoproteins that act to mediate immune responses through antiviral, antiproliferative, and immunoregulatory activities. Although in use for a number of years, the potential use of interferons for a number of different malignancies is still being explored. In the advanced disease setting, single agent interferon has no documented activity (58). Preclinical tumour models have suggested synergy between 5-FU and interferon (59,60), and have prompted the testing of the combination in the clinical setting. In a phase II study conducted at the MD Anderson Cancer Centre (Texas, USA) in 30 previously treated patients, PRs were reported in 30% of patients, with a median duration of response at just over 5 months (61). In a subsequent trial from the same institution in 28 chemoresistant patients, cisplatin was added to the combination, with a decrease in the 5-FU dose. The overall response rate was 61% (7% CR) (62). The use of an identical regimen in 24 previously untreated patients yielded a 71% response rate including five CRs (63). A trial organized by the European Organization for Research and Treatment of Cancer is currently in progress aiming to confirm these results. It seems quite likely though, that the potential of interferon is more likely to be realized in superficial bladder cancer.

THE APPLICATIONS OF MONOCLONAL ANTIBODIES IN THE TREATMENT OF BLADDER CANCER

Bladder cancer, although exhibiting heterogeneity between patients and between different tumours arising in the same patient (64) has, nevertheless, some characteristics that make it suitable for studies using monoclonal antibodies (mAbs). At least 75% of bladder cancers present as superficial disease, many of them multifocal, requiring treatment of the bladder as a whole (65). Furthermore, when instilled intravesically, the antibody is in direct contact with the tumour and is not diluted in the circulation, therefore cross-reactivity of mAbs is less of a concern. Finally, as mAbs are not absorbed systemically from the bladder (66,67), a human anti-mouse response is unlikely to occur. All the above make bladder cancer patients ideal candidates for immunotherapy, using tumour-associated antigens as targets.

Over the past two decades several efforts have been made for the therapeutic use of mAbs against various malignancies. Most therapeutic strategies have employed the systemic administration of tumour-associated mAbs, either used alone ('naked' mAbs), or conjugated to a cytotoxic agent (radionuclides, conventional chemotherapeutic drugs, toxins). Unfortunately their application has been associated with poor tumour uptake (<0.01% of the injected dose), the binding of the mAb to normal tissues and the development of human antimouse antibodies (HAMA) (68).

As access to the tumour site may be a limiting factor in the targeting of solid tumours, other routes of administration, in addition to the systemic one, have been considered for the regional delivery of the mAbs (i.e. intraperitonealy for ovarian carcinoma, intrathecally for meningeal carcinomatosis). Intravesical treatment of superficial bladder cancer with conventional chemotherapeutic agents or with BCG is a long established practice and this tumour seemed appropriate for local, intravesical application of mAbs conjugates.

Cytotoxic drug conjugates

Conventional cytotoxic drugs used for the treatment of bladder cancer, such as doxorubicin and mitomycin C, have been conjugated to mAbs and administered intravesically. Although the toxicity was considerably reduced, the therapeutic results were very poor, mainly because of the inadequate uptake of the conjugate by the tumour cells and the consequent failure to administer a cytotoxic dose to the tumour (69).

Radioimmunotherapy

Over the last decade the use of mAbs as carriers of high activity radionuclides for the treatment of malignant diseases (radio-immunotherapy—RIT) spurred an unprecedented effort in oncology and nuclear medicine research. The mAb–isotope conjugate, after binding to the target cell and delivering a lethal radiation dose, could offer the advantage of killing many untargeted cells through 'cross-fire irradiation' (70). This distribution of the cytotoxic activity by the radiolabelled mAb could, in theory, be the solution to the considerable problem of tumour heterogeneity in antigen expression.

Clinical studies with intravesical administration of radiolabelled antibodies in patients with bladder cancer confirmed a high absolute uptake of the antibody in the tumour and a favourable tumour : non-tumour ratio, although the antigens used as targets were also expressed by some normal epithelial cells. Unfortunately, these studies showed that, while intravesical administration of radiolabelled mAbs in patients with bladder cancer would not produce local or systemic toxicity, it is, nevertheless, unlikely that a cytotoxic dose of radiation could be delivered to the tumour with this technique (66,67).

Toxins

mAbs have been used as carriers of toxins from plants (ricin, abrin), or bacteria (*Diphtheria*, *Pseudomonas*) that inhibit protein synthesis, for cancer therapy. *In vitro* data showed encouraging results with the use of a ricin A chain immunotoxin conjugated to the mAb 486P3/12 (71), while *in vivo* studies, through the intravenous route of administration, have shown high toxicity, mainly hepatotoxicity and vascular leak syndrome (72,73). *In vitro* and animal studies on human bladder cancer cell lines showed considerable therapeutic effect, using the immunotoxins ricin (74–77), *Pseudomonas* exotoxin A (78–80) and saporin (81). There is only one study with the intravesical use of a recombinant form of *Pseudomonas* exotoxin A/transforming growth factor-α (TGF-α) protein (78). The results are not encouraging, mainly because, in addition to the tumour heterogeneity and the poor tumour uptake, the mAb–toxin conjugate needs to be internalized after binding to the antigen in order to exert its cytotoxic effect.

Liposomes

The anticancer activity of immunoliposomes containing chemotherapeutic agents (such as doxorubicin) and targeting a tumour-associated antigen has already been demonstrated. In bladder cancer in particular, doxorubicin-containing immunoliposomes directed against the c-erbB-2 gene product showed some toxicity *in vitro* against bladder cancer cells (82). It has also been demonstrated that the encapsulation of a chemotherapeutic agent (methotrexate, cis-platinum) or immunomodulator (IFN-α) augments its therapeutic effect against human bladder cancer cells (83–87). *In vivo* studies showed that intravesical administration of radiolabelled liposomes did not yield significant systemic absorption and deposition in distant organs (85), but clinical trials have not been performed yet.

Antibody-directed enzyme prodrug therapy

As the use of a tumour-associated antibody as carrier of a prodrug was not satisfactory, Philpott exploited the idea of using the antibodies to carry enzymes at the tumour sites (88,89). This concept was further developed and described by Bagshawe (90,91) and Senter (92,93). This two-step approach, is known as antibody-directed enzyme prodrug therapy (ADEPT) (Fig. 20.1). Tumour-associated antibodies are conjugated with enzymes, delivered to tumour sites and allowed to clear from the rest of the tissues. Subsequently, a prodrug is administered. This is converted by the enzyme into an active cytotoxic agent. The interval between the two administrations is optimized to achieve minimal systemic toxicity by accomplishing satisfactory accumulation of the conjugate in the tumour and clearance from blood and normal tissues. In

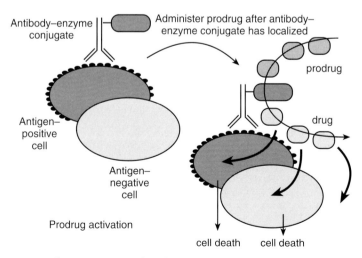

Fig. 20.1 Selective activation of prodrugs at tumour sites by applying antibody-directed enzyme prodrug therapy (ADEPT).

addition, as the active drug diffuses in the tumour, it provides a bystander effect. This approach has the advantages of reduced toxicity and amplification, compared with other applications of mAbs in oncology.

The above therapeutic strategy has already been tried *in vitro* in bladder cancer cell lines and has been proved to be highly cytotoxic, while preliminary biodistribution studies in bladder cancer patients has shown successful localization of the mAb–enzyme conjugate on the malignant cells and selective activation of the prodrug at the tumour sites. Clinical trials are in progress to test the effectiveness of the above system *in vivo*, after intravesical administration (94,95).

Key Points

1. Although advanced bladder cancer is a relatively chemosensitive disease, nevertheless established chemotherapeutic regimens appear to have reached a therapeutic plateau.
2. New agents are continuously being evaluated in the advanced disease setting; their introduction in new combination regimens could provide a hope for improving the therapeutic results in this group of patients.
3. Bladder cancer provides an ideal model for the study of regional immunotherapy, using tumour-associated antigens as targets.
4. Several strategies have been developed for the intravesical treatment of bladder cancer, with the application of mAbs, as carriers of a cytotoxic agent, while drug delivery systems, which amplify the tumour : non-tumour uptake ratio are the most likely candidates for therapeutic intervention.

References

1 Sternberg CN, Yagoda A, Scher HI *et al.* Preliminary results of methotrexate, vinblastine, adriamycin and cisplatin (M-VAC) in advanced urothelial tumours. *J Urol* 1985, **133**, 403–7.
2 Harker W, Meyers FJ, Freiha FS *et al.* Cisplatin, methotrexate, and vinblastine (CMV); an effective chemotherapy regimen for metastatic transitional cell carcinoma of the urinary tract a Northern California Oncology Group study. *J Clin Oncol* 1985, **3**, 1463–70.
3 Sternberg C, Yagoda A, Scher HI *et al.* Methotrexate, vinblastine, doxorubicin and cisplatinum for advanced transitional cell carcinoma of the urothelium: efficacy and patterns of response and relapse. *Cancer* 1989, **64**, 2448–58.
4 Wakisaka S, Miyahara S, Nonaka A *et al.* Brain metastasis from transitional cell carcinoma of the bladder: case report. *Neuro Med Chir* 1990, **30**, 188.
5 Slavati M, Cervoni L, Orlando ER *et al.* Solitary brain metastases from carcinoma of the bladder. *J Neurooncol* 1993, **16**, 217–8.
6 Fossa SD, Sternberg CN, Scher HI *et al.* Post-chemotherapy survival of patients with advanced urothelial cancer. *Br J Cancer* 1996, **74**, 1655–9.
7 Barnes J, Calvert AH, Freedman LS *et al.* A phase II study of carboplatin in metastatic transitional cell carcinoma of the bladder. *Eur J Cancer Clin Oncol* 1987, **23**, 375–7.
8 Arena MG, Sternberg CN, Zeuli M *et al.* Carboplatin and 5-fluorouracil in poor performance status patients with advanced urothelial cancer. *Ann Oncol* 1993, **4**, 241–4.
9 Dogliotti L, Bertetto O, Berutti A *et al.* Combination chemotherapy with carboplatin and methotrexate in the treatment of advanced urothelial carcinoma. *Am J Clin Oncol (CCT)*, 1995, **18**, 78–82.
10 Waxman J, Abel P, Farah JN *et al.* New combination chemotherapy programme for bladder cancer. *Br J Urol* 1989, **63**, 68–71.
11 Waxman J, Barton C. Carboplatin-based chemotherapy for bladder cancer. *Cancer Treat Rev*, 1993, **19**, 21–5.
12 Tashiro R, Kawada Y, Sakuri Y *et al.* Antitumour activity of a new platinum complex, oxalato (trans-I-1,2-diaminocyclohexane) platinum (II): New experimental data. *Biomed Pharmacother*, 1989, **43**, 251–60.
13 Myers TG, Paull KD, Fojo AT *et al.* Multivariate analysis of high-flux screening data using the DISCOVER computer program package: integrated analysis of activity patterns and molecular structure features of platinum complexes. *Proc Am Assoc Cancer Res* 1994, **35**, 371A (abstract).
14 Pendyala L, Creaven PJ. In vitro cytotoxicity, protein binding, red blood cell partitioning, and biotransformation of oxaliplatin. *Cancer Res* 1993, **53**, 5970–6.
15 Alvarez M, Ortuzar W, Rixe O *et al.* Cross resistance patterns of cell lines selected with platinum suggest differences in the activities and mechanisms of resistance of platinum analogues. *Proc Am Assoc Cancer Res* 1994, **35**, 439A (abstract).

16 Mathe G, Chenu E, Bourut C *et al*. Experimental study of three platinum complexes: CDDP, CBDCA and L-OHP on L1210 leukemia. Alternate or simultaneous association of two platinum complexes. *Proc Am Assoc Cancer Res* 1989, **30**, 872A (abstract).

17 Ortuzar W, Paull K, Rixe O *et al*. Comparison of the activity of cisplatin (CP) and oxaliplatin (oxali) alone or in combination in parenteral and drug resistant sublines. *Proc Am Assoc Cancer Res* 1994, **35**, 332A (abstract).

18 De Gramont A, Vignoud J, Tournigand C *et al*. Oxaliplatin with high-dose leucovorin and 5-fluorouracil 48-hour continuous infusion in pretreated metastatic colorectal cancer. *Eur J Cancer* 1997, **33**, 214–19.

19 Levi F, Zidani R, Misset JL. Randomised multicentre trial of chronotherapy with oxaliplatin, fluorouracil, and folinic acid in metastatic colorectal cancer. International Organization for Cancer Chronotherapy. *Lancet* 1997, **350**, 681–6.

20 Hayes RL. Radioisotopes of gallium. In: *Radioactive pharmaceuticals* (ed. Andrews GA, Knisesky RM, Wagner HN). AEG Conf, 1966, p. 603–11.

21 Edwards CL, Hayes RL. Tumor scanning with 67Ga-citrate. *J Nuclear Med* 1969, **10**, 103–5.

22 Hayes RL, Nelson B, Swartzendruber DC *et al*. Gallium-67 localization in rat and mouse tumors. *Science*, 1970, **167**, 289–90.

23 Edwards CL, Nelson B, Hayes RL. Localization of gallium in human tumors. *Clin Rep* 1970, **18**, 89.

24 Rosenberg B, Vancamp L, Trosko JE *et al*. Platinum compounds: a new class of potent antitumour agents. *Nature*, 1969, **222**, 385–6.

25 Foster BJ, Clagget-Carr K, Hoth D *et al*. Gallium nitrate: the second metal with clinical activity. *Cancer Treat Rep* 1986, **70**, 1311–19.

26 Annual Report to the Food and Drug Administration on Gallium Nitrate (NSC 15200; IND 10123). Division of Cancer Treatment, NCI Oct., 1987.

27 Crawford ED, Saiers JH, Baker LH *et al*. Gallium nitrate in advanced bladder carcinoma: Southwest Oncology Group study. *Urology*, 1991, **38**, 355–77.

28 Seligman PA, Crawford ED. Treatment of advanced transitional cell carcinoma of the bladder with continuous infusion gallium nitrate. *J Natl Cancer Inst*, 1991, **83**, 1582–4.

29 Seidman AD, Scher HI, Heinemann MH *et al*. Continuous infusion gallium nitrate for patients with advanced refractory urothelial tract tumours. *Cancer* 1991, **68**, 2561–5.

30 McCaffrey J, Hilton S, Bajorin D *et al*. Gallium nitrate and 5-fluorouracil combination versus M-VAC in patients with advanced urothelial tract tumours: A phase II randomized trial. *J Clin Oncol* 1997, **15**, 2449–55.

31 DeHaven JI, Traynelis CT, Riggs D *et al*. Taxol with or without cisplatin reduces the growth of transitional cell carcinoma and prostatic carcinoma cell lines in vitro. *Proc Am Assoc Cancer Res* 1995, **36**, 297A (abstract).

32 Niell HB, Rangel C, Miller A *et al*. The activity of antimicrotubular agents in human bladder tumour cell lines. *Proc Am Ass Cancer Res* 1993, **34**, 202A (abstract).

33 Keung A, Kaul S, Pinedo H *et al*. Pharmacokinetics of Taxol given by 3-hr or 24-hr infusion to patients with ovarian carcinoma. *Proc Am Soc Clin Oncol* 1993, **12**, 321A (abstract).

34 Schilder L, Egorin M, Zuhowski E *et al*. The pharmacokinetics of taxol in a dialysis patient. *Proc Am Soc Clin Oncol* 1994, **13**, 338A (abstract).

35 Roth BJ, Dreicer R, Einhorn LH *et al*. Significant activity of Paclitaxel in advanced transitional-cell carcinoma of the urothelium: a phase II trial of the Eastern Cooperative Oncology Group. *J Clin Oncol* 1994, **12**, 2264–70.

36 Papamichael D, Gallagher CJ, Oliver RTD. Phase II study of Paclitaxel in pretreated patients with locally advanced/metastatic cancer of the bladder and ureter. *Br J Cancer* 1997, **75**, 606–7.

37 McCaffrey JA, Hilton S, Mazdumar M *et al*. A phase II trial of ifosfamide, paclitaxel and cisplatin in patients with transitional cell carcinoma. *Proc Am Soc Clin Oncol* 1997, **16**, 324A (abstract).

38 Redman B, Hussain M, Smith D *et al*. Phase II evaluation of paclitaxel and carboplatin in advanced urothelial cancer. *Proc Am Soc Clin Oncol* 1997, **16**, 325A (abstract).

39 McCaffrey J, Hilton S, Mazumdar M *et al*. Phase II trial of Docetaxel in patients with advanced or metastatic transitional cell carcinoma. *J Clin Oncol* 1997, **15**, 1853–7.

40 de Wit R, Stoter G, Blanc C et al. Phase II study of first-line docetaxel (taxotere) in patients with metastatic urothelial cancer. *Ann Oncol* 1994, **5** (8), 67–71.

41 Kamen BA, Eibl B, Cashmore A et al. Uptake and efficacy of trimetrexate, a non-classical antifolate in methotrexate resistant leukemia cells in vitro. *Biochem Pharmacol*, 1984, **33**, 1697–9.

42 Witte RS, Elson P, Khandaker J et al. An Eastern Cooperative Oncology Group phase II trial of trimetrexate in the treatment of advanced urothelial carcinoma. *Cancer* 1994, **73**, 688–91.

43 Feun LG, Savaraj N, Benedetto P et al. Phase I trial of piritrexim capsules using prolonged, low-dose oral administration for the treatment of advanced malignancies. *J Natl Cancer Inst*, 1991, **83**, 51–5.

44 De Wit R, Kaye SB, Roberts JT et al. Oral piritrexim; An effective treatment for metastatic urothelial cancer. *Br J Cancer* 1993, **67**, 388–90.

45 Storniolo AM, Allerheiligen SR, Pearce HL. Preclinical, pharmacologic, and phase I studies of gemcitabine. *Semin Oncol* 1997, **24** (7), 77–87.

46 Pollera CF, Ceribelli A, Crecco M et al. Weekly gemcitabine in advanced bladder cancer: A preliminary report from a phase I study. *Ann Oncol* 1994, **5**, 182–4.

47 Von der Maase H, Andersen L, Crino L et al. A phase II study of gemcitabine and cisplatin in patients with transitional cell carcinoma (TCC) of the urothelium. *Proc Am Soc Clin Oncol* 1997, **16**, 324A (abstract).

48 Moore MJ, Tannock IF, Ernst DS et al. Gemcitabine: a promising new agent in the treatment of advanced urothelial cancer. *J Clin Oncol* 1997, **15**, 3441–5.

49 Einhorn LH. Phase II study of gemcitabine plus cisplatin in non-small cell lung cancer: a Hoosier Oncology Group study. *Semin Oncol* 1997, **27** (8), 24–38.

50 Abratt RP, Hacking DJ, Goedhals L et al. Weekly gemcitabine and monthly cisplatin for advanced non-small cell lung carcinoma. *Semin Oncol* 1997, **24** (8), 18–23.

51 Degardin M, Bonnetterre J, Hecquet B et al. Vinorelbine (navelbine) as a salvage treatment for advanced breast cancer. *Ann Oncol* 1994, **5**, 423–6.

52 Crawford J, O'Rourke M, Schiller JH et al. Randomized trial of vinorelbine compared with fluorouracil plus leucovorin in patients with stage IV non-small cell lung cancer. *J Clin Oncol* 1996, **14**, 2627–30.

53 Mahjoubi M, Kattan J, Droz JP et al. Feasibility trial of a combination of vinorelbine, ifisfamide, fluorouracil and folinic acid (VIF regimen) in advanced urothelial cancer. *Eur J Cancer* 1993, **29A**, 285–6.

54 Sobecks RM, Stadler WM, Daugherty CK et al. Vinorelbine and paclitaxel in relapsed metastatic bladder carcinoma. *Proc Am Soc Clin Oncol* 1997, **16**, 344A (abstract).

55 Rougier P, Bugat R, Douillard JY et al. Phase II study of irinotecan in the treatment of advanced colorectal cancer in chemotherapy-naive patients and patients pretreated with fluorouracil-based chemotherapy. *J Clin Oncol* 1997, **15**, 251–60.

56 Keane T, McGuire W, Petros J et al. CPT-11/cisplatin: an effective preclinical combination in the therapy of advanced human bladder cancer (TCC). *Proc Am Soc Clin Oncol* 1995, **14**, 491.

57 Witte RS, Propert KJ, Burch P et al. An ECOG phase II trial of topotecan in previously treated advanced urothelial carcinoma. *Proc Am Soc Clin Oncol* 1997, **16**, 324a.

58 Niijima T. Phase II study of interferon-a 2A for tumors of urogenital tract. *Jpn Clin Med Pharmacol*, 1985, **1**, 395–406.

59 Elias L, Crissman HA. Interferon effects upon the adenocarcinoma 38 and HL-60 cell lines: Antiproliferative responses and synergistic interactions with halogenated pyrimidine antimetabolites. *Cancer Res* 1988, **48**, 4868–73.

60 Wadler S, Schwartz EL, Wersto R et al. Interferon modulates the activity of 5-fluorouracil against two human colon cancer cell lines. *Proc Am Assoc Cancer Res* 1989, **30**, 569A (abstract).

61 Logothetis CJ, Hossan E, Sella A et al. Fluorouracil and recombinant human interferon alfa-2A in the treatment of metastatic chemotherapy-refractory urothelial tumours. *J Natl Cancer Inst*, 1991, **83**, 285–8.

62 Logothetis C, Dieringer P, Ellerhorst J et al. A 61% response rate with 5-fluorouracil, interferon-α2b and cisplatin in metastatic chemotherapy refractory transitional cell carcinoma. *Proc Am Assoc Cancer Res* 1992, **33**, 221A (abstract).

63 Bacoyiannis C, Skarlos D, Aravantinos A *et al.* 5-Fluorouracil, interferon-alpha-2b and cisplatin (FAP) for advanced urothelial cancer. A phase II study. *Ann Oncol* 1997, **8**, 373–8.

64 Raghavan D, Shipley WU, Garnick MB *et al.* Biology and management of bladder cancer. *N Engl J Med* 1990, **322**, 1129–31.

65 Heney NM, Nocks BN, Daly JJ *et al.* Ta and T1 bladder cancer: location, recurrence and progression. *Br J Urol* 1982, **54**, 152–7.

66 Yu LZ, Gu FL, Zhang CL. Radioimmunoimaging diagnosis of human bladder carcinoma. *Scand J Urol Nephrol*, 1994, **157**, 13–17.

67 Kunkler RB, Bishop MC, Green DJ *et al.* Targeting of bladder cancer with monoclonal antibody NCRC48: a possible approach for intravesical therapy. *Br J Urol* 1995, **76**, 81–6.

68 Syrigos KN, Epenetos AA. Radioimmunotherapy of ovarian cancer. *Hybridoma*, 1995, **14**, 121–4.

69 Li L, Zhang Y, Lin Q *et al.* Clinical application of monoclonal antibody-drug conjugate to immunotargeting chemotherapy of bladder cancer. *Chin Med J Engl*, 1995, **108**, 764–8.

70 Britton KE, Mather SJ, Granowska M. Radiolabelled monoclonal antibodies in oncology. III. *Radioimmunother Nuclear Med Commun*, 1991, **12**, 333–47.

71 Thiesen HJ, Juhl H, Arndt R. Selective killing of human bladder cancer cells by combined treatment with A and B chain ricin antibody conjugates. *Cancer Res* 1987, **47**, 419–23.

72 Vitetta ES, Thorpe PE. Immunotoxins containing ricin or its A chain. *Semin Cell Biol*, 1991, **2**, 47–58.

73 Vitetta ES, Thorpe PE, Uhr JW. Immunotoxins: magic bullets or misguided missiles? *Immunol Today* 1993, **14**, 252–9.

74 Wawrzynczak EJ, Cumber AJ, Henry RV *et al.* Pharmacokinetics in the rat of a panel of immunotoxins made with abrin A chain, ricin A chain, gelonin, and momordin. *Cancer Res* 1990, **50**, 7519–26.

75 Wawrzynczak EJ, Cumber AJ, Henry RV, Parnell GD. Comparative biochemical, cytotoxic and pharmacokinetic properties of immunotoxins made with native ricin A chain, ricin A1 chain and recombinant ricin A chain. *Int J Cancer* 1991, **47**, 130–5.

76 Wawrzynczak EJ, Henry RV, Cumber AJ *et al.* Biochemical, cytotoxic and pharmacokinetic properties of an immunotoxin composed of a mouse monoclonal antibody Fib75 and the ribosome-inactivating protein alpha-sarcin from *Aspergillus giganteus. Eur J Biochem* 1991, **196**, 203–9.

77 Timar J, McIntosh DP, Henry R *et al.* The effect of ricin B chain on the intracellular trafficking of an A chain immunotoxin. *Br J Cancer* 1991, **64**, 655–62.

78 Theuer CP, FitzGerald DJ, Pastan I. A recombinant form of *Pseudomonas* exotoxin A containing transforming growth factor alpha near its carboxyl terminus for the treatment of bladder cancer. *J Urol* 1993, **149**, 1626–32.

79 Sarosdy MF, Hutzler DH, Yee D, Von Hoff DD. In vitro sensitivity testing of human bladder cancers and cell lines to TP-40, a hybrid protein with selective targeting and cytotoxicity. *J Urol* 1993, **150**, 1950–5.

80 Siegall CB. Targeted therapy of carcinomas using BR96 sFv-PE40, a single-chain immunotoxin that binds to the Le (y) antigen. *Semin Cancer Biol*, 1995, **6**, 289–95.

81 Battelli MG, Polito L, Bolognesi A *et al.* Toxicity of ribosome-inactivating proteins-containing immunotoxins to a human bladder carcinoma cell line. *Int J Cancer* 1996, **65**, 485–90.

82 Suzuki S, Uno S, Fukuda Y *et al.* Cytotoxicity of anti-c-erbB-2 immunoliposomes containing doxorubicin on human cancer cells. *Br J Cancer* 1995, **72**, 663–8.

83 Bassett JB, Anderson RU, Tacker JR. Use of temperature-sensitive liposomes in the selective delivery of methotrexate and cis-platinum analogues to murine bladder tumor. *J Urol* 1986, **135**, 612–15.

84 Bassett JB, Tacker JR, Anderson RU, Bostwick D. Treatment of experimental bladder cancer with hyperthermia and phase transition liposomes containing methotrexate. *J Urol* 1988, **139**, 634–6.

85 Frangos DN, Killion JJ, Fan D *et al.* The development of liposomes containing interferon alpha for the intravesical therapy of human superficial bladder cancer. *J Urol* 1990, **143**, 1252–6.

86 Killion JJ, Fan D, Bucana CD *et al.* Augmentation of antiproliferative activity of interferon alfa against human bladder tumor cell lines by encapsulation of interferon alfa within liposomes. *J Natl Cancer Inst* 1989, **81**, 1387–92.

87 Killion JJ, Fishbeck R, Bar-Eli M, Chernajovsky Y. Delivery of interferon to intracellular pathways by encapsulation of interferon into multilamellar liposomes is independent of the status of interferon receptors. *Cytokine* 1994, **6**, 443–9.

88 Philpott GW, Bower RJ, Parker CW. Selective iodination and cytotoxicity of tumor cells with an antibody-enzyme conjugate. *Surgery* 1973, **74**, 51–8.

89 Philpott GW, Shearer WT, Bower RJ, Parker CW. Selective cytotoxicity of hapten-substituted cells with an antibody-enzyme conjugate. *J Immunol* 1973, **111**, 921–9.

90 Bagshawe KD. Antibody directed enzymes revive anti-cancer prodrugs concept. *Br J Cancer* 1987, **56**, 531–2.

91 Bagshawe KD, Springer CJ, Searle F *et al.* A cytotoxic agent can be generated selectively at cancer sites. *Br J Cancer* 1988, **58**, 700–3.

92 Senter PD, Saulnier MG, Schreiber GJ *et al.* Anti-tumor effects of antibody-alkaline phosphatase conjugates in combination with etoposide phosphate. *Proc Natl Acad Sci USA* 1988, **85**, 4842–6.

93 Senter PD, Schreiber GJ, Hirschberg DL *et al.* Enhancement of the in vitro and in vivo antitumor activities of phosphorylated mitomycin C and etoposide derivatives by monoclonal antibody-alkaline phosphatase conjugates. *Cancer Res* 1989, **49**, 5789–92.

94 Syrigos KN, Rowlinson-Busza G, Epenetos AA. In vitro cytotoxicity following specific activation of amygdalin by β-glucosidase conjugated to a bladder cancer-associated monoclonal antibody. *Int J Cancer*, 1998, **78**, 712–9.

95 Syrigos KN, Kawaza M, Williams G, Epenetos AA. Intravesical administration of radiolabelled tumour associated monoclonal antibody in bladder cancer. *Acta Oncol*, 1998, **38**, 529–32.

21. GENE THERAPY OF BLADDER CANCER

Christian T.F. Freund and Seth P. Lerner

INTRODUCTION

What is gene therapy?

Gene therapy is a novel treatment approach based on direct genetic modification of gene expression in somatic cells to treat both acquired and inherited diseases (1). Gene therapy is also referred to as 'molecular medicine' because it attempts to correct or eliminate the specific molecular reason for disease on a cellular level rather than to treat its symptoms in an overall and non-specific manner (2). Gene therapy applies the principles we have learned from studying disease on a molecular level and integrates techniques derived from molecular biology, genetics, and virology to form a new treatment modality. Gene therapy is a new form of pharmacology, and we are in the earliest stages of drug development. In this chapter we present a rationale for applying gene therapy to the treatment of bladder cancer, give a brief introduction to the complex field of vector systems for delivery of genes, and review the abundant preclinical data providing proof of principle in bladder cancer cell lines and animal models. The first human clinical phase I trials are currently under way and will provide the basis for establishing the safe and effective application of gene therapy to human bladder cancer.

Why gene therapy and bladder cancer?

Despite advances in intravesical chemotherapy and immuno-therapy, recurrence rates for Ta tumours are 30–70% in the first 12 months after resection and at least 60% over a period of 10 years (3). While these tumours infrequently progress to invasive cancer, enormous resources are consumed in their treatment with frequent cystoscopy, urine cytology, chemotherapy, and immunotherapy. T1 tumours and carcinoma *in situ* (CIS) are high risk cancers and progress in 15–25% of patients to muscle invasive, potentially life-threatening cancers (4,5). Radical cystectomy provides excellent long-term local control for muscle invasive cancers. Despite advances in surgical and anaesthetic techniques and systemic chemotherapy, the 5-year survival for patients with

T2–T4 NX M0 tumours is 50–60% (6). Durable complete responses in patients with visceral metastatic disease are achieved in only 10–15% of patients with multi-agent chemotherapy. Among urological organs, the bladder is uniquely accessible through cystoscopy and easily visualized with a variety of radiological modalities. The need for novel therapies and the unique accessibility of bladder cancer create an enormous opportunity to apply the principles of gene therapy for this disease.

VECTOR SYSTEMS AND GENE TRANSFER TECHNOLOGY

Overview

Therapeutic results for any form of gene therapy directly depend upon the availability of powerful gene expression systems. Currently, no single vector system expresses genes of interest in an entirely efficient, durable, and safe way at a specific, defined target site. Based on its underlying biology, each vector system has distinct advantages and limitations so that for each gene therapy strategy, the most appropriate expression system has to be determined. For each therapeutic situation, the following issues must be carefully considered before a vector system is chosen and an appropriate gene of interest is expressed.

Target tissue considerations

(i) The type and biology of the target cell population; (ii) The temporal expression of the gene of interest and the intensity and duration of gene expression; (iii) The spatial expression of the gene of interest and the extent of transduction in the target tissue; (iv) The gene expression targeted to a specific cell population and inside the target cell genome.

Vector system options and limitations (7):

1. The type and biology of the vector system.
2. The size of the gene to be delivered and the vector's accommodation capacity.
3. Dosage, technical availability, and cost of the vector.
4. Routes of vector administration.
5. The use of replication-competent or replication-deficient vector systems.
6. Risks and side-effects:
   (a) direct vector-related toxicity;

(b) risk of insertional mutagenesis with subsequent malignant transformation of target cells;

(c) the potential for environmental spread of genetically modified viruses, including the possibility of recombination with endogeneous virus particles with release of a new agent with an unknown level of public health risk.

7. The extent of the host immune response towards the vector and transgene products.

8. The degree of preimmunization against the vector in the target population.

Principles of gene transfer

For successful gene transfer, both viral and non-viral vectors must maintain the ability to: (i) access target cells; (ii) bind to structures on the cell surface; (iii) accomplish cell entry; (iv) undergo cytoplasmic transport; (v) avoid degradation by lysosomal enzymes; (vi) manage transport of genetic material into the nucleus; and (vii) achieve strong and long-lasting expression of functional gene product (8).

Vector systems

We briefly summarize the features of some of the most important vectors used in gene therapy of bladder cancer. Vector systems can be divided into two broad categories: viral and non-viral.

Viral vectors

The vector is the transport vehicle that facilitates entry into the cell. The therapeutic gene is inserted into the viral genome, and a specific promoter, such as the Rous sarcoma virus long terminal repeat (RSV) or the cytomegalovirus promoter (CMV), is inserted into the viral genome to drive production of the therapeutic gene. In general, viral vectors are more efficient than non-viral vectors in terms of transduction efficiency, but they also raise more questions about the safety of the gene therapy treatment. Because of the unique life cycle of viruses that depends on inserting genetic material into host cells, taking over the cell metabolism, and propagating offspring, viruses have evolved efficient strategies to accomplish these goals. Many of the complex interactions between virus and host cell are not yet understood, but viral vectors are the most commonly used vectors in human clinical trials today. The two most widely used vector systems are adenoviruses and retroviruses.

Adenoviral vectors are DNA viruses and mild pathogens in humans. Adenovirus vectors have become very popular gene transfer vehicles because they are easy to handle, easy to produce in large quantity, have a broad range of cellular hosts, promote high level of gene expression, and they do not cause insertional mutagenesis (9). Substitution of the gene of interest into a genomic site important for virus replication renders adenoviruses replication-defective and provides an additional margin of safety (10). Importantly, adenoviruses infect not only proliferating but also quiescent cells, and thus enormously extend their usage in gene therapy (11). Their natural tropism for epithelial cells is helpful in transducing tumour cells of genitourinary epithelial origin (12). The adenovirus genome is maintained in an extra-chromosomal state inside the host cell nucleus. Because of concomitant expression of viral proteins, a strong immune response is raised against the vector and transduced cells. Although this immune response could well be advantageous in some settings of cancer gene therapy, it limits duration of gene expression so that initially very high levels of gene expression are lost over time in immunocompetent hosts (13). Currently, attempts are being made to delete more, if not all, of the viral backbone genome, thereby increasing vector accommodation capacity, decreasing viral protein expression and minimizing immune response. Replication competent vectors have been designed and tested recently in other tumour model systems (1,7,14,15).

Retroviral vectors are RNA viruses, derived mainly from the Moloney-Murine Leukaemia Virus (MMLV) and rendered replication-defective. Retroviral-mediated gene transfer is the most commonly used in clinical trials to date, and several limitations have been identified (9,16). Retroviral vectors are unable to infect non-dividing cells. The tropism of retroviruses is dependent upon the type of envelope protein for which their genome is encoded and the presence or absence of the respective receptor protein on the target cell surface. The retrovirus genome after being converted to DNA by the viral enzyme reverse transcriptase, is stably and irreversibly integrated into the host genome at random locations and passed on to progeny cells. This introduces safety concerns about insertional mutagenesis, whereby the process of inserting genetic material could potentially trigger subsequent malignant transformation by itself. Unfortunately, retroviral vectors can be produced only at low titres, and infectious particles are quite unstable. This has limited their direct *in vivo* use. Instead, packaging cells, which release retroviral particles over time without themselves being killed, are being grafted into the tumour tissue. Currently, researchers are trying to learn how to extend the range and extent of gene delivery *in vivo* as well as how to increase the production of retroviral vectors (15,17).

Other viral vector systems have been used in pre-clinical and human phase I bladder cancer gene therapy, including vaccinia virus, a type of pox virus, and this is discussed later in this chapter.

Non-viral vector systems

Non-viral vector systems are an important alternative because they do not carry the risks implicit in the use of viral vectors. However, these systems are generally less efficient in terms of gene transfer. Nevertheless, strategies used by viruses to accomplish gene transfer can be borrowed and used in the construction of non-viral vectors. The following methods currently are being used (18): (i) direct DNA-plasmid injection into target tissue, (ii) particle bombardment of target tissue with DNA-coated gold beads using an accelerator ('gene gun'); (iii) injection of cationic liposomes, which encapsulate DNA, absorb to cell membranes and release DNA into the cell cytoplasm; and (iv) introduction of DNA-polylysine conjugates, which facilitate DNA uptake and transport into cells.

Targeting gene transfer

Gene therapy strategies frequently warrant restricted gene expression only to target tissue (18–21). There are various methods of targeting gene expression and these are described in Table 21.1.

Table 21.1

STRATEGIES FOR TARGETING GENE THERAPY FOR TISSUE SPECIFIC EXPRESSION
Physically targeted
Inject/instill/perfuse vector at desired location (20)
Particle mediated transfer with 'gene gun'
Ligand-directed
Receptor-mediated (changes to adenovirus-fibre protein/cell receptor modulations)
Antibody-targeted immunoliposomes with incorporated antibodies specific for target cell membrane determinants
Genetically targeted (19)
Use of tumour-/tissue-specific promoters (preferentially express genes of interest in target tissue by employing constructs with specific enhancers and promoters)
Radiation-inducible promoters (induce gene expression in transduced cells by selectively radiating target tissue areas) (21)
Drug-inducible constructs (gene expression depends upon presence or absence of drugs (e.g. tetracycline system), thereby switching gene expression on or off)

Strategies in bladder cancer gene therapy

Overview

Cancer is a genetic disease and represents a multistep process of multiple genetic and epigenetic alterations to the genomic material of a given cell. The process eventually leads to malignant transformation. Over time, the transformed cell continues to grow, produces a cluster of identical cells which, together, progress to a premalignant lesion finally to reach the stage of clinical cancer. Genetic lesions in cancer are extremely varied and involve many different proteins. Because of the intense complexity of processes such as cell growth regulation and malignant transformation, processes that are understood only marginally if at all, cancer gene therapy encompasses a wide variety of treatment strategies, many of which are based on previously established anti-tumour principles. The following strategies are currently being used in bladder cancer gene therapy:

Marker genes

As a first step in gene therapy, one must prove that transfer of foreign genetic material into target cells is at all possible. In order to evaluate the transduction efficiency of a system, it is necessary to determine the level of gene product expressed in transduced cells after specifically designed reporter genes have been inserted. Reporter genes encode for a protein product that is innocuous to the host cell in which it is being expressed, and is readily detectable even when present in small quantities. The amounts of reporter gene product correlate with the transduction efficacy of a given vector system for a specific host cell type. Two of the most widely used reporter genes are the *Escherichia coli lacZ* gene (β-gal) and the firefly luciferase gene (luc). The *Escherichia coli lacZ* gene encodes for an enzyme, galactosidase, which converts a colourless substrate, galactoside, into a deep blue coloured product that can be measured in various ways. Firefly luciferase catalyses the oxidation of beetle luciferin with the concomitant production of light, which is quantified with a luminometer.

We and others have demonstrated that both murin and human transitional cell carcinoma cell lines are transducible *in vitro* by adenoviral vectors and that the marker gene is expressed in a dose-dependent fashion (20,22). Bass *et al.* transduced one mouse and three human bladder cancer cell lines at MOI 1000 with an adenoviral vector encoding for luc and assayed for luc expression after 48 h (22). All four cell lines could be successfully transduced, although the absolute transduction efficacy varied. Peak expression occurred at day 1 for human and day 4 for mouse cell lines and was detectable for up to 7 days. After instillation of an adenovirus encoding for luc into mouse bladders, evidence of gene transfer was seen for up to 7 days, although it varied considerably between animals and gene expression decreased with time. Thus gene expression in the MBT-2 murine bladder cancer cell line is both time and dose-dependent (20).

In order to demonstrate *in vivo* gene transfer, Morris *et al.* directly instilled an adenoviral vector encoding for β-gal ($1 \times 10e^9$ p.f.u. in 500 lu) intravesically into rat bladders (23). Sporadically transduced cells were observed in superficial layers of the epithelium and smooth muscle of the bladder. Transduced cells were detected at their highest level 24 h after vector instillation and persisted for at least 7 days. No toxicity or other deleterious effects were seen.

Similar results have been achieved with other vectors including vaccinia virus and herpes simplex virus (24,25). Transitional epithelium, both benign-appearing and malignant, is susceptible to transduction by viral vectors and capable of expressing foreign genes, making bladder cancer a rational target for a variety of gene therapy strategies.

Prodrug-activating systems (suicide gene therapy)

Prodrug-activating systems cause the expression of genes encoding for enzymes that convert a prodrug to an active toxic drug in order to kill target cells selectively and specifically. To qualify as a prodrug, a substance must permeate the cell and be specifically converted by the expressed enzyme. Because these enzymes are expressed intracellularly, they may avoid the non-specific and deleterious effects on normal tissues or organs commonly observed with conventional antitumour therapies. Although at least 15 different suicide systems are under development, herpes simplex thymidine kinase/ganciclovir (HSV-tk/GCV) is the best established of these systems (26,27).

The herpes simplex thymidine kinase gene (HSV-*tk*) plus ganciclovir (GCV) is a simple strategy for suicide gene therapy. Ganciclovir is an acyclic nucleoside analogue that is not normally metabolized by mammalian cell thymidine kinases. However, herpes simplex thymidine kinase is able to monophosphorylate the relatively non-toxic prodrug ganciclovir, which is subsequently metabolized by endogenous mammalian kinases into ganciclovir triphosphate. Ganciclovir triphosphate is a purine analog that competes with normal nucleotides and can inhibit DNA polymerase and thus lead to cell death, possibly by apoptosis (28–30). A characteristic feature of suicide systems is the so-called bystander effect, whereby non-transduced neighbouring tumour cells undergo cell death. Several mechanisms have been proposed, including direct transfer of toxic products, metabolic cooperation via gap junctions, disruption of tumour blood supply, apoptosis, and cell-mediated immune response (8,26,31–38). Culver *et al.* have shown that transduction of ≤10% of tumour cells with HSV-*tk* results in >50% tumour ablation in the presence of ganciclovir (39).

We have demonstrated proof of principle with this approach in a murine model of bladder cancer using the MBT-2 cell line to establish subcutaneous or orthotopic tumours in syngeneic C3H female mice (20,40). We initially transduced MBT-2 cells *in vitro* with an adenovirus encoding for HSV-*tk* at MOIs ranging from 1.8 to 4000 (20). Either ganciclovir or phosphate-buffered saline (PBS) was added to the wells and after 72 h, numbers of surviving cells were assayed. Adenovirus-*tk* plus GCV demonstrated 95% cell killing at a MOI of 61 or greater, while little or no effect was seen at comparable MOIs with adenovirus-*tk* plus PBS. Indirect evidence of the bystander effect was found by demonstrating that a relatively low-efficiency marker gene transfer transduced 95% of cells at MOI 3000, but high-efficiency killing with adenovirus-tk was achieved at MOIs as low as 61.

We established efficacy *in vivo* by directly injecting established subcutaneous tumours with single doses of ADV/RSV-*tk* ranging from $3 \times 10e^7$ to $2 \times 10e^9$ p.f.u. followed by intraperitoneal injection of ganciclovir 20 mg/kg b.i.d. for 6 days. While control tumours increased in size 8.5–10-fold, tumours injected with $3 \times 10e^8$ p.f.u. of adenovirus-*tk* only doubled in size. In animals injected with doses of $1 \times 10e^9$ p.f.u. or more, hepatitis-like toxicity was observed. In a larger experiment, using the same dose of $3 \times 10e^8$ p.f.u. of adenovirus-*tk*, a fourfold reduction in tumour growth was boserved without any evidence of toxicity. Direct intratumoral injection of adenovirus-*tk*resulted in survival significantly better than that of control groups, as survival was prolonged by 59% from 35 to 59 days. Histological evaluation of tumours consistently demonstrated viable tumour cells in the periphery of the tumour with variable amounts of central necrosis. We have demonstrated similar efficacy and survival benefit with direct injection of established orthotopic tumours (40).

On the basis of these experiments, we have designed a phase I clinical trial to treat patients prior to cystectomy by direct injection of invasive of transitional cell cancer with ADV/RSV-*tk* followed by intravenous ganciclovir. Patients with Ta or T1 tumours that are refractory to standard intravesical therapy who do not require cystectomy will also be included. We will assess local and systemic toxicity, the distribution of HSV-*tk* in the cancer and surrounding tissues, the biological effects on the cancer, and the immune response to this treatment.

Immunomodulation systems (tumour immunology/tumour vaccination)

For immune control of tumours to be possible, the malignant cells must express determinants, so-called tumour antigens, which are potentially capable of being recognized by components of the immune system ('antigenicity') and against which an effective immune response can be mounted ('immunogenicity'). In addition, these determinants must be sufficiently different from normal cell determinants to ensure that any subsequent immunity raised against them does not lead to autoimmune destruction of normal cells.

The current aim of molecular immunotherapy is to increase the immunogenicity of tumour cells above the threshold at which effective immune reactions are generated and thus to allow the host to mount an anti-tumour immune response. However, in some instances, tumours have been shown to evade destruction by the immune system by relying on various mechanisms such as down-regulation of major histocompability complex (MHC) I molecules, inhibition of functions of lymphocytes or antigen-presenting cells, and selection for non-immunogenic clones. Because of the immense complexity of the immune system, there are several treatment options designed to augment an immune response to tumours. These options include transferring genes encoding for cytokines, co-transfer of accessory molecules for T-cell recognition/activation, and transferring antigens and suicide genes into either tumour cells, T cells or antigen-presenting cells (41).

In bladder cancer, increased effort has been focused on modification of tumour and/or host immunogenicity. Gene therapy approaches have been developed to enhance the immune system's recognition of tumour cells by inducing MHC expression with the immunomodulators interferon-gamma (IFN-γ) or interleukin-2 (IL-2) (42,43).

Connor *et al.* developed a retroviral vector construct to express the cytokines IL-2 and IFN-γ in murine MBT-2 bladder cancer cells (44). Transduced cells that were stably expressing IL-2 and IFN-γ failed to grow after intradermal injection in syngeneic mice. In a second experiment, animals were injected intradermally with either $1 \times 10e^5$ MBT-2/IL-2 cells, $1.5 \times 10e^5$ MBT-2/IFN-γ, or cell culture medium and challenged 3 weeks later with $2 \times 10e^4$ unmodified tumour cells instilled intravesically. The cytokine secreting cells provided specific immunity, and no tumours formed intravesically. Finally they demonstrated efficacy in the treatment of 7-day established intravesical tumours with multiple intraperitoneal injections of irradiated cytokine-producing cells. In 60% of mice treated with cells secreting IL-2, tumours completely regressed, while controls and animals treated with IFN-γ died. There was no added benefit of combined treatment with both IL-2 and IFN-γ.

Hiura *et al.* demonstrated induction of tumor-specific cytotoxic lymphocytes after subcutaneous injection of $1.5 \times 10e^5$ MBT-2 cells stably transduced by a retrovirus vector to express the cytokine IFN-γ (42). No tumour growth was observed with cells expressing IFN-γ in 28 of 29 animals, while tumours grew progressively in animals injected with parental cells or cells transduced with a control vector. However, while tumour-forming capacity of tumour cells expressing IFN-γ was almost abrogated, a single administration of IFN-γ producing cells in animals with established tumours was of no therapeutic benefit.

Saito *et al.* demonstrated attraction of CD4+ and CD8+ T lymphocytes after injection of retrvirally transduced MBT-2 cells expressing various cytokines (45). Cells expressing IL-2 failed to grow, while other cells, including those expressing IFN-γ grew as well as unmodified control cells. It appeared that IL-2, but not the other cytokines tested, induced a cellular infiltrate and rejection of the tumour cells. IL-2 was also the only cytokine to recruit natural killer (NK) cells. IL-2 secreting cells injected intraperitoneally caused regression of established intravesical tumours, and cured animals were resistant to a second intravesical tumour challenge. The presence of tumour-specific cytotoxic lymphocytes could be demonstrated.

These studies demonstrate that experimental bladder cancer is sensitive to modulation of the host immune response by direct modification of bladder cancer cells to facilitate high titre cytokine expression. They thus provide a rationale for direct modification of human bladder cancer cells for use as a vaccine to prevent new tumour formation and for the treatment of established bladder cancer when conventional therapy has failed.

Vaccinia virus is a double-stranded pox virus and has been well characterized since its successful use as a live vaccine to prevent smallpox. The pox viruses have the largest gene capacity; they do not require a replicating cell, and the passenger genes are not integrated into the genome (9). Temporal gene expression is short but can be maintained with repeated exposure. The disadvantage is that replication-competent vaccinia can result in a fatal infection in an immunocompromised host (9).

Lee *et al.* used a replication-competent, recombinant vaccinia virus to locally insert and express foreign antigenic proteins including haemagglutinin (HI) and nucloprotein (NP) from an unrelated influenza virus into bladder cancer cells *in vitro* and *in vivo* in order to induce systemic anti-tumour immunity (46). Intravesical instillation of $1 \times 10e^4$ p.f.u. of vaccinia virus into mice with established bladder tumours induced a systemic anti-tumour immune response that was specific for the MB-49 tumour cells. However, intravesical instillation with a single dose of greater than $1 \times 10e^5$ p.f.u. of the replication-competent vaccinia virus apparently led to systemic infection and was lethal for previously non-immunized mice, while mice previously immunized by intraperitoneal injection of $1 \times 10e^7$ p.f.u. demonstrated no signs of toxicity. Histological analysis revealed virus-infected urothelial cells lining the bladder lumen. With intravesical instillation of $2 \times 10e^6$ p.f.u. of vaccinia recombinants into pre-immunized mice, significant gene expression 22 h after transduction could be demonstrated in established tumours.

Lee *et al.* constructed a recombinant vaccinia virus containing the murine GM-CSF gene (47). Murine melanoma and bladder tumours (MB-49) infected with the therapeutic virus produce high levels of the active cytokine. They have recently completed a phase I human clinical trial of intravesical vaccinia in patients with invasive transitional cell carcinoma prior to cystectomy (48). Patients received escalating doses of intravesical vaccinia vector at 4-day intervals for a total of three doses. Cystectomy was performed 1 day after the third dose, and the tissues were subjected to histological evaluation for inflammation and viral infection. Significant mucosal and submucosal inflammation was observed in patients receiving at least $100 \times 10e^6$ p.f.u. These changes were observed in both normal and malignant urothelial cells, and there was no systemic toxicity. These data provide the basis for proceeding with additional human studies to determine the efficacy of this approach.

Systems restoring disturbed cellular growth control mechanisms by providing normal copies of genes (corrective gene therapy) or by silencing gene expression of cancer-promoting genes (ribozymes, anti-sense oligos, anti-sense oncogenes)

With corrective gene therapy, a defective gene that has allowed the uncontrolled growth of a tumour is replaced by its wild type, normally functioning, counterpart (49). An example is the p53 tumour suppressor gene, which is mutated in a high percentage of carcinoma *in situ* and invasive bladder tumours. The strategy for anti-sense oncogene therapy is to suppress or modulate the activated oncogenes. Both strategies aim at restoration of normal control of cell growth and differentiation by suppressing malignant phenotype of tumour cells (4,50).

Tumour suppressor gene therapy

Because cancer-related defects of tumour-suppressor genes are usually mutations or deletions at various locations throughout the gene, it is necessary to replace the mutated gene with a normal copy in order to restore the normal function. Although tumours develop multiple changes in various genes, a single normal copy of one suppressor gene may be able to overcome the effects of multiple cytogenetic changes on tumour progression.

Mutations of the p53 tumour suppressor gene are among the most frequent genetic alterations identified in human malignancies. The p53 protein is involved in the control of the cell cycle and other key cell metabolism pathways, is highly conserved throughout evolution, and is expresses in most normal tissues. Of all known tumour suppressor genes with therapeutic potential, p53 is the most extensively studied. p53 mutations are demonstrated in at least one-half of high grade bladder transitional cell carcinomas and are associated with a high rate of progression to invasive cancer and decreased survival with radical cystectomy (51–53).

Human and murine bladder cancer cell lines are transducible with adenoviral vectors at high titres, and adenoviral-mediated transduction of human bladder cancer cell lines by wild-type p53 results in reversal of the tumorigenic phenotype *in vitro* and *in vivo* (54,55). Werthman *et al.* used $5 \times 10e^9$ p.f.u. of adenoviral constructs expressing wild-type p53 or a reporter gene (β-gal) to transduce $1 \times 10e^6$ MBT-2 bladder cancer cells growing either intravesically or intraperitoneally in mice (55). After 36 h successful tumour transduction was confirmed by PCR and p53 recombinant gene product detected by immunohistochemical staining and Western blot analysis. Superficial luminal cell layers expressed the transgene protein, but penetration of the bladder tumour was not demonstrated. Intraperitoneal vector injection resulted in hepatic, splenic, peritoneal, and tumoral transduction, although diffuse hepatic transduction was the primary finding. Gotoh *et al.* demonstrated a significant reduction in tumour growth rate and tumour volume with direct injection of subcutaneous experimental bladder tumours in mice using adenoviral-mediated p53 under control of the CMV promoter. Survival was significantly improved over that in control animals (56).

A phase I trial has been approved at MD Anderson Cancer Centre (Texas, USA) for intravesical delivery of adenoviral-mediated p53 in patients with unresectable muscle invasive or metastatic transitional cell carcinoma. This is a dose escalation study and group 1 patients will receive Ad-p53 on days 1 and 4; group 2 on days 1 through 4, and group 3 on days 1 through 4 and days 8 through 11. The primary goals of this study are to determine the safety and toxicity of the vector; to measure infection and confirm expression of p53; and to characterize the response of measurable disease.

The Rb (retinoblastoma) tumour suppressor gene is inactivated in at least one-quarter to one-half of bladder cancers (57,58). The unphosphorylated Rb gene product appears capable of blocking the cell cycle in the G1 phase, thereby maintaining cells in a quiescent state. Loss of the normal Rb protein can remove a residual checkpoint of cell-cycle control, thereby further promoting the growth and/or malignant progression of cancer cells. Recent studies suggest that prognosis in T1 and muscle invasive bladder cancer is adversely affected if either p53 or Rb is altered, and there may be an additive adverse effect if both of these tumour suppressor genes are altered (59,60). These studies emphasize the potential importance of altered Rb function and support a rationale for the application of gene therapy strategies to restore normal function of the Rb tumour suppressor gene in bladder cancer.

Xu *et al.* used a recombinant adenovirus to express either the N-terminal truncated form of the Rb protein, the full length Rb protein, or a marker gene (β-gal) in the Rb-defective human bladder cancer cell lines 5637 and HT 1376 (61). After transduction of 5637 and HT 1376 cells *in vitro* with various MOIs ranging from 0.5 to 50, the cell lines expressed high levels of exogenous, mostly unphosphorylated Rb protein. Transduced 5637 and HT 1376 cells demonstrated morphological changes as well as growth inhibition in a dose- and cell-type-dependent fashion. Transduced cells expressing the Rb protein were non-tumorigenic in nude mice in a dose-dependent fashion.

In order to establish whether these recombinant adenoviruses could also transduce tumour cells in established solid tumours *in vivo*, either $1 \times 10e^7$ 5637 Rb-negative cells or Rb-reconstituted, Rb-positive 5637 cells were injected subcutaneously into nude mice, and tumours were allowed to develop for 2-3 weeks (61,62). Control $5 \times 10e^8$ p.f.u. or the therapeutic vector were then administered intratumorally twice weekly for a total of six doses to tumour-bearing animals. Repeated injection resulted in widespread Rb immunohistchemical staining of the tumours and, compared with control vector, most small tumours (target volume 15 mm³) injected with Rb vectors grew at a reduced rate. However, the same treatment was less effective with well-established and larger tumours in nude mice. The effect was independent of whether the tumour's Rb status was normal or mutated.

Anti-sense oncogene therapy

Along the pathway for genetic information from DNA to protein, several interventions have been developed to modulate and regulate gene expression and to restrict expression of oncogenes. The following strategies have been used:

Anti-sense oligonucleotides specifically inhibit the activities of various oncogenes and proto-oncogenes, presumably by binding to mRNA and inducing translation arrest. Still, the exact mechanism(s) by which oligonucleotides exert their action has not yet been clearly demonstrated by *in vivo* evidence.

Anti-sense RNA in their DNA template forms can be delivered very efficiently into target cells and be expressed in a controllable manner. A set of mechanisms of action has been proposed that is very similar to that of oligonucleotides.

Anti-oncogene ribozymes are RNA molecules that exhibit specific catalytic activities, thereby destroying RNA translation templates for 'unwanted' gene products. The most clearly characterized subgroup is the hammerhead ribozymes, which can perform true enzymatic reactions and are named for their hammerhead-like structure.

Feng *et al.* used a hammerhead ribozyme to abrogate the aberrant expression of a dominant oncogene, H-ras (63). The ribozyme was designed to cleave the mutant sequence in codon 12 of the activated, transforming H-ras oncogene transcript. The EJ human bladder carcinoma cell line contains the activated, transforming H-ras gene. Transduction of EJ cells with a recombinant adenovirus encoding for the H-ras ribozyme resulted in a specific decrease in the relative levels of the H-ras mRNA which was associated with significant growth suppression *in vitro*. Heterotopic implantation of control-vector transduced EJ cells into nude mice resulted in the rapid development of progressive tumour nodules, while use of the H-ras ribozyme encoding virus resulted in complete abrogation of tumorigenicity.

Eastham *et al.* transfected EJ cells expressing H-ras with a plasmid encoding for a ribozyme that specifically cleaved the mRNA product of the ras gene (64). Transfected tumour cells

$(2 \times 10e^6)$ were instilled intravesically into mice, and the animals were assessed for presence of tumour and survival. Tumours containing the anti-ras ribozyme showed a reduction in tumorigenicity (35% vs. 45%) and prolonged survival (74 days vs. 65 days) for controls. However, loss of ribozyme expression over time in 60% of animals, suggested problems in ribozyme stability. Animals that maintained ribozyme expression had a longer mean survival than animals that lost expression. These experiments demonstrated that expression of an anti-ras ribozyme could blunt the invasive phenotype and delay, but not abolish, the metastatic phenotype.

Inactivation of oncogenes

Activation of ras oncogenes is one of the representative genetic stages of the process of malignant transformation and one frequently observed in human tumours. The ras gene protein product p21 is an essential signal transducer for cellular proliferation and differentiation and acquires the transforming capacity by single point mutations. Inactivation of ras oncogenes is one potential method for reverting neoplastic phenotypes.

Ogiso *et al.* reported that a dominant negative ras mutant suppressed the transformed phenotypes of NIH3T3 cells induced by overexpression of the H-ras proto-oncogene and possibly induced apoptotic cell death (65,66). They subsequently transfected T24 human bladder cancer cells with a plasmid vector into which a dominant negative H-ras mutant was cloned (67). Compared with a control plasmid, the transduced T24 cells demonstrated about 20% of colony-forming efficiencies relative to the control transfection, suggesting that growth suppression was associated with this inactiviation of the cellular ras function.

Other strategies

Cell adhesion molecules (CAM) are important mediators for cell–cell interaction and communication and are required for both morphogenesis and ontogenesis in multicellular organisms. Neoplastic transformation is considered a dedifferentiation process, and loss of cell communication signifies an early event leading to neoplastic transformation. E-cadherin is a calcium-dependent, homotypic cell adhesion molecule, found circumferentially in squamous and transitional epithelium. Loss of expression is frequently observed in human transitional cell cancers and is associated with advanced tumour stage and decreased survival (68–70). It is likely that re-establishment of cell communication between malignant cells will restore their normal differentiation pathway.

Kleinerman *et al.* employed a gene encoding for a cellular adhesion molecule called C-CAM 1 and demonstrated that intravesical injection of $1 \times 10e^6$ adenovirally transduced human bladder cancer cells (MOI 20) expressing C-CAM 1 into nude mice had a tumour-suppressing effect (71). Compared with unmodified cells and cells transduced with a control vector, animals injected with cells expressing C-CAM 1 demonstrated smaller tumour sizes and lower bladder tumour weights after 4 weeks. In this experiment, 15 animals were mock-infected and 16 animals were treated with a recombinant adenovirus expressing C-CAM 1. However, no animals exhibited complete or long-lasting regression.

Summary

The novel and exciting strategies for treatment of bladder cancer that we have reviewed here are made possible by an entirely new treatment approach called gene therapy. Further studies are required to confirm and expand upon results of the initial studies and to prepare human clinical trials in bladder cancer. Despite encouraging results in early studies of cancer gene therapy, this new technology is still is in its infancy. Before gene therapy can become a true fourth treatment arm in oncology, or even replace conventional tumour treatments, we must develop strategies to: (i) direct gene expression in a durable and safe way specifically to the target tissues; (ii) understand more of the key mechanisms of the immune system in states of health and disease; and (iii) elucidate more details of the structure and regulation of the complex pathways of cell growth and malignant transformation.

A few years ago, it would have been hard to envision the emergence of the science of gene therapy as it exists today. However, considering the tremendous progress made in the last few years in basic and clinical research, the likelihood seems great that we will finally overcome the technical and biological hurdles of cancer gene therapy to the benefit of future patients.

References

1 Kozarsky KF, Wilson JW. Gene therapy: adenovirus vectors. *Curr Opin Genet Dev* 1993, **3**, 499–503.
2 Wilson JM. Molecular medicine: adenoviruses as gene-delivery vehicles. *N Engl J Med*, 1996, **334**, 1185–7.
3 Lamm DL. Long-term results of intravesical therapy for superficial bladder cancer. *Urol Clin North Am*, 1992, **19**, 573–80.
4 Zhang GK, Uke ET, Sharer WC, Borkon WD, Bernstein SM. Reassessment of conservative management for stage T1N0M0 transitional cell carcinoma of the bladder. *J Urol*, 1996, **155**, 1907–9.

5 Amling CL, Thrasher JB, Frazier HA *et al.* Radical cystectomy for stages Ta, Tis and T1 transitional cell carcinoma of the bladder. *J Urol*, 1994, **151**, 31–36.

6 Lerner SP, Skinner DG. Radical cystectomy for bladder cancer. In *Comprehensive textbook of genitourinary oncology* (ed. Vogelgang NJ, Shipley WU, Scardino PT, Coffey DS), Williams and Wilkins, Philadelphia, 1996.

7 Blaese M, Blankenstein T, Brenner M *et al.* Vectors in cancer therapy: how will they deliver? *Cancer Gene Ther*, 1995, **2**, 291–7.

8 Vile RG, Nelson JA, Castleden S *et al.* Systemic gene therapy of murine melanoma using tissue specific expression of the hsv-tk gene involves an immune component. *Cancer Res*, 1994, **54**, 6228–34.

9 Mastrangelo MJ, Berd D, Nathan FE, Lattime EC. Gene therapy for human cancer: an essay for clinicians. *Semin Oncol*, 1996, **23**, 4–21.

10 Graham FL, Prevec L. Manipulation of adenovirus vectors. In: *Methods in molecular biology: gene transfer and expression protocols* (ed. Murray EJ) The Humana Press Inc.; Clifton NY, 1991, 109–28.

11 Mulligan RC. The basic science of gene therapy. *Science*, 1993, **260**, 926–32.

12 Mutsen MA, Belshe RB. A review of adenoviruses in the etiology of acute hemorrhage. *J Urol*, 1976, **115**, 191–4.

13 Kass-Eisler A, Leinwand L, Gall J *et al.* Circumventing the immune response to adenovirus-mediated gene therapy. *Gene Ther*, 1996, **3**, 154–62.

14 Horwitz MS. Adenoviruses. In *Fields virology* (ed. Fields BN), 3rd edn. Raven; Philadelphia, 1996, 2149–71.

15 Jolly D. Viral vector systems for gene therapy. *Cancer Gene Ther*, 1994, **1**, 51–64.

16 Hermann F. Cancer gene therapy: principles, problems, and perspectives. *J Mol Med*, 1995, **73**, 157–63.

17 Patel PM, Collins MKL. Gene therapy. In: *Immunotherapy in cancer* (ed. Gore MPR) Wiley, London, 1996, 221–34.

18 Nakanishi M. Gene introduction into animal tissue. Critical reviews in therapeutic drug carrier systems, 1995, **12**, 263–310.

19 Miller N, Whelan J. Progress in transcriptionally targeted and regulatable vectors for genetic therapy.(Review.) *Hum Gene Ther*, 1997, **8**, 803–15.

20 Sutton MA, Berkman SA, Chen S-H *et al.* Adenovirus-mediated suicide gene therapy for experimental bladder cancer. *Urology*, 1997, **49**, 173–180.

21 Tang D-C, Jennelle RS, Shi Z, Garver RI, Carbone DP, Loya F, Chang C-H. Overexpression of adenovirus-encoded transgenes from the cytomegalovirus immediate early promoter in irradiated tumor cells. *Human gene therapy*, 1997, **8**, 2117–24.

22 Bass C, Cabrera G, Elgavish A *et al.* Recombinant adenovirus-mediated gene transfer to genitourinary epithelium in vitro and in vivo. *Cancer Gene Ther*, 1995, **2**, 97–104.

23 Morris BD Jr., Drazan KE, Csete ME *et al.* Adenoviral-mediated gene transfer to bladder in vivo. *J Urol*, 1994, **152**, 506–9.

24 Lee SS, Eisenlohr LC, McCue PA *et al.* Intravesical gene therapy: vaccinia virus recombinants transfect murine bladder tumors and urothelium. *Proc Annu Meet Am Assoc Cancer Res*, 1993, **34**, A2005.

25 Saito S, Fong Y, Yoshimura I *et al.* Herpes simplex virus as a vector for gene transfer to established gene modified bladder tumor cells. *Proc Annu Meet Am Assoc Cancer Res*, 1995, **36**, A2489.

26 Culver KW, Ram Z, Walbridge S *et al. In vivo* gene transfer with retroviral vector-producing cells for treatment of experimental brain tumors. *Science*, 1992, **256**, 1550–52.

27 Deonarain MP, Spooner RA, Epenetos AA. Genetic delivery of enzymes for cancer therapy. *Gene Ther*, 1995, **2**, 235–44.

28 Moolten FL. Tumor chemosensitivity confused by inserted herpes thymidine kinase genes: paradigm for a prospective cancer control strategy. *Cancer Res*, 1986, **46**, 5276–81.

29 Matthews T, Boehme R. Antiviral activity and mechanisms of action of ganciclovir. *Rev Infect Dis*, 1988, **10**, S490–4.

30 Samejima Y, Meruelo D. 'Bystander killing' induces apoptosis and is inhibited by forskolin. *Gene Ther*, 1995, **2**, 50–8.

31 Barba D, Hardin J, Sadelain M, Gage FH. Development of anti-tumor immunity following thymidine kinase-mediated killing of experimental brain tumors. *Proc Natl Acad Sci USA*, 1994, **91**, 4348–52.

32 Caruso M, Panis Y, Gagandeep S *et al*. Regression of established macroscopic liver metastases after in situ transduction of a suicide gene. *Proc Natl Acad Sci USA*, 1993, **90**, 7024–6.

33 Chen S-H, Chen XHL, Wang Y *et al*. Combination gene therapy for liver metastasis of colon carcinoma *in vivo*. *Proc Natl Acad Sci USA*, 1995, **92**, 2577–81.

34 Elshami AA, Saavedra A, Zhang H *et al*. Gap junctions play a role in the 'bystander effect' of the herpes simplex virus thymidine kinase/ganciclovir system in vitro. *Gene Ther*, 1996, **3**, 85–92.

35 Moolten FL, Wells JM. Curability of tumors bearing herpes thymidine kinase genes transferred by retroviral vectors. *J Natl Cancer Inst*, 1990, 297–300.

36 Ram Z, Culver KW, Walbridge S *et al*. In situ retroviral-mediated gene transfer for the treatment of brain tumors in rats. *Cancer Res*, 1993, **53**, 83–8.

37 Perez-Cruet MJ, Trask TW, Chen S-H *et al*. Adenovirus-mediated gene therapy of experimental gliomas. *J Neurosci*, 1994, **39**, 506–11.

38 Ram Z, Walbridge S, Shawker T *et al*. The effect of thymidine kinase and ganciclovir therapy on vasculature and growth of 9L gliomas in rats. *J Neurosurg*, 1994, **81**, 256–60.

39 Culver KW, Lamsam J, Stratton J *et al*. Molecular surgery for solid tumors. In: *Gene therapy and molecular medicine* (ed. Woo SLC, Blaese M, Glorioso J) Steamboat Springs, Colorado, March 26–April 1, 1995.

40 Sutton MA, Freund CTF, Berkman SA *et al*. The treatment of orthotopic murine bladder tumors with adenovirus-mediated suicide gene therapy. *J Urol*, 1997, **157**, 306 (Abstract 1194).

41 Schirrmacher V. Biotherapy of cancer-perspectives of immunotherapy and gene therapy. *J Cancer Res Clin Oncol*, 1995, **121**, 443–51.

42 Hiura M, Hashimura T, Watanabe Y *et al*. Induction of specific anti-tumor immunity by interferon-gamma gene-transferred murine bladder carcinoma MBT-2. *Folia Biol*, 1994, **40**, 49–61.

43 Nouri A, Hussain R, Oliver R. The frequency of major histocompatability complex antigen abnormalities in urological tumors and their correction by gene transfection or cytokine stimulation. *Cancer Gene Ther*, 1994, **1**, 119–23.

44 Connor J, Bannerji R, Saito S *et al*. Regression of bladder tumors in mice treated with interleukin 2 gene-modified tumor cells. *J Exp Med*, 1993, **177**, 1127–34.

45 Saito S, Bannerji R, Gansbacher B *et al*. Immunotherapy of bladder cancer with cytokine gene-modified tumor vaccines. *Cancer Res*, 1994, **54**, 3516–20.

46 Lee SS, Eisenlohr LC, McCue PA *et al*. Intravesical gene therapy : in vivo gene transfer using recombinant vaccinia virus vectors. *Cancer Res*, 1994, **54**, 3325–8.

47 Lee SS, Eisenlohr LC, McCue PA *et al*. In vivo gene therapy of murine tumors using recombinant vaccinia virus encoding GM-CSF. *Proc Annu Meet Am Assoc Cancer Res*, 1995, **36**, 248 (Abstract 1481).

48 Gomella LG, Mastrangelo MJ, Eisenlohr LC *et al*. Phase I study of intravesical vaccinia virus as a vector for gene therapy of bladder cancer. *Proc Annu Meet Am Assoc Cancer Res*, 1997, **38**, 9 (Abstract 61).

49 Sanda M, Simmons J. Gene therapy for urologic cancer. *Urology*, 1994, **44**, 617–24.

50 Friedmann T. Gene therapy of cancer through restoration of tumor-suppressor functions. *Cancer*, 1992, **70**, 1810–17.

51 Sarkis AS, Dalbagni G, Cordon-Cardo C *et al*. Association of p53 nuclear over-expression and tumor progression in carcinoma in situ of the bladder. *J Urol*, 1994, **152**, 388–92.

52 Esrig D, Spruck CH III, Nichols PW *et al*. p53 nuclear protein accumulation correlates with mutations in the p53 gene, tumor grade, and stage in bladder cancer. *Am J Pathol*, 1993, **143**, 1389–97.

53 Esrig D, Elmajian D, Groshen S *et al*. Accumulation of nuclear p53 and tumor progression in bladder cancer. *N Eng J Med*, 1994, **331**, 1259–64.

54 Harris MP, Sutjipto S, Wills FN *et al*. Adenovirus mediated p53 gene transfer inhibits growth of human tumor cells expressing mutant p53 protein. *Cancer Gene Ther*, 1996, **3**, 121–30.

55 Werthman PE, Drazan KE, Rosenthal JT *et al*. Adenoviral—p53 gene transfer to orthotopic and peritoneal murine bladder cancer. *J Urol*, 1996, **155**, 753–6.

56 Gotoh A, Shirakawa T, Okada H *et al*. Gene therapy for bladder cancer using adenoviral vector. *J Urol*, 1997, **157**, 307 (Abstract 1197).

57 Cordon-Cardo C, Wartinger D, Petrylak D *et al.* Altered expression of the retinoblastoma gene product: Prognostic indicator in bladder cancer. *J Natl Cancer Inst*, 1992, **84**, 1251–6.

58 Logothetis CJ, Xu HJ, Ro JY *et al.* Altered expression of retinoblastoma protein and prognostic variables in locally advanced bladder cancer. *J Natl Cancer Inst*, 1992, **84**, 1256–61.

59 Grossman HB, Liebert M, Dinney CPN *et al.* p53 and pRB expression predict progression in T1 bladder cancer. *Clin Cancer Res*, 1998, **4**, 829–34.

60 Cote RJ, Dunn MD, Stein JP *et al.* Level of pRB expression and cooperative effects of p53 and pRB alterations in bladder cancer progression. *Cancer Res*, 1998, **58**, 1090–4.

61 Xu H, Zhou Y, Seigne J *et al.* Enhanced tumor supressor gene therapy via replication-deficient adenovirus vectors expressing an N-terminal truncated retinoblastoma protein. *Cancer Res*, 1996, **56**, 2245–9.

62 Signe JD, Hu S-X, Kong K-T *et al.* Rationale and development of retinoblastoma (RB) tumor supressor gene therapy for bladder cancer. *J Urol*, 1996, **155**, 320A (Abstract 38).

63 Feng M, Cabrera G, Deshane J *et al.* Neoplastic reversion accomplished by high efficiency adenoviral-mediated delivery of an anti-ras ribozyme. *Cancer Res*, 1995, **55**, 2024–8.

64 EAstham JA, Ahlering TA. Use of an anti-ras ribozyme to alter the malignant phenotype of a human bladder cancer cell line. *J Urol*, 1996, **156**, 1186–8.

65 Ogios Y, Gutierrez L, Wrathall LS *et al.* Trans-Dominant suppressor mutations of the H-ras oncogene. *Cell Growth Different*, 1990, **1**, 217–24.

66 Sakai N, Ogiso Y, Fujita H *et al.* Induction of apoptosis by a dominant negative H-RAS mutant (116Y) in K562 cells. *Exp Cell Res*, 1994, **215**, 131–6.

67 Ogiso Y, Sakai N, Watari H *et al.* Suppression of various human tumor cell lines by a dominant negative H-ras mutant. *Gene Ther*, 1994, **1**, 403–7.

68 Byrne RR, Chakraborty S, Brown RW *et al.* An immunohistochemical study of E-cadherin in transitional cell carcinoma and carcinoma *in situ* in frozen adn paraffin sections. *J Urol*, 1996, **155**, 614A (Abstract 1212).

69 Bringuier PP, Umbas R, Schaafsma E *et al.* Decreased E-cadherin immunoreactivity correlates with poor survival in patients with bladder tumors. *Cancer Res*, 1993, **53**, 3241–5.

70 Syrigos KN, Krausz T, Waxman J *et al.* E-cadherin expression in bladder cancer using formalin-fixed, paraffin-embedded tissues: Correlation with histopathological grade, tumor stage and survival. *Int J Cancer*, 1995, **64**, 367–70.

71 Kleinerman DI, Dinney CP, Zhang WW *et al.* Suppression of human bladder cancer growth by increased expression of C-CAM1 gene in an orthotopic model. *Cancer Res*, 1996, **56**, 3431–5.

22. LOCALLY INDUCED HYPERTHERMIA IN BLADDER CANCER

Patrizio Rigatti, Avidgor Lev, Luigi Filippo Da Pozzo, Andrea Salonia, and Renzo Colombo

INTRODUCTION

For long time now local hyperthermia (LHT) has appeared to be a promising approach for treating solid tumours, particularly those located on the surface of the body or within a natural body cavity. Unfortunately, lack of a suitable and safe technology has prevented so far the implementation of this therapeutic solution. Based on advances in technology and on knowledge regarding the pathophysiology of the neoplastic diseases, recently acquired, many interesting clinical applications concerning hyperthermia alone or in combination with chemo- and/or radiotherapy in tumour ablation and prevention have been documented. A supra-additive, or at least additive antitumoral effect induced by the associated administration of local hyperthermia and radiation or cytostatic drugs has been indeed demonstrated *in vitro*, in animal models, as well as in many clinical trials.

Owing to its peculiar intracavitary location, superficial transitional cell carcinoma of the bladder is best suited to a combined approach with local hyperthermia and intravesical chemotherapy (ICT). An advanced apparatus, specifically designed to deliver intravesical hyperthermia alone or in combination with cytostatics in superficial bladder tumour patients has been recently developed and clinically tested in the Department of Urology, Scientific Institute H. San Raffaele, Milan, Italy.

HISTORICAL EXCURSUS AND RATIONALE

The chance of treating tumours by hyperthermia was first sustained by Busch (1) who observed the disappearance of a sarcoma after a febrile episode caused by streptococcic toxin during the clinical course of erysipelas. Based on this observation Coley (2) tested some pyretogenic bacterial toxins in order to induce voluntarily an hyperpyretic condition, expecting to obtain a remission of the neoplastic disease. Many therapeutic applications of hyperthermia in the oncological field have been organized enthusiastically during the following decades but the results were disappointing, mainly due to technical limitations. In the last two decades, several experimental investigations *in vivo* and *in vitro*, showing the high thermo-susceptibility of the malignant cells and an increase of the tumour cell killing when heated over 40°C, kept on supporting utilization of hyperthermia in the anticancer treatment (3–13). In 1974 Hall (14) proposed, for the first time, the possibility to use an isotonic solution heated at 45°C and instilled via the transurethra into the bladder for superficial tumour ablation. This experiment had poor results in terms of tumour response but demonstrated that bladder cancer, due to its localization into a natural closed cavity easily accessible through the urethra, could represent an excellent field for local hyperthermia clinical application. Afterwards, various techniques for local hyperthermia delivering have been proposed. Among these ultrasounds and electromagnetic non-ionizing radiations as radiofrequencies have also been clinically tested by different authors (15–18) and also by ourselves. Many criticisms, including the non-homogeneous heating achieved, the risk of an urethral overwarming, and an excessive transparietal gradient involving the perivesical structures, dramatically reduced the clinical implementation of HT for bladder cancer. On the other hand, microwaves (MW) appeared as a very reliable physical source for LHT implementations in clinical trials (19,20). Since 1988, several studies have verified feasibility, safety, and efficacy of local MW-induced hyperthermia (LMWHT) in the treatment of superficial transitional cell carcinoma of the bladder (STCCB). We are, therefore, able to present a wide collection of both laboratory and clinical information.

PRECLINICAL STUDIES

Two sets of experiments were conducted to examine the ability of designed applicator to heat the bladder wall. In the first, liquid and solid phantoms were constructed and in the second, female pigs were treated.

With the use of the liquid phantom we demonstrated that the electromagnetic (e.m.) radiation is transmitted from the applicator in a cylindrical symmetrical mode, that there is no e.m. radiation in undesired zones, that e.m. radiation energy has a typical shape, with higher energy transmitted towards distant bladder wall and lower energy to near bladder wall. The particular radiation pattern would allow for more homogeneous energy deposition in all bladder wall once bladder is inflated in a controlled manner. Finally, it could be demonstrated that the e.m. radiation propagating from the applicator does not decay exponentially, because, as expected, the whole volume of interest is in the near field.

The solid phantom simulated a bladder embedded in a special material equivalent to the muscle tissue to study the dielectric properties of the specific e.m. frequency (21). With this phantom, we simulated treatments with the use of a catheter (Fig. 22.1 and Plate 5). We measured the heat deposition in the vicinity of the bladder wall in area corresponding to the lamina propria, muscle as well as in areas of the 'urethra'. The measurements were done also to verify heat deposition further in depth.

We demonstrated that the heat absorption rate to the e.m. radiation from our applicator, in the circumstances resembling treatment, gave indeed homogeneous heating of bladder wall surface, decayed rapidly with depth—typically at 5 mm—and that there was no potentially harmful heating in undesired areas, such as in the urethra.

Finally, we treated female pigs with catheters having the applicator loaded in it inserted through the urethra and thermocouples (t.c.) measured the temperature on the external surface of the bladder. Having such a thin bladder wall, the pigs bladders were surgically exposed (under complete anaesthesia with ethical committee approval for the experiments) and the t.c. attached to them.

We were able to demonstrate that the heating mechanism was directly heating the bladder wall with the e.m. radiation, and not due to heating the medium (distilled water) in the bladder, which in turn heated the bladder wall. We also compared the t.c. values

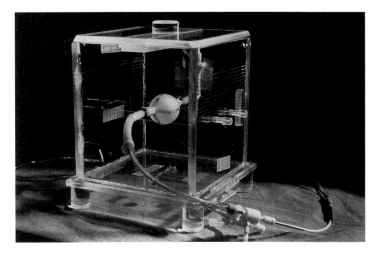

Fig. 22.1 Phantom simulating treatment including balloon catheter for the heat deposition measurement at different distances from the microwaves applicator

which are part of the operative catheter and demonstrated that the internal t.c. were measuring the bladder wall temperature correctly and were not influenced by the e.m. radiation or by the medium temperature.

THE SB-TS 101 *SYNERGO® SYSTEM*

Based on the abovementioned investigations, a novel apparatus specifically designed for delivering intravesical hyperthermia alone or in combination with cytostatic solution was constructed. The SB-TS 101 *Synergo® System*, consists of two integrated parts: a peculiar transurethral catheter, which represents the peripheral operative arm and a computerized central unit for the treatment monitoring (Fig. 22.2). The operative catheter is a 20 Fr silicon

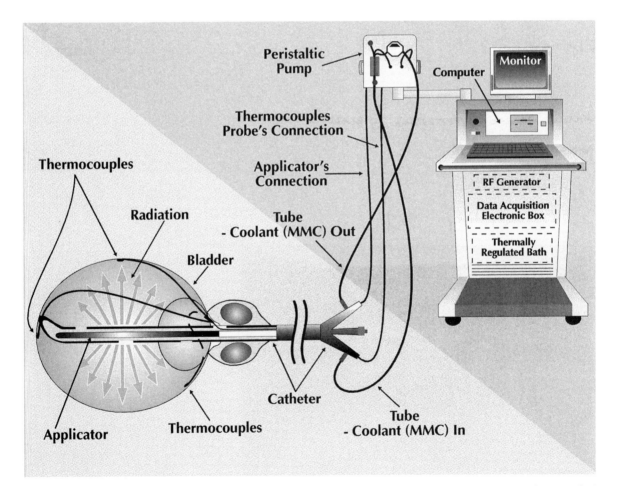

Fig. 22.2 *Schematics of the* Synergo® System *showing the computerized unit for treatment monitoring and the special transurethral catheter during the operative session*

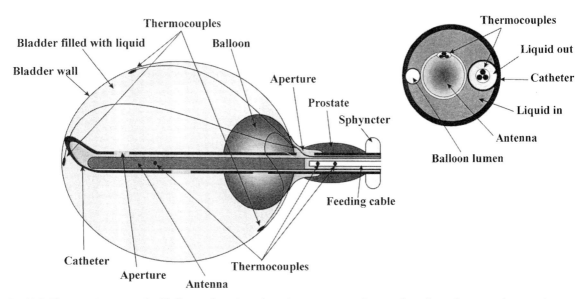

Fig. 22.3 *The operative transurethral balloon catheter in a schematic representation during a chemothermotherapy application. The cross-section shows the ways for the applicator insertion, the thermocouples location, and the closed circulatory circuit*

balloon catheter. The lumen of catheter includes many separate parts (Figs 22.3 and 22.4 and Plate 6) allowing for residual urine voiding, MW applicator insertion, intracavitary t.c. set introduction, and cytostatic solution intravesical instillation. In addition, a closed circulatory circuit which allows the solution pumping in and out of the bladder, is placed into the same catheter. The intravesical applicator is a centrally fed, asymmetric dipole type antenna connected to a 915 MHz MW source which is located into

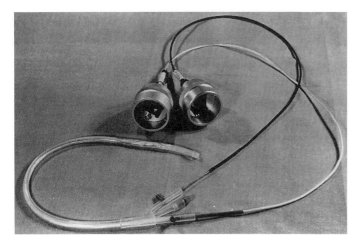

Fig. 22.4 *Ultimate version of the* Synergo® System *operative catheter ready for treatment. The lure cone connections for closed loop circulation of cytotoxic solution and the connections of microwaves applicator to central unit are shown*

the central unit. The thermocouple set includes six elements: one of them is placed in the applicator feeding point, which during the application is the hottest zone. Two other thermocouples are placed on the cable of the applicator in the prostatic urethral zone. Only one of these thermocouples is needed in female patients and is used to measure the temperature in the urethral sphincter zone. The feeding cable, the MW applicator and the t.c. are covered by a thin poly(tetrafluoroethene) (Teflon) layer. In a separate lumen of the catheter a set of three additional thermocouples are loaded to record the temperature in different areas of bladder walls. With the exception of the terminal part, they are bundled together; in the last 10 cm only they are separated into three distinct sensors. When the catheter is ready for the insertion, the bundled part lies in the lumen, while the separated part of the thermocouples project out from the lumen just before the balloon. These are pushed back to special predetermined holes further down in the catheter, so that when the balloon is inflated inside the bladder, the thermocouples spread out from the holes and are pushed against the bladder wall. Owing to special reinforcement inserted along the thermocouples, giving them a special mechanical force resembling a spring, constant mechanical contact is maintained within the tissue. The entire thermocouples structure is coated with a thin poly(tetrafluoroethene) layer. Owing to the fact that the tips of these thermocouples are thin, when pushed against the tissue they conform to it and, therefore, they are thermally isolated from the buffer in the bladder. This configuration ensures reliable temperature measurement of the first cell layers of the bladder wall. The cytostatic solution flows out through one of the aforementioned lumens and, after thermal treatment (cooling or heating), flows back in through the other lumen. Then, the solution flows in an external closed circuit where the thermal treatment is performed in a heat exchanger. To avoid the risk of urethral overheating, the solution is pumped out from the bladder and then pumped in after being cooled. This circulatory system is closed and allows control of the urethral temperature and of the solution in the bladder. The location of the operative catheter during the application can be observed by suprapubic ultrasounds. During the application, all physical parameters are registered and monitored by the computerized unit.

Our schedule of treatment administration generally included 8 weekly sessions lasting 40–60 min. In some cases the weekly sessions were followed by 4 monthly sessions performed as inductive and maintenance cycles, respectively. The entire treatment is conducted on an outpatient basis using an urethral gel containing 2.5 mg lignocaine. The bladder is first emptied of residual volume, the transurethral operative catheter is inserted, and the balloon is inflated with 15 ml of distilled water. The three thermocouples are spread out to touch the bladder walls. The solution of cytostatic drug dissolved in distilled water is then instilled. Owing to their different length, these thermocouples generally come into contact with the posterior, lateral wall and bladder neck, respectively. However, their location, as well as the general bladder configuration, can be observed by means of ultrasound scanning. A cytostatic drug, mitomycin C at a dose of 20–40 mg in 40–60 ml of distilled water was then used. In patients refractory or allergic to mitomycin C, a solution of epirubicin at a dose of 50 mg was employed. LHT delivered for at least 40 min at 42.5–44.5°C was necessary for considering every session successful.

CLINICAL STUDIES

Local hyperthermia and chemotherapy for superficial bladder tumour ablation

From 1988 to 1998 over 150 superficial bladder tumour patients have been treated for ablation using thermochemotherapy applied with the use of the *Synergo® System*. All patients had STCCB recurrent after transurethral resection (TUR) for Ta/T1 transitional tumours and most were recurrent in spite of chemo- and or immunoprophylaxis. Before the combined treatment each patient underwent complete clinical assessment including excretory urography, pelvic computerized tomography (CT) and/or nuclear magnetic resonance and bone scan and cystoscopy. During rigid cystoscopy biopsies of visible tumours, suspect areas and normal looking mucosa were taken. Uroflowmetry with residual urine and compilation of detailed questionnaire regarding subjective symptomatology completed the pretreatment evaluation. Before starting treatment all patients were required to sign an informed consent form defined according to the Helsinki Committee and approved by the ethical committee of our institute. The combined regimen was administered on native bladder tumours as neoadjuvant approach before TUR. The schedule of administration included six sessions given once a week with an overall treatment period no longer than 8 weeks. Patients suffering from high-risk STCCB (highly recurrent and with extensive tumoral mass) underwent also maintenance therapy of 4 monthly sessions. The effect of the treatment was evaluated after four sessions and 7–10 days after the treatment completion by means of cystoscopy and biopsies, uroflowmetry, and subjective questionnaire compilation. Patients underwent TUR no later than 3 weeks after treatment completion. In terms of tumour response we defined complete response when no residual tumour cells could be observed after treatment in any biopsy specimen and partial response when an overall endoscopic reduction of more than 50% of the initial tumour mass was seen.

In general the combined administration of local HT and intravesical chemotherapy using the *Synergo® System* was subjectively well tolerated according to the comparison of the pre- and postoperative questionnaires. Cystitic symptoms including nocturia, urge, and mild urethral pain were generally referred. However, in few cases only these disturbances required stopping of the treatment before the scheduled time and always spontaneously disappeared within 1 week after the last session. No systemic side-effects were observed, with the exception of three cases of cutaneous rash reaction. One case of urethral stricture, two cases of vesico-ureteral reflux, and one case of bladder contracture were registered as delayed complications. It cannot be excluded, however, that these events were due to the repeated TUR or previous intravesical chemotherapy. The cystoscopic evaluation during and after local combined treatment showed a progressive flattening and a dramatic reduction of tumour dimensions, which was related to the number of sessions. In cases of complete response after treatment, the vegetations totally disappeared leaving only a fibrinous coating. In cases of partial response, degenerative changes such as exfoliation, erosion, and necrosis of vegetations were observed. On the contrary the non-neoplastic mucosa in all cases showed only minimal modifications attributable to oedema and erythema. The selective antitumoral effect of combined approach was also confirmed by histological evaluations, which affirmed as the most evident features the extensive necrosis of malignant lesions and the minimal inflammatory reaction of non-tumoral areas. In cases of complete response massive calcification, sclerohyaline necrosis extended to the lamina propria in T1 tumours, and thrombosis of vascular structure at the tumoral basis were constantly documented (Fig. 22.5 and Plate 7). Residual viable neoplastic cells showing evident degenerative and/or irreversible changes such as vacuolization, ballooning of cytoplasm and nuclear pyknosis were constantly detected in cases of partial response. Histological changes could never be observed in the detrusal layer. TUR after treatment was technically easy in all cases. Overall, according to our previously defined criteria, histological examination on TUR specimens after treatment documented a tumour complete response in about 65% and partial response in 25% of patients respectively. All tumours on the posterior bladder wall were completely eradicated, while residual disease was mainly found in the lateral walls or trigone.

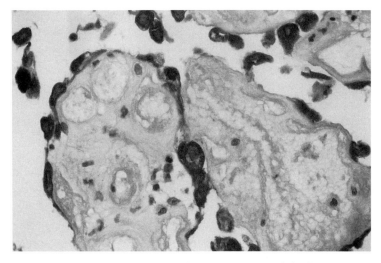

Fig. 22.5 Massive calcification and sclerohyaline necrosis extended to lamina propria in T1 tumours after chemo-thermotherapy treatment. Thrombosis of vascular structure at the tumoral basis are also evident. Haematoxylin and eosin, × 400

Seven patients in whom the disease superficially involved the prostatic urethra, had complete eradication of these tumours too. The response rate seemed to be independent from stage or grade of tumours, the complete remission being documented in both Ta and T1 as well as in GI and GII cases. Complete response was also registered in high recurrent chemo- or immunorefractory tumours. Location and size of vegetations appeared to be the main factors conditioning the tumour response rate. However, many tumours larger than 2 cm could be totally eradicated.

From February 1989 to December 1993, 52 patients with Ta-T1 intact bladder tumours entered a prospective randomized neo-adjuvant study (22) in order to compare the tumour ablative power of local thermochemotherapy delivered using the *Synergo® System* versus standard intravesical chemotherapy alone. Of the patients included, 29 were randomly assigned to receive thermochemotherapy, while 23 intravesical chemotherapy alone. Mitomycin C at 40 mg diluted in distilled water was used as cytostatic solution in both groups and LHT was delivered at 43.5°C temperature in the *Synergo® System* group. All patients completed the scheduled administration and 10 days after treatment underwent TUR of residual tumours and/or suspected areas. Our study proved the high superiority of the thermochemotherapy approach when compared with the standard intravesical chemotherapy as the complete responses in this group of patients were as high as 66% versus 22% of the control group ($P < 0.01$). The most interesting results have been documented when the *Synergo®*

treatment was administered to a special subset of patients who, in spite of superficial stage tumours, were candidates for radical cystectomy (23,24). We refer to 19 patients suffering from high recurrent, chemorefractory, multifocal, and extensive disease. Seventeen of them were Ta–T1 low grade and two were T1 GIII tumours. The disease-free interval was generally less than 6 months for all patients. The preoperative tumour dimension ranged from a few millimetres to 3 cm in diameter and the overall extension of the disease measured at cystoscopy ranged from 30% to 70% of the whole bladder surface. Five patients had vegetation both at the bladder neck and prostatic urethra. For all of them TUR was considered technically not feasible or not curative and radical cystectomy was suggested. As radical surgery was refused, these patients underwent Synergo® treatment as a neoadjuvant organ sparing programme. Mitomycin C at 40 mg was used as cytostatic in 16 patients while in three, allergic to mitomycin C, epirubicin at 50 mg was administered. In this set of patients in an effort to potentate the effectiveness and to stabilize the drug concentration into the bladder throughout the entire session, the cystostatic solution was replaced after 30 min of every application. After treatment all patients underwent cystoscopy which demonstrated the complete disappearance of all tumours in eight patients. In the remaining 11 cases, cystoscopy showed an extensive necrosis of some tumours together with residual vegetations involved in evident regressive degenerative changes. In these cases, the necrosis selectively occurred in the neoplastic areas sparing the normal mucosa. TUR of residual tumours or areas of doubt was considered feasible and easy in 15 cases. Histological examination on TUR specimens confirmed eight (42%) complete responses and seven (37%) partial responses. Surprising all vegetations located in the prostatic urethra were totally eradicated while residual tumours were observed in the lateral wall and rarely in the bladder neck. In the remaining four patients due to extensive residual tumours, TUR was still considered unfeasible and radical cystectomy was performed. In the 15 patients who had their bladder spared after Synergo® System treatment and TUR, in a medium 16-month follow-up only eight overall superficial relapses occurred and were easily removed by TUR or laser therapy.

Local hyperthermia and chemotherapy for prophylaxis of recurrence of superficial bladder tumours

Based on safety, selectivity and synergistic antitumour effect proved in clinical neoadjuvant ablative trials, the local thermochemotherapy appeared a promising method also for prophylaxis of recurrences after TUR. Reducing the recurrence rate and improving the disease-free interval remain the crucial targets of every approach to superficial bladder tumour due to the high prevalence and the social cost of the disease. Most patients who underwent ablative trials as previously reported, were only followed-up after TUR without adjunctive prophylactic regimen. For over 50 of them, the follow-up is at present longer than 5 years. For these patients, the overall recurrence rate was ranged from 16% to 33%. These data are generally better than those reported in literature for the standard treatments irrespectively of the kind of drugs or schedules administered. Furthermore, when each patient treated by thermochemotherapy was used as their own control, a clear preventive efficacy of the combined regimen was evident in both reduction of number of relapses and increase of disease-free interval. It seems that both ablation of tumours and prevention of recurrences could be performed. In order to verify the efficacy of local thermochemotherapy in STCCB prophylaxis after TUR, since January 1994 a prospective randomized multicentric study is ongoing. Until now 60 patients entered the study. Of them 29 were randomly assigned to the combined approach and 31 to the intravesical chemotherapy using mitomycin C, 40 mg alone. The schedule of administration includes 8 weekly and 4 monthly sessions. Follow-up includes cytology, cystoscopy, and biopsies every 3 months up to 24 months. At a mean follow-up of 26.2 months only two recurrences were registered in the combined group while in the chemotherapy alone group we recorded 18 recurrences ($P < 0.01$). Although preliminary, these results are encouraging but longer follow-up and more patients are certainly needed to substantiate these findings.

CONCLUSIONS

Epidemiology and social cost proclaim that superficial bladder tumour remains of crucial interest for the development of novel therapeutic strategies. About 40 000 new cases of bladder tumour per year have been registered in the USA during the last decade (25,26). Approximately 75% of them are superficial at first observation. Among these, 30–40% will recur in spite of intravesical chemo- or immunoprophylaxis, and nearly 35% will progress in stage or in grade (27–37). These data confirm that at present we certainly need to enhance our ability in STCCB management.

LHT is of recent interest in oncology as a potential minimally invasive procedure for treating solid tumours in both curative and palliative situations. Many studies showed that when hyperthermia is used alone a clinical evident antitumoral effect can be obtained (38). However, the complete response rate achieved using LHT alone is only in the range of 10–15% mainly due to the fact that the uniform elevation of tumour temperature to curative levels can only rarely be achieved safely using current devices. Thus, at present time it appears that LHT can be satisfactory used in clinical situations only in combination with other effective antitumoral treatments. Literature suggests that, when LHT is used in conjunction with selected anticancer agents, a synergistic antitumour effect can be expected (39). The mechanism of this interaction between LHT and cytostatics could be explained by an increase in drug uptake, an alteration in intracellular distribution and metabolism of drug, an increase in drug reaction rate with DNA or heat-induced inhibition of DNA repair. Unfortunately, the clinical implementation of this rationale has been prevented so far by evident technological limitations. A prototype system, designed to deliver intravesical hyperthermia by means of a MW applicator which directly irradiates both the bladder wall and the cytostatic solution filling the bladder cavity, was recently developed and clinically tested (40,41). Tests were carried out in both animals and humans and showed that this technology enables heating of the superficial layers of the bladder within a range of 42.5–46°C. In this way, the heat can be quite homogeneously delivered to the entire bladder surface with an expected maximum gradient between different areas, which is generally lower than 1°C. The risk of overheating the urethral or prostatic mucosa is prevented by a closed transurethral circulatory system allowing for the cooling of the solution as necessary. The same circulatory closed circuit also allows the concentration of the cytostatic solution to be modified in the bladder, for example by adding a concentrated drug, in order to ensure optimum performance during the treatment session. Since 1989, over 150 patients affected by STCCB have been treated in a pre-TUR regimen using a combination of LMW-induced hyperthermia and ICT. The schedule of treatment administration generally included 6 weekly sessions lasting 40–60 min. Temperature was delivered at medium 43.5°C and mitomycin at 40 mg in 50 ml normal saline was used as a cytostatic solution in most cases. The treatment, administered in outpatient basis without anaesthesia was, in general well tolerated by all patients. Further clinical investigations are needed to define the role of this regimen in the management of superficial bladder cancer.

Key Points

1. Owing to its intracavitary location, STCCB is an ideal model for a combined approach with LHT and ICT.
2. Based on safety, selectivity, and synergistic antitumour effect the combined administration of LHT and ICT using the *Synergo® System* is a promising method, which reduces the recurrence rate and improves the disease-free interval.
3. At present we cannot state to what extent the results observed are due to hyperthermia and whether or not there is a true synergism with chemotherapy. The most adequate schedule of administration has also to be defined. It is hoped that randomized clinical trials presently in progress, will satisfactorily address the above issues.

References

1 Busch W. Uber den Einfluss, welchen heitigere Erysipeln zuweilen auf organisierte neubildungen ausuben. In: *Verhandl Naturh*. Preuss Rhein, Westphal, 1866, pp. 23–8.

2 Coley WR. The treatment of malignant tumours by repeated inoculation of erysipelas. With a report of ten original cases. *Am J Sci*, 1893, **105**, 487–9.

3 England HR, Anderson JD, Minasian H *et al*. The therapeutic application of hyperthermia in the bladder. *Br J Urol* 1976, **47**, 849–52.

4 Gerner EW, Boone R, Connor WG *et al*. A transient thermotollerant survival response produced by single thermal doses in He LA cells. *Cancer Res* 1976, **36**, 1035–40.

5 Giovannella BC, Stehlin JS, Morgan AC. Select lethal effect of supranormal temperatures on human neoplastic cell. *Cancer Res* 1976, **36**, 3944.

6 Dewey WC, Hopwood LE, Sapareto SA, Gerweck LE. Cellular responses to combinations of hyperthermia and radiation. *Radiation*, 1977, **123**, 463–74.

7 Bhunyan BK, Day KJ, Edgerton CE, Ogunbase O. Sensitivity of different cells lines and of different phases in the cell cycle to hyperthermia. *Cancer Res* 1977, **37**, 3780–4.

8 Bhunyan BK. Kinetics of cell kill by hyperthermia. *Cancer Res* 1979, **39**, 2277–84.

9 Henle KJ. Sensitization to hyperthermia below 43°C in Chinese hamster ovary cells by stepdown heating. *J Natl Cancer Inst* 1980, **64**, 1479–81.

10 Henle KJ, Roti Roti J. Time-temperature conversion in biological applications of hyperthermia. *Radiat Res* 1980, **82**, 138–45.

11 Dewhirst MW, Sim DA, Gross J, Kundrat MA. Effect of heating rate in tumor and normal tissue microcirculatory function. In: *Hyperthermic oncology* (ed. Overgaard J). Taylor and Francis, London, 1984, 1, 77–180.

12 Luk KH, Pajak TF, Perez CA *et al*. (1984). Prognostic factors for tumor response after hyperthermia and radiation. In: *Hyperthermic oncology* (ed. Overgaard J). Taylor and Francis, London, 1984, 1, 353–356.

13 Oleson JR, Calderwood SK, Coughlin CT *et al*. Biological and clinical aspects of hyperthermia in cancer therapy. *Am J Clin Oncol* 1988, **11** (3), 368–80.

14 Hall RR, Schade ROK, SwinneyY. Effects of hyperthermia on bladder cancer: preliminary communication. *Br Med J*, 1974, **2**, 593–4.

15 Le Veen H, Wapnick Piccone V *et al*. Tumor eradication by radiofrequency theraphy. Response 21 patients. *JAMA* 1976, **235**, 2198–200.

16 Marmor JB, Pounds D, Hahn GM. Clinical trial of ultrasound induced hyperthermia. *Proceedings of the Fourteenth Annual Meeting of the American Society of Clinical Oncology*, 1978, 19, 330.

17 Bichler KH, Fluchter SH, SteimannJ, Strhmaier WL. Combination of hyperthermia and cytostatics in the treatmentof bladder cancer. *Urologia Intis*, 1989, **44**, 10–4.

18 Debicki P, Okoniewska E, Okoniewski M. Superficial and intraurethral applicators for microwave hyperthermia. *Adv Exp Med Biol*, 1990, **267**, 321–6.

19 Yerushalmi A, Fishelovitz Y, Singer D *et al*. Localized deep microwave hyperhermia in the treatment of poor operative risk patients with benign prostatic hyperplasia. *J Urol* 1985, **133**, 873–7.

20 Servadio C, Leib Z, Lev A. Disease of prostate treated by local microwave hyperthermia. *Urology*, 1987, **30**, 97–9.

21 Chou CK, Chen GW, Guy AW, Luk KH. Formula for preparing phantom muscle tissue at various radiofrequencies. *Bioelectromagnetics*, 1984, **5**, 435–41.

22 Colombo R, Da Pozzo LF, Lev A *et al*. Neoadjuvant combined microwave induced local hyperthermia and topical chemotherapy versus chemotherapy alone for superficial bladder cancer. *J Urol* 1996, **155**, 1227–32.

23 Colombo R, Da Pozzo LF, Lev A *et al*. Local microwave hyperthermia and intravesical chemotherapy as bladder sparing treatment for select multifocal and unresectable superficial bladder tumors. *J Urol* 1998, in press.

24 Colombo R, Lev A, Da Pozzo LF *et al*. A new approach using local combined microwave hyperthermia and chemotherapy in superficial transitional bladder carcinoma treatment. *J Urol* 1995, **153**, 959–63.

25 Kiemeney LA, Witjes JA, Verbeek AL *et al*. The clinical epidemiology of superficial bladder cancer. Dutch South-East Cooperative Urol Group. *Br J Cancer* 1993, **67** (4), 806–12.

26 Ross RK, Jones PA, Yu MC. Bladder cancer epidemiology and pathogenesis. *Semin Oncol* 1996, **23**, 536–45.

27 Soloway MS, Jordan AM, Murphy WM. Rationale for intravesical chemotherapy in the treatment and prophylaxis of superficial transitional cell carcinoma. *Prog Clin Biol Res* 1989, **310**, 215–36.

28 Soloway MS. Intravesical therapy for bladder cancer. *J Urol* 1994, **152**, 379–81.

29 Lamm DL. BCG in perspective: advances in the treatment of superficial bladder cancer. *Eur Urol* 1995, **27** (1), 2–8.

30 Lamm DL. BCG immunotherapy for transitional-cell carcinoma in situ of the bladder. *Oncology*, 1995, **9** (10), 947–52.

31 Lamm DL, Van der Meijden AP, Akaza H *et al.* Intravesical chemotherapy and immunotherapy: how do we assess their effectiveness and what are their limitations and uses? *Int J Urol* 1995, **2** (2), 23–35.

32 Morales A. Intravesical therapy of bladder cancer: an immunotherapy success story. *Int J Urol* 1996, **3**, 329–33.

33 Nseyo UO, Lamm DL. Therapy of superficial bladder cancer. *Semin Oncol* 1996, **23**, 598–604.

34 Soloway MS. Bladder cancer. *Urology* 1996, **48** (4), 631–8.

35 Hall RR. Application of clinical trials to the care of patients with bladder cancer. *Eur Urol* 1997, **31** (1), 42–6.

36 Martinez-Pineiro JA, Martinez-Pineiro L. BCG update: intravesical therapy. *Eur Urol* 1997, **31** (1), 31–41.

37 Witjes JA. Current recommendations for the management of bladder cancer. Drug therapy. *Drug* 1997, **53** (3), 404–14.

38 Overgaard J. Rationale and problems in design of clinical studies. In: *Hyperthermic oncology* 1984 (ed: Overgaard J). Taylor and Francis, London, 1985, 2, 325–338.

39 Herman TS, Teicher BA, Jochelson M *et al.* Rationale for use of local hyperthermia with radiation therapy and selected anticancer drugs in locally advanced human malignancies. *Int J Hyperthermia*, 1988, **4**, 143–58.

40 Rigatti P, Lev A, Colombo R. Combined intravesical chemotherapy with Mytomicin C and local bladder microwave-induced hyperthermia as a preoperative therapy for superficial bladder tumors. A preliminary clinical study. *Eur Urol* 1991, **20**, 204–10.

41 Colombo R, Da Pozzo LF, Lev A *et al.* Local microwave hyperthermia and intravesical chemotherapy with Mytomicin C as neoadjuvant treatment for selected multifocal and unresectable superficial bladder tumors. *Acta Urol Italica*, 1995, **4**, 167.

23. ALTERNATIVE URINARY RESERVOIRS AND CONDUITS: STATE OF THE SCIENCE

Francois Desgrandchamps and Donald P. Griffith

INTRODUCTION

Bladder augmentation or bladder replacement is required in some patients with malignancies or other advanced pathological problems. Conduits and reservoirs constructed from reconstituted autologous large and small intestine have worked reasonably well for the past 75+ years. A robust literature thoroughly documents the advantages, disadvantages, and limitations of the many variations of intestinal alternatives. Common to all intestinal alternatives is a need for: (i) a general anaesthetic; (ii) a major operation with attendant stress, morbidity, and convalescence; (iii) significant expense; and (iv) significant recurrent medical problems in managing the conduit or reservoir. Despite the successful use of bowel many investigators have dreamed and worked toward other alternatives.

The purpose of this chapter is to review selected historical initiatives and present new technologies which may contribute to development of alternative 'conduits' or 'reservoirs' to augment or replace the diseased urinary bladder.

HISTORICAL EXPERIENCE WITH ALLOPLASTIC BLADDER REPLACEMENT

Modern historical initiatives that attempted to develop alternative conduits and reservoirs began in the 1950s and 1960s, although there were many earlier attempts. Historically, investigations focused on four strategies. One initiative was the use of a foreign body or alloplast to act as a 'patch' for bladder augmentation (1). A second initiative was the use of an alloplast as a scaffold for 'growth of a neo-bladder' from residual urothelial and smooth muscle tissues (2–5). A third strategy was the use of alloplastic materials to create a 'distensible reservoir' (6–11). A fourth strategy focused on the development of a fixed volume, rigid wall reservoir that utilized gravity drainage for filling and evacuation (12).

Alloplastic patches

Alloplastic augmentation of the small native bladder was attempted several times (1) using Dacron, poly(tetrafluoroethene) (PTFE) and perhaps other porous alloplasts. These materials were probably chosen because of the successful use of such materials in replacement of diseased arteries. Alloplastic augmentation of the bladder was invariably a failure. Failure occurred because intraluminal bacteriuria eroded anastomotic union of the alloplast with native collecting system tissues. When the porous alloplast was maintained outside the urinary tract the 'patch' healed but within months the 'patch' extruded intraluminally.

Alloplastic scaffolds

Collecting system tissues (smooth muscle and urothelium) have a long history of regenerative ability. Several investigators have tried to 'grow a new bladder' by placing a spherical alloplast in the pelvis following cystectomy (2–5). The bladder neck, urethra, and the distal ureters were left 'in situ' in the pelvis in close proximity to the spherical alloplast. The investigators thought that smooth muscle and urothelium would regenerate from the bladder neck and ureters and form a neo-bladder around the alloplastic sphere. The sphere was to be removed several months after implantation by which time the neo-bladder was to have regenerated.

This strategy demonstrated some success inasmuch as there was growth of some residual smooth muscle and urothelium but the neo-bladder contracted had little or no innervation and was not functional in the normal sense. In summary this strategy also failed and has been abandoned.

Though the historical 'alloplastic scaffold theory' has been abandoned the notion of 're-growth' of a neo-bladder has had resurgent interest using modern 'tissue engineering' principles. New initiatives which look very promising- will be summarized later in this chapter.

Expansile–contractile bladder prostheses

Numerous investigators (6–11) have tried to make a distensible prosthetic bladder that expands and contracts much like native human bladders. Such a model requires anastomotic union with the collecting system (ureter, renal pelvis, and/or urethra). It commonly employed features to effect reduced or negative pressures intraluminally, to facilitate filling, and increased or positive pressures to effect evacuation. The most sophisticated of these models was the one described by Barrett and Donovan (7,8) in 1992 and

O'Sullivan and Barrett in 1994 (9) (e.g. the Mayo Clinic model). The most successful of these models is the one described by Rohrman *et al.* in 1996 (11) (e.g. the Aachen, Germany model).

The Mayo model is composed of a reservoir that contains a rigid polysulphone shell inside of which is a distensible silicone shell. The two shells are connected only at the bladder neck. A system of springs and mechanical pumps creates negative pressure within the lumen of the silicone shell to facilitate filling. A similar mechanical pressurized pump facilitates evacuation. Renal pelvic urine drains into the prosthetic reservoir through two 8F silicone tubes place into the native ureters. The reservoir drains under positive pressure into a silicone tube inserted into the urethra. Watertight closure of silicone tubes is achieved by wrapping the ureterosilicone interface and the urethrosilicone interface with a porous Dacron™ cuff. Reflux was prevented via a 'duckbill' valve. This sophisticated device when implanted intraperitoneally in canines, however, suffered the same fate as virtually

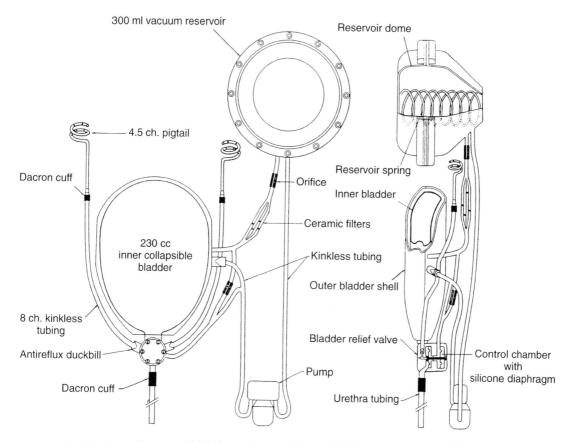

Fig. 23.1 Expansile–contractile bladder prosthese: the Mayo model (9) schematic anterior and lateral view

all of the prior initiatives. It failed within a few weeks due to:
(i) mechanical failure of the device components; (ii) leakage
of urine at the prosthesis-collecting system anastomoses; and
(iii) infection exterior to the device leading to loss of tissue
bonding and abscess formation.

The Aachen model which has been in development for many
years utilizes a subcutaneous reservoir rather than an intraperitoneal reservoir (e.g. the Mayo model). The latest version of the
Aachen model used an elastic reservoir that was compressible by
extracorporeal manual pressure. Compression provided positive
pressure to evacuate the reservoirs and created negative pressure
within the reservoir to enhance filling. Separate reservoirs drained
each kidney via Dacron-covered silicone tubes placed through the
renal parenchyma as prosthetic ureters. Fibroblasts within the
renal parenchyma bonded with the Dacron to effect watertight
union of the silicone ureters to the renal collecting system. Both
subcutaneous reservoirs drained into the urethra via a Dacron
reinforced Y-tube of silicone. This model worked effectively for
18 or more months in two animals that had no mechanical problems. Urinary leakage occurred in three animals owing to anastomotic or material failures. These studies demonstrated 'proof of

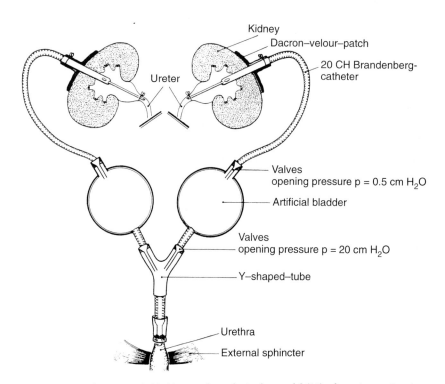

Fig. 23.2 Expansile–contractile bladder prosthese: the Aachen model (11) schematic anterior view

principle' that a subcutaneous reservoir could effectively drain the upper tracts without hydronephrosis and that reservoir urine could be manually expressed into the urethra if watertight anastomoses could be made, reliably.

In both the Mayo and the Aachen initiatives watertightness of alloplast-collecting system anastomoses depended upon Dacron bonding to the collecting system. It is not entirely clear why Dacron a porous alloplast was chosen. However, as Dacron had a long history as a successful vascular prosthesis it was an obvious candidate material. Fibroblasts grow into the pores of porous alloplasts to effect tissue bonding. The greater the in-growth the more robust the tissue alloplast union. Experimental studies suggest that large pore size favours a more robust union than small pores (13). Failure of the Mayo and Aachen models could be the result of the failure of Dacron as a tissue-bonding material in the urinary tract.

Conduits and anastomoses

Desgrandchamps *et al.* (14) have used porous PTFE clinically to effect watertight bonding of bladder and renal parenchyma to silicone tubes with near uniform success. These prosthetic ureters which were composed of silicone rubber and coated externally with PTFE have been used for up to 4 years in some patients and have been tolerant of intraluminal bacteriuria in many cases.

Gleeson and Griffith (12) and Gurpinar and Griffith (14) studied bonding of urethra, bladder, and ureter to PTFE-coated silicone in several animal species. In these studies no anastomotic leaks occurred. Moreover, mature PTFE-collecting system anastomoses were tolerant of chronic intraluminal bacteriuria for more than 4 years (14). These studies used large-pore PTFE. Preliminary tissue culture experiments demonstrated deeper penetration of fibroblasts into pores than occurred with small pore alloplasts.

The Desgrandchamps experience with prosthetic ureters show that fixed wall conduits drain the upper tracts by gravity successfully. Negative pressure in the prosthetic bladder may not be needed to drain the upper tracts. Gleeson suggested that a fixed volume prosthetic bladder could be designed to drain by gravity (12). Simple designs are attractive in that they may be less likely to undergo mechanical failure.

INFECTION AND ENCRUSTATION

Extravasation of infected urine around all types of alloplastic implants causes loss of the implant. Thus, development of reliable watertight alloplast-collecting system anastomoses is of paramount importance. Chronic bacteriuria in the absence of extravasation has not necessarily been problematic as demonstrated by Desgrandchamp's clinical experience (14) and experimental experience (12,14). Bacteria that produce urease are of greater risk than are non-urease-producing bacteria because of the propensity for such organisms to induce struvite ($MgNH_4PO_4$) encrustations and stones on the intraluminal components (16).

Encrustation of foreign bodies (tubes and reservoirs, etc.) remains the principal unsolved or non-preventable problem. Urine is supersaturated with calcium phosphate and calcium oxalate more or less continuously in all persons (17). Intermittent crystalluria is also almost universal in healthy humans with sterile urine (18). Foreign bodies such as silicone devices act as a nidus for heterogeneous nucleation and adherence of crystals. Thus, intraurinary devices, such as catheters, stents, conduits, or reservoirs are constant candidates for encrustation and stone formation. High fluid intake and special diets and drugs may be helpful in reducing the risks of encrustation, but these modalities alone are unlikely to prevent the problem. Improvements in the surface composition of devices might make encrustation less problematic. Potential improvements are in development and are reviewed later in this essay.

From the foregoing experimental studies a list of principles have evolved. They are shown in Table 23.1.

Table 23.1

PRINCIPLES OF ALLOPLASTIC RECONSTRUCTION OF THE URINARY TRACT
1. Two types of reservoirs are possible: a dynamic expansile–contractile reservoir and a fixed volume rigid wall reservoir.
2. Muscularis grows into some porous alloplasts and makes an effective and durable watertight anastomosis.
3. Porous alloplasts if colonized with bacteria harbour and perpetuate bacterial growth leading to disruption and failure of fibroblastic in-growth into the pores of the alloplast.
4. Fibroblasts from collecting system muscularis grow into porous alloplasts and make a mature collagen-rich, watertight anastomosis with the pores of the alloplast in the absence of motion or bacteria. Motion of the alloplast (during body movement) or bacterial colonization of the pores will prevent and erode fibroblastic bonding.
5. Mature porous alloplast–urothelial anastomoses are tolerant of intraluminal bacteriuria.
6. Alloplastic patches used for bladder augmentation usually result in the patch being extruded intraluminally within 12–24 months.
7. Solid (non-porous) alloplasts like silicone rubber do not make watertight anastomoses with any organ.
8. Solid (non-porous) alloplasts induce a fibroblastic reaction that surrounds the alloplast as a fibrous capsule and which may be as much as a centimetre thick.
9. Bacteriuria and encrustation of intraluminal alloplasts will occur in time. Replaceable, renewable or exchangeable intraluminal alloplasts would be helpful in minimizing the risks and/or morbidity of bacteriuria and encrustation.
10. Large pore alloplasts bond quicker and more extensively than small pore alloplasts.
11. Anastomotic leakage of urine, material failure, and encrustation are the problems that must be solved to effect useful prosthetic urological organs.

ALLOPLASTS

Non-biological materials (called alloplasts) have a long and successful history in the rehabilitation or replacement of diseased organs (19).Successful organ development is highly dependent upon the characteristics of the alloplastic material.

Egyptians used urethral catheters made from papyrus several hundred years BC (20). Latex rubber was used to make relatively soft and flexible indwelling urethral catheters during the past two centuries. In the last two decades reports of urethral strictures induced by noxious agents leaking from latex catheters prompted a search for less irritating alternatives to latex (21–23). Polyethylene has been used to make ureteral catheters but polyethylene is thought to be too stiff to be an effective and comfortable urethral catheter. Polyvinyl chloride is another plastic that has been tried as a urological device but like polyethylene it is fairly stiff and has been largely replaced by newer and better-suited alloplasts. All of these alloplasts are solid, e.g. non-porous. Vascular surgeons were among the first to demonstrate that porous alloplasts like woven or knitted Dacron became bound to native tissues by fibroblastic ingrowth. Second generation solid alloplasts include silicone rubber and polyurethane. Second generation porous alloplasts also include polyurethane and PTFE. These second-generation materials offer significant advantages and seem destined for additional enhancement.

Silicone rubber

Silicone rubber is a solid alloplast. It has been used in permanent and temporary urological devices and has low tissue reactivity and less risk of encrustation than many other alloplasts (24–27). It is the most experienced candidate for intraluminal alloplastic conduits or reservoirs. Silicone prostheses engender a vigorous fibroblastic reaction from surrounding tissue. This reaction creates a thick fibrous capsule around the silicone prosthesis. The fibrous capsule may limit expansion and contraction of a distensible reservoir over time. All solid alloplasts engender similar fibrous encapsulation. All solid alloplasts within the urinary tract act as sites of heterogeneous nucleation and thereby promote formation of urinary stones. Bacteria adhere to catheter surfaces and embed in a biofilm layer that consists of host factors such as fibrin, fibronectin, and microbial exopolysaccharide material (25–28). Bacteria that become so embedded are resistant to glycopeptide antibiotics and normal host defences such as antibodies and phagocytic polymorphonuclear cells (25–26). New technologies may be added to silicone to make the surface resistant to crystal and bacterial adhesion (28–39). Additionally, silicone may be coated on its external surface with porous alloplasts that bond the device to autologous tissues and eliminate the fibrous encapsulation that occurs with native silicone polymers.

Solid polyurethane

Polyurethane can be fabricated in both porous and non-porous forms. Solid polyurethane is a good candidate for an intraluminal alloplast inasmuch as it is almost as soft and flexible as silicone. It is subject to the same risks of bacterial adherence and encrustation as previously detailed for silicone rubber. Like silicone it offers the potential for surface coatings that retard bacterial and crystal adhesion.

Porous polyurethane

Polyurethane can also be formulated as a porous material to stabilize permanent implants. Porous polyurethane can be synthesized in many different forms and in many differ pore sizes. It is a good candidate for an external coating used to effect fibroblastic union between alloplasts and the muscularis layer of the urinary collecting system.

Poly(tetrafluoroethene)

PTFE can be fabricated in both non-porous and porous forms. The non-porous form is most commonly marketed under the trade name Teflon. Porous PTFE has been used in medical implants both as Gore-Tex and as Proplast. Gore-Tex contains small pores which are typically $<20~\mu$m in diameter. Proplast contains much larger pores which typically are $>100~\mu$m in diameter. Both Gore-Tex and Proplast are candidates to be external porous coatings that are useful in permanently bonding alloplastic implants to autogenous tissues. Experimental studies with Proplast (12,15,40) and clinical trials with Gore-Tex (14) document efficacy in bonding prosthetic ureters, bladders, and urethras to the urinary tract in a watertight fashion.

Polyester (Dacron)

Dacron is a synthetic filament. It is also called polyester and polyethylene terephthalate. Dacron prostheses are typically prepared for vascular applications. Prostheses can be woven, knitted, or made into a velour. Porosity and thickness can vary widely depending upon the manufacturer and the intended application. Dacron grafts for vascular replacement typically have small pores to minimize bleeding.

The experimental data previously reviewed suggest that PTFE may be more effective than Dacron, although no statistical significant studies have compared the materials. We are not aware of studies involving porous polyurethane to achieve watertight bonding in the urinary tract. Head to head comparisons of the strength, integrity, watertightness, and durability of the porous alloplasts have not been reported. Collective experimental data suggest that any contact of the porous material with bacteria will lead to colonization of the alloplast and erosion and loss of fibroblastic tissue in-growth. Experimental experience dictates that porous alloplasts be used only external to the urinary tract. Anecdotal data suggest that movement of a porous alloplast within tissue retards or inhibits effective tissue bonding. Solid alloplasts will be used within the lumen of the urinary tract. To date, there is no compelling data in the literature to demonstrate superiority of one solid alloplast over another. Silicone rubber and/or polyurethane or some proprietary materials similar to these are likely candidates. Selection of the optimum solid alloplast is likely to hinge on the effectiveness of antimicrobial or anti-adhesive coatings, which will be discussed below.

DESIGN CONSIDERATIONS

Chronic bacteriuria and encrustation are the limiting factors that currently complicate and thwart prosthetic urinary reservoirs and conduits. Designs that incorporate an exchangeable or renewable lumenal surface (with minimal morbidity and expense) should overcome the encrustation problem. A closed system that is not exposed to skin or other colonized sites is desirable to minimize bacterial contamination. A closed system with a renewable lumenal component which is impregnated or coated with antimicrobials or anti-adhesive materials should optimize development of alloplastic urinary organs.

NEW TECHNOLOGIES

Several new technologies may decrease and/or resolve the infection and encrustation problems that currently plague prosthetic urinary devices.

Lipid-coated alloplasts

Many biological cells contain a derivative of phosphorylcholine (PC) on their external surface. This lipid membrane prevents adherence of other cells including bacteria and crystals. Alloplasts like the ones mentioned above can now be surface-coated with PC (41–45). Studies of fibrinogen and platelet binding have shown significant reductions in adsorption on the PC-coated alloplasts (41) as compared with non-PC coated controls. PC-coated PTFE vascular grafts reduced neo-intimal hyperplasia and cell proliferation on the PC-coated surfaces as compared with controls (43). Preliminary studies in the urinary tract show that bacterial adhesion and crystal adhesion to alloplastic catheters are much reduced on PC-coated surfaces as compared with non-PC-coated surfaces (41). Thus, PC-coated solid silicone or polyurethane tubes offer the potential for reducing intraluminal attachments of bacteria or crystals.

Antibiotic coated solid alloplasts

Bacteria that adhere to catheter surfaces and embed in a biofilm of host factors are the basis for the chronic bacteriuria that invariably attend use of alloplasts within the urinary tract. Antimicrobial coating of catheters has resulted in significant reduction of the colonization of these devices *in vitro* and *in vivo*. Cefazolin, chlorhexadine gluconate, silver sulphadiazine, and quinolones have demonstrated effectiveness (31–34). In an *in vitro* comparative trial catheters coated with chlorhexadine gluconate (CHG) and silver sulphadiazine (SS) were compared with catheters coated with minocycline and rifampicin (MR). The MR coating was significantly superior to the CHG–SS combination (35,36). In a rabbit model the MR coated catheters were also significantly superior to the CHG–SS-coated catheters. In an *in vitro* comparison of efficacy the MR combination was superior to vancomycin, clindamycin, novobiocin, and minocycline alone or in combination with rifampicin. The MR-coated urinary urethral catheters are currently in evaluation in FDA monitored clinical trials and may soon be marketed by a major international urological device manufacturer.

Tissue bonding cystostomy (TBC)

From the foregoing discussion it is apparent that special coatings of solid alloplasts offer the prospect of minimizing or preventing bacterial and crystal attachment. However, the passing of time and urine will gradually erode the surface coating. A replaceable or renewable intraluminal surface is therefore desirable. From the foregoing it is also apparent that porous alloplastic materials grafted to the external surface of a solid alloplast creates a permanent fibroblastic, watertight bonding of the implant with native tissues, and the porous alloplast prevents formation of a constricting fibrous capsule around the implant. These principles will be evaluated in forthcoming clinical trials of a TBC (46).

The TBC is an implantable device made of a permanently implanted component and a replaceable or renewable transcutaneous component.. The device embraces the concepts of: (i) a porous external alloplast grafted to a solid alloplast to effect a watertight tissue anastomosis, and (ii) a replaceable and renewable lumenal component that is coated with one or more technologies to prevent bacterial growth and/or crystal adherence. Prototyping of a TBC device is in progress and FDA and Institutional Review Boards have approved phase I clinical trials.

The TBC is designed for the treatment of the permanently dysfunctional bladder like that found in paraplegics and quadriplegics. The TBC can drain the bladder continuously as does a conventional suprapubic tube or it can be closed with a simple manually actuated valve to effect use of the native bladder as a reservoir. The native bladder can then be evacuated volitionally by opening the drainage valve. The TBC should be useful in patients with chronic retention like that caused by detrusor-sphincter dysynergia and/or patients with chronic incontinence. The TBC will effect watertight closure of the bladder so that there will be no urine doors, no skin spillage with urine, and no migration of skin bacteria into the native bladder. The TBC will be small (~12 F diameter), cosmetically attractive and non-irritating. Drugs can be introduced directly into the bladder lumen via a self-sealing injection port. The TBC is expected to maintain sterile urine in patients who have sterile urine prior to implantation. The intraluminal component which is coated with antimicrobials and/or anti-adherence materials will be changed in the clinic at periodic intervals which are anticipated to be quarterly or semi-annually.

The TBC is intended to be a functional and useful device. However, it will also evaluate the clinical effectiveness of the principles cited above. If the TBC is clinically effective and stands the test of time then clinical proof of principle will have been demonstrated in humans. Development of prosthetic urethras, prosthetic bladders, and prosthetic ureters using the same principles can be anticipated.

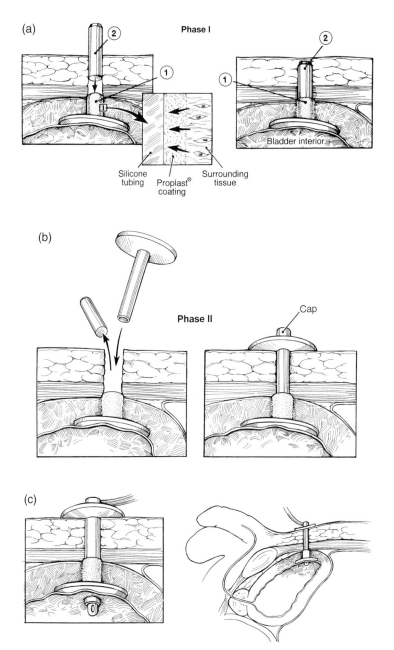

Fig. 23.3 *(a) Phase I. The tissue-bonding permanent implant (1) is 'sandwiched' between and secured with sutures to the rectus abdominis and detrusor muscles. A space occupying silicone plug (2) 'locks' (reversibly) into the permanent implant. Both components are buried beneath skin to allow fibroblastic bonding of the deep implant to the adjacent muscles. A fibrous 'capsule' typically forms around the silicone plug (2). (b) Phase II. Three or more months after the phase I implant the phase II procedure is performed. A circle of skin approximately 5 mm diameter is removed. The plug is 'unlocked' from the deep implant and removed. The flanged transcutaneous tube is customized (e.g. the extra length is cut-off) and the transcutaneous tube which is impregnated with antimicrobial agents is 'locked' into the deep implant as shown. The lumen of the transcutaneous tube is capped with a plug. (c) Phase III. One or more months after the phase II procedure the phase III procedure is performed. The time delay is to ascertain whether there has been any bacterial colonization of the deep implant. The cap is removed and an 18 gauge needle is passed through the transcutaneous tube into the bladder. The transcutaneous tube is 'unlocked' from the deep implant and removed. The bladder opening is dilated with a dilating balloon and conical 'Amplatz' dilators. A longer transcutaneous tube is customized (e.g. length adjusted) and is inserted into the bladder and 'locked' into the deep implant. The transcutaneous tube and flange are impregnated with antimicrobials. A right angle drainage tube is attached to the cap. The drainage tube has a 'built-in' manual valve for drainage. The cap on the transcutaneous drainage tube contains a 'self-sealing' port for injection of drugs into the bladder. The transcutaneous drainage tube will be changed in the clinic at periodic intervals estimated to be quarterly or semiannually*

Tissue engineering

During the past decade much investigational attention has focused upon cell biology, genetic engineering, and tissue engineering. At least three and perhaps more initiatives are in progress whereby urological investigators are attempting to grow functional urological organs using tissue engineering technology.

Submucosal small intestine xenografts

Kropp *et al.* (47–50) have prepared cell-free small intestine submucosa (SIS) from several species and used this material as a xenograft for augmentation of the urinary bladder. The SIS does not induce an immune response and is readily transferable between species. The SIS graft is prepared as a flat sheet and can be used to augment and possibly replace native collecting system. Neovascularization of the SIS graft occurs early. SIS stimulates epithelialization on its lumenal surface with normal-appearing urothelium 3–4 weeks after grafting. Smooth muscle regeneration and neural regeneration are histologically present 8–10 weeks after implantation. Canine survival studies of up to 15 months after bladder augmentation show normal upper tracts, normal urodynamics, and normal bladder histology.

Bladder acellular matrix graft

Investigators (51–53) are evaluating the usefulness of acellular matrix derived from bladder or ureter to act as scaffolds for the re-growth of function organs. This approach involves removing the epithelial cells and smooth muscle cells from host tissues of bladder and ureter. Removal of the cells seems to eliminate immunogenicity. The remaining matrix is composed of collagen fibres and elastin fibres. Success in experimental animals has been achieved with bladder augmentation using acellular matrix grafts (BACG). Twelve weeks postgrafting the histological appearance of the augmented bladder graft was almost indistinguishable from normal bladder wall. Smooth muscle and nerve regeneration was present.

Ureteral replacement has been similarly successful in rats using acellular homologous ureteral segments. The success of these homograft studies is thought to be related to the expression of multiple growth factors in an immune state leading to proliferation of urothelium and smooth muscle from adjacent normal tissues. The acellular matrix serves as a scaffold which is subsequently populated with normal cells that grow into the matrix from adjacent normal tissues.

Organ biopsy, cell expansion *in vitro* and auto-grafting

Atala and colleagues (54–61) seek to augment and/or replace urological organs using autologous cells expanded *in vitro*, grafted on to absorbable alloplastic scaffolds, and then reimplanted into the original host.

In this approach urothelial cells and smooth muscle cells are obtained by biopsy and the cells are expanded *in vitro* in tissue culture media over several weeks. Very large quantities of cells can be obtained. Thereafter the urothelial cells are seeded on to biodegradable polyglycolic acid mesh. The implanted mesh is maintained in a sterile tissue culture environment. Several days later the expanded smooth muscle cells are seeded on the opposite side of the polyglycolic acid mesh. The seeding cell density approaches 10^7 cells/cm^2. The doubly seeded mesh is returned to cell culture media for approximately 5 days. Thereafter the doubly seeded mesh is used surgically to augment or replace urological organs. The technique has successfully replaced the supra-trigonal bladder (55,57) and ureteral segment (58), and a segment of urethra (60). The technique has also been used to reconstruct experimentally created extrophy (61). Organ anatomy (gross and histological) and function in these experimental studies has been normal radiographically and functionally normal.

In summary, multiple tissue engineering approaches are being intensely investigated. Each approach has its own inherent advantages, disadvantages, and limitations. Successful clinical use of one or more of these technologies to augment or replace a urological organ is likely in the very near future. If one organ can be augmented or replaced then it is quite likely that other organs can be similarly reconstructed and/or replaced.

There are an array of new technologies that open the door to alternative urological organs. New alternatives to traditional forms of bladder augmentation and/or replacement are likely in the near future.

References

1   Ashkar L, Heller E. The silastic bladder patch. *J Urol* 1967, **98**, 679–83.
2   Bohne AW, Urwiller KL. Experience with urinary bladder regeneration. *J Urol* 1957, 77, 725–32.
3   Abbou C, Leandri J, Auvert J, Rey P. New prosthetic bladder. *Trans Am Soc Artif Intern Organs* 1977, **23**, 371–4.
4   Apoil A, Grange A, Sausse A, Stern A. Experimental and clinical studies of prosthetic bladder replacement. In: *Genito-urinary reconstruction with prostheses* (ed. Wagenknecht LV, Furlow WL, Auvert J). Georg Thieme Verlag, Stuttgart, 1981, pp. 75–80.
5   Auvert J. Trends in alloplastic replacement of segments of the urinary tract. *Urol Res* 1976, **4**, 143–5.

6 Bogash M, Kohler FP, Scott RH, Murphy JJ. Replacement of the urinary bladder by a plastic reservoir with mechanical valves. *Surg Forum*, 1960, **10**, 900–3.

7 Barrett D, Donovan MG. Prosthetic bladder augmentation and replacement. *Semin Urol II*, 1984, **3**, 167–75.

8 Barrett D, O'Sullivan D, Parulkar BG, Donovan MG. Artificial bladder replacement: a new design concept. *Mayo Clin Proc*, 1992, **67**, 215–20.

9 O'Sullivan DC, Barrett DM. Prosthetic bladder: in vivo studies on an active negative-pressure-driven device. *J Urol* 1994, **151**, 776–80.

10 Hannapel J, Rohrman D, Heinrichs B *et al.* Long term implantation from artificial bladder implantation in animals. *J Urol* 1987, **137** (4 part 2), A16.

11 Rohrman D, Albrecht D, Hannapel J *et al.* Alloplastic replacement of the urinary bladder. *J Urol* 1996, **156**, 2094–7.

12 Gleeson MJ, Anderson S, Homsy C, Griffith DP. Experimental development of a fixed volume, gravity draining, prosthetic urinary bladder. *ASAIO Trans* 1990, **36**, 429–32.

13 Weslowski SA, Fries CC, Karlson KE *et al.* Porosity: Primary determinant of ultimate fate of synthetic vascular grafts. *Surgery*, 1961, **50**, 91–6.

14 Desgrandchamps F, Cussenot O, Meria P *et al.* Subcutaneous urinary diversions for palliative treatment of pelvic malignancies. *J Urol* 1995, **154**, 367–70.

15 Gurpinar T, Griffith DP. The prosthetic bladder. *World J Urol* 1996, **14**, 47–52.

16 Griffith DP, Musher DM, Itin C. Urease: the primary cause of infection-induced urinary stones. *Invest Urol* 1976, **13**, 346–50.

17 Robertson WG, Peacock M, Nordin BEC. Activity products in stone-forming and non-stone forming urine. *Clin Sci*, 1968, **34**, 579–94.

18 Robertson WG, Peacock M, Nordin BEC. Calcium oxalate crystalluria and urine saturation in recurrent stone formers. *Clin Sci*, 1971, **40**, 365–74.

19 Canby TY, O'Rear CO. Advanced materials—Reshaping our lives. *Natl Geographic*, 1989, **176**, 746.

20 Bitschai J, Brodny ML. *A history of urology in Egypt.* Riverside Press, New York, 1976, p. 76.

21 Nacey JN, Delahunt B. Urinary catheter toxicity. *NZ Med J*, 1991, **104**, 355–6.

22 Ruutu M, Alfthan O, Talja M, Andersson LC. Cytotoxicity of latex urinary catheters. *Br J Urol* 1985, **57**, 82–7.

23 Reid G, Busscher HJ. Importance of surface properties in bacterial adhesion to biomaterials, with particular reference to the urinary tract. *Int Biodeter Biodegrad*, 1992, **30**, 105–22.

24 Ruutu ML, Talja MT, Andersson LC, Alfthan OS. Biocompatibility of urinary catheters—present status. *Scand J Urol Nephrol*, 1991, **138**, 235–8.

25 Roberts JA, Fussell EN, Kaack MB. Bacterial adherence to urethral catheters. *J Urol* 1990, **144**, 264–9.

26 Ferrie BG, Groone J, Sethia B, Kirk D. Comparison of silicone and latex catheters in the development of urethral stricture after cardiac surgery. *Br J Urol* 1986, **58**, 549–50.

27 Nickel JC, Costerton JW, McLean RJC, Olson M. Bacterial biofilms: Influence on the pathogenesis, diagnosis and treatment of urinary tract infections. *J Antibio Chem*, 1994, **33A**, 32–41.

28 Holmes SAV, Cheng C, Whitfield HN. The development of synthetic polymers that resist encrustation on exposure to urine. *Br J Urol* 1992, **69**, 651–5.

29 Choong S, Fry C, Whitfield H. The effect of biomaterial surface properties on encrustation of urological devices. *J Endourol*, 1997, **11** (1), S50.

30 Nickel JC, Downey JA, Costerton JW. Ultrastructural study of microbiological colonization of urinary catheters. *Urology*, 1990, **34**, 284–91.

31 Johnson JR, Roberts PL, Olsen RJ *et al.* Prevention of catheter-associated urinary tract infection with a silver oxide-coated urinary catheter: Clinical and microbiologic correlates. *J Infect Dis*, 1990, **162**, 1145–50.

32 Liedberg H, Lundberg T. Silver coating of urinary catheters prevents adherence and growth of pseudomonas aeruginosa. *Urol Res* 1989, **17**, 357–8.

33 Wilcox MH, Spencer RC. Ciprofloxin to prevent catheter-associated urinary tract infection. *Lancet* 1992, **339**, 1421–2 (letter).

34 Langer R. New methods of drug delivery. *Science*, 1990, **249**, 1527–33.

35 Raad I, Darouiche R, Hachem R *et al.* The broad-spectrum activity and efficacy of catheters coated with minocycline and rifampin. *J Infect Dis*, 1996, **173**, 418–24.

36 Raad I, Darouiche R, Hachem R *et al.* Antibiotics and prevention of microbial colonization of catheters. *Antimicrob Agents Chemother* 1995, **39**, 2397–400.

37 Darouiche RO, Dhir A, Miller AJ *et al.* Vancomycin penetration into biofilm covering infected prostheses and effect on bacteria. *J Infect Dis* 1994, **170**, 720–3.

38 Schierholz JM, Pulverer G. Developement of a new CSF-shunt with sustained release of an antimicrobial broad-spectrum combination. *Zentralbl Bakteriol* 1997, **286**, 107–23.

39 Schierholz JM, Rump A, Pulverer G. Drug delivery concepts for the efficacious prevention of foreign-body infections. *Zentralbl Bakteriol*, 1996, **284**, 390–401.

40 Gleeson MJ, Griffith DP. The use of alloplastic biomaterials in bladder substitutions. *J Urol* 1992, **148**, 1377–82.

41 Campbell EJ, O'Byrne V, Stratford PW *et al.* Biocompatible surfaces using methacryloylphosphorylcholine. *ASAIO J* 1994, **40**, M853–7.

42 Yu J, Lamba NM, Courtney JM *et al.* Polymeric biomaterials: influence of phosphorylcholine polar groups on protein adsorption and complement activation. *Int J Artif Organs* 1994, **17**, 499–504.

43 Chen C, Lumsden AB, Ofenlock JC *et al.* Phosphorylcholine coating of PTFE grafts reduces neointimal hyperplasia in canine model. *Ann Vasc Surg* 1997, **11**, 74–9.

44 Heaton RJ, Harris PL, Russell JC, Chapman D. Application of SPR and FTIR spectroscopy to the study of protein–biomaterial interactions. *Biochem Soc Trans* 1995, **23**, 502S.

45 Nishida K, Sakakida M, Ichinose K *et al.* Development of a ferrocene-mediated needle-type glucose sensor covered with newly designed biocompatible membrane, 2-methacrylaoyloxyethyl phosphorylcholine-co-n-butyl methacrylate. *Med Prog Technol* 1995, **21**, 91–103.

46 Griffith DP, Gleeson MJ. Tissue bonded iontophoretic cystostomy: conceptual and experimental considerations. *J Endourol* 1993, **7**, 169–77.

47 Kropp BP, Rippy MK, Badyla SF *et al.* Regenerative urinary bladder augmentation using small intestine submucosa: urodynamic and histopathologic assessment in long-term canine bladder augmentations. *J Urol* 1996, **155**, 2098–104.

48 Kropp BP, Badylak S, Thor KB. Regenerative bladder augmentation: a review of the initial pre-clinical studies with porcine small intestine mucosa. *Adv Exp Med Biol* 1995, **385**, 229–35.

49 Pope JC, 4th Davis MM, Smith ER Jr *et al.* The ontogeny of canine small intestinal submucosa regenerated bladder. *J Urol*, 1997, **158**, 1105–10.

50 Kropp BP, Sawyer BD, Shannon HE *et al.* Characterization of the small intestinal submucosa regenerated canine detrusor: assessment of re-innervation, in vitro compliance and contractility. *J Urol* 1996, **156**, 599–607.

51 Sutherland RS, Baskin LS, Hayward SW, Cunha GR. Regeneration of bladder urothelium, smooth muscle, blood vessels and nerves into an acellular tissue matrix. *J Urol* 1996, **156**, 571–7.

52 Dahms SE, Piechota HJ, Nunes L *et al.* Free ureteral replacement in rats: regeneration of ureteral wall components in the acellular matrix graft. *Urology* 1997, **50**, 818–25.

53 Probst M, Dahiya S, Tanagho EA. Reproduction of functional smooth muscle tissue and partial bladder replacement. *Br J Urol* 1997, **79**, 505–15.

54 Atala A, Vacanti JP, Peters CA *et al.* Formation of urothelial structures in vivo from dissociated cells attached to biodegradable polymer scaffolds in vitro. *J Urol* 1992, **148** (2 part 2), 658–62.

55 Yoo JJ, Atala A. Bladder augmentation using a new biomaterial composed of allogenic bladder submucosa. *Pediatrics*, 1996, **98S**, 615.

56 Yoo JJ, Atala A. A novel gene delivery system using urothelial tissue engineered neoorgans. *J Urol* 1997, **158**, 1066–77.

57 Satar N, Yoo JJ, Atala A. Bladder augmentation using biodegradeable polymer scaffolds seeded with urothelial and smooth muscle cells. *J Urol* 1996, **155** (5), 336A.

58 Yoo JJ, Satar N, Retik AB, Atala A. Ureteral replacement using biodegradeable polymer scaffolds seeded with urothelial and smooth muscle cells. *J Urol* 1995, **153** (4) 375A.

59 Yoo JJ, Meng J, Oberpenning F, Atala A. Bladder augmentation using allogenic bladder submucosa seeded with cells. *Urology*, 1998, **51**, 221–5.

60 Cilento BJ, Retik AB, Atala A. Urethral reconstruction using a polymer mesh. *J Urol* 1995, **153**, 4 371A.

61 Fauza DO, Fishman SJ, Mehegan K, Atala A. Videofetoscopically assisted fetal tissue engineering: bladder augmentation. *J Pediatr Surg* 1998, **33**, 1–7.

24. PALLIATIVE CARE FOR PATIENTS WITH BLADDER CANCER

K.J. Harrington and K.N. Syrigos

INTRODUCTION

To many the term palliative care is synonymous with the treatment of patients in the terminal phase of a disease process, usually cancer. However, this is a narrow view and fails to embrace the wide variety of clinical scenarios which can justifiably be included under this heading. It is more useful to consider that palliative care is the specific treatment given to patients with incurable disease with the aim of relieving disease-related symptoms and promoting physical, psychological, and spiritual well-being. In the sphere of malignant disease, palliative care legitimately includes active therapeutic manoeuvres such as the use of surgery, chemotherapy, and radiotherapy, as well as the more widely recognized palliative therapies such as pain relief. Many patients present with disease too advanced to allow for the possibility of cure and others may have concomitant medical conditions that preclude the use of aggressive therapy which might, under different circumstances, have offered the chance of a cure. In these patients the aim of treatment from the very outset is to achieve symptom palliation and, if possible, prolongation of their lives. Therefore, palliative care of patients with cancer is a challenging and diverse discipline in which palliative care physicians, oncologists, and surgeons can play an important part. In addition, the involvement of a variety of healthcare professionals including nurses, social workers, counsellors, physiotherapists, and occupational therapists as part of a multidisciplinary team allows important psychosocial issues to be addressed as part of the overall care package.

Most patients with muscle invasive bladder will die of their disease. Failure to achieve a cure results mainly from the occurrence of distant metastatic disease, although in a significant proportion of patients local pelvic disease remains uncontrolled or recurs. During the course of such patients' illnesses, a wide variety of manifestations of the disease may arise, both locally in the pelvis and at more distant sites. In this chapter an attempt will be made to review the most frequently encountered clinical situations and to give guidelines as to their most appropriate management. Those problems common to patients with a number of different tumour types will be reviewed initially, followed by a detailed discussion of problems particularly related to bladder cancer.

GENERAL SYMPTOMS OF CANCER

Pain

Pain can be defined as an unpleasant sensory and emotional experience associated with actual or potential damage or described in terms of such damage (1). It is the most feared symptom of cancer and occurs at some time in the majority of patients. Many patients are afraid to tell their carers about new or increasing pain because it may signify recurrent or progressive disease. This may prove to be a considerable obstacle to the accurate diagnosis and treatment of cancer-related pain. However, with appropriate assessment and therapy this symptom can be successfully controlled in most patients (2).

The cornerstones of provision of adequate pain relief are careful diagnosis of the cause of each individual pain and selection of the most appropriate class of analgesic medication. Evaluation of pain should begin with an adequate pain history, including the site, speed of onset, quality, radiation, and modifying factors, including the effect of previous analgesic medication. In addition, the effect of the pain on the patient's life-style should be assessed. Certain distinct types of pain can be recognized by their clinical features (e.g. burning or shooting pains due to nerve compression or infiltration) (Table 24.1). Once these details are known, it is possible to decide what analgesic medication and adjuvant therapy should be prescribed.

Table 24.1

CANCER-RELATED PAIN: TYPE OF PAIN AND ASSOCIATED SYMPTOMS	
Type of pain	**Associated symptoms**
Nerve compression or invasion	Continuous ache Burning or stinging Episodic stabbing (lancinating) pain Hyperaesthesia/anaesthesia
Bone metastases	Continuous ache Worsened by movement Sudden increase with pathological fracture
Obstruction of hollow viscus	Intermittent Colicky/cramping
Capsular/fascial stretch	Continuous dull ache Associated tenderness over the organ

The WHO analgesic ladder

This is a well-established and validated approach to the treatment of cancer-related pain (Table 24.2). The recommendations are that analgesic medication is administered by mouth (if possible), regularly, and according to an escalating response to the pain ('by mouth, by the clock, by the ladder'). There are three rungs to the analgesic ladder (and the appropriate reaction to failure to control pain with medication from one level is to move up the ladder to a higher level, not to prescribe a different drug at the same analgesic level. In addition to the conventional analgesic drugs, a number of adjuvant agents are available which can be particularly useful in helping to control atypical pain. If these general guidelines are adhered to, pain can be adequately controlled in up to 90% of cases (2).

Level 1

Drugs in this level are non-opioids. The most commonly used drugs in this class are paracetamol, aspirin, and the non-steroidal anti-inflammatory drugs (NSAIDs) which, in addition to their analgesic properties, may also benefit symptoms by virtue of the fact that they are capable of modifying the inflammatory response. When prescribing NSAIDs to this group of patients, it is important to ask about symptoms of dyspepsia or a prior history of peptic ulcer disease, in which case a prophylactic H_2-receptor antagonist (e.g. cimetidine or ranitidine) should also be prescribed. Drugs at this level of the analgesic ladder are useful in controlling mild to moderate pain but, in patients with advanced disease, their main role is in conjunction with weak or strong opioid medication.

Level 2

Drugs at this level are the weak opioid analgesics, such as codeine, dihydrocodeine, and dextropropoxyphene. These agents are effective against moderately severe pain which is not controlled by simple analgesics and/or NSAIDs. They should be used at full doses and as regular medication before they can be considered to have failed.

Table 24.2

THE WORLD HEALTH ORGANIZATION ANALGESIC LADDER	
First level	Non-opioid ± adjuvant therapy
Second level	Weak opioid and non-opioid ± adjuvant therapy
Third level	Strong opioid and non-opioid ± adjuvant therapy

Level 3

Drugs at this level are the strong opioids, of which morphine is the drug of choice (2). Oral morphine is available in a number of different preparations which aim to facilitate the use of this drug. In the initial phase of converting a patient from a weak opioid to a strong opioid, it is usual to prescribe an instant release formulation which ensures prompt delivery of pain control. Such preparations include oramorph liquid and sevredol tablets. The usual starting dose is 10 mg every 4 h. The patient must be encouraged to take the medication regularly and should be reassured that this is a starting dose and that there is scope for altering the dose to tailor the delivery of analgesia to his individual needs. Furthermore, at this stage the patient should be told that if the pain persists or returns before the 4 h interval they can take extra doses of morphine (so-called breakthrough doses), which should be the same as the 4-hourly regular doses. If the starting dose of morphine has failed to control the pain after 24 h, the regular 4-hourly doses should be increased (e.g. doubled), as should the breakthrough doses. Using this approach, if the pain is opiate-responsive, it should be possible to arrive at a dose of morphine which controls the pain within a short space of time. A stable dose of morphine can be considered to be one which controls pain for 2 consecutive days with only two breakthrough doses needed in each 24-h period. Once pain control has been stabilized, it is possible to convert the morphine to a sustained release preparation which can be given once or twice daily. This is achieved by assessing the 24 h requirement of the instant relief morphine preparation and converting on a 1 : 1 basis to a sustained release preparation such as MST Continus, MXL and Morcap SR, and oramorph SR. For example, a patient requiring 120 mg of instant release oramorph could be treated with MST Continus 60 mg twice daily or MXL 120 mg once daily.

When prescribing morphine for the first time, it is important that the patient is made aware of the possible adverse effects of the drug and given appropriate medication to ameliorate such reactions. Otherwise, there is a serious risk that the patient will take insufficient amounts of the drug and will suffer unnecessary uncontrolled pain and anxiety. Constipation, which can sometimes be severe, is almost invariable with the doses of morphine employed in a palliative setting. Furthermore, this effect of the drug is not subject to tolerance and, therefore, will persist for as long as morphine is prescribed. Patients should be prescribed prophylactic laxatives with the aim of increasing bowel motility (e.g. senna, bisacodyl) and softening the stool (e.g. docusate sodium). Bulk-forming (e.g. ispaghula husk) and osmotic (e.g. lactulose) laxatives should not be used routinely in the prophylaxis of opiate-induced constipation. In patients with intractable opiate-induced constipation, oral naloxone may be of use (3). Naloxone does not antagonize the analgesic effects of morphine but is able to attenuate its local action on gut motility. Nausea and vomiting, induced by stimulation of the chemoreceptor trigger zone, are relatively common in the first few days of morphine therapy, occurring in approximately 30% of patients (4). This unpleasant side-effect frequently settles spontaneously within the first week of therapy, with or without short-term use of anti-emetics (e.g. metoclopramide 10 mg thrice daily, haloperidol 1–2 mg at night). Occasionally, opiate-sensitive patients may require more prolonged use of prophylactic anti-emetics. Rarely, a patient may be unable to tolerate morphine despite the above measures, in which case a trial of an alternative opiate is indicated. Many patients experience sedation as an early side-effect of morphine medication, an effect that is exacerbated by alcohol consumption. Therefore, patients should be warned of the risks of driving or operating heavy machinery in this situation. The sedative effect of morphine tends to wear off after a week or so. Other adverse effects of morphine include xerostomia in approximately 40% of patients (5), urinary retention in approximately 5% (6), and myoclonic jerks in patients receiving high doses of the drug.

In addition to morphine, there are a number of alternative opiate drugs. These agents are generally used when the patient is unable to tolerate oral morphine or when administration by a different route (subcutaneous, transdermal, rectal) may improve efficacy and compliance. Perhaps the most commonly used of these drugs is diamorphine. This drug is often used by the subcutaneous route (usually using a continuous infusion via a syringe driver) when patients are unable to receive morphine by mouth because of nausea and vomiting, dysphagia, general debility, or unconsciousness. This situation is a typical feature of the final days or hours of a patient's life. Diamorphine is a very convenient agent to use because of its high solubility and compatibility with other agents which can be administered concomitantly in the same syringe driver. When converting a patient from oral morphine to subcutaneous diamorphine, a conversion factor of 3 : 1 applies i.e. 3 mg of morphine is equivalent to 1 mg of diamorphine. Other alternative opiates include fentanyl, that can be delivered by transdermal patch, phenazocine, which can be useful in patients who are morphine intolerant, and dextromoramide, which can be useful as a short-acting analgesic when patients are undergoing unpleasant procedures such as regular dressing changes.

Nausea and vomiting

This distressing symptom occurs in as many as 50% of patients with advanced cancer. The aetiology of nausea and vomiting in this group of patients is often complex and may include factors relating to progression of the primary disease and its metastatic spread or the consequences of therapeutic manoeuvres aimed at treating the disease or disease-related symptoms (Table 24.3).

Vomiting may be induced by a number of stimuli acting at different receptor sites, both in the brain and peripherally. The chemoreceptor trigger zone, which lies in the region of the area postrema, lies outside the blood–brain barrier and is, therefore, exposed to circulating toxic chemicals. The vomiting centre lies within the blood–brain barrier and may be stimulated directly (e.g. cranial irradiation) or through signals from higher cortical centres or from vagal afferents from the gastrointestinal and genitourinary tracts. Direct stimulation of peripheral receptors, including those in the gastric antrum, can lead to stimulation of vagal afferents and release of mediators of vomiting directly into the bloodstream. The complexity of the whole system is increased further by the wide range of interconnections of neural pathways within the brain. One such connection to the so-called higher centres has a significant effect on the response of individuals to emetogenic stimuli. As yet, the detailed mechanisms underlying the causation of nausea and vomiting remain unclear, despite considerable improvements in knowledge in recent times.

Table 24.3

CAUSES OF NAUSEA AND VOMITING IN PATIENTS WITH ADVANCED CANCER

Metabolic derangement
    Hypercalcaemia
    Uraemia
    Hepatic failure
Drug-induced
    Cytotoxic chemotherapy
    Opiates (strong > weak)
Radiotherapy
    Abdomino-pelvic radiotherapy
    Cranial radiotherapy
Gastrointestinal disturbance
    Bowel obstruction
    Constipation
    Gastric stasis
Central nervous system metastases
    Intracranial metastases
    Carcinomatous meningitis
Pain
Anxiety and fear

The management of nausea and vomiting should be based initially on an attempt to define a reversible cause such as metabolic disturbance, intestinal obstruction, brain metastases, etc. Specific treatment aimed at the individual cause may alleviate the symptoms without recourse to anti-emetic therapy. For example, patients with hypercalcaemia of malignancy usually respond very well to rehydration and treatment with intravenous bisphosphonates. Similarly, the use of high dose steroids and whole brain irradiation (see below) can often relieve nausea and vomiting due to cerebral metastases and raised intracranial pressure.

If a specific cause can not be pin-pointed, as is often the case, treatment with anti-emetic medication should be commenced immediately. A large number of drugs from different pharmacological classes (antidopaminergic, anticholinergic, antihistaminergic, antiserotoninergic, and cannabinoids) will prevent nausea and vomiting. Some examples are provided in Table 24.4, along with guidelines to appropriate dose and frequency of administration.

As in the case of analgesic medication, the preferred route of administration should be by mouth. However, uncontrolled vomiting can prevent effective dosing and many of the agents are available in a range of alternative formulations for delivery by other routes, including subcutaneous, intravenous, rectal, and buccal administration. Subcutaneous infusions of anti-emetics via

Table 24.4

COMMONLY PRESCRIBED ANTI-EMETIC MEDICATION			
Class of drug	**Examples**	**Dose and route of administration**	**Specific uses**
Antidopaminergic	Metoclopramide	10 mg t.i.d.; p.o., s.c., i.v. 30 mg over 24 h via s.c. syringe driver	Gastric stasis
	Domperidone	10–20 mg t.i.d.; p.o. 30–60 mg t.i.d.; p.r..	Gastric stasis
	Haloperidol	1.5–3.0 mg o.d.; p.o., s.c., i.v. 3–10 mg over 24 h via s.c. syringe driver	Opiate-induced nausea Bowel obstruction
	Prochlorperazine	5–10 mg t.i.d.; p.o., p.r. 3–6 mg b.i.d.; buccal.	Vertigo
	Methotrimeprazine	6.25–12.5 mg o.d./b.i.d.; p.o., s.c. 12.5–150 mg over 24 h via s.c. syringe driver	Sedative Bowel obstruction
Antihistaminergic	Cyclizine	50 mg t.i.d.; p.o., s.c., i.v. 150 mg over 24 h via s.c. syringe driver	Vertigo Bowel obstruction
Anti-5HT$_3$	Ondansetron	4–8 mg b.i.d.; p.o., i.v.	Drug-induced nausea
	Granisetron	1 mg b.i.d.; p.o. 3 mg o.d.; i.v.	Bowel obstruction
Anticholinergic	Hyoscine	400 µg t.i.d.; s.c. 500 µg q 3 days; transdermal 600–1200 µg over 24 h via s.c. syringe driver	Bowel obstruction
Steroid	Dexamethasone	2–8 mg b.i.d.; p.o., i.v., s.c. 4–16 mg over 24 h via s.c. syringe driver	Brain metastases Hepatic capsular stretch
Cannabinoid	Nabilone	1–2 mg b.i.d.; p.o.	Drug-induced nausea

a syringe driver are particularly useful, especially in the setting of the final days and hours of a patient's illness when oral medication may not be tolerated or accepted.

Anorexia and weight loss

Cancer cachexia is a familiar feature of advanced stage disease. Patients are often pitifully thin and literally waste away as the disease progresses. Most patients do not have a clearly identifiable cause for their anorexia, they simply have a markedly decreased appetite and eat only small quantities despite encouragement. In some patients direct local tumour progression, leading to bowel obstruction or restriction of the capacity of the stomach, may be responsible. In others, ill-defined changes in the sense of taste and smell can lead to an aversion to food and drink. Iatrogenic causes include opioid medication, palliative chemotherapy, and radiotherapy. In the absence of identifiable causes, the syndrome is usually ascribed to circulating products from the tumour or altered levels of endogenous cytokines.

As yet, no specific treatment has been described to address this problem. Therapy involves provision of appetizing food and drink whenever the patient feels up to eating it, even if this involves unconventional menus and mealtimes. Dietetic support with high calorie supplements may be accepted and certainly has the benefit of seeming to provide a specific solution. Appetite stimulation with progestogens (e.g. medroxyprogesterone acetate or megesterol acetate) or corticosteroids (dexamethasone) can occasionally be of benefit but the adverse effects are often excessive. Despite these measures, most patients with the cancer cachexia syndrome will continue to lose weight and gradually become bedbound. Under these circumstances, death usually occurs due to intercurrent infection. Enteral (e.g. nasogastric or gastrostomy) or parenteral nutrition is entirely inappropriate in these patients.

Constipation

Constipation occurs in as many as 50% of patients with advanced cancer (7) and can cause severe discomfort to patients. Misdiagnosis of symptoms such as abdominal fullness, loss of appetite, nausea and vomiting, pain, diarrhoea, and confusional states can result in subjecting the patient to unnecessary investigations, therapy, and physical and mental stress. The unfortunate, but not uncommon, situation of a patient with morphine-induced constipation being given ever-increasing doses of morphine to combat the pain of constipation is one that should be avoidable.

Constipation in patients with disseminated malignant disease can have a number of different causes, including dietary changes (e.g. low residue diet and reduced fluid intake), metabolic derangement (e.g. hypercalcaemia), drug-induced reduction in bowel contractility, tumour-induced partial mechanical obstruction, and neurogenic constipation in patients with spinal cord lesions. In general, the commonest and most predictable cause of constipation in patients with terminal cancer is the use of medication. The opioid analgesics are a frequent cause of constipation which can become severe if adequate aperients are not prescribed prophylactically (see above). Other drugs which can cause constipation include drugs with an anticholinergic action, such as the tricyclic antidepressants, hyoscine hydrobromide, methotrimeprazine, and cyclizine. In patients receiving constipating drugs, prophylactic laxatives should be used regularly rather than waiting for constipation to occur and then instituting treatment. In most cases one or two co-danthrusate (danthron 50 mg, docusate sodium 60 mg) capsules nocte will suffice, although the precise dose required will depend on the dose of the constipating agents and may vary widely between different patients.

For patients with metabolic derangement, such as hypercalcaemia, effective treatment with rehydration with intravenous fluids (typically 4–6 litres over the first 24 h) and intravenous bisphosphonates if the calcium level is greater than 3.0 mmol/l can lead to clinical improvement in bowel function. However, many of these patients will be profoundly constipated and may need short-term treatment with laxatives that will soften the stool (e.g. docusate sodium) and increase bowel motility (e.g. senna). Patients with neurogenic constipation due to spinal cord lesions will need regular laxatives, but even with these measures they may remain severely constipated. Such patients can often be managed successfully by intermittent manual evacuation of faeces. The management of constipation due to bowel obstruction is discussed in the next section.

Bowel obstruction

Malignant bowel obstruction can occur due to local spread of disease in the pelvis, nodal metastatic disease in the pelvis or abdomen, or large liver metastases. It is most common in patients with ovarian and colorectal cancers, but does occur in patients with locally advanced bladder cancer. The typical symptoms will depend on the level of the obstruction but usually include nausea and vomiting, constipation, colicky abdominal pain, and abdominal bloating. The obstruction usually comes on slowly and the patient may describe previous episodes which resolved spontaneously. Alternatively, the condition may present as acute bowel obstruction with no preceding symptoms. The diagnosis rests with the history, physical examination, and the aid of plain abdominal X-rays. Contrast studies may be of use in delineating the level of obstruction and are of particular importance if a palliative surgical procedure is contemplated. It must be borne in mind that not all cases of bowel obstruction in patients with advanced cancer will be due to the malignant process. Patients who have undergone prior cystectomy or who have received radical radiotherapy may develop adhesions or benign strictures.

In most cases of bowel obstruction in the palliative setting, surgical intervention is not appropriate. However, patients with a single site of obstruction and the option of further palliative anti-cancer therapy may benefit from either a defunctioning procedure (e.g. defunctioning colostomy or ileostomy) or from excision of the obstructed segment and re-anastomosis. Similarly, patients with intractable symptoms which cannot be controlled by medical means may be palliated effectively by a limited surgical approach. However, this group of patients has a poor prognosis and surgical procedures are often complicated by infection, anastomotic leak, the development of fistulae and wound complications. Therefore, a surgery should only be contemplated after very careful consideration of each individual case.

Most patients will be managed successfully by conservative means. The standard approach should be to make the patient 'nil by mouth' and provide intravenous hydration. The use of a nasogastric tube (drip and suck) may be useful in patients with upper gastrointestinal obstruction and high-output vomiting. Nausea and vomiting is relieved by regular anti-emetics which are best given by the parenteral route, usually as a continuous subcutaneous infusion by syringe driver. Cyclizine, haloperidol and hyoscine are suitable agents (Table 24.5). The visceral pain of obstruction, which is usually a dull ache, along with episodes of severe spasm, can generally be controlled by the use of a level 3 analgesic with or without the aid of an antispasmodic such as hyoscine. It is common to use a continuous subcutaneous infusion of diamorphine, titrating the dose upwards to control symptoms. All of the drugs which are used to treat this condition can be given via a single syringe driver which improves compliance and ease of administration for the patient and staff. Where peri-tumour oedema is thought to be a contributing factor to the obstructive process, the addition of high dose dexamethasone can yield a therapeutic benefit, although the evidence in support of this therapy is somewhat anecdotal. Constipation may also exacerbate (or even cause)

Table 24.5

CAUSES OF DYSPNOEA IN PATIENTS WITH ADVANCED CANCER
Pulmonary metastases
Gross metastatic deposits
Lymphangitis carcinomatosa
Pulmonary emboli
Anaemia
Secondary to haematuria
Secondary to palliative chemotherapy
Secondary to bone marrow infiltration
Serous effusion
Pleural
Pericardial
Respiratory infection
Superior vena caval obstruction
Anxiety

bowel obstruction and should be managed with suppositories and enemas. Using this approach, an episode of subacute or acute bowel obstruction will often settle but recurrence is frequent within a short period of time.

If the above measures fail and surgery is not a palliative option, the prognosis is usually extremely bleak. Attempts to control the symptoms with escalating doses of analgesia and more powerful anti-emetics (e.g. methotrimeprazine) can be successful, often at the expense of heavy sedation. If vomiting is a persistent and distressing symptom, symptomatic relief can be gained from placement of a nasogastric tube or, if this is poorly tolerated, insertion of a percutaneous gastrostomy tube may allow drainage of the stomach contents at intervals (8–10). This latter approach has the added advantage of allowing patients to eat and drink a little which can be a major addition to the quality of life. The use of octreotide, a long-acting analogue of the hypothalamic release-inhibiting hormone somatostatin, to reduce gastrointestinal secretions has been reported as an effective means of palliating unresponsive obstructive symptoms in a number of cases (10–12). The usual starting dose is 300 μg as a subcutaneous infusion over 24 h and this can be increased up to 600 μg if indicated.

Oedema

Leg, perineal, and abdominal oedema are a frequent complication of locally advanced bladder cancer. The cause can be complex with contributions due to general malnutrition and hypoalbuminaemia, pelvic venous obstruction, thrombosis (see below), and obstruction of the pelvic lymphatics. Efforts should be made to identify the cause of the oedema correctly as this has a direct bearing on the choice of therapy.

The treatment of cancer-related thrombosis is discussed in detail below. Peripheral oedema due to a low albumin state in patients with advanced disease can be managed effectively by low pressure support stockings which should be designed to provide an even but graduated pressure. Lymphoedema should be managed actively by means of massage, skin care, support, and movement (13). Skin discomfort and pain should be treated with effective analgesia. Low dose oral diuretics (e.g. frusemide 40 mg, amiloride 5 mg) may relieve the perception of skin tightness but are unlikely to affect the degree of swelling. High dose steroids are sometimes of use if the lymphoedema is secondary to lymphatic obstruction due tumour infiltration and swelling. However, they should be prescribed only in the form of a short trial course and should be withdrawn promptly if they prove to be ineffective. It should be remembered that steroid-induced fluid retention and procoagulant activity have the potential to exacerbate rather than relieve symptoms. Massage, even at sites distant from the oedema, may have a beneficial effect on lymphatic return and can be useful. Skin care is of enormous importance. Regular moisturizers (e.g. E45 cream) should be used and infection should be treated vigorously with appropriate antibiotics (e.g. amoxycillin and flucloxacillin). Recurrent episodes of cellulitis in a lymphoedematous limb are an indication for prophylactic antibiotic use. Low pressure compression hosiery may be of benefit but may succeed only in moving fluid from one place to another without promoting its resorption. If the patient is able to keep the limb moving this is likely to promote lymphatic flow. If not, passive movement may be of benefit.

Cancer-related thromboembolic disease

Thromboembolic disorders have been reported in 1–11% of patients with malignant disease, and a further 10% of patients suffer haemorrhagic episodes, although only 1 in 10 of these is directly related to disordered clotting function (14,15). Disseminated intravascular coagulation (DIC), with its attendant risks of thrombosis and/or haemorrhage, occurs in 9–15% of patients to a degree sufficient to require intervention. These figures underlie the status of thromboembolic disease and haemorrhage as the second commonest cause of mortality in patients with cancer (14).

Venous obstruction and thrombosis should be sought actively. This complication of malignant disease is very common and can give rise to considerable morbidity and mortality. In a recent study, Harrington *et al.* (16) assessed the incidence and resource implications of cancer-related thromboembolic disease over a 2-year period in a single, large cancer centre. One in eight of these patients had locally advanced or relapsed bladder cancer. This study highlighted a number of important issues: (i) cancer-related thromboembolic disease occurred frequently and accounted for approximately 6% of inpatient bed occupancy; (ii) most patients with this condition had advanced or relapsed/incurable disease; (iii) nearly half of the patients suffered additional thromboses, despite maintenance warfarin anticoagulation; and (iv) a significant number of patients experienced anticoagulation-induced haemorrhage. Similar results were reported by Chan and Woodruff (17) who detailed major bleeding in 35% and further thromboembolism despite therapeutic levels of anticoagulation in 13% of patients. Specific data relating to patients cared for in a hospice setting are not available, but it is likely that cancer-related thromboembolic disease is at least as common as in a cancer centre.

It is difficult to make general statements regarding the most appropriate management of patients with cancer-related thromboembolic disease in the context of terminal cancer. If the patient's life expectancy is very short, active management is likely to be inappropriate and compression hosiery and analgesia may be all that is required. However, if the patient's life expectancy is measured in weeks or months, anticoagulant treatment may provide significant symptom palliation. Where possible, patients should be investigated with Doppler ultrasound as this is less traumatic than contrast venography. V/Q scanning is justified if there is a suspicion of recurrent symptomatic pulmonary emboli. Patients with confirmed thrombosis should be managed with intravenous heparin and oral warfarinization, aiming to achieve an International Normalized Ratio of 2.5–3.5. However, as mentioned above, oral anticoagulation can be particularly difficult to manage in this group of patients. A delicate balance must be struck between the risks of further thromboembolism in inadequately anticoagulated patients and the haemorrhagic complications of excessive therapy. Disease progression in the form of bone marrow, hepatic or vascular invasion may increase the chance of bleeding, while immobilization due to general debility, pathological fractures, or paralysis may accentuate the prothrombotic state. The situation is rendered even more complex by the observation that some patients with cancer-related thromboembolic disease appear to be relatively refractory to conventional heparin and warfarin-based anticoagulation regimens, which can lead to a situation in which either recurrent cancer-related thromboembolic disease or haemorrhagic sequelae of high dose anticoagulation may occur. The use of low molecular weight

heparins (LMWH) given as a single daily subcutaneous injection
may offer improved efficacy with fewer complications and reduced
morbidity. Further studies are required to elucidate the role of these
agents in the prevention and treatment of cancer-related thromboembolic disease (18).

Dyspnoea

Shortness of breath is an extremely frequent and distressing symptom of end-stage malignant disease (7). There are a variety of possible causes of this symptom (Table 24.5). It should be remembered
that patients may often have more than one of these conditions
contributing to the sensation of breathlessness. Careful assessment
is important as specific measures may be available against each of
the individual problems. A chest X-ray will reveal the presence
of gross metastatic deposits, lymphangitis carcinomatosa, pleural
fluid, pulmonary infections, and pulmonary emboli. Measurement
of the arterial oxygen tension by sampling of arterial blood or
pulse oximetry may give a useful index of the degree of hypoxia
and can also guide the provision of oxygen therapy. It must be
remembered that a large number of patients with bladder cancer
are also heavy smokers and may have an element of chronic
obstructive airways disease and the risk of carbon dioxide retention and respiratory suppression with excessive oxygen therapy.
Dyspnoea is a frightening symptom and in many cases the patient
may gain considerable symptomatic benefit from the regular pre-
scription of drugs aimed at reducing the stress of this sensation.
Useful agents include diazepam at a dose of 2 mg twice or thrice
daily and morphine elixir at a dose of 5 mg every 4 h.

Gross pulmonary metastatic disease or lymphangitis carcinomatosa are rarely suitable for specific antitumour therapy in the
palliative setting. Instead, management should focus on relieving
the symptoms of breathlessness by provision of oxygen with or
without the addition of a trial of intermediate dose dexamethasone 4 mg twice daily. Respiratory infections are often the immediate cause of death in patients with end-stage cancer and the
issue of whether, or not, to treat them is often a difficult one. In
general, if a patient has reached the phase of their illness herald-
ing a terminal decline, active treatment of a chest infection with
antibiotics is inappropriate unless such treatment may potentially
relieve unpleasant symptoms such as fever and pleuritic chest
pain. In fact, these symptoms may be palliated far better by the
use of physical means of cooling and antipyretic drugs to control
fever and analgesia to control pain. Similarly, the treatment of
symptomatic pulmonary emboli is a matter for careful clinical

judgement. Anticoagulation does not guarantee effective prevention of further emboli and carries with it the risk of severe side-effects (16). The placement of vena caval filters is associated with a number of potential complications and requires the use of maintenance anticoagulation. Most patients are unlikely to gain a net benefit from this procedure.

The management of malignant pleural effusions depends on the degree of symptoms caused by the fluid and the availability of systemic therapeutic manoeuvres. The option of treating malignant effusions with specific anti-cancer therapies is seldom available in the palliative care of patients with advanced cancer. In general, pleural effusions of a sufficient size to cause dyspnoea should be managed by drainage. This can be achieved as a simple palliative procedure with a 22 G intravenous cannula inserted under local anaesthesia through the intercostal space allowing drainage of the fluid by direct suction via a 50 ml Luer lock syringe. A 3-way tap arrangement allows preservation of an air tight seal with the fluid being voided into a measuring cylinder. It is usually possible to drain up to 1000 ml of pleural fluid safely over 10–20 minutes using this set-up. Attempts to drain more than this by direct suction over a short space of time can be accompanied by coughing, a feeling of chest tightness, and paradoxical worsening of the shortness of breath. These symptoms are thought to be due to the development of pulmonary oedema secondary to the rapid re-expansion of collapsed lung tissue and accompanying mediastinal shift. Contrary to popular belief, this procedure can provide a significant improvement in symptoms without rapid reaccumulation of the pleural fluid. In patients with a limited life expectancy, this may be all that is required to control symptoms before death occurs by other disease-related processes. In the presence of recurrent or very large pleural effusions, it may be necessary to insert a chest drain. This should be done using a medium bore tube (16–18 F) under local anaesthesia. After placement of the tube, 500–1000 ml can be drained immediately via a system with an underwater seal. Thereafter, the tube should be clamped for 60 min and then 500 ml can be drained each hour until the rate of flow decrease to less than 500 ml per hour, after which time the tube can be left on free drainage. Once the chest has been drained to dryness, it is common to attempt to achieve a chemical pleurodesis using a range of agents including tetracycline (1 g mixed with bupivicaine) and bleomycin (60 mg) (19,20). In patients in whom this procedure fails, it may be worthwhile to attempt a talc pleurodesis at mini-thoracotomy or insertion of a pleuroperitoneal shunt (21), although, in the palliative setting, this should be considered carefully before it is undertaken.

Bone metastases

Pain due to bone metastases is a common feature in patients with advanced cancer. The pattern of metastasis of bladder cancer is not typically to the bones, but this event occurs frequently enough to merit consideration here. Bone pain generally arises due to erosive metastases and can present as a gradually worsening pain over a number of weeks or as a sudden pain arising from the occurrence of a pathological fracture. Mild to moderate pain may be controlled by simple analgesia from levels 1 and 2 of the analgesic ladder, such as an NSAID. However, if this medication fails to give symptomatic relief within 1 week it should be discontinued because of the risk of adverse effects such as gastric irritation. For more severe pain, a combination of morphine and an NSAID can be effective. Evaluation of the cause of the bone pain is very important. X-rays of the affected area should be performed and patients with osteolytic deposits at risk of fracture should be considered for a prophylactic surgical approach if their underlying illness suggests that they have a reasonable life expectancy. In the presence of demonstrable bony metastatic disease, palliative radiotherapy is extremely effective and gives pain relief in approximately 80–90% of cases (22). The optimal dose and schedule of palliative radiotherapy in this situation have not been defined clearly. The available data from randomized studies suggest that short course or single fraction radiotherapy is well-tolerated and as effective as more protracted irradiation schedules(23–27). Therefore, most patients will be palliated by a dose of 8 Gy as a single fraction or 20 Gy in five fractions. However, there is an apparent reluctance on the part of many physicians to use single fraction or short course radiotherapy, especially in sites of disease where there is a perceived risk of pathological fracture or in patients with a good performance status and a life expectancy measured in months rather than weeks (28,29). In such patients, a schedule of 30 Gy in 10 fractions is frequently employed. In patients with recurrent bone pain in a site that has previously been irradiated with good effect, there is a very high response rate to repeated irradiation (22).

Cerebral metastases

The diagnosis of brain metastases should be considered in patients presenting with new neurological symptoms and should be confirmed by computed tomography scanning if further palliative treatment is contemplated. During the period of investigation, it is usual to commence treatment with high dose dexamethasone 8 mg twice daily and this treatment, in itself, may lead to a considerable improvement in symptoms by virtue of its effect on peri-tumour vasogenic oedema (30). Patients with confirmed brain metastases should be considered as candidates for palliative radio-therapy. Palliative treatment of brain metastases accounts for approximately 5% of the workload of UK radiotherapy depart-ments (31). This form of treatment can be very effective at reliev-ing the symptoms of raised intracranial pressure and may restore motor and sensory function in certain circumstances. The optimal radiotherapy schedule remains to be defined. In the 1970s the Radiation Therapy Oncology Group (RTOG) conducted a number of studies in which patients received doses of radiotherapy ranging from 20 Gy in 1 week to 50 Gy in 4 weeks. The studies showed no difference between the different fractionation regimens in terms of neurological improvement (approximately 80%), time to disease progression (median 2–3 months) or overall survival (median 3.5–5 months) (32,33). Thereafter, the emphasis switched towards assessment of abbreviated courses of radiation in an attempt to provide effective palliation without the need for pro-longed and intensive treatment. The RTOG conducted a pilot study in which patients were treated with either 10 Gy as a single fraction or 12 Gy in two fractions (34). The results of this study demonstrated no significant difference between the rate of onset of improvement, the median survival and the morbidity for the two abbreviated fractionation regimens, and the more prolonged treatments delivering 30–40 Gy which had been used in the earlier studies. There was a difference in the duration of symptom relief in favour of the higher radiation dose, but this effect was considerably attenuated by the use of further single fraction brain irradiation in patients with recurrent symptoms. In a recent prospective randomized trial, 544 patients with symptomatic cere-bral metastases were treated with whole brain radiotherapy to a dose of either 12 Gy in two fractions on consecutive days or 30 Gy in 10 fractions over 2 weeks (35). The median survival was 11 weeks for the two-fraction treatment and 12 weeks for the 10-fraction treatment. The short duration of survival hampered an adequate assessment of the response rates, but overall responses were seen in 39% and 44% of those treated with two and 10 frac-tions, respectively.

Brain metastases from bladder cancer are uncommon. In a large single institution study, Anderson *et al.* (36) reported nine patients with brain metastases among a cohort of 293 patients. In seven of the patients, there was only one brain metastasis and in three patients this was the only site of disease. These three patients were treated aggressively with surgery and high dose fractionated radio-therapy to 40–50 Gy, with an average survival of 2.5 years. Those patients with multiple central nervous system deposits or evidence of metastases in other organ systems were treated with whole brain radiotherapy to a dose of 30 Gy in 10 fractions and fared very poorly, with an average survival of 7 weeks. Rosenstein *et al.* (37) retrospectively identified 28 patients with brain metastases from bladder cancer. Data were available for analysis for only 19 patients. The median survival of the whole group was 4 months, although this was considerably longer for patients with a single metastasis treated by a combination of surgery and postoperative radiotherapy.

SPECIFIC UROLOGICAL SYMPTOMS

Neuropathic pain syndromes in pelvic malignancy

Neuropathic pain arises as a result of damage to nerves of the peripheral or central nervous system. Such pains may present in a number of different ways including shooting or stabbing, burning or dull aching pains. Certain recognizable syndromes exist in which patients present with reproducible symptoms and signs. Recognition of these types of pelvic pain allows the physician to commence appropriate therapy immediately. This is of considerable importance as these conditions are rarely responsive to opiates alone and usual require the addition of one or more adjuvant drugs (Table 24.6).

Uncontrolled local pelvic disease frequently presents with a constant, dull, aching or, dragging pain which radiates to the

Table 24.6

DRUGS COMMONLY USED AS ADJUVANTS TO CONVENTIONAL ANALGESICS		
Nature of pain	**Class of drug**	**Typical examples, dose and schedule**
Neuropathic	Tricyclic antidepressants	Amitryptiline 25–150 mg at night
	Anticonvulsant	Valproate 100–400 mg b.d., Carbamazepine 100–200 mg t.i.d.
	Local anaesthetic (oral)	Flecainide 100–200 mg b.d., Mexilitine 150 mg b.d.
	Corticosteroid	Dexamethasone up to 8 mg b.d.
	Calcium channel blocker	Nifedipine—start 5mg t.i.d., maximum 20 mg t.i.d.
	Others	Baclofen—start 5 mg t.i.d., maximum 100 mg per day
Bone	Bisphosphonates	Clodronate 800 mg b.d./q.i.d., Pamidronate 60–90 mg i.v. q3–4 wk
	Corticosteroid	Dexamethasone 2–4 mg b.d.
Muscle spasm		
Skeletal muscle	Benzodiazepine	Diazepam 2–5 mg b.d.
	GABA antagonist	Baclofen—start 5 mg t.i.d., maximum 100 mg per day
Smooth muscle	Anticholinergic	Hyoscine butylbromide up to 20 mg q.i.d.
	Calcium channel blocker	Nifedipine—start 5 mg t.i.d., maximum 20 mg t.i.d.

lower back. This pain may occur in conjunction with the pain of lumbosacral plexus involvement which causes pain in the lower back, which may radiate to the buttock and down the leg. It may also be associated with weakness and numbness in the distribution of the affected nerve roots. Similarly, disease involving the perineal nerve roots can cause a very unpleasant perineal sensation of stabbing or burning perineal pain. This pain can be exacerbated by sitting and patients with this problem often appear to be unable to keep still as they constantly shift their position in an attempt to gain respite from their discomfort. Such pelvic, lumbosacral, and perineal pains can be extremely difficult to control completely but most patients will gain some benefit from opiate analgesia, an antineuropathic agent such as amitryptiline or sodium valproate, and an NSAID. In patients who have not already received full-dose radiotherapy, palliative irradiation of bulk disease may lead to a degree of tumour shrinkage and relief of pressure on the affected nerves.

Tenesmus describes a feeling of fullness of the rectum which is associated with the desire to evacuate, which often exacerbates the discomfort rather than relieving it. Tenesmus can result from direct tumour infiltration of the rectum or involvement of sacral nerve roots. Opiate analgesia often gives some relief, although additional adjuvant agents such as amitryptiline, sodium valproate, and calcium channel antagonists are frequently needed.

Haematuria

While painless haematuria is frequently the presenting symptom of bladder cancer, its reappearance later in the course of the disease process generally signals the presence of recurrent disease. This should be confirmed in all cases by repeat cystoscopy and biopsy. Patients with recurrent bladder haemorrhage may suffer recurrent episodes of clot retention and symptomatic anaemia requiring multiple blood transfusions. The principal aim of palliative treatment should be to secure haemostasis, if possible. The presence of infection, which can exacerbate haematuria, should be sought actively and treated appropriately. In patients who have already been treated with radical bladder conserving therapy at their initial presentation, palliation of this distressing symptom can be very difficult to achieve because radical radiation doses will already have been used. However, if there is scope within the limits of normal tissue tolerance, further doses of radiotherapy (e.g. 8 Gy single fraction or 30 Gy in 10 fractions) can be very effective. The ability of two different radiotherapy fractionation regimens to palliate the symptoms of bladder cancer has been evaluated in prospective study (38). Patients were treated in a non-randomized fashion with either 17 Gy in two fractions over 3 days or 45 Gy in 12 fractions over 26 days. Patient selection was based on the clinician's assessment of their general condition and performance status. The two-fraction treatment was more effective at palliating pain and haematuria than the more protracted conventional fractionation, although the survival was shorter in this group of patients. Further randomized evaluation of the most appropriate fractionation schedule for the palliation of bladder cancer is under way.

Patients who have already received maximal doses of radiotherapy can be treated in other ways. Ethamsylate is a non-hormonal agent which decreases capillary exudation and blood loss. It is thought to act by increasing capillary vascular resistance and platelet adhesiveness in the presence of vascular lesions. It has no direct action on the normal coagulation mechanism. It can be used at a dose of 500 mg, four times daily, in patients with intractable haematuria (7). The antifibrinolytic agent, tranexamic acid, should be avoided in this situation as the formation of very hard clots can cause clot retention and even ureteric obstruction(7). Bladder irrigation with a 1% alum solution can also be of benefit (39). Similarly, intravesical instillation of a 4% solution of formalin has been reported with good results (40). Physical measures such as balloon distension, diathermy, and embolization should be used with great caution (7,41).

Recurrent urinary tract infections

Patients with either primary locally advanced bladder cancer or locally recurrent disease are prone to repeated episodes of urinary tract infection. This tendency may be increased by the need for catheterization in patients with bladder outflow obstruction, incontinence, fistulae, or clot retention due to haematuria. Patients with an indwelling urinary catheter will almost always have evidence of bacteriuria which does not require specific therapy in the absence of local or systemic symptoms of infection. Patients presenting with dysuria, frequency, suprapubic discomfort, loin pain, or fever should have a specimen of urine taken for microbiological analysis. If the symptoms are mild to moderate it may be possible to wait for the result of this test before commencing therapy. If the symptoms are more severe, or if there is constitutional upset, it is reasonable to treat patients with a single dose of 400 mg of trimethoprim by mouth. This treatment is especially effective in the case of urinary tract infections in females. Patients with indwelling urinary catheters should receive a more prolonged course of antibiotics for 5–7 days according to the drug sensitivities demonstrated by the microbiological culture. In the case of repeated infections, it may be necessary to give a 2-week course of antibiotics and repeat the culture of the urine to ensure eradication of the responsible pathogen.

Fistulae

The development of urinary fistulae can be extremely distressing and frightening to patients. Locally advanced bladder cancers can infiltrate the bowel in males and either the bowel or vagina in females leading to persistent leakage of urine. Less commonly, skin involvement and subsequent breakdown can also lead to leakage of urine through the skin. In certain instances complex fistulae can arise with leakage of urine and faeces per rectum, per urethra, or per vagina. Uncontrolled fistulae may have a dramatic impact on a patient's quality of life and may result in an otherwise relatively well patient remaining virtually housebound. Active palliative therapy of a malignant fistula can lead to considerable improvements in quality of life and should be pursued vigorously.

The optimal management of a malignant fistula is dictated by the clinical situation. The standard surgical approach of excision of the fistula (42) and repair is often impossible in these patients. Therefore, the aim of treatment is more usually directed towards limiting the extent of leakage, minimizing the deleterious effects of constant perineal irritation due to leakage of urine and/or faeces over the skin of the perineum and attempting to maintain the quality of life of the patient. Leakage can be reduced by inserting an indwelling urinary catheter or by using a vaginal tampon. If appropriate, in patients with good performance status and a reasonable life expectancy, urinary diversion with percutanous nephrostomy tubes or formation of an ileal conduit offers an alternative. Skin care is of considerable importance as, unless it is protected by barrier creams and/or protective dressings, it can become severely excoriated and infected. Malodorous lesions can be effectively treated by the use of topical metronidazole gel (43).

Bladder instability

Patients with uncontrolled local tumours in the bladder will often experience symptoms of an unstable bladder, including suprapubic discomfort, frequency of micturition, nocturia, urgency, and incontinence of urine. Whenever feasible, reduction of the local tumour mass should be attempted. This is most easily attempted by means of palliative hypofractionated radiotherapy (see above). In the event that local therapeutic manoeuvres are not possible, drugs with anti-cholinergic (antimuscarinic) actions which have the ability to increase bladder capacity and reduce unstable detrusor contractions should be used. Agents such as imipramine at a dose of 10–20 mg nocte (increasing to a maximum of 100 mg) may improve symptoms. Newer drugs, including oxybutinin (5 mg twice a day to four times a day) and flavoxate (200 mg three times a day), also have activity in this situation but are associated with a significant incidence of adverse effects, including xerostomia and blurred vision. These agents are contra-indicated in patients with glaucoma.

Urinary incontinence

Urinary incontinence is a particularly distressing symptom and has an enormous impact on the patient's quality of life. It is frequently caused by locally advanced disease within the pelvis causing disruption of the intrinsic sphincter. However, reversible causes such as urinary tract infection and overflow incontinence due to bladder outflow obstruction should be sought and treated appropriately. Local hypofractionated radiotherapy at a dose of 30 Gy in 10 fractions may lead to a reduction in tumour bulk which may restore the functional anatomy of the urinary sphincter. Where no reversible cause can be isolated, urinary catheterization is effective. An indwelling catheter is frequently employed, but the technique of intermittent self-catheterization may also be very useful, especially in patients who are unable to tolerate a urinary catheter on a permanent basis due to local symptoms such as bladder or trigone irritation or for patients with a hypotonic bladder. A catheter is inserted under clean conditions (strict asepsis is not necessary) at least four times a day and the bladder is emptied. The same catheter can be used repeatedly so long as it is sterilized between insertions.

Obstructive nephropathy

Locally uncontrolled bladder cancer frequently causes life-threatening urinary obstruction. This condition can be treated relatively easily by insertion of percutaneous nephrostomy tubes followed by internalization of urinary drainage with J–J ureteric stents. However, in recent years there has been considerable controversy surrounding the ethics of such treatment. Some authors have proposed that urinary diversion is not in the patient's best interest as a peaceful death from uraemia may be prevented, with only a short-term extension of life span of poor quality ending in death from another, potentially more symptomatic, complication of the malignant disease (44). The contrary view has also been advanced, based on the observation of improvement in quality and quantity of life following percutaneous nephrostomy and insertion of J–J stents (45,46).

The importance of clinical criteria which can assist in selection of patients for appropriate use of nephrostomies has been demonstrated in a number of studies. Fallon *et al.* (45) summarized the features predicting for a beneficial outcome of urinary diversion as being undiagnosed malignant disease, prostatic and cervical primary tumours, patients for whom there is an available treatment modality with a reasonable chance of a response and patients who request urinary diversion as a means of prolonging life for legal or financial reasons. Feuer *et al.* (46) concluded that the following criteria contra-indicated the insertion of drainage tubes: progression of disease while on therapy, potentially life-threatening co-incidental medical problems, poor performance status, no available effective salvage therapy, non-compliance with treatment, and uncontrolled pain.

The role of urinary diversion has been investigated in a prospective study in 42 patients who presented with renal failure secondary to malignant obstructive nephropathy (47). Twenty-one of the patients had locally advanced bladder cancer. The obstructive nephropathy was relieved in 33 of the 42 patients by insertion of percutanous nephrostomies. The median survival of the entire group was 133 days (range 7–712 days). Survival of 6 months or more was seen in 17 patients, nine of whom had bladder cancer. However, five patients died within 30 days of undergoing urinary diversion, three of whom had bladder cancer. This point exemplifies the importance of careful selection of patients for treatment. Analysis of patients by the number of therapeutic modalities that they had received prior to urinary diversion revealed that patients who had been heavily pretreated with combinations of surgery, radiotherapy, and chemotherapy had a short median survival following urinary diversion, whereas the availability of an effective therapeutic option was associated with a greater probability of prolonged survival. In another study of patients treated by surgical urinary diversion, Fallon *et al.* (1980) reported a median survival of 4.5 months for patients with bladder cancer among 100 patients with a variety of malignant diseases.

MANAGEMENT OF THE DYING PATIENT

The management of the dying patient presents a number of specific problems. When a stage at which a terminal decline has been reached, it is important that the medical staff recognize this fact and communicate it to the family. Unnecessary treatment should be withdrawn and investigations, including blood tests, should be discontinued. Strenuous efforts must be made to ensure that the patient has adequate provision of analgesics and anti-emetics. At this stage, all medication is usually delivered by sub-cutaneous syringe driver. Assessment of the presence of pain may be difficult and it is important to heed the advice of family members and nursing staff who have greater contact with the patient at this time. If there is doubt, it is wise to err on the side of caution in providing increased doses of analgesia, rather than leaving a patient with suboptimal pain control. Terminal agitation is frequently part of the natural process, but it is important to exclude and treat reversible causes such as pain, urinary retention or bowel obstruction. In the absence of these causes, sedation with a benzodiazepine (e.g. midazolam 10–30 mg over 24 h) or methotrimeprazine (25–100 mg over 24 h) can be very effective. Retained secretions can cause noisy breathing, the so-called 'death rattle', which can be effectively relieved by fluid restriction and subcutaneous hyoscine. Wherever possible, provision of a quiet side-room to allow the patient and family members a measure of privacy is an important consideration.

Key Points

1. The majority of patients with muscle-invasive bladder cancer will die of the disease.
2. The provision of effective palliative treatment of patients with incurable bladder cancer is an essential part of the management of this disease.
3. A multidisciplinary approach aids the provision of optimal physical, psychological, and social support.
4. Specific symptoms should be assessed individually and addressed by specific therapies.
5. The side-effects of some commonly prescribed drugs can mimic the symptoms of cancer. The possibility of 'iatrogenic symptoms' should always be considered.

References

1 International Association for the Study of Pain (IASP). Subcommittee on the taxonomy classification of chronic pain. *Pain* 1986, **3**, 216–21.
2 World Health Organisation (WHO). *Cancer pain relief.* WHO, Geneva, 1986.
3 Sykes NP. Oral naloxone in opioid-associated constipation. *Lancet* 1991, **337**, 1475.
4 Campora E, Merlini L, Pace M. The incidence of narcotic-induced emesis. *J Pain Symptom Manage* 1991, **6**, 428–30.
5 White ID, Hoskin PJ, Hanks GW, Bliss JM. Morphine and dryness of the mouth. *Br Med J* 1989, **298**, 1222–3.
6 Schug SA, Zech D, Grond S. A long term survey of morphine in cancer pain patients. *J Pain Symptom Manage* 1992, **7**, 259–66.
7 Regnard CFB, Tempest S. *A guide to symptom relief in advanced cancer*, 3rd edn. Haigh and Hochland Ltd, Manchester, 1991.
8 Baines M, Oliver DJ, Carter RL. Medical management of intestinal obstruction in patients with advanced malignant disease. A clinical and pathological study. *Lancet* 1985, **ii**, 990–3.
9 Ashby MA, Game PA, Devitt P. Percutaneous gastrostomy as a venting procedure in palliative care. *Palliative Med* 1991, **5**, 147–50.
10 Campagnutta E, Cannizzaro R, Zarrelli A *et al.* Palliative treatment of upper intestinal obstruction by gynecological malignancy: The usefulness of percutaneous endoscopic gastrostomy. *Gynecol Oncol* 1996, **62**, 103–5.
11 Khoo D, Hall E, Motson R *et al.* Palliation of malignant intestinal obstruction using octreotide. *Eur J Cancer* 1994, **30**, 28–30.
12 Mangili G, Franchi M, Mariani A *et al.* Octreotide in the management of bowel obstruction in terminal ovarian cancer. *Gynecol Oncol* 1996, **61**, 345–8.
13 Badger C, Twycross RG. *Management of lymphoedema—guidelines.* Sobell Study Centre, Oxford, UK, 1988.
14 Ambrus JL, Ambrus CM, Mink IB, Pickren JW. Causes of death in cancer patients. *J Med* 1975, **6**, 61–71.

15 Belt RJ, Leite C, Haas CD, Stephens RL. Incidence of haemorrhagic complications in patients with cancer. *JAMA* 1978, **239**, 2571–4.

16 Harrington KJ, Bateman AR, Syrigos KN *et al.* Cancer-related thromboembolic disease in patients with solid tumours: a retrospective analysis. *Ann Oncol* 1997, **8**, 1–5.

17 Chan A, Woodruff RK. Complications and failure of anticoagulation therapy in the treatment of venous thromboembolism in patients with disseminated malignancy. *Aust NZ J Med* 1992, **22**, 119–22.

18 Kakkar VV. Prevention and management of venous thrombosis. *Br Med Bull* 1994, **50**, 871–903.

19 Tattersall MHN, Boyer MJ. Management of malignant pleural effusions. *Thorax* 1990, **45**, 81–2.

20 Ruckdeschel JC. Management of malignant pleural effusions. *Semin Oncol* 1995, **22** (3), 58–63.

21 Petrou M, Kaplan D, Goldstraw P. Management of recurrent malignant pleural effusions: The complementary role of talc pleurodesis and pleuroperitoneal shunting. *Cancer* 1982, **75**, 801–5.

22 Mithal NP, Needham PR, Hoskin PJ. Retreatment with radiotherapy for painful bone metastases. *Int J Radiat Oncol Biol Phys* 1994, **29**, 1011–14.

23 Price P, Hoskin PJ, Easton D. Prospective randomised trial of single and multi-fractional radiotherapy schedules in the treatment of painful bony metastases. *Radiother Oncol* 1986, **6**, 247–55.

24 Price P, Hoskin PJ, Easton D *et al.* Low dose single fraction radiotherapy in the treatment of metastatic bone pain: A pilot study. *Radiother Oncol* 1988, **12**, 297–300.

25 Hoskin PJ, Price P, Easton D *et al.* A prospective randomised trial of 4 Gy or 8 Gy single doses in the treatment of metastatic bone pain. *Radiother Oncol* 1992, **23**, 74–8.

26 Cole DJ. A randomised trial of a single treatment versus conventional fractionation in the palliative radiotherapy of painful bone metastases. *Clin Oncol* 1989, **1**, 59–62.

27 Niewald M, Tkocz HJ, Abel U *et al.* Rapid course radiation therapy vs more standard treatment: a randomised trial for bone metastases. *Int J Radiat Oncol Biol Phys* 1996, **36**, 1085–9.

28 Bates T. A review of local radiotherapy in the treatment of bone metastases and cord compression. *Int J Radiat Oncol Biol Phys* 1992, **23**, 217–21.

29 Booth M, Summers J, Williams MV. Audit reduces the reluctance to use single fractions for painful bone metastases. *Clin Oncol* 1993, **5**, 15–18.

30 Kirkham SR. The palliation of cerebral tumours with high dose dexamethasone: a review. *Palliative Med* 1989, **2**, 27–33.

31 Maher EJ, Dische S, Grosch E. Who gets radiotherapy? *Health Trends* 1990, **22**, 78–83.

32 Borgelt B, Gelber R, Kramer S *et al.* The palliation of brain metastases: Final results of the first two studies by the Radiation Therapy Oncology Group. *Int J Radiat Oncol Biol Phys* 1980, **6**, 1–9.

33 Kurtz JM, Gelber R, Brady LW *et al.* The palliation of brain metastases in a favourable patient population: A randomised clinical trial by the Radiation Therapy Oncology Group. *Int J Radiat Oncol Biol Phys* 1981, **7**, 891–5.

34 Borgelt B, Gelber R, Larson M *et al.* Ultra-rapid high dose irradiation schedules for the palliation of brain metastases: The final results of the first two studies by the Radiation Therapy Oncology Group. *Int J Radiat Oncol Biol Phys* 1981, **7**, 1633–8.

35 Priestman TJ, Dunn J, Brada M *et al.* Final results of the Royal College of Radiologists' trial comparing two different radiotherapy schedules in the treatment of cerebral metastases. *Clin Oncol* 1996, **8**, 308–15.

36 Anderson RS, El Mahdi AM, Kuban DA, Higgins EM. Brain metastases from transitional cell carcinoma of the urinary bladder. *Urology* 1992, **39**, 17–20.

37 Rosenstein M, Wallner K, Scher H, Sternberg CN. Treatment of brain metastases from bladder cancer. *J Urol* 1993, **149**, 480–3.

38 Srinivasan V, Brown CH, Turner AG. A comparison of two radiotherapy regimens for the treatment of symptoms from advanced bladder cancer. *Clin Oncol* 1994, **6**, 11–13.

39 Bullock N, Whittaker RH. Massive bladder haemorrhage. *Br Med J* 1985, **291**, 1522–3.

40 Vicente J, Rios G, Caffaratti J. Intravesical formalin for the treatment of massive haemorrhagic cystitis: Retrospective review of 25 cases. *Eur Urol* 1990, **18**, 204–6.

41 Muefti GR, Virdi JS, Singh M. Reappraisal of hydrostatic pressure treatment for intractable postradiotherapy vesical haemorrhage. *Urology* 1990, **35**, 9–11.

42 Holmes SAV, Christmas TJ, Kirby RS, Hendry WF. Management of colovesical fistulae associated with pelvic malignancy. *Br J Surg* 1992, **79**, 432–4.

43 Newman V, Allwood M, Oakes RA. The use of metronidazole gel to control the smell of malodorous lesions. *Palliative Med* 1989, **3**, 303–5.

44 Kerby IJ. Strive to keep alive? *Clin Oncol* 1993, **5**, 192–8.

45 Fallon B, Olney L, Culp DA. Nephrostomy in cancer patients: To do or not to do? *Br J Urol* 1980, **52**, 237–42.

46 Feuer GA, Fruchter R, Seruri E. Selection for percutaneous nephrostomy in gynecologic cancer patients. *Gynecol Oncol* 1991, **42**, 60–3.

47 Harrington KJ, Pandha HS, Kelly SA *et al*. Palliation of obstructive nephropathy due to malignancy. *Br J Urol* 1995, **76**, 101–7.

25. THE ROLE OF THE RESEARCH NURSE IN THE MANAGEMENT OF BLADDER CANCER PATIENTS

M.M. Bowerbank

INTRODUCTION

As previous chapters have already suggested, the treatment of bladder cancer depends on the extent of the patient's disease, as does the overall aim of treatment. For some, one treatment modality is enough, for others, a combination of surgery, chemotherapy or radiotherapy will be needed. Although advances have been made in the treatment of bladder cancer, overall management of this disease in all its stages, remains controversial. Unless current treatment modalities for this disease are evaluated within the auspices of large scale, prospective, randomized clinical trials, treatment is likely to remain controversial (1,2).

Despite most oncologists, radiotherapists, and urolologists being committed to the concept of prospective trials, there are a number of logistical and perceptual problems which can act as deterrents to trials being taken on board by clinicians. The expense of running trials, problems with recruiting and consenting patients, organizing burdensome data collection, may all deter the clinician. For the patient, there may be the inconvenience of extra visits and tests, scepticism over the nature and intention of research. All are potential barriers to the success of clinical trials and therefore to the progress of bladder cancer management generally (3–5). This is where the role of the research nurse can make a significant impact. Nurses, perhaps more than any other health care professional, are ideally placed to promote strategies to overcome these difficulties. Their involvement in clinical trials is pivotal to both the prospective development of new treatment modalities for patients with bladder cancer and to the actual care of the bladder cancer patient. One of the biggest hurdles in running a trial, however, is actually recruiting enough patients.

RECRUITMENT

Accrual and retention of patients is critical to the successful completion of a clinical trial. Relatively speaking, only small numbers of patients are actually entered into trials, despite many being eligible. Only about 25 000, (2%) of approximately 1 million newly diagnosed cancer patients in the USA are actually enrolled in clinical trials, despite estimates that some 12–44% are eligible (6). Evaluation of different bladder cancer therapies has thus far been very difficult as there have not been any randomized trials offering sufficient numbers of patients who have been followed up for sufficiently long periods of time to allow for definitive results. For example, to detect a 5% increase in 2 year survival rate from 50% in the control arm to 55% in the experimental arm, some 3500 patients would need to be recruited, 1000 patients for a 10% increase, 400 patients for a 15% increase. Few cancer centres approach these sorts of accrual rates.

Isaaacman and Reynolds found that the addition of a research nurse increased recruitment of patients and that both doctor and research nurse demonstrated equivalent judgement regarding patient eligibility for a trial (7). The research nurse can help to optimize recruitment by simply trawling out-patient clinic notes, both in urology and oncology clinics, and cross-checking eligibility criteria for potentially eligible bladder cancer patients (8). These patients can then be put forward for consideration by the investigator for the trial. The clinician can then introduce the idea of the trial to the patient alongside the research nurse. Once the patient has been deemed eligible by the investigator and research nurse, the process of informed consent begins.

INFORMATION GIVING AND INFORMED CONSENT

The recognition that formal ethical guidance was needed for clinical research was originally born out of concern and outrage at the atrocities carried out during the second world war by the Nazis. Some years later, the Declaration of Helsinki set minimal ethical standards for research, stating that all patients considering entering clinical trials should be informed of the aims of the treatment, benefits and hazards of the research (9). More specifically, there are now guidelines for good clinical practice (GCP) laid down by the European Union, clearly stipulating the 'gold standard' for the conduct of clinical trials (10). These guidelines describe the package of procedures needed to ensure that clinical studies meet the required international standards. They set out the obligations of the sponsor, the monitor, and the investigator in the form of standard operating procedures.

The whole process of informed consent has evolved substantially since then, as part of the broader framework of the consumer rights movement. The UK government promulgated initiatives such as Working for Patients (11) and the Patients Charter (12), as a means to try and increase patient participation in the whole treatment decision-making process generally. Such participation has been related to better outcomes in terms of patient care, better quality of life for the cancer patient, and a more satisfactory relationship with doctors (13–15). However, it is important to note here that not all patients wish to be involved in treatment decisions of such gravity. They may feel that they do not have the requisite knowledge upon which to base such a decision. However, research suggests that cancer patients still have a strong desire for information, even though this does not necessarily translate into a desire to participate in the actual decision making (16). Where the bladder cancer patient has made a conscious decision to defer the ultimate treatment decision onto the doctor, then this so-called 'negative' right must be respected. Research actually supports the notion that such behaviour reflects a rational response on their part to a situation which feels totally outside their realm of knowledge or experience (17). Tabak and others found that the more severe the patient's illness, the less of a role they wished to have in their treatment decision-making (18,19).

Patients with bladder cancer are frequently asked to consider entering a clinical trial at a time when they are experiencing considerable physical and/or emotional stress. The visit to the outpatient clinic is often approached with fear and trepidation. The patient is confronted not only with the initial diagnosis of cancer, recurrent cancer, or cancer that is not responding to treatment, but also with the need to make a major treatment decision. Some 80% of those diagnosed with advanced metastatic bladder cancer have no prior history of the disease. As such, the diagnosis comes as a great shock (20). Such emotionally fraught situations may well hinder the patient's decision-making capacity and ability to assimilate all the information given to him/her at that specific time. Research has indicated that as many as 40% of patients could not recall the purpose and nature of a trial despite reading information sheets about the trial and receiving verbal information (21). In a study of 100 breast cancer patients, about a quarter were unable to name any of their drugs, and although the purpose of their adjuvant treatment was cure, only 29% were actually aware of this intent (22). Moreover, patients in this study were often unable to trace and explain the process by which they arrived at their decision in consenting to a trial. The urology research nurse is there to help the patient and family navigate their way through this process by mediating the flow of information between the doctor and the patient.

During the initial consultation, the doctor presents treatment options to the patient, including information about other treatment options as well as the trial treatment. The research nurse should ideally sit in on this, assuming the role of active listener, noting carefully how the clinician presents the treatment options, the purposes of the trial, and what treatment entails. The research nurse also notes the questions the patient and family are raising and their response to the answers. After the consultation, the patient and family spend time with the research nurse to clarify and discuss matters further. The patient is then at liberty to evaluate these options based on their own particular values and priorities in life. The research nurse is ideally placed to bridge the gap, wherever possible, between what the patient does not understand and what the clinician has not included in this initial consultation. It is not uncommon for the patient to ask the research nurse things that they were too embarrassed to ask the doctor. The research nurse can then provide anticipatory guidance, focusing on practical issues such as timing and duration of treatment, side-effects and the likely effect on both the patient's and family's quality of life. Very often, education at this stage of the patient's treatment experience can prevent problems with non-compliance in the future as patients feel well prepared for whichever treatment they have. It is also at this stage that the research nurse needs to identify any physical or psychosocial limitations that would interfere with the patient's ability to participate in the proposed treatment plan. The patient and family can discuss issues such as other health problems that they are having to cope with alongside their bladder cancer treatment. This is where the research nurse needs to liaise with allied health professionals such as the urology nurse specialist and the stoma therapist in order to provide a holistic service for the patient and his/her family.

By providing the opportunity for the bladder cancer patient to gather information that is of importance to them, the patient's sense of control is more likely to be enhanced. Achieving this during the initial stages of treatment discussions should theoretically make it easier for the patient to develop a sense of commitment to, and control over, the whole treatment plan and, ultimately, their whole treatment experience. Such strategies should hopefully minimize post-decisional regret (23).

As patients who experience difficulties understanding information tend to be less likely to participate in their treatment decision-making, it is imperative that the doctor and the research nurse work as a team throughout, with the patient at the heart of that team (24–26). This collaborative model recognizes that it takes more than medical expertise to determine what is best for the patient and is respectful of the patient's autonomy. If a patient does not feel able to ask questions during the initial consultation, perhaps because of intimidation or shock following bad news, then this may then set a precedence for all other consultations. The doctor may assume from then on that the patient does not wish to acquire information or participate in decisions. A pattern of dominance is established, essentially by default (27). The research nurse should try to maximize that element of reciprocity within the doctor-patient relationship and narrow the knowledge gap between them. Interestingly, research has indicated that consent forms have become increasingly lengthy and unreadable over time and have not improved patient's overall level of comprehension at all (28,29). It is therefore important for the research nurse to ascertain the patient's recall and understanding of the trial, before the actual consent form is signed, and indeed thereafter. Informed consent should ideally be viewed as a multi-stage process which continues on past the actual signing of the consent form, rather than as an isolated event.

The different phases of a clinical trial pose some specific problems.

Consenting for Phase I Trials

Consenting patients for phase I trials pose particular challenges to both the clinician involved and the research nurse. Generally speaking, little pre-clinical toxicology and limited efficacy data are available before a new drug is used in patients. During the initial stages of a dose escalation study, for example, the doctor is faced with the prospect of giving treatment at relatively low doses which is unlikely to hold any therapeutic benefit for the patient, in terms of disease response. Difficulties inevitably arise when consenting patients to this sort of trial tend to hold on to the expectation that treatment may help them, despite full and honest disclosure as to the purpose of such trials, on the part of the doctor. There is much research to support the fact that altruistic motives play a limited role in patients' willingness to participate in early phase trials and that less than half of patients consenting to phase I studies actually understand their purpose. Indeed, patients may derive psychological benefit from having the chance at what they perceive as their last option. Yoder et al. (30), using a structured questionnaire approach, found that the majority of patients entered phase I trials because they perceived that they would be receiving 'state of the art' treatment.

This is where the role of the research nurse becomes increasingly important. S/he needs to ensure that the present effectiveness of experimental drugs or schedules are presented to the patient and family in a meaningful way. According to Stetz (31), people with advanced cancer engage in what he called 'survival work', whereby the patient tends to chose active treatment over letting the disease take its course. The research nurse must act as the patient's advocate in the face of often unreal expectations on the part of the patient, family, and sometimes the doctor. Optimism and hope are integral to the psychological framework of patients entering phase I trials (20). Essentially, the research nurse's role is to skilfully coach the patient through their decision-making in an atmosphere of openness and honesty, whilst trying to maintain that element of hope and support. No mean task!

Consenting for Phase II Trials

Consenting patients for phase II trials present similar problems. Although the doctor is able to tell the patient more about the side-effects of the treatment and he may feel more assured about the dosages involved, there is an increased likelihood of toxicity as treatment is given at or near the maximum tolerated dose. There is still an overall low response rate in phase II trials (32), providing either unrealistically hopeful expectations or going along with such unreal expectations are not an appropriate basis for truly informed decision-making. Numerous reviews indicate that the quality of clinical trial reporting in journals is generally poor, with results often being exaggerated (33–35). The research nurse needs, again, to ensure that the chances of therapeutic benefit are presented in an honest and realistic light. S/he needs to be able to translate the current expected outcomes of treatment, in terms of survival expectations, response rates, toxicities, and impact on quality of life, into words that are meaningful to the patient and family.

Consenting for Phase III Trials

When consenting patients for phase III randomized trials, the research nurse needs to explain the rationale behind randomization whilst reassuring the patient and family that they will receive the best care possible whichever treatment arm they draw.

Patients often find it difficult to accept this concept as it seems to be leaving treatment decisions in the hands of chance. The research nurse needs to help the patient understand that randomization is justified when the clinician truly does not know which treatment would be best for the patient. Again, this is often hard for the patient to accept as they may well expect the doctor to know which treatment is best and want them to recommend a particular treatment. Trust in the doctor in fact constitutes a major component in patients' ultimate decision-making. It can be equally hard for the doctor and research nurse to openly acknowledge that they do not know which treatment is best. However, it is important to maintain an open and honest dialogue throughout. The research nurse can reassure the patient and family by emphasizing the extent of research that has gone before such trials.

Notably, there has been a lot of research carried out on those who consent patients for phase III trials. Simes *et al.* (36), studied how clinical investigators in Europe consented their patients for randomized trials. Their results indicated that 12% of these investigators never actually informed their patients about the trial before they actually randomized them. 38% did not tell the patient that their treatment would be assigned randomly and 42% provided information about the experimental arm of the trial only. Perhaps this is because of the inherent difficulties associated with explaining such concepts to patients. Certainly, research has found that oncologists find the whole process of informed consent difficult fearing that it will have an adverse affect on their relationship with the patient (37–40). If the research nurse and clinician work together with the patient and family, many of these issues can be overcome, or at least made a little easier for all concerned.

When a patient has formally consented to a trial and has officially been enrolled onto a study, their treatment plan can begin. The research nurse will oversee their care thereafter.

Protocol compliance

In a clinical trial, the protocol is essentially the detailed plan outlining the logistics for the study treatment. Adherence to this protocol is vital to the success of the study and, as such, the research nurse should ideally be involved in the development of these protocols so as to ensure that the practicalities of caring for the patient and collecting the data are in place before the trial is activated. The investigator needs to be able to depend on the research nurse to ensure that everyone adheres to this protocol. This is crucial if one is to preserve the reliability and validity of the study.

Most trials in bladder cancer will involve frequent tests for screening and assessing the disease. The patient and family need support both practically and emotionally throughout the various blood tests, urine tests for cytology, cystoscopies, CT scans etc. The research nurse is ideally placed to organize the appropriate protocol-specified tests for the patient whilst ensuring that the patient understands the rationale for these tests and that they receive results in a timely and supportive fashion. It is sometimes difficult for the research nurse to justify to patients why so many tests are needed, but with explanation and reassurance, the nurse can minimize the discomfort and inconvenience caused by these extra commitments.

MONITORING PATIENT TOXICITY

Toxicity monitoring and reporting are important aspects of the care of patients in bladder cancer trials. Continuity of care is absolutely crucial, not only from the patient's point of view, but for accurate data collection over time. A comprehensive review of all the patient's symptoms, side-effects and any changes in social and psychological status must be carried out pre-treatment through to follow-up, to detect any that may be due, or thought to be due, to the particular drug or way of giving the treatment. The research nurse is responsible for monitoring symptoms and side-effects closely, so that dose modifications can be made safely, in line with protocol recommendations. Good interviewing skills and the ability to actively listen are clearly the most important skills of the research nurse. Patients often use ambiguous terms to describe their symptoms, the research nurse must try to decipher these terms by encouraging the patient to clarify so that she is able to record the information accurately and as objectively as possible. The patient needs to be encouraged and continually reminded to report any known or suspected toxicities and other unusual symptoms or events following their treatment. Careful monitoring and recording of these events, alongside their timing is essential if for example, two regimens are being compared which are equally effective but turn out to have quite different toxicities, the degree and type of toxicity may be the basis for selecting one regime over another. The research nurse is responsible for anticipating such toxicity and organizing subsequent support to manage it.

As bladder cancer tends to manifest in later life, the patient may well be suffering from co-morbid conditions such as cardiovascular disease, urinary problems, prostate problems etc. Such conditions complicate the symptomatic picture further for the research nurse and clinician. The patient undergoing intravesical therapy is likely to experience chemical cystitis resulting in irritative symptoms, fever, malaise, and hematuria, all of which the patient may associate with symptoms of their disease or progression of their disease. For the patient with a long history of superficial bladder cancer that has been repeatedly treated with endoscopic resection or diathermy, the syndrome of malignant cystitis is likely to be severe. Again, there may be debilitating urinary symptoms of dysuria, nocturia, frequency, hematuria, and perineal pain. It is therefore imperative that the research nurse documents these symptoms and discuss them with the trial investigator or co-investigator. The use of immunotherapies such as interleukin-2 are currently being used in trials for superficial bladder cancer. Some of the associated side-effects may seem non-specific and not worth mentioning. However, the research nurse needs to encourage detail from the patient if s/he is to accurately collate data for a trial. This information is crucial if the research nurse is to make recommendations for a patient to come off a study. Decisions need to be based on sound clinical evidence and as the research nurse is the primary contact for the patient, their evaluation of the patient can profoundly influence team decisions. Monitoring laboratory reports is part and parcel of this information gathering process and is the primary responsibility of the research nurse. S/he must understand their significance as potential measures of drug toxicity.

Many bladder cancer patients may not tolerate the significant toxicity associated with particular cytotoxic drugs and/or radiotherapy regimens precisely because of their bladder disease, their age, and concurrent medical problems. Indeed, there are many changes in organ function in older patients generally and as many of the cytotoxic drugs have a relatively narrow therapeutic index, any factors that potentially alter the pharmacokinetics of the drug may increase toxicity. For some trial treatments, for example, MVAC for advanced bladder cancer, toxicity can be severe.

Serious adverse events, i.e. those involving hospitalization or prolonging hospitalization, need to be reported promptly by the research nurse if the pharmaceutical company is to assess early signs of a trend.

Follow-up of any symptoms and side-effects should be carried out by the same research nurse upon each visit to the hospital or clinic. Such one-to-one contact makes for more accurate and efficient data collection. This continuity of care also provides a sense of stability in patients' lives at a difficult and stressful time. Research supports the view that patients benefit from this type of personalized care system as they tend to feel more able to share their worries and concerns with someone they have had the opportunity to develop a close relationship with (41). They tend to feel that they are being closely monitored and looked after. However, the early provision of support links for the patient back in the community, e.g. Macmillan nurses, is extremely important so that the patient does not feel abandoned once the actual treatment has stopped.

QUALITY OF LIFE ASSESSMENT

As bladder cancer is predominantly a disease of the elderly, quality of life becomes an increasingly important endpoint for consideration in the search for new and more tolerable therapies for bladder cancer patients. This is particularly so for trials in the advanced or metastatic setting, in which treatment may offer only small gains in survival or disease control but is likely to have debilitating side-effects. Ultimately, any treatment discussions and subsequent decision-making will be influenced by quality of life assessments as well as predictions of tumour response and disease control (42). Although patients may often exchange quality for quantity, it is important to maintain a distinction between a decrease in quality where there is an attempt at cure and one where palliation is the main aim.

Certainly over the years, the patient's perspective with regard to quality of life has gained considerable credibility alongside a shift in the objectives of health care to more socially relevant outcomes (43). With many bladder cancer patients being elderly as already stated, quality of life assessments can refute previously held beliefs that particular treatment modalities adversely affects this group of patients in terms of quality of life; or conversely, treatment protocols may be changed if it is found that the quality of life of the bladder cancer patient is adversely affected by the treatment. The research nurse is responsible for collecting such quality of life data from bladder cancer trial patients in a way which optimizes its reliability and validity. Most phase III trials now incorporate self-administered instruments, acknowledging the subjective nature of quality of life assessments. However, there is more to collecting this data than simply giving it to the patient to complete. Patients need somewhere quiet and private to complete a questionnaire properly. The research nurse needs to ensure that the patient can actually read the questionnaire and understand how to answer the questions. The patient must be given time in which to complete it otherwise they may respond erroneously or incompletely generating unusable, inaccurate data. This information is important if new treatment modalities are to be compared with standard treatment in a holistic and meaningful way. The research nurse also needs to ensure that quality of life is assessed during follow-up as this provides vital information into the natural history of the quality of life relative to the course of the cancer and its treatment. This however, can be difficult as many patients may be lost to follow-up and drop out of studies at a time when their assessments are most crucial. It is important for the research nurse to try to re-establish follow up with these patients where possible. Doctors or spouses should not attempt to complete these questionnaires as this compromises validity and reliability of the research.

FOLLOW-UP

When the patient has actually finished treatment, s/he will still need the continued support of the research nurse. Close follow-up of patients with carcinoma *in situ* is particularly essential because of the high possibility of recurrent tumour with invasion (44). In view of the fact that patients who have had one recurrence are more likely to have another, this support becomes increasingly important for the patient. Since the primary endpoints for phase II and III trials are disease response, careful follow-up is essential to determine the degree and duration of response in patients with accuracy. Again, the patient will need to undergo repeated investigations, blood tests, urinalysis, cystoscopies, CT scans, etc., so that any recurrence can be detected promptly and treated accordingly. If the research nurse explains the rationale for these tests and repeated out-patient visits, the patient is more likely to feel well prepared and supported and therefore more likely to comply with the study requirements.

CONCLUSION

Clinical trials are becoming increasingly important for our understanding of different treatment modalities in bladder cancer. The urology research nurse can make a significant contribution to the overall management of these trials by maximizing recruitment opportunities, facilitating the whole decision-making process and, ultimately, by ensuring that data is complete, accurate, and meaningful. More specifically, by providing direct, expert care and support for the patient and family, throughout consent and treatment, their whole experience of participating in a trial should hopefully be a positive one.

Key Points

1. Large-scale randomized trials are needed to improve current treatment outcomes for bladder cancer patients.
2. Research nurse is integral to successful trial co-ordination.
3. Research nurse acts as patient's advocate. Facilitates decision-making and informed consent.
4. Bladder cancer patient and family receive specialist expert care and support throughout treatment and follow-up.

References

1 Fillingham S, Douglas J. *Urological nursing.* 2nd Edn. Ballière-Tindall, London, 1997.

2 DeVita V, Hellman S, Rosenburg SA. *Cancer: principles and practices of oncology.* Lippincott JB, 4th ed, Philadelphia, 1993, pp. 1052–72.

3 Morrow G, Hickok J, Burish T. Behavioural aspects of clinical trials. An integrated framework from behaviour theory. *Cancer Supplement*, 1994, **74**, 2676–91.

4 Mansour E. Barriers to clinical trials. Part III: knowledge and attitudes of health care providers. *Cancer Supplement*, 1994, **74**, 2672–75.

5 Schain W. Barriers to clinical trials. Part II: knowledge and attitudes of potential participants. *Cancer Supplement*, 1994, **74**, 2666–71.

6 Byrd W, Clayton L. Cancer clinical trials. Presented to National Cancer Control Research Network Committee Meeting. Harvard School of Public Health, 1–13. Boston, Massachusetts, 1992.

7 Isaacman D, Reynolds E. Effect of a research nurse on patient enrolment in a clinical study. *Paed Emerg Care*, 1996, **12**, 340–2.

8 Fillingham S, Douglas J. Urological nursing, 2nd Ed, Ballière-Tindall, London, 1997, pp. 17.

9 World Medical Association. Declaration of Helsinki. 41st World Medical Assembly, Hong Kong. Ferney-Voltaire, World Medical Association, 1989.

10 CPMP Working Party on Efficacy of Medicinal Products. Good Clinical Practice for Trials on Medicinal Products. EEC Note for Guidance, 1990, 361–72.

11 Department of Health. *Working for Patients: the health service caring for the 1990s.* HMSO, London, 1989.

12 HMSO. *The Patients' Charter.* HMSO, London, 1995.

13 Horder J, Moore G. The consultation and health outcomes. *Br J Health Practice*, 1990, Nov, 442–3.

14 Roter D. Patient participation in the patient provider interaction: the effect of patient question asking on the quality of interaction, satisfaction and compliance. *Health Education Monograph*, 1977, **5**, 281–315.

15 Greenfeld S, Kaplan S, Ware J. Expanding patient involvement in patient care. *Ann Int Med*, 1985, **102**, 520–8.

16 Cassileth B, Zudkis R, Sutton-Smith K. Information and participation preferences among cancer patients. *Ann Int Med*, 1980, **92**, 832–6.

17 Bowerbank M. Treatment decision-making: a qualitative study of elderly cancer patients' consultation experiences. Unpublished MMedSci Theses, 1997.

18 Tabak N. Decision-making in consenting to experimental cancer therapy. *Cancer Nursing*, 1994, **18**, 89–96.

19 Ende J, Lews K, Moscowitz M. Measuring patients' desire for autonomy: decision-making and information preferences among medical patients. *J Gen Int Med*, 1989, **4**, 23–30.

20 Kaye K, Lange P. Mode of presentation of invasive bladder cancer: Reassessment of the problem. *J Urol*, 1982, **128**, 31–9.

21 Cassileth B, Zupkis R, Sutton-Smith K *et al.* Informed Consent: why are its goals imperfectly realised? *N E J Med*, 1980, **302**, 896–900.

22 Muss HB, White DR, Michielutte R *et al.* Written informed consent in patients with breast cancer. *Cancer*, 1979, **43**, 1549.

23 Nuefeld K, Degner L, Dick J. A nursing intervention strategy to foster patient involvement in treatment decisions. *Oncology Nursing Forum*, 1993, **20**, 631–5.

24 Palmer A, Whole J. Voluntary admissions forms: does the patient know what he's signing? *Hospital Community Psychiatry*, 1972, **32**, 200–52.

25 Busby A, Gilchrist B. The role of the nurse in the medical ward round. *J Adv Nurs*, 1992, **17**, 339–46.

26 Rintald D, Hanover D, Alexander J. Team care: an analysis of verbal behaviour during patient rounds in a rehabilitation hospital. *Arch Phys Med and Rehabilitation*, 1986, **67**, 118–22.

27 Schain W. Patient's rights in decision-making: the case for personalism versus paternalism in health care. *Cancer*, 1980, **46**, 1035–41.

28 Baker MT, Taub HA. Readability of informed consent forms for research in a Veterans Administration medical centre. *JAMA*, 1983, **250**, 2646.

29 Grossman SA, Piantadosi S, Covahey C. Are informed consent forms that describe clinical oncology research protocols readable by most patients and their families? *J Clin Onc*, 1994, **12**, 2211.

30 Yoder L, O' Rourke J, Etnyre A *et al*. Expectations and experiences of patients with cancer participating in phase I clinical trials. *Oncology Nursing Forum*, 1997, **24**, 891–96.

31 Stetz K. Survival work: the experience of the patient and the spouse involved in experimental treatment for cancer. *Seminars in Oncology Nursing*, 1993, **9**, 121–26.

32 Marsoni S, Hoth D, Simon R *et al*. Clinical drug development: an analysis of phase II trials, 1970–1985. *Cancer Treat Reports*, 1987, **71**, 71.

33 Hellman S, Hellman DS. Of mice but not men. Problems of the randomised clinical trial. *N E J Med*, 1991, **324**, 1585.

34 Markman M. Ethical difficulties with randomised clinical trials involving cancer patients: examples from the field of gynaecological oncology. *J Clin Ethics*, 1992, **3**, 193.

35 Freedman B, Fuks A, Weijer C. Demarcating research and treatment: a systematic approach for the analysis of the ethics of clinical research. *Clin Res*, 1992, **40**, 655.

36 Simes RJ, Tattersall MHN, Coates AS *et al*. Randomised comparison of procedures for obtaining informed consent in clinical trials of treatment for cancer. *Br Med J*, 1986, **293**, 1065.

37 Taylor KM, Margolese RG, Soskolne CL. Physicians' reasons for not entering eligible patients in a randomised clinical trial of surgery for breast cancer. *N Eng J Med*, 1984, **310**, 136.

38 Taylor KM, Shapiro M, Soskolne CL *et al*. Physician response to informed consent regulation for randomised clinical trials. *Cancer*, 1987, **60**, 1415.

39 Taylor KM, Kelner M. Informed consent: the physician's perspective. *Social Science and Medicine*, 1987, **24**, 135.

40 Taylor KM, Feldstein ML, Skeel RT *et al*. Fundamental dilemmas of the randomised clinical trial process: results of a survey of 1,737 Eastern Co-operative Oncology Group investigators. *J Clin Oncol*, 1987, **12**, 1796.

41 Cox K, Avis M. Psychosocial aspects of participation in early anticancer drug trials. *Cancer Nursing*, 1996, **19**, 177–86.

42 Moody H. Ageing, meaning and allocation of resources. *Ageing and Society*, 1995, **15**, 163–84.

43 McGregor S. Quality of life in advanced cancer. *J Cancer Care*, 1994, **3**, 144–52.

44 Skinner D. Current state of classification and staging of bladder cancer. *Cancer Res*, 1977, **37**, 2838–42.

INDEX

Note: References in **bold** indicate chapter extents. Those in *italics* denote photographic plates. There may also be textual references on these pages.